Lasers in Dentistry

To God, without whom my life would have no direction and my projects would not be successful

To my husband – Alessandro, and my kids – Felipe and Clara, for making my days always special. Love you.

Patrícia

To God and to his only son Jesus, for all the guidance until this moment.

To the loves of my life…my parents Sonia and Antonio Carlos, my husband Ricardo and my daughter Manuella, my greatest love!

To my eternal mentor, Professor José Nicolau, who believed in my choice, and to Dr Sidney Luiz Stabile Junior, representing all of those who saved my life.

Alyne

Lasers in Dentistry
Guide for Clinical Practice

Edited by

Patrícia M. de Freitas DDS, PhD

Associate Professor
Special Laboratory of Lasers in Dentistry (LELO)
Department of Restorative Dentistry
School of Dentistry
University of São Paulo (USP)
São Paulo, SP, Brazil

Alyne Simões DDS, PhD

Assistant Professor
Department of Biomaterials and Oral Biology
School of Dentistry
University of São Paulo (USP)
São Paulo, SP, Brazil

Foreword by Marcia Martins Marques DDS, PhD

Full Professor
Department of Restorative Dentistry
School of Dentistry
University of São Paulo (USP)
São Paulo, SP, Brazil

WILEY Blackwell

Editorial Offices

1606 Golden Aspen Drive, Suites 103 and 104, Ames, Iowa 50010, USA

The Atrium, Southern Gate, Chichester, West Sussex, PO19 8SQ, UK

9600 Garsington Road, Oxford, OX4 2DQ, UK

For details of our global editorial offices, for customer services and for information about how to apply for permission to reuse the copyright material in this book please see our website at www.wiley.com/wiley-blackwell.

Library of Congress Cataloging-in-Publication Data

Lasers in dentistry (Freitas)

   Lasers in dentistry : guide for clinical practice / edited by Patricia M. de Freitas, Alyne Simoes.

      p. ;   cm.

   Includes bibliographical references and index.

   ISBN 978-1-118-27502-3 (paperback)

I. Freitas, Patricia M. de, editor.   II. Simoes, Alyne, editor.   III. Title.

[DNLM: 1. Laser Therapy–methods.   2. Oral Surgical Procedures–instrumentation.   3. Dentistry–methods.

4. Stomatognathic Diseases–therapy. WU 26]

   RK501

   617.6′058–dc23

                                                 2015000698

Set in 9.5/12pt Minion by SPi Publisher Services, Pondicherry, India

Printed and bound in Singapore by Markono Print Media Pte Ltd

1 2015

Contents

List of contributors

Lucio Frigo
Laser in Dentistry Program
Cruzeiro do Sul University
São Paulo, SP, Brazil

Luciana Almeida-Lopes
Research and Education Center for Photo Therapy
in Health Sciences
São Carlos, SP, Brazil

Patricia Aparecida Ana
Center for Engineering, Modeling and Applied Social Sciences
Federal University of ABC (UFABC)
Santo André, Brazil

Akira Aoki
Department of Periodontology
Graduate School of Medical and Dental Sciences
Tokyo Medical and Dental School
Tokyo, Japan

Victor Elias Arana-Chavez
Department of Biomaterials and Oral Biology
School of Dentistry
University of São Paulo (USP)
São Paulo, SP, Brazil

Ana Cecilia Corrêa Aranha
Special Laboratory of Lasers in Dentistry (LELO)
Department of Restorative Dentistry
School of Dentistry
University of São Paulo (USP)
São Paulo, SP, Brazil

Luciane Hiramatsu Azevedo
Dentistry Clinic
University of São Paulo (USP)
São Paulo, SP, Brazil

Vanderlei Salvador Bagnato
São Carlos Institute of Physics
University of São Paulo (USP)
São Carlos, SP, Brazil

Artur Felipe Santos Barbosa
Center of Biophotonics
School of Dentistry
Federal University of Bahia (UFBA)
Salvador, BA, Brazil
National Institute of Optics and Photonics
São Carlos, SP, Brazil
Laboratory of Immunomodulation and New Therapeutic
Approaches (LINAT)
Recife, PE, Brazil

Marina Stella Bello-Silva
Center for Research and Innovation in Laser
University Nove de Julho
São Paulo, SP, Brazil

Leticia Mello Bezinelli
Oncology, Hematology and Bone Marrow Transplantation Program
Hospital Israelita Albert Einstein
São Paulo, SP, Brazil

Jan Magnus Bjordal
Physiotherapy Research Group
Department of Global and Public Health
University of Bergen
Bergen, Norway

Mariana Minatel Braga
Department of Pediatric Dentistry
School of Dentistry
University of São Paulo (USP)
São Paulo, SP, Brazil

Aldo Brugnera Jr
Federal University of Rio de Janeiro (UFRJ)
Rio de Janeiro, RJ, Brazil
Master and PhD course at Federal University of Bahia (UFBA)
Salvador, BA, Brazil
Private Dental Practice – Brugnera & Zanin Institute
São Paulo, SP, Brazil
Masters and Doctoral Courses of Biomedical Engineering
University of Camilo Castelo Branco – Technological Park
São José dos Campos, SP, Brazil

Luana de Campos
Department of Biomaterials and Oral Biology
School of Dentistry
University of São Paulo (USP)
São Paulo, SP, Brazil

Mariana Torres Carvalho
São Carlos Institute of Physics
University of São Paulo (USP)
São Carlos, SP, Brazil

Paulo Francisco Cesar
Department of Biomaterials and Oral Biology
School of Dentistry
University of São Paulo (USP)
São Paulo, SP, Brazil

Maria Cristina Chavantes
Laser Medical Center of the Heart Institute
General Hospital
Medical School
University of São Paulo (USP)
São Paulo, SP, Brazil

Roberta Chow
Nerve Research Foundation
Brain and Mind Institute
The University of Sydney
Camperdown, Australia

Rosely Cordon
Center for Excellence in Prosthesis and Implants (CEPI)
School of Dentistry
University of São Paulo (USP)
São Paulo, SP, Brazil

Luciana Corrêa
General Pathology Department
School of Dentistry
University of São Paulo (USP)
São Paulo, SP, Brazil

Alessandro Cosci
Department of Physics and Materials Science
São Carlos Institute of Physics
University of São Paulo (USP)
São Carlos, SP, Brazil

Caroline Maria Gomes Dantas
Private Dental Practice
São Paulo, SP, Brazil

Elodie Debefve
Swiss Federal Institute of Technology (EPFL)
Lausanne, Switzerland

Christopher Deery
School of Clinical Dentistry
University of Sheffield
Sheffield, UK

Danilo Antônio Duarte
Pediatric Dentistry
University of Cruzeiro do Sul (UNICSUL)
São Paulo, SP, Brazil

Carlos de Paula Eduardo
Special Laboratory of Lasers in Dentistry (LELO)
Department of Restorative Dentistry
School of Dentistry
University of São Paulo (USP)
São Paulo, SP, Brazil

Fernanda de Paula Eduardo
Oncology, Hematology and Bone Marrow
Transplantation Program
Hospital Israelita Albert Einstein
São Paulo, SP, Brazil

Marcella Esteves-Oliveira
Department of Operative Dentistry
Periodontology and Preventive Dentistry
RWTH Aachen University
Aachen, Germany

Juliana Ferreira-Strixino
University of the Vale of Paraíba
São José dos Campos
São Paulo, SP, Brazil

Leila Soares Ferreira
Biodentistry Master Program
School of Dentistry
Ibirapuera University (UNIB)
São Paulo, SP, Brazil

Patrícia M. de Freitas
Special Laboratory of Lasers in Dentistry (LELO)
Department of Restorative Dentistry
School of Dentistry
University of São Paulo (USP)
São Paulo, SP, Brazil

Lucio Frigo
Laser in Dentistry Program
Cruzeiro do Sul University
São Paulo, SP, Brazil

Aguinaldo S. Garcez
São Leopoldo Mandic Dental Research Center
Campinas, SP, Brazil

Valdir Gouveia Garcia
Research and Study on Laser in Dentistry Group (GEPLO)
Department of Surgery and Integrated Clinic
Division of Periodontics
University Estadual Paulista (UNESP)
Araçatuba, SP, Brazil

Maria Garcia-Diaz
Wellman Center for Photomedicine
Massachusetts General Hospital
Boston, MA, USA
Molecular Engineering Group
IQS School of Engineering
University of Ramon Llull
Barcelona, Spain

Marcelo Giannini
Department of Restorative Dentistry
Piracicaba Dental School
State University of Campinas (UNICAMP)
Piracicaba, SP, Brazil

Thais Gimenez
Department of Pediatric Dentistry
School of Dentistry
University of São Paulo (USP)
São Paulo, SP, Brazil

Sheila C. Gouw-Soares
School of Dentistry
University of Cruzeiro do Sul (UNICSUL)
São Paulo, SP, Brazil

Clóvis Grecco
São Carlos Institute of Physics
University of São Paulo (USP)
São Carlos, SP, Brazil

Luiz Alcino Guerios
Maurício de Nassau University Center
Recife, PE, Brazil
Department of Clinic and Preventive Dentistry
Pernambuco Federal University
Recife, PE, Brazil

Michael R. Hamblin
Department of Dermatology
Harvard Medical School
Boston, MA, USA
Wellman Center for Photomedicine
Massachusetts General Hospital
Boston, MA, USA
Harvard–MIT Division of Health Sciences and Technology
Cambridge, MA, USA

Liyi Huang
Department of Dermatology
Harvard Medical School
Boston, MA, USA
Wellman Center for Photomedicine
Massachusetts General Hospital
Boston, MA, USA
Department of Infectious Diseases
First Affiliated College & Hospital
Guangxi Medical University
Nanning, China

Ying-Ying Huang
Department of Dermatology
Harvard Medical School
Boston, MA, USA
Wellman Center for Photomedicine
Massachusetts General Hospital
Boston, MA, USA
Aesthetic and Plastic Center of
Guangxi Medical University
Nanning, China

Tiina I. Karu
Institute of Laser and Information Technologies of the
Russian Academy of Sciences
Troitsk, Moscow Region
Russian Federation

Vivian Cunha Galletta Kern
Special Laboratory of Lasers in Dentistry (LELO)
School of Dentistry
University of São Paulo (USP)
São Paulo, SP, Brazil

Cristina Kurachi
Department of Physics and Materials Science
São Carlos Institute of Physics
University of São Paulo (USP)
São Carlos, SP, Brazil

Dalva Cruz Laganá
Center for Excellence in Prosthesis and Implants (CEPI)
School of Dentistry
University of São Paulo (USP)
São Paulo, SP, Brazil

José Luiz Lage-Marques
Discipline of Endodontics
Department of Restorative Dentistry
School of Dentistry
University of São Paulo (USP)
São Paulo, SP, Brazil

Jair Carneiro Leão
Department of Clinic and Preventive Dentistry
Pernambuco Federal University
Recife, PE, Brazil

Attilio Lopes
Research and Education Center for Photo Therapy
in Health Sciences
São Carlos, SP, Brazil

Rodrigo Alvaro Brandão Lopes-Martins
Institute of Biomedical Sciences
Pharmacology Department
University of São Paulo (USP)
São Paulo, SP, Brazil

Ana Claudia Luiz
Cancer Institute of São Paulo (ICESP)
São Paulo, SP, Brazil

Aparecida Maria Cordeiro Marques
Center of Biophotonics
School of Dentistry
Federal University of Bahia (UFBA)
Salvador, BA, Brazil
National Institute of Optics and Photonics
São Carlos, SP, Brazil

Juliana Marotti
Department of Prosthodontics and Biomaterials
Center for Implantology
Medical School of the RWTH Aachen University
Aachen, Germany

Andrea Malluf Dabul de Mello
Herrero Faculty
Curitiba, PR, Brazil

Fabiano Augusto Sfier de Mello
Herrero Faculty
Curitiba, PR, Brazil

Fausto Medeiros Mendes
Department of Pediatric Dentistry
School of Dentistry
University of São Paulo (USP)
São Paulo, SP, Brazil

Daiane Thais Meneguzzo
São Leopoldo Mandic Dental Research Center
Campinas, SP, Brazil

Dante Antonio Migliari
Department of Stomatology
School of Dentistry
University of São Paulo (USP)
São Paulo, SP, Brazil

Cesar A. Migliorati
Department of Diagnostic Sciences
and Oral Medicine
College of Dentistry
University of Tennessee Health Science Center
Memphis, TN, USA

Simone Gonçalves Moretto
Special Laboratory of Lasers in Dentistry (LELO)
Department of Restorative Dentistry
School of Dentistry
University of São Paulo (USP)
São Paulo, SP, Brazil

Lilian Tan Moriyama
Department of Physics and Materials Science
São Carlos Institute of Physics
University of São Paulo (USP)
São Carlos, SP, Brazil

Edgar Kazuyoshi Nakajima
Special Laboratory of Lasers in Dentistry (LELO)
School of Dentistry
University of São Paulo (USP)
São Paulo, SP, Brazil
Private Dental Practice
São Paulo, SP, Brazil

José Nicolau
Department of Biomaterials and
Oral Biology
School of Dentistry
University of São Paulo (USP)
São Paulo, SP, Brazil

Marinês Nobre-dos-Santos
Department of Pediatric Dentistry
Piracicaba Dental School
State University of Campinas (UNICAMP)
Piracicaba, SP, Brazil

Silvia C. Núñez
São Leopoldo Mandic Dental Research Center
São Paulo, SP, Brazil

Mario Pansini
Private Dental Practice
Curitiba, PR, Brazil

Nivaldo Parizotto
Department of Dermatology
Harvard Medical School
Boston, MA, USA
Wellman Center for Photomedicine
Massachusetts General Hospital
Boston, MA, USA
Department of Physiotherapy
Federal University of São Carlos
São Carlos, SP, Brazil

Antonio Luiz Barbosa Pinheiro
Center of Biophotonics
School of Dentistry
Federal University of Bahia (UFBA)
Salvador, BA, Brazil
National Institute of Optics and Photonics
São Carlos, SP, Brazil

Nathali Cordeiro Pinto
Cardiovascular and Thoracic Surgery Department of
the Heart Institute
General Hospital, Medical School
University of São Paulo (USP)
São Paulo, SP, Brazil

Karen Müller Ramalho
Biodentistry Master Program
School of Dentistry
Ibirapuera University (UNIB)
São Paulo, SP, Brazil

Martha Simões Ribeiro
Center for Lasers and Applications
Institute for Nuclear and Energy Research
IPEN-CNEN/SP
São Paulo, SP, Brazil

David N. J. Ricketts
Dundee Dental Hospital and School
University of Dundee
Dundee, UK

Lidiany Karla Azevdo Rodrigues
Faculty of Pharmacy
Dentistry and Nursing
Federal University of Ceará
Fortaleza, CE, Brazil

Georgios E. Romanos
Stony Brook University
School of Dental Medicine
Stony Brook, NY, USA

Daniel Simões A. Rosa
Private Dental Practice
São Paulo, SP, Brazil

Caetano P. Sabino
Wellman Center for Photomedicine
Massachusetts General Hospital
Boston, MA, USA
Center for Lasers and Applications
IPEN-CNEN/SP
São Paulo, SP, Brazil

Giselle Rodrigues de Sant'Anna
Pediatric Dentistry
University Cruzeiro do Sul (UNICSUL)
São Paulo, SP, Brazil

Lucia de Fátima Cavalcanti dos Santos
Real Center of Systemic Dentistry
Real Hospital Português de Pernambuco
Recife, PE, Brazil

Mark Schubert
Oral Medicine – UW School of Dentistry
Seattle, WA, USA
Oral Medicine – Seattle Cancer Care Alliance
Seattle, WA, USA

Igor Henrique Silva
Maurício de Nassau University Center
Recife, PE, Brazil

Alyne Simões
Department of Biomaterials and Oral Biology
School of Dentistry
University of São Paulo (USP)
São Paulo, SP, Brazil

Luiz Guilherme Pinheiro Soares
Center of Biophotonics
School of Dentistry
Federal University of Bahia (UFBA)
Salvador, BA, Brazil
National Institute of Optics and Photonics
São Carlos, SP, Brazil

Ana Maria Aparecida de Souza
Private Dental Practice
São Paulo, SP, Brazil
Special Laboratory of Lasers in Dentistry (LELO)
School of Dentistry
University of São Paulo (USP)
São Paulo, SP, Brazil

Marinês Vieira S. Sousa
Department of Orthodontics
Bauru Dental School
University of São Paulo (USP)
Bauru, SP, Brazil

Felipe F. Sperandio
Wellman Center for Photomedicine
Massachusetts General Hospital
Boston, MA, USA
Department of Pathology and Parasitology
Institute of Biomedical Sciences
Federal University of Alfenas
Alfenas, MG, Brazil
Department of Dermatology
Harvard Medical School
Boston, MA, USA

Cláudia Strefezza
Faculdades Metropolitanas Unidas (FMU)
São Paulo, SP, Brazil

Junji Tagami
Department of Cariology and Operative Dentistry
Faculty of Dentistry
Tokyo Medical and Dental University
Tokyo, Japan

Leticia Helena Theodoro
Research and Study on Laser in Dentistry Group (GEPLO)
Department of Surgery and Integrated Clinic
Division of Periodontics
University Estadual Paulista (UNESP)
Araçatuba, SP, Brazil

Marines Sammamed Freire Trevisan
Private Dental Practice
São Paulo, SP, Brazil
Special Laboratory of Lasers in Dentistry (LELO)
School of Dentistry
University of São Paulo (USP)
São Paulo, SP, Brazil

Jan Tunér
Private Dental Practice
Grängesberg, Sweden

Daniela Vecchio
Department of Dermatology
Harvard Medical School
Boston, MA, USA
Wellman Center for Photomedicine
Massachusetts General Hospital
Boston, MA, USA

Rodrigo Ramos Vieira
Special Laboratory of Lasers in Dentistry (LELO)
School of Dentistry
University of São Paulo (USP)
São Paulo, SP, Brazil
Private Dental Practice
São Paulo, SP, Brazil

Carolina Lapaz Vivan
Private Dental Practice
São Paulo, SP, Brazil

José Dirceu Vollet-Filho
São Carlos Institute of Physics
University of São Paulo (USP)
São Carlos, SP, Brazil

Mateus Cóstola Windlin
Private Dental Practice – Brugnera & Zanin Institute
São Paulo, SP, Brazil

Fátima Zanin
Federal University of Rio de Janeiro (UFRJ)
Rio de Janeiro, RJ, Brazil
Master and PhD course at Federal University
of Bahia (UFBA)
Salvador, BA, Brazil
Private Dental Practice – Brugnera & Zanin Institute
São Paulo, SP, Brazil

Denise Maria Zezell
Center for Lasers and Applications
Institute for Nuclear and Energy Research
IPEN-CNEN/SP
São Paulo, SP, Brazil

Foreword

It is an honor to write the foreword for this book that has brought together the most important researchers in the field around the world. Lasers are no longer just a promising therapeutic tool in dentistry; they have become one of the most important advances in dental care. From the chapters in this book, the reader will also realize that the use of lasers in dentistry is a strongly evidence-based science.

To write a book is a noble and hard task and the editors have done a very good job. They have picked very special authors for each chapter, each giving personal clinical experience and/or the scientific evidence. The chapters give a broad view of the issues from their basic concepts, to safety management, to clinical applications; from prevention to treatment of several oral pathologies; and of the different lasers available today.

The editors are dental school professors who have followed the growth of the use of lasers in dentistry from early in their academic lives. It has been a wonderful experience to follow this process. Patrícia was introduced to the research and clinical use of lasers during her PhD course, whereas Alyne entered the field earlier in her undergraduate course. Both were enchanted with different lasers applications. For Patrícia, a professor of Restorative Dentistry, the high power lasers were the most useful. On the other hand, Alyne has been in love with low power lasers. Both are brilliant and dedicated clinicians and researchers and this book certainly reflects their effort in disseminating their own knowledge and that of others.

I hope the reader will take advantage of this book's contents and can realize the importance this technology has in improving the quality of the lives of their patients.

I congratulate Patrícia and Alyne in this achievement.

Marcia Martins Marques

Preface

"And God said: Let there be light, and there was light. God saw that the light was good..."

(Holy Bible, Genesis 1:3)

The knowledge that light is beneficial and may lead to cure does not belong exclusively to our time; Greek and Ancient Egyptian doctors practiced cures by exposure to sunlight. However, it was in the past century that one of the great technological advancements was made: the development of laser appliances for use in fields ranging from CDs and DVDs to performing surgeries and treating diseases.

Taking into consideration the scope and importance of the subject, coordinating this book, in which renowned researchers and clinicians who work with lasers in dentistry have participated, has certainly been a great responsibility. With love, belief in our ideals, and enthusiasm, we accepted the challenge.

At this time, in seeking knowledge and intellectual preparation to deal with the different situations in which life places us, our major ally has certainly been God. With Him, challenges have been overcome and limits transformed into actions to bring our readers all the latest information concerning the use of lasers and LEDs in dentistry.

There is no longer any doubt that therapies with lasers and LEDs have positive results; nevertheless, there is still no consensus about the best manner of application of these therapies in each clinical situation for optimal results. The incessant search for effective clinical protocols was the starting point for this extensive work, with the aim of opening the clinical professional's eyes to the various possibilities for the use of this new technology in dentistry. These protocols are not immutable, but they are supported by basic and clinical research. These are protocols that open various doors to other new protocols and clinical applications of lasers and LEDs in the diverse specialties of dentistry. They are protocols designed to enable you to explore this world, in which light interacts with soft and hard oral tissues, bringing benefits to our patients.

Explore, question, innovate... We challenge you, the reader, to become part of this work, to make use of the broad body of knowledge that has so honorably been shared with us by our collaborators!

Good reading!

Patrícia M. de Freitas and Alyne Simões

Basic principles of lasers and LEDs

CHAPTER 1

Physics of lasers and LEDs: Basic concepts

Clóvis Grecco, José Dirceu Vollet-Filho, Mariana Torres Carvalho, and Vanderlei Salvador Bagnato

São Carlos Institute of Physics, University of São Paulo (USP), São Carlos, SP, Brazil

Lasers

Laser light has very specific properties, thanks to the way that electromagnetic radiation is generated, and these properties are especially useful in science and technology. A special process produces laser light and this depends on some aspects of the interaction between the atoms that constitute matter and the electromagnetic radiation. To understand why laser light has unique properties, comprehension of the basic concepts of physics is required and these are explained in this chapter.

Key points to be understood include atomic structure, and how light originates and the path it takes through matter. The concept of the atom can be traced back to the ancient philosophers. They defined the "atom," from the Greek for "not divisible," as the smallest possible portion of a rock that could be formed by repeatedly splitting a rock until it could not be split further and without changing the basic properties of the original rock. They believed the atom was indestructible, a belief that has been disproved by scientific advances.

In 1808, the British scientist John Dalton scientifically defined the atom: "The atom is the smallest matter particle. It is indestructible. Its mass and size cannot be changed. Atoms may combine with each other, creating other species of matter." The current definition of the atom diverges from that of Dalton. Unlike in current models, Dalton viewed the atom as a rigid sphere. Nevertheless, Dalton's simplified model may still be used in describing situations such as chemical reactions and the law of definite proportions (Proust's law), in which atoms may be considered as rigid spheres.

Later in the 18th century, Ernest Rutherford, a British scientist, introduced new concepts about atomic structure (the reader is referred to basic chemistry and physics texts for a detailed description of his model). His main concept was that "the atom would be constituted of a central part, called nucleus, and it has positive electric charge. The nucleus's size would be smaller than the atom's size (100 000–10 000 times smaller)." The question then was: if the atom has a nucleus with an expressive positive charge, how is it that matter is usually neutral? Rutherford answered the question by proposing that the positive charge of the nucleus is balanced by particles with a negative charge, called "electrons," which revolve around the nucleus. He proposed a dynamic balance, as illustrated in Figure 1.1, because if electrons were not moving, they would be attracted to the nucleus.

However, there was a problem with Rutherford's model of an electric charge revolving around the nucleus. Electromagnetic theory at that time had already determined that electrically charged particles (such as electrons) emit energy when they accelerate. Therefore, in Rutherford's model, electrons should emit energy constantly (since a curved trajectory implies acceleration according to Newton's laws) and as a result, the radius of their circular trajectory will reduce as kinetic energy, which sustains their movement, is lost. According to this theory, matter would quickly collapse as electrons fall inwards and onto the nucleus.

The Danish physician Niels Bohr (1885–1962) used the basic ideas of Max Planck (1858–1947) to solve the problem of why matter does not collapse. He made certain propositions, known as "Bohr's postulates," to explain the electron–nucleus dynamics:

1 The electrons revolving around the nucleus follow well-defined circular orbits, under the influence of the Coulomb attraction.
2 The radii of the orbits of the electrons around the nucleus can only assume certain values, proportional to $h/2\pi$ (where h is Planck's constant).
3 The energy of the atom has a definite value when the electrons are in a given stationary orbit. When an electron moves to a new orbit, energy is absorbed or emitted. The amount of absorbed/emitted energy can be obtained from the expression $\Delta E = hf$, where ΔE is the energy absorbed or emitted, h is Planck's constant, and f is the frequency of radiation (see later in this chapter). Note that ΔE is the energy difference between the two stationary orbits involved in the process.

The energy emitted or absorbed by an electron when it changes its orbit was named a "photon." A photon can be viewed as a small energy "packet" or "quantum." Therefore, when the

Lasers in Dentistry: Guide for Clinical Practice, First Edition. Edited by Patrícia M. de Freitas and Alyne Simões.

electron moves to an orbit closer to the nucleus, it emits a photon; when it moves to an orbit that is farther from the nucleus, it absorbs a photon (Fig. 1.2). Bohr assumed that the angular momentum ($\vec{L} = \vec{r} \times m\vec{v}$, where $\vec{r}$ is the radius vector, m is the scalar mass, and $\vec{v}$ is the velocity vector) of the electron revolving around the nucleus was an integral multiple of Planck's constant h divided by 2π. This is called Bohr's quantization rule.

Bohr's ideas were not pulled out of the hat, but based on experimental studies of the emission spectrum of hydrogen. To understand what is meant by "spectrum," think about white light passing through a prism (Fig. 1.3). It is decomposed into all the colors that constitute the visible light spectrum. This same phenomenon creates rainbows, where water droplets act as spherical prisms and the sun is the light source. Bohr used this technique to decompose the light spectrum emitted by a hydrogen gas lamp.

The frequency of each light wave (which our eyes interpret as different colors) is associated with its length (the so-called "wavelength"). A light wave oscillates in time and space. If we stop it in time, its wavelength is the distance at which the wave shape repeats itself. If we stop it in one specific position, its frequency is the number of times the wave repeats itself (cycles) per second. Several, hardly distinguishable wavelengths constitute what we call the "white" color, and the observed effect is called a "continuum spectrum."

Bohr observed discrete lines of emission in the spectrum of the hydrogen lamp. The word "discrete" here means that there are separated, very specific lines, which are observed instead of a continuum spectrum composed of photons carrying a specific amount or quantum of energy (Fig. 1.4). These discrete lines in the spectrum from the hydrogen lamp are composed of a few specific wavelengths only; this is referred to as a "discrete spectrum." However, how is the emission generated?

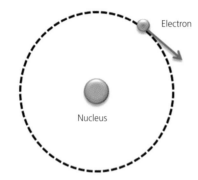

Figure 1.1 Schematic of the atom according to Bohr.

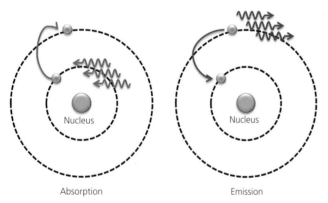

Figure 1.2 Representation of absorption and emission of photons by an electron, with transition to an energy level farther from (absorption) or closer to the nucleus (emission).

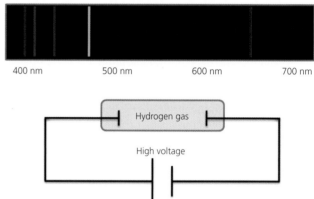

Figure 1.4 Schematic of the hydrogen gas lamp (bottom) and the specific lines (wavelengths) obtained form the emission of that gas (top).

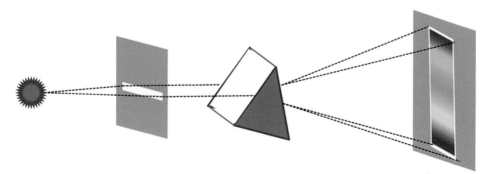

Figure 1.3 A beam of white light may be diffracted into different colors when passed through a prism. Each wavelength has a specific angle of diffraction, which "bends" light more or less, separating the colors (the colors of the rainbow are seen because of this phenomenon when water droplets diffract light).

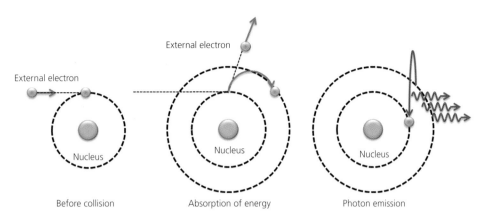

Figure 1.5 Example of an external electron interacting with an electron in an atom: the incoming electron collides with the internal electron, transfering energy to it; the incoming electron can then move to an orbit farther from the nucleus; this new orbit can accommodate an electron with this new amount of energy. Later, this excited electron emits energy (e.g. as photons) and "relaxes" back to a lower energy level.

When a gas, such as hydrogen, at low pressure is subjected to a high voltage between two electrodes, an electrical field is generated in the tube and the free electrons in the ionized gas are accelerated from the cathode to the anode. On their path, the free electrons may collide with hydrogen atoms and transfer energy to the latter. The "ground" state electron (i.e. the one having the minimum possible energy) in the hydrogen atom absorbs the energy and moves to an orbit farther from the nucleus. This process is called "excitation"; it is said that the electron moves to an "excited" state.

An excited state is unstable as the most stable atomic configuration is the one with the lowest possible energy. Therefore, shortly after absorbing this energy, the atom "expels" it (which may happen in many different forms) and the electron returns to its most stable orbit. Therefore, as illustrated in Figure 1.5, a photon can emit energy equivalent to the energy difference between the two orbits. Different photons, with different energies, may be emitted by the atom because following the collision between an electron and an atom, the atom's electron might be excited to different orbits depending on the amount of energy absorbed. However, only certain photon energies can be observed and these make up the discrete spectrum observed by Bohr. The spectrum provides a "fingerprint" of the atom, where each photon represents emission from a different orbit.

Electrons within a given orbit have a specific energy. The orbits are called "energy levels." Each energy level is assigned an integer number (n = 1, 2, 3…), which is called the "principal quantum number" and corresponds to the number obtained from Bohr's quantization rule. This number characterizes the energy for an electron in a specific orbit and the "leaps" between two energy levels are called "electronic transitions". The wavelength for a photon emitted when an electron moves to an orbit closer to the nucleus will not be observed if it falls outside the visible spectrum.

The above may appear to be a long explanation, but understanding how electrons allow atoms and molecules to absorb and emit light is critical to understanding how the laser works.

Laser light generation

So far, we have discussed two main processes: absorption and emission. When an atom (or molecule) absorbs a photon, this energy promotes an electron to a more energetic state. When emitting a photon, an atom (or molecule) expels energy corresponding to the difference between the excited and the more stable state involved.

A third and equally important process for atomic systems needs to be considered: the *stimulated emission*. Suppose that an atom is in an excited state. As has already been discussed, this is not a stable condition and the atom will eventually return to its fundamental state. In fact, any disturbance in its equilibrium may result in decay from the excited state, with consequent emission. Therefore, the amount of time that the system stays in the excited state, called the "lifetime" of the excited state, is an essential characteristic of the atomic system for the generation of laser light. In stimulated emission, if a photon "passes nearby" an excited atom, it can induce an electrical perturbation (which works as a "seed") that stimulates the system to emit an identical photon, but only if the lifetime of the excited state is long enough to allow the photon to pass by the atom, therefore increasing the "probability" of the event occurring. Also, the photon energy has to correspond to a permitted (i.e. highly probable) electronic transition of the atomic system. The stimulated photon may be seen as the "twin" of the seed photon. They both have the same energy; therefore, their frequencies and wavelengths are identical and they leave the atomic system with the same direction and "phase" (i.e. they propagate in unison in space).

Figure 1.6 shows the three processes that have been described. The schematic on the left represents the absorption process, where a photon interacts with the atomic system and is absorbed. In the middle schematic, emission is represented, where the atomic system, which is in the excited state, emits a photon and an electron is demoted to a lower energy level. On the right, stimulated emission is represented, where a photon stimulates the emission of a second, identical photon.

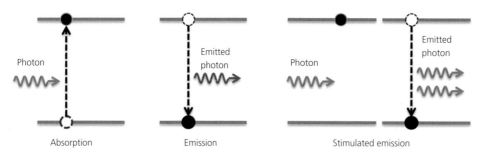

Figure 1.6 Schematic comparing absorption, simple emission, and stimulated emission of radiation. The latter processes both start with the first one (absorption), but the last one needs an excited electron to be disturbed by its interaction with a photon with the same energy as the one to be emitted. When this happens, a photon is emitted in phase with the incoming photon, and with the same energy (i.e. wavelength).

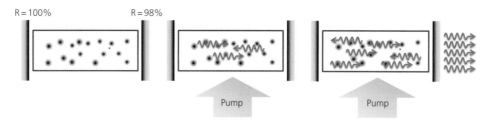

Figure 1.7 Schematic showing the generation of laser light. The active medium (rectangle) has a mirror at each end: one is a 100% reflector and the other is a partial reflector (e.g. 98%; the remaining light leaves the medium). An energy source (electricity, another laser, etc.) is used to "pump" electrons to the excited states so that photons can be stimulated. Those photons are reflected backwards and forwards inside the cavity and stimulate new photons. Part of the energy is emitted as the laser beam.

If the conditions are correct, each of the two resulting photons from the stimulated emission will disturb other excited atoms, promoting more stimulated emissions. Therefore, there is a cascade of stimulated emissions. These stimulated emissions are later amplified by the laser device design, and it is this amplification of the stimulated emission that results in laser light generation.

Consider a material medium (active medium) where most of the atoms are in excited states (this is known as "inversion of population," because under normal conditions, the majority of the atoms will not be excited). Suppose a photon stimulates the emission of a second photon in this medium. Each of those photons may stimulate new emissions if they interact with other already excited atoms. This generates four photons, then eight, and so on. Very quickly there will be a great number of photons emitted in the same direction, since each stimulated photon is released in the direction of its seed. Then, if all those photons are redirected back to the active medium (using mirrors, for example) and the medium is maintained in the inversion of population condition (i.e. if electrons are constantly excited), in a very short time a huge number of photons with the same characteristics will be generated. This is the basis of the technique known as "**L**ight **A**mplification by **S**timulated **E**mission of **R**adiation" – or just LASER.

Laser devices must include an optical cavity to produce the laser beam (or "ray"). It is usually composed of the active medium (composed of atoms and molecules whose electrons will be excited to obtain the stimulated photons) plus two mirrored surfaces at the extremities: one must be a complete reflector, and the other a semi-reflector. These are necessary to keep a positive gain of photons inside the optical cavity (i.e. more photons are emitted than absorbed by the active medium) and also to emit part of the beam (generated photons) out of the cavity. The complete reflector surface ensures generated and stimulated photons repeatedly travel back and forth through the cavity, stimulating even more photons, and the semi-reflector surface emits part of the generated beam.

However, if the generation of new photons is to be maintained, electrons must be continuously excited, or "pumped" to the excited state. If most electrons have returned to their ground states, no stimulated or spontaneous emissions will be achieved. This pumping is achieved by connecting an external energy source (such as a light source – sometimes other lasers, electrical discharges, chemical reactions, etc.) to the cavity. If excited electrons emit radiation, spontaneous or stimulated, they can be returned to the excited state.

With appropriate parameters, the probability of stimulated emission can be kept very high within the cavity and a laser beam will be produced. Thus, to create and sustain the optimum conditions within the cavity, it is necessary to feed the active medium with energy so that the inversion of population remains, and to keep redirecting the photons to the active medium, to maintain a positive feedback and sustain the stimulated emission. Figure 1.7 represents one possible configuration for a laser. The atoms/molecules in the medium form the active medium; the 100% and the 98% mirror complete the laser cavity.

From the moment the pump is turned on (low input energy), the atomic systems are excited and start to emit spontaneously; only a few atoms may be stimulated to emit. Once energy input reaches a certain level (the threshold), the stimulated emissions outnumber the spontaneous emissions; the former are suppressed and almost all the atoms in the active medium are stimulated to emit. Hence, the output light beam, which is released from the cavity by the semi-reflector mirror, is composed of photons that share the same characteristics: energy (wavelength and frequency), direction, and phase coherence.

The active medium may be solid, liquid or gaseous. Common materials are sapphire or ruby crystals (a ruby crystal rod was the active medium for the first laser ever constructed), dye solutions, and argon ion, nitrogen or neon gases. Active media should maintain electrons in the excited state for as long as possible (10^{-10} seconds is the usual lifetime – the duration of the excited state before decay), so that as many electrons as possible may achieve the excited state, allowing the stimulated emission of a massive number of photons. This is also necessary to compensate for photons absorbed by the medium and maintain a positive balance of photons in the laser cavity.

Since light wavelength is related to the photon energy, to obtain a laser beam with a specific wavelength, the active medium must allow energy transitions corresponding exactly to the energy of the desired photons. Additionally, the length of the cavity must be a multiple of the desired wavelength if light is to be released from the cavity and control of the coherence is to be maintained within the cavity. If it is not, light will repeatedly be reflected within the cavity and photons will lose their relative phase coherence; thus, the positive balance within the cavity will be lost. The reasons why this happens will not be discussed in detail, but briefly it should be appreciated that a light wave propagates as continuous cycles of its wavelength, and if a wavelength is not a multiple of the length of the cavity, light will not be emitted. From this it follows that the length of the cavity is a determinant of the wavelengths of the output.

In summary, a laser device needs to achieve an inversion of population and start spontaneous emission. Each spontaneous photon then promotes the stimulated emission of another identical photon. A cascade of photons is obtained as mirrors at the extremities of the optical cavity deflect photons back into the active medium. Electrons are constantly pumped back to excited states by an external energy source. Millions of cycles of this process produce a huge number of identical photons (light amplification). Finally, the semi-reflective mirror releases part of the light from the cavity – the laser beam.

This complex process is worthwhile because a laser beam is not "just" light: it is a very special kind of light! A laser beam has important characteristics that give it several technological and scientific applications. The light emitted by lasers is different from that produced by more common light sources such as incandescent bulbs, fluorescent lamps, and high power arc lamps. Laser light is nearly monochromatic, coherent, and its beam has directionality; a very high power output is achieved as a result.

All common light sources emit light of many different wavelengths. As mentioned previously, white light contains all, or most, of the colors of the visible spectrum. Ordinary colored light, such as that emitted by colored lamps, consists of a broad range of wavelengths covering a particular portion of the visible light spectrum. The beam of a laser, on the other hand, is a very pure color. It consists of an extremely narrow range of wavelengths. It is said to be nearly "monochromatic."

Monochromaticity (or near monochromaticity) is a unique property of laser light. This characteristic is associated with photon frequency and hence photon energy, and is unique because it reflects the specific transitions of the electrons that are excited to obtain those photons. Perfectly monochromatic light cannot be produced even by a laser, but laser light is many times more monochromatic than the light from any other source.

Why is monochromaticity important? As discussed earlier, both atomic absorption and emission have an intrinsic relationship with the photon energy (color). If one needs to excite a specific electronic transition within a medium, the effect will be much more efficient if the photon used has the same energy as (or is very close to) the energy of the transition, because otherwise a great amount of energy is wasted in generating photons that are not used for the desired transition. The efficiency will impact on the amount of power necessary to obtain the desired effect. If excitation can be efficiently achieved, less power is needed to obtain the same results. For example, when comparing a colored lamp and a laser, both in the same color range, to obtain excitation of the transition for 633 nm (red photons), a laser emitting at a wavelength of 633 nm will be fully utilized in excitation, while only a very small portion of light from a lamp's emission spectrum (hundreds of wavelengths between, say, 610 and 660 nm) will achieve the same effect, requiring much more energy to be provided by the lamp for 633-nm emission.

Conventional light sources, such as an incandescent bulb, usually emit light in all directions. Even though one can use lenses, reflectors, and other kinds of optical systems to collimate the emitted light, such that it is emitted in a directed beam, this beam always diverges (spreads) more rapidly than the beam generated by a laser. This leads to a decrease in light intensity with increasing distance from the light source.

Directionality is the characteristic of laser light that makes it travel in a single direction, with only a narrow cone of divergence. Collimated light, that is a perfectly parallel beam of directional light, cannot be produced even by a laser, but laser light is many times more collimated than the light from any other source. Because of the intrinsic characteristic of the stimulated photons (twin photons), they are almost all emitted in the same direction; therefore all photons in the beam deviate minimally from the beam axis. A laser device can produce a light beam that is approximately collimated for kilometers! This is the property which makes laser light suitable for so many uses, from telecommunications to medical applications, due to the possibility of delivery through optical fibers. Because the output photons of a laser travel mostly in the same direction, laser light may be many times more efficient when compared to a usual light source in terms of power output. The high power output of a laser (the amount of energy generated in a certain time interval, which is proportional to the number of photons generated in that time) is a very important feature, since high power lasers can be used to destroy or modify structures. Pulsed lasers can achieve power outputs in the order of tera-watts (10^{12} W).

As illustration, consider the red light generated by a red bulb lamp compared to a diode laser (for simplicity, assume that both sources produces the same number of photons per second). The red lamp will emit photons in all directions – in a sphere around the source (isotropic emission), while the laser will emit these in a single direction with a very small cone of divergence. The physical quantity that describes this effect is the intensity, which is the amount of power per area. Therefore, a laser device can achieve very high intensities, which is extremely important in some technological applications.

However, coherence is an entirely different concept from intensity. To understand the coherence property of laser light, we must remember that light waves behave like water waves: if a rock is dropped into a lake, it produces subsequent waves that can be observed propagating from the center in all directions; each crest is followed by a trough, which is followed by a crest, and so on. However, if many rocks are dropped simultaneously but randomly into the lake, the interference between the many waves will mean that the crests and troughs of the individual waves will probably not be recognized. With this picture in mind, think of coherence as the property of waves that behave just like the ones generated by the single rock dropped into the lake: they move continuously and are synchronized.

The photons generated by stimulated emission are equal, which means they are also "in phase" with each other: they are synchronized and, if represented as a wave, this means their crests and troughs are aligned, both in time and space. This is the case because during the stimulated emission, the photons "drag" other photons with them, forcing them to "behave" in the same way. Remember also that stimulated emission generates a cascade effect, which means that the photon that starts the process dictates the behavior of all the subsequent photons, and they are synchronized with it. With that in mind, we can introduce new concepts: *coherence length* and *coherence time*.

For the same reasons it is not possible to construct a perfectly monochromatic or collimated source, it is not possible to have a perfectly coherent laser. All these concepts are connected, but it is beyond the scope of this chapter to provide further discussion. The photons that exit a laser can only be synchronized for a certain amount of time – the "coherence time." The light is traveling during that time and the distance covered during that time is the "coherence length." In other words, the coherence time/length is the time/distance between two photons generated by the same source during which they will be synchronized; after this time/distance, they no longer "recognize" that they were generated by the same source and will no longer be synchronized.

Light emitting diode

You certainly use a light emitting diodes (LEDs) many times in your daily life. They are in TV remote controls, clock displays, and TV screens. LEDs were first used as an electronic component in the 1960s. Later, with the development of electronic systems and materials, it was possible to construct high power LEDs, allowing their use as efficient light sources.

To explain how LEDs work, we need to discuss the interaction between atoms in a crystalline array. When atoms are close enough, such as in a crystalline structure, the energy levels of one atom will be slightly disturbed by its neighbors. This effect may result in a near continuum of energy levels. In solids, the ground state corresponds to the electrons occupying the lowest possible energy level. The energy gaps determine whether the solid is an insulating material or a conductor (Fig. 1.8). This is a very simplistic description, since it is the wave nature of the electrons in the crystal that is responsible for generating the energy band; the reader is referred to more detailed books for further insights into this subject if desired.

Conducting materials, such as metals, have high conductivity at the last occupied band as they have a small gap between the electronic bands. Consequently, changes in the electrons states are possible when an electric field is applied, promoting conduction. Some materials, known as semi-metals, have a slightly higher resistance than normal metals. Materials that do not conduct electric current are known as insulators.

It is also possible for enough electrons to be excited thermally so that an applied electric field can produce a modest current; these materials are known as semi-conductors.

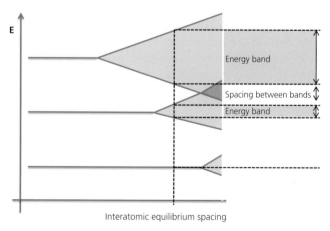

Figure 1.8 Recombination between electrons and holes, which releases energy as emitted photons.

The band structures of insulators and semi-conductors are qualitatively similar. Normally there exists in both insulators and semi-conductors a filled energy band (referred to as the valence band) separated from the next higher band (referred to as the conduction band) by an energy gap. For a semi-conductor, the energy gap is usually smaller than about 1 electron volt. In general, the gap in insulators is at least several electron volts; overcoming this large energy gap to promote sufficient numbers of electrons to the conduction band cannot be achieved with an applied field or by thermal excitation. Therefore, there is high resistance to changing the total electron momentum and allow the electrons to move as they would in a conductor.

In a semi-conductor, the valence band is full at very low temperatures (close to 0 K), but when the temperature increases, electrons acquire sufficient thermal energy to be promoted to the conduction band, which was empty initially. This effect creates the so-called "holes" in the valence band, which correspond to the "vacancies" left by the electrons that leave for the conduction band. These holes are able to generate an electric current when an external electric field is applied, because they represent the absence of negative charges – it is helpful to think of them as positive charges. The conductivity of a material depends on the number of electrons that can be transferred to the conduction band and therefore are "free" to move within the crystalline arrangement.

The main difference between semi-conductors and insulators is the energy gap. The number of electrons in the conduction band changes with temperature. Pure semi-conductors are called "intrinsic," and because of their dependence on temperature, they are not used in the manufacture of electrical devices (a device that only worked under a specific range of temperature would have limited utility). In order to use semi-conductor materials, manufacturers usually use a technique called "doping," which means modifying the conductivity of a material by incorporating "impurities." This enables tighter control of the conduction conditions and allows different electronic devices to be made using the semi-conductor. In the absence of an external electric field, the band gap is large enough for these semi-conductors to act as insulators, but when an external field is applied, the balance of energy changes and the electrons and holes acquire some degree of freedom. In this way, the behavior of semi-conductors can be controlled. Doped materials are usually called "extrinsic" materials.

LEDs are made from two types of extrinsic material. The characteristics of the semi-conductor will change depending on the impurities added. If impurities that can donate electrons are added, an "n-type" semi-conductor ("n" for negative) is formed. These are usually made by introducing atoms with five electrons in their valence band, with the fifth electron weakly bound; consequently, these electrons are free to move around the crystal. Impurities in n-type materials are called donor atoms. The other kind of material is called a "p-type" semi-conductor ("p" for positive), which is made by the addition of impurities that

have only three valence electrons. In this case, the number of electrons is insufficient to make covalent bonds, creating holes in the crystalline array. Impurities with incomplete covalent bonds are called acceptor atoms.

The transition processes in semi-conductors, either from photon emissions or absorptions, are more efficient when impurities have been added. The impurities facilitate electrons and holes to recombine in the process of photon emission. In LEDs, whenever an electron makes a transition from the conduction band to the valence band (effectively recombining electron and hole) there is a release of energy in the form of a photon. In some materials, the spacing of the energy levels is such that the emitted photon is in the visible part of the spectrum. Figure 1.9 represents the recombination of electrons and holes, which leads to the emission of photons.

The "p–n" junction is at the base of the LED. The junction between a p-material and an n-material forms a semi-conductor diode. The electrons in the "n" side move to the junction and will be projected into the "p" side to produce a high electron concentration in the conduction band, which is larger than when in thermal equilibrium. The same happens on the other side, with the holes. When an electron combines with a hole, energy is released, a fraction as thermal energy and another as a photon (Fig. 1.10a). When an external field is applied to the junction, the electrons and holes have sufficient energy to recombine and eventually emit a photon

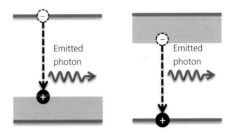

Figure 1.9 Schematic of the overlap of the energy bands, with energy versus interatomic equilibrium spacing. Not all energy levels overlap, only specific ones, depending on the material characteristics.

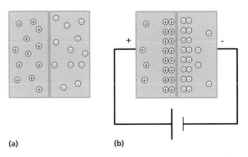

Figure 1.10 P–n junction in an LED. (a) Electrons (material "n") and holes (material "p", vacancies of electrons that behave as positive charges) are found in specific materials. (b) If a voltage is applied across the material, electrons and vacancies try to follow the electric field and the energy transfers involved promote light emission.

Table 1.1 Some common materials used in LED, with their characteristic wavelength and color.

Material	Wavelength (nm)	Color
GaAs (gallium–arsenide)	904	Infrared
InGaAsP (indium–gallium–arsenide–phosphide)	1300	Infrared
AsGaAl (gallium–aluminum–arsenide)	750–850	Red
AsGaP (arsenic–gallium–phosphorus)	590	Yellow
InGaAlP (indium–gallium–aluminum–phosphide)	560	Green
CsI (caesium iodide)	480	Blue

(Fig. 1.10b). The wavelengths of the emitted photons depend on the materials from which the LED is manufactured. Table 1.1 lists some semi-conductor materials (their names also indicate the impurity used in the manufacture of the device), with the corresponding wavelength (color) of the light they generate.

LED light is neither coherent nor collimated, but it is much more monochromatic than other light sources, excluding laser devices. In contrast to lasers, LEDs consume very little energy to produce light. Additionally, they are durable and, depending on the desired wavelengths, may be very cheap and easily sourced. As such, when light of specific wavelengths is required, they are a better option than lamps, which make them an important tool in science and technology development.

CHAPTER 2

High power lasers and their interaction with biological tissues

Denise Maria Zezell[1] and Patricia Aparecida Ana[2]

[1]Center for Lasers and Applications, Institute for Nuclear and Energy Research, IPEN-CNEN/SP, São Paulo, SP, Brazil
[2]Center for Engineering, Modeling and Applied Social Sciences, Federal University of ABC (UFABC), Santo André, Brazil

Introduction

The biological effects of coherent light have been the subject of scientific interest since the development of the first laser system in the early 1960s.[1] With the commercial availability of new laser technologies, efforts have been made to understand the interaction of these lasers with biological tissues and also the effects promoted by each wavelength, in order to establish an effective and efficient protocol for their clinical use.

In recent decades, it has been demonstrated that laser irradiation can be a useful tool for many procedures in medicine, dentistry, biology, physiotherapy, and other life sciences. In dentistry, lasers have become an attractive instrument for many procedures, including soft tissue surgery,[2,3] decontamination,[4,5] assuring anti-inflammatory effects,[6,7] cavity preparation,[8,9] caries prevention,[10-12] caries decontamination,[13] and caries removal.[14,15] The clinical use of laser irradiation is based on a wide range of physical phenomena of light interaction with biological tissues, cells, and fluids. Understanding of the concepts of absorption, scattering, transmission, and reflection is required by professionals in order to validate any protocol for a clinical procedure that uses laser irradiation. Also, this knowledge is indispensable in choosing the best equipment and to avoid deleterious effects on irradiated tissue. Each of the processes of laser interaction with biological tissues depends on the characteristics of the laser system, such as wavelength, pulse duration, pulse energy, repetition rate, beam spot size, delivery method, laser beam characteristics,[16] and optical properties of tissue, such as the refractive index, scattering coefficient (μ_s), absorption coefficient (μ_a), and anisotropy factor.[17-19]

In life sciences, the most commonly studied laser systems are those that involve thermal interaction. When high power lasers, or high intensity lasers, are used, heat is generated in almost all irradiation conditions, which can be converted into controlled temperature rises in a small and specific area of biological tissues.[20] Depending on the temperature rises and the interaction of laser irradiation with these tissues, it is possible to produce microstructural and/or physical changes in biological tissues. With high power lasers, it is possible to vaporize, coagulate, and ablate biological tissues, allowing clinical procedures to be performed with safety, little bleeding, and asepsis.[21] The intense thermal action of high power lasers makes them suitable as coadjutants in tumors excision in oncology, for example, as well as it in the execution of conservative cavity preparation in dentistry.

In dentistry, the most frequently used high power laser systems are the Nd:YAG (1064 nm),[5,10,11] argon (488 nm),[12] Ho:YLF (2065 nm),[22] Ho:YAG (2100 nm),[23] Er:YAG (2940 nm),[8,15] Er,Cr:YSGG (2780 nm),[9,16,20,24] diode (810 nm),[4,25] and CO_2 9300 nm, 9600 nm or 10600 nm).[11,26-28] With the exception of the argon laser, these lasers emit light in the infrared range of the electromagnetic spectrum, and most equipment operates in the free running mode, with a pulse duration of tens of hundreds of microseconds (μs).

More recently, researchers have reported the use of other type of laser systems in dentistry, in which non-linear interactions with biological tissues take place. These systems have extremely short pulse lengths (femtoseconds, fs) and are called *ultrashort pulsed lasers* (USPLs).[29-31] Due to this fact, these systems cut precisely and can achieve well-defined cavities and controlled caries removal.[32] Efforts have been made to understand their interaction with biological tissues and to determine safe and appropriate parameters for their future clinical application in dentistry.[33-37]

This chapter will focus on recent developments in the use of high power laser irradiation in dentistry, as well summarizing the main interactions of these lasers with biological tissues.

High power lasers

Since the development of the first lasers, the most studied applications of lasers in health sciences are those determined by thermal effects (when the absorbed energy is subsequently transformed into heat).[21,29] The thermal effects are necessary for clinical procedures such as cutting, coagulation, vaporization, and ablation of biological tissues, and to achieve these, high

Lasers in Dentistry: Guide for Clinical Practice, First Edition. Edited by Patrícia M. de Freitas and Alyne Simões.
© 2015 John Wiley & Sons, Inc. Published 2015 by John Wiley & Sons, Inc.

Table 2.1 Commercially available high power lasers used in dentistry and their main clinical applications.

Laser	Wavelength (nm)	Emission mode	Typical pulse width	Main interaction	Main clinical applications
CO_2	10600	CW or PW	Continuous or O (50 ms)	Water and hydroxyapatite (PO_4^- radical)	Soft tissue surgery, caries prevention, coagulation
Er:YAG	2940	PW	100–150 μs	Water	Hard tissue ablation (cavity preparation, caries removal, bone surgery), caries prevention, soft tissue surgery, decontamination, endodontics
Er,Cr:YSGG	2780	PW	140 μs	Water and hydroxyapatite (OH^- radical)	Hard tissue ablation (cavity preparation, caries removal, bone surgery), caries prevention, soft tissue surgery, decontamination, endodontics
Nd:YAG	1064	CW or PW	100 μs	Melanin, hemoglobin	Soft tissue surgery, caries prevention, dentin hypersensitivity, decontamination, endodontics
Argon	488 or 514	CW or PW	50–500 ms	Melanin, hemoglobin, hemosiderin	Soft tissue surgery, polymerization of composite resins, dental whitening, illumination of caries
Diode	810 or 940	CW or PW	Continuous or O (50 ms)	Melanin, hemoglobin	Soft tissue surgery, decontamination, endodontics

CW, continuous wave; PW, pulsed wave

power lasers are used. However, recently, the use of laser irradiation for biostimulation of tissues has become popular and, in this case, the effects are based on cellular mechanisms other than an increase in temperature[38] and low power lasers can then be used. It is important to distinguish between low power lasers and high power lasers in order to appreciate their possible effects.

Exposure of body tissue to irradiation at a power density, or intensity, of a few mW/cm^2 excludes the possibility of thermal effects.[29] Lasers that emit in this range of intensities are identified as low power lasers. Therapy with lasers that emit low intensities relies on non-thermal effects (photophysical, photochemical, and photobiological) and the temperature of biological tissue does not exceed 37.5 °C.[21,29,38,39]

In contrast, high power lasers are those that generate a power equal to or higher than $1 W/cm^2$; these lasers increase tissue temperature by 1 °C or more and, in this way, promote coagulation, cutting, vaporization or ablation of tissues.[21,29,38]

As well as the power, some other characteristics of laser systems are essential n determining the specific effects on biological tissues. Among these, the most important ones are the wavelength, emission mode (i.e. continuous or pulsed), peak power, energy density, repetition rate, and pulse duration.[40]

The correct choice of wavelength is important to assure the expected interaction with the chromophores present in biological tissues; the photons of the laser beam must be absorbed by a biological tissue in order for the local thermal effect to be achieved. The emission mode, the peak power, and the energy density establish the amount of energy delivered to a tissue – the higher the energy delivered, the higher the temperature rise in the irradiated tissue. Depending on the temperature increases, distinct clinical effects can be achieved.

The repetition rate and pulse duration also influence the manner in which the energy is delivered. Lasers that operate in pulsed wave (PW) have more advantages than continuous wave

(CW) lasers, since they assure the correct thermal relaxation time of irradiated tissue even when operating at extremely high peak power.[29] The adjustment of repetition rate is important to assure that the inter-pulse period is longer than the thermal relaxation time of tissues, as then the temperature of the irradiated tissues decreases between laser pulses.[41] Depending on the pulse length and repetition rate, it is possible to increase the temperature of a small area of the tissue without thermal side effects to both irradiated and surrounding tissues.[21,29]

Table 2.1 lists the most commonly used commercially available high power lasers in dentistry, as well as their main clinical applications.

Interaction of high power lasers with biological tissues

The interaction of laser light with biological tissues results in the following phenomena: reflection, scattering, absorption, and transmission.[21,29,39,40] It should be pointed out that refraction occurs each time light changes its propagation medium; the light path bends. These effects are illustrated in Figure 2.1 and must be understood in order for the clinician to be able to choose the best equipment and irradiation conditions for a specific clinical application and to avoid thermal and mechanical damage to the target and surrounding tissue. Depending on the case, the dentist may need to use different laser wavelengths and irradiation parameters during the course of laser treatment, or to obtain different effects in the same tissue.

The type of biological tissue, as well as the laser wavelength, are important in determining the predominant type of interaction during laser irradiation. The main phenomena that can occur in the interaction between high power lasers and biological tissues are described below, as well as the factors that influence the occurrence of each type of interaction.

Reflection and refraction

Reflection occurs when electromagnetic radiation that is focused on the surface of a medium is returned at this surface. In general, the reflecting surface is a physical interface between two materials of different refractive indexes, such as air and tissue.[21]

The angle of incidence (θ) is that between the normal surface (the surface of the tissue) and the incident beam. The angle of

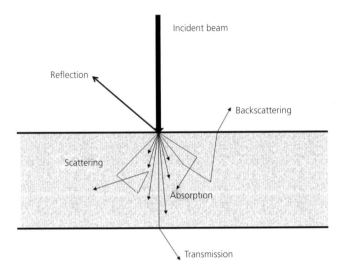

Figure 2.1 Schematic of the laser–tissue interactions: reflection, scattering, absorption, and transmission.[40]

reflection (θ') is that between the normal surface and the reflected beam (Fig. 2.2). When the surface is smooth, it is assumed that any irregularities are small compared to the wavelength of the incident radiation and, as a result, *specular reflection* occurs. On the other hand, when the surface irregularities are equal to or greater than the wavelength of the incident radiation, *diffuse reflection* occurs. The latter is a common phenomenon with biological tissues.[29]

Refraction occurs when a reflective surface separates two media with different refractive indexes. This phenomenon occurs as a result of changes in the velocity of the incident light (Fig. 2.2). Like reflection, refraction depends on the angle of incidence, polarization of the radiation, and refractive indexes of the media involved. The relationship between reflection and refraction is known as *Fresnel's law*.

Absorption and transmission

The absorption phenomenon occurs when the electromagnetic radiation is not returned from the incident surface nor propagates in the tissue. *Absorbance* is the ratio of the intensity of absorbed to incident light.[21]

Considering the concept of absorption, it is also possible to define the concepts of *transparency* and *opacity*. A transparent medium allows all incident light to pass without absorption; the incident radiant energy equals the energy that exits the medium. Incident light is transmitted through the medium (Fig. 2.3).

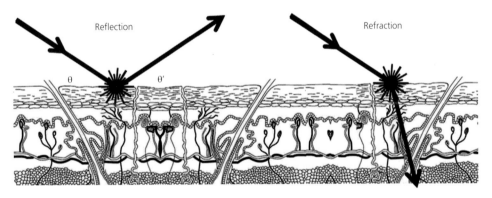

Figure 2.2 Schematic of reflection and refraction of light incident on skin (Zezell et al. 2011. Reproduced with pen access permission of In Tech Europe).

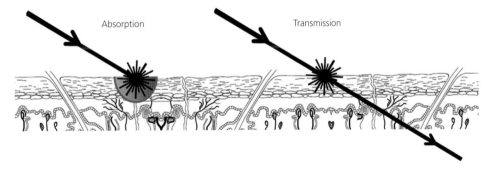

Figure 2.3 Schematic of absorption and transmission of light incident on skin.

On the other hand, an opaque medium reduces the energy of the incident radiation to close to zero (Fig. 2.3). Thus the "transparency" or "opacity" of a medium depends on the wavelength of the incident light.

During absorption, part of the radiation is converted into heat or kinetic energy (vibration of the molecules of the biological tissue). The ability of a tissue to absorb electromagnetic radiation depends on several factors, such as the electronic constitution of atoms or molecules, wavelength of the radiation, thickness of the absorbing layer, and internal parameters such as temperature and concentration of absorbing agents. The effect of thickness on absorption is defined by *Beer–Lambert's law*:

$$I_{(z)} = I_0 e^{-\alpha z}$$

and of concentration by *Beer's law*:[29]

$$I_{(z)} = I_0 e^{-k'cz}$$

where z = optical axis, $I_{(z)}$ = light intensity at distance z, I_0 = initial intensity of light, α = absorption coefficient of the medium, c = concentration of absorbers, and k' = internal parameters.

Water and macromolecules, such as proteins and pigments, are largely responsible for absorption by biological tissues. There is a "therapeutic window" between 600 nm and 1200 nm,[21] as outside this range there is no strong absorption by macromolecules or water (Fig. 2.4). Within this range of the electromagnetic spectrum, the radiation penetrates more deeply into biological tissues and these wavelengths are frequently used for LLLT (low level laser therapy).

Scattering

When the charged particles of a tissue are elastically confined and exposed to electromagnetic waves, their movements change according to the incident electric field. If the frequency of the incident wave is equal to the natural frequency of vibration of free particles of irradiated tissue, the phenomenon of resonance occurs. The resonance is accompanied by considerable absorption.[21,29]

The scattering phenomenon occurs when the frequency of incident light does not correspond to the natural frequency of the vibration of particles of irradiated tissue. The resultant oscillation is determined by the induced vibration of particles. In general, the vibration will have the same frequency and direction as the electrical field of the incident radiation; however, its magnitude is much smaller than that when resonance occurs. Furthermore, the phase of the induced vibration differs from the phase of the incident wave, reducing the velocity of the photons that penetrate a dense medium. Therefore, scattering can be considered as the basic source of the dispersion (Fig. 2.5).

Depending on the conversion of energy of the incident photon, it is possible to observe *elastic* or *inelastic* scattering. In the former case, the incident and scattered photons have the same energy. A special case of elastic scattering is *Rayleigh scattering*. Its limitation is that the scattered particles must be smaller than the wavelength of the incident radiation. In this type of phenomenon, there is a relationship between scattered intensity and refractive index – the scattering is inversely proportional to the wavelength of the incident beam to the fourth, and this relationship is known as *Rayleigh´s law* ($\sim 1/\lambda^4$). When the scattered particles have a dimension comparable to the wavelength of the incident beam, Rayleigh scattering does not

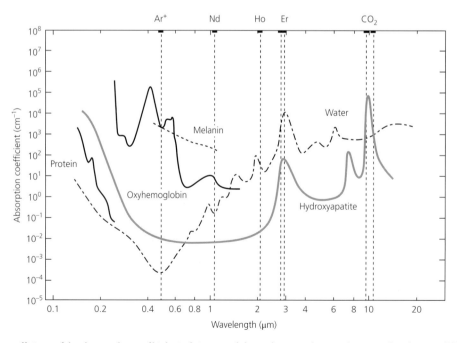

Figure 2.4 Absorption coefficients of the chromophores of biological tissues and their relation to the main lasers used in dentistry.[16,21]

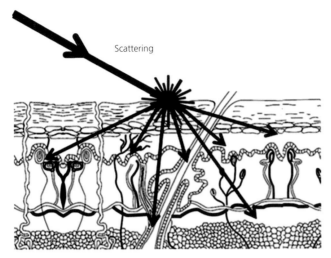

Figure 2.5 Schematic of scattering of light incident on skin.

Table 2.2 Effects of temperature on soft tissues.[21]

Temperature (°C)	Primary effect	Secondary effect
37	None	None
42	Tissue heating	Destruction of some chemical bonds; changes in cellular membranes; necrosis of small areas
50	Reduction of enzymatic activity	Ablation of cells
60	Tissue denaturation	Coagulation, necrosis, bleaching of tissue
80	Changes in permeability of membranes	Destruction of chemical bond
100	Cutting, vaporization	Thermal decomposition
150	Carbonization	Darkening of the tissue (this can be avoided by the use of a coolant)
400	Melting	Fast incision

occur; instead, *Mie scattering* occurs. Mie scattering shows weak dependence on the wavelength of the incident beam compared with Rayleigh scattering.[21]

In biological tissues, photons are likely scattered in the direction of the incident beam. This phenomenon cannot be explained by Rayleigh scattering, but the dependence on the wavelength is stronger than can be predicted by Mie scattering. As neither Rayleigh nor Mie scattering can completely explain the scattering in biological tissues, it is necessary to define a probability function $p(\theta)$ of a photon to be scattered at an angle θ. If the probability function does not depend on the θ angle, the scattering is defined as *isotropic*. Otherwise, the scattering is defined as *anisotropic*.[21,29]

Thermal effects of laser irradiation in biological tissues

Consideration of the thermal effects when applying high power lasers to biological tissues is extremely important. A rise in the temperature of a tissue promotes several changes in its structure, such as denaturation of proteins, water evaporation, coagulation, etc. In dental hard tissues, a temperature rise can change the crystallographic characteristics of the mineral matrix, such as the crystalline lattice, size of hydroxyapatite crystals, and formation of new composites.[16,22,24,42] Thus, when establishing safe and effective protocols it is important to consider the expected temperature rises in irradiated tissue during laser irradiation.

Parameters such as wavelength, energy density, power, peak power, average power, repetition rate, and pulse length are extremely important in determining the heat generation due to irradiation on any biological tissue. The amount of heat generated inside the tissue is highly dependent on the tissue's optical properties, such as absorption and scattering coefficients. Also, heat transfer is dependent on some properties of

biological tissues, such as thermal diffusivity and thermal conductivity.[43–45]

Considering the interaction of a laser wavelength with the main chromophores of biological tissues,[29,39] it can be noted that:

1. In the ultraviolet (<400 nm) and infrared (>1500 nm) regions of the electromagnetic spectrum, absorption prevails and scattering has less influence; light does not penetrate deeply into biological tissue (limited to a few micrometers);
2. In the visible region of the spectrum (400–600 nm), both absorption and scattering occur and light penetrates to a depth of 0.5–2.5 mm;
3. In the red to near infrared region (600–1500 nm), scattering prevails and light penetrates to a depth of 8–10 mm.

Effects on soft tissues

Table 2.2 summarizes the main effects of temperature rises on biological soft tissues. It can be noted that a temperature increase of about 5 °C is enough to change some chemical bonds and to alter cellular membranes, and there is a linear relation between temperature and the tissue changes.[21,29,40]

The increase in local temperature is important for clinical effects such as coagulation, healing, and precise cutting. These effects can also be used for the decontamination of irradiated tissue: temperatures higher than 44 °C are necessary to assure killing of some bacteria.[46] Laser irradiation for this purpose usually leads to a local increase in temperature of tens, even hundreds, of degrees Celsius during the laser pulse.

Lasers that emit in the visible and near infrared regions of the spectrum are useful in treating soft tissues. The higher absorption by hemoglobin of argon, Nd:YAG, and diode laser irradiation achieves precise cutting and as such these lasers are less invasive, with better hemostasis and facilitated visualization. CO_2 lasers are strongly absorbed by water, which achieves shallower cutting than the above mentioned lasers.[29] The erbium lasers (Er:YAG and Er,Cr:YSGG) are also effectively absorbed by water and they can be used to cut soft tissues, but their cutting is more superficial and as a consequence they are less effective in achieving hemostasis.[21]

Effects on hard tissues

The tooth is composed of enamel, dentin, pulp, and cementum, and the main constituent is hydroxyapatite.[47,48] Dentin and cementum have a higher water and organic compound percentage compared to enamel and are thus more susceptible to heat storage than enamel.[49] Dentin has low thermal conductivity values, which can lead to significant rises in local tissue temperature. When lasers are used to irradiate deeper regions, where dentin tubule area and density are increased, the risk to the pulp and periodontal tissues is greater.[50] As an example, considering the use of CO_2 lasers, the absorption coefficient for dentin is lower than that for enamel due to its low inorganic content; also, the thermal diffusivity is approximately three times smaller, which means less heat dissipation and, as a consequence, higher pulp heating.[51] Dental pulp is a connective and vital tissue, and its higher vascularization makes it susceptible to thermal changes. A small change in pulp temperature ($\Delta T \leq 5\,°C$) is sufficient to alter the microvascularization, and cellular activation and capacity for hydration and defense.[40,52,53]

The majority of high power lasers used to irradiate dental hard tissues cause photothermal and photomechanical effects.[44] Photons emitted at wavelengths in the visible and near infrared regions of the electromagnetic spectrum are poorly absorbed by dental hard tissues and thus heat is easily diffused to the pulp. In this way, lasers such as the Nd:YAG, diode or argon should be used with care when irradiating dental hard tissues. In clinical application, the chosen parameters for laser irradiation must promote significant temperature increases on enamel and dentin surfaces, to produce mechanical and/or thermal effects on these structures, but limit side effects to pulp or adjacent tissues.[20]

Table 2.3 shows the effects of temperature on dental hard tissues. It can be noted that the temperature rise can strongly interfere with enamel and dentin composition[54-56] and, as a consequence, their mechanical properties. These changes can influence several clinical applications, such as adhesive procedures in restorative dentistry[57] or caries prevention.[10,16,17,22,39,42]

Due to the composition of hard tissues, lasers that emit in the infrared region, such as CO_2 (9600 nm), Er:YAG (2940 nm), and Er,Cr:YSGG (2780 nm), are the best candidates for cutting enamel, dentin, and bone. However, the CO_2 laser is not commercially available. Comparing the absorption of Er:YAG with Er,Cr:YSGG lasers by dental hard tissues, Er:YAG lasers have a stronger interaction with OH^- in water molecules in the teeth, while Er,Cr:YSGG lasers are better absorbed by water and the OH^- in hydroxyapatite (Fig. 2.2).[44,58] Due to this fact, Er:YAG lasers achieve surface temperatures of up to 300\,°C at the ablation threshold, and Er,Cr:YSGG lasers 800\,°C during ablation of enamel.[58] These differences in temperature promote distinct effects in hard tissues (Table 2.3).

Table 2.3 Effects of temperature on dental hard tissues[54-56] (Fowler et al. 1986. Reproduced with permission of Springer).

Temperature (°C)	Primary effect
100–140	Evaporation of water
250–400	Oxidation and pyrolysis of organic compounds
100–650	Conversion of phosphate to pyrophosphates
500–900	Carbon oxidation of organic matrix and decomposition of carbonate of inorganic phase
700–850	Total decomposition of carbonate of inorganic phase
1000–1100	Formation of tricalcium phosphates, tetracalcium phosphate, and bruxite
1280	Melting of enamel and natural hydroxyapatite

Erbium lasers cut dental hard tissues by a mechanism called thermal ablation.[21,29] This process is also known as explosive (water-mediated) tissue removal. This process is the result of the fast heating of the sub-surface water confined by the hard tissue matrix, which absorbs infrared laser irradiation. The heating of these water molecules increases their molecular vibration and, consequently, the sub-surface pressures; the latter can exceed the strength of the hard tissue. Finally, an "explosion" of tissue due to material failure can occur, resulting in the removal of material. This process takes place at temperatures below the melting point of dental hard tissues (1200\,°C), and varies according to the laser wavelength (e.g. Er:YAG lasers achieve temperatures of 300\,°C at the ablation threshold, Er,Cr:YSGG lasers 800\,°C, and CO_2 lasers 1000\,°C).

The ablation process has been studied for the past 30 years, with the intention of choosing the best laser wavelength and parameters to promote effective removal of tissue, selective removal of caries, and minimum thermal side effects such as cracks or carbonization. For this, continuous emission lasers or lasers pulsed at longer than 1 picosecond should be well absorbed by the main components of teeth (i.e. water and hydroxyapatite).[29,59] For shorter pulses, such as femtosecond laser pulses, ablation occurs due to non-linear interactions with the tissue, resulting in a plasma-mediated ablation.

Non-linear interactions

Even at higher repetition rates and with the use of air–water coolant during the cutting procedure, commercially available high power infrared lasers cannot cut dental hard tissues with the same speed or the same precision as drills.[60,61] Studies have been performed to determine the possibility of using ultrashort pulsed lasers (USPLs) to cut dental hard tissues, given that these have been used successfully for precise cutting in ophthalmology.[29]

According to Niemz,[62] lasers with pulse durations in the range of milliseconds (10^{-3} s), microseconds (10^{-6} s) or nanoseconds (10^{-9} s) generate considerable heat during ablation of dental hard tissues. On the other hand, lasers with pulse durations of picoseconds (10^{-12} s) and femtoseconds (10^{-15} s) ablate tissues by forming ionizing plasma.[21]

USPLs interact with tissues by a mechanism called *plasma-induced ablation* or *plasma-mediated ablation*, in which the phenomenon of *optical breakdown* occurs.[29] Briefly, the ablation is caused by plasma ionization, in which laser irradiation produces an extremely high electric field that leads to the ionization of molecules and atoms, promoting breakdown and, then, the ablation or ejection of the target tissue.[29] During the cutting, it is possible to observe the formation of a bright plasma spark, and a noise of low tone, characteristic of plasma formation.

These lasers operate at very high repetition rates (>15 kHz) and energy per pulse typically of hundreds of microJoules.[63] The main characteristics of these complex systems[37,64] are their very low pulse duration and high precision (extremely small focus area).

Several systems have been tested for applications in dentistry, such as the Nd:YLF,[29] Ti:Al$_2$O$_3$,[37] and Cr:LiSAF (Alexandrite) lasers.[65] The literature reports the possibility of cavity preparation in enamel and dentin with good precision and virtual absence of thermal damage when compared with cavities prepared using lasers operating with pulse lengths of microseconds and nanoseconds. Researches have confirmed that the application of USPLs with pulse lengths of a few femtoseconds almost completely avoid thermal damage and the formation of microcracks in irradiated and surrounding tissues.[29,33–37] Further studies have demonstrated the possibility of selective removal of restorative material, including amalgam.[37]

USPLs appear to be a promising alternative for assuring precise and selective cutting of biological tissues without side effects.[66,67] However, although commercially available equipment is available for ophthalmic application, the cost and complexity of these systems still represent a barrier to their application in dentistry.[68]

Conclusion

The effects of high power laser irradiation on biological tissues are based on heat generation. Understanding the mechanisms of interaction of these lasers with biological tissues is important in determining safe and effective protocols for their use in clinical practice. Depending on the laser wavelength, the chromophores of the tissue, and the characteristics of laser system, it is possible to achieve faster cutting, good hemostasis, decontamination, and several other applications in both soft and hard tissues.

References

1 Stern RH, Sognnaes RF. Laser beam effect on dental hard tissue. *J Dent Res* 1964; 43: 873.

2 Yang SW, Tsai CN, Lee YS, et al. Treatment outcome of dysplastic oral leukoplakia with carbon dioxide laser-emphasis on the factors affecting recurrence. *J Oral Maxillofac Surg* 2011; 69: 78–87.

3 Sperandio FF, Meneguzzo DT, Ferreira LS, et al. Different air-water spray regulations affect the healing of Er,Cr:YSGG laser incisions. *Lasers Med Sci* 2011; 26: 257–265.

4 Benedicenti S, Cassanelli C, Signore A, et al. Decontamination of root canals with the gallium-aluminum-arsenide laser: an in vitro study. *Photomed Laser Surg* 2008; 26: 367–370.

5 Koba K, Kimura Y, Matsumoto K, et al. A histopathological study of the morphological changes at the apical seat and in the periapical region after irradiation with a pulsed Nd:YAG laser. *Int Endod J* 1998; 31: 415–420.

6 Kato IT, Pellegrini VD, Prates RA, et al. Low-level laser therapy in burning mouth syndrome patients: a pilot study. *Photomed Laser Surg* 2010; 28: 835–839.

7 Lang-Bicudo L, Eduardo FP, Eduardo CP, et al. LED phototherapy to prevent mucositis: a case report. *Photomed Laser Surg* 2008; 26: 609–613.

8 De Moor RJ, Delme KI. Laser-assisted cavity preparation and adhesion to erbium-lased tooth structure: part 2. Present-day adhesion to erbium-lased tooth structure in permanent teeth. *J Adhes Dent* 2010; 12: 91–102.

9 Obeidi A, McCracken MS, Liu PR, et al. Enhancement of bonding to enamel and dentin prepared by Er,Cr:YSGG laser. *Lasers Surg Med* 2009; 41: 454–462.

10 Zezell DM, Boari HG, Ana PA, et al. Nd:YAG laser in caries prevention: a clinical trial. *Lasers Surg Med* 2009; 41: 31–35.

11 Rechmann P, Fried D, Le CQ, et al. Caries inhibition in vital teeth using 9.6-μm CO$_2$-laser irradiation. *J Biomed Opt* 2011; 16: 071405.

12 Nammour S, Rocca JP, Pireaux JJ, et al. Increase of enamel fluoride retention by low fluence argon laser beam: a 6-month follow-up study in vivo. *Lasers Surg Med* 2005; 36: 220–224.

13 Nammour S, Zeinoun T, Bogaerts I, et al. Evaluation of dental pulp temperature rise during photo-activated decontamination (PAD) of caries: an in vitro study. *Lasers Med Sci* 2010; 25: 651–654.

14 White JM, Goodis HE, Setcos JC, et al. Effects of pulsed Nd:YAG laser energy on human teeth: a three-year follow-up study. *J Am Dent Assoc* 1993; 124: 45–51.

15 Neves AA, Coutinho E, De Munck J, et al. Caries-removal effectiveness and minimal-invasiveness potential of caries-excavation techniques: a micro-CT investigation. *J Dent* 2011; 39: 154–162.

16 Ana PA, Bachmann L, Zezell DM. Lasers effects on enamel for caries prevention. *Laser Phys* 2006; 16: 865–875.

17 Featherstone JDB. The science and practice of caries prevention. *J Am Dent Assoc* 2000; 131: 887–899.

18 Cheong WF, Prahl SA, Welch AJ, A review of the optical properties of biological tissues. *IEEE J Quantum Electronics* 1990; 26: 2166–2185.

19 Fried D, Glena RE, Featherstone JDB, et al. Nature of light scattering in dental enamel and dentin at visible and near-infrared wavelengths. *Appl Optics* 1995; 34: 1278–1285.

20 Ana PA, Blay A, Miyakawa W, et al. Thermal analysis of teeth irradiated with Er,Cr:YSGG at low fluences. *Laser Phys Lett* 2007; 4: 827–834.

21 Zezell DM, Ribeiro MS. *Interação da Luz com tecidos biológicos – aplicações*. São Paulo: Mestrado Profissionalizante Lasers em Odontologia IPEN-FOUSP, 2007.

22 Bachmann L, Craievich AF, Zezell DM. Crystalline structure of dental enamel after Ho:YLF laser irradiation. *Arch Oral Biol* 2004; 49: 923–929.

23 Gouw-Soares S, Gutknecht N, Conrads G, et al. The bactericidal effect of Ho:YAG laser irradiation within contaminated root dentinal samples. *J Clin Laser Med Surg* 2000; 18: 81–87.

24 Botta SB, Ana PA, de Sa Teixeira F, et al. Relationship between surface topography and energy density distribution of Er,Cr:YSGG beam on irradiated dentin: an atomic force microscopy study. *Photomed Laser Surg* 2011; 29: 261–269.

25 Ribeiro AC, Nogueira GE, Antoniazzi JH et al. Effects of diode laser (810 nm) irradiation on root canal walls: thermographic and morphological studies. *J Endod* 2007; 33: 252–255.

26 Marraccini TM, Bachmann L, Wigdor HA, et al. Morphological evaluation of enamel and dentin irradiated with 9.6 µm CO2 and 2.94 µm Er:YAG lasers. *Laser Phys Lett* 2005; 2: 551–555.

27 Staninec M, Darling CL, Goodis HE, et al. Pulpal effects of enamel ablation with a microsecond pulsed lambda = 9.3-microm CO_2 laser. *Lasers Surg Med* 2009; 41: 256–263.

28 Esteves-Oliveira M, Zezell DM, Ana PA, et al. Dentine caries inhibition through CO(2) laser (10.6 µm) irradiation and fluoride application, in vitro. *Arch Oral Biol* 2011; 56: 533–539.

29 Niemz MH. *Laser-Tissue Interactions – Fundamentals and Applications*, 3rd edn. Berlin: Springer, 2004.

30 Strickland P, Mourou G. Compression of amplified chirped optical pulses. *Opt Commun* 1985; 56: 219.

31 Bloembergen N. From nanosecond to femtosecond science. *Rev Mod Phys* 1999; 71: 283–287.

32 Serbin J, Bauer T, Fallnich C, et al. Femtosecond lasers as novel tool in dental surgery. *Appl Surface Sci* 2002; 197: 737–740.

33 Altshuler GB, Belashenkov NR, Karasev VB, et al. Application of ultrashort laser pulses in dentistry. *SPIE* 1993; 2080: 77–81.

34 Kruger J, Kautek W, Newesely H. Femtosecond-pulse laser ablation of dental hydroxyapatite and single-crystalline fluoroapatite. *Appl Phys A-Mater Sci Proc* 1999; 69: S403–S407.

35 Lizarelli RFZ, Costa MM, Carvalho-Filho E, et al. Selective ablation of dental enamel and dentin using femtosecond laser pulses. *Laser Phys Lett* 2008; 5: 63–69.

36 Strassl M, Wieger V, Brodoceanu D, et al. Ultra-short pulse laser ablation of biological hard tissue and biocompatibles. *J Laser Micro Nanoeng* 2008; 3: 30–40.

37 Freitas AZ, Freschi LR, Samad RE, et al. Determination of ablation threshold for composite resins and amalgam irradiated with femtosecond laser pulses. *Laser Phys Lett* 2010; 7: 236–241.

38 Karu T. *The Science of Low-Power Laser Therapy*. Amsterdam: Gordon and Breach Science Publishers,1998.

39 Kishen A, Asundi A. *Fundamentals and Applications of Biophotonics in Dentistry*. London: Imperial College Press, 2007.

40 Zezell DM, Ana PA, Pereira TM, et al. Heat generation and transfer on biological tissues due to high-intensity laser irradiation. In: Bernardes MAS (ed). *Developments in Heat Transfer*. Rijeka: In Tech, 2011: 227–246.

41 McDonald A, Claffey N, Pearson G, et al. The effect of Nd:YAG pulse duration on dentine crater depth. *J Dent* 2001; 29: 43–53.

42 Bachmann L, Rosa K, Ana PA, et al. Crystalline structure of human enamel irradiated with Er,Cr:YSGG laser. *Laser Phys Let* 2009; 6: 159–162.

43 Brown WS, Dewey WA, Jacobs HR. Thermal properties of teeth. *J Dent Res* 1970; 49: 752–755.

44 Seka W, Featherstone JDB, Fried D, et al. Laser ablation of dental hard tissue: from explosive ablation to plasma-mediated ablation. *SPIE* 1996; 2672: 144–158.

45 Yu D, Powell GL, Higuchi WI, et al. Comparison of three lasers on dental pulp chamber temperature change. *J Clin Laser Med Surg* 1993; 11: 119–122.

46 Nermela SI, Sivela C, Luoma T, et al. Maximum temperature limits for acidophilic, mesophilic bactéria in biological leaching systems. *Appl Environ Microbiol* 1994; 60: 3444–3446.

47 Chadwick DJ, Cardew G. *Dental Enamel*. Chichester: Wiley, 1997.

48 Gwinnett AJ. Structure and composition of enamel. *Oper Dent* 1992; Suppl 5: 10–17.

49 Craig RG, Peyton FA. Thermal conductivity of tooth structure, Dental cements, and amalgam. *J Dent Res* 1961, 40: 411.

50 Srimaneepong V, Palamara JEA, Wilson PR. Pulpal space pressure and temperatura changes from Nd:YAG laser irradiation of dentin. *J Dent* 2002; 30: 291–296.

51 Fried D, Zuerlein MJ, Featherstone JDB, et al. Thermal and chemical modification of dentin by pulsed CO_2 laser irradiation at 9–11 µm. *SPIE* 1997; 2973: 94–100.

52 Nyborg H, Brännström M. Pulp reaction to heat. *J Prosthet Dent* 1968; 19: 605–612.

53 Zach L, Cohen G. Pulp response to externally applied heat. *Oral Surg* 1965; 19: 515–530.

54 Fowler BO, Kuroda S. Changes in heated and in laser-irradiated human tooth enamel and their probable effects on solubility. *Calcif Tissue Int* 1986; 38: 197–208.

55 Kuroda S, Fowler BO. Compositional, structural, and phase changes in in vitro laser-irradiated human tooth enamel. *Calcif Tissue Int* 1984; 36: 361–369.

56 Oho T, Morioka T. A possible mechanism of acquired acid resistance of human dental enamel by laser irradiation. *Caries Res* 1990; 24: 86–92.

57 Botta SB, Ana PA, Zezell DM, et al. Adhesion after erbium, chromium:yttrium-scandium-gallium-garnet laser application at three different irradiation conditions. *Lasers Med Sci* 2009; 24: 67–73.

58 Fried D, Featheastone JDB, Visuri SR, et al. The caries inhibition potential of Er:YAG and ErCr:YSGG laser irradiation. *SPIE* 1996; 2672: 73–77.

59 Fried D. IR laser ablation of dental enamel. Lasers in dentistry VI. *Proc SPIE* 2000; 1: 136–148.

60 White JM, Goodis HE, Hennings D, et al. Dentin ablation rate using Nd:YAG and Er:YAG lasers. *J Dent Res* 1996; 73: 318.

61 Kim BM, Feit MD, Rubenchik AM, et al. Influence of pulse duration on ultrashort laser pulse ablation of biological tissue. *J Biomed Opt* 2001; 6: 332–338.

62 Niemz MH. Cavity preparation with the Nd:YLF picosecond laser. *J Dent Res* 1995; 74: 1194–1199.

63 Wieger V, Strassl M, Wintner E. Pico- and microsecond laser ablation of dental restorative materials. *Laser Particle Beams* 2006; 24: 41–45.

64 Beaud PA, Rucharson M, Miesak EJ. Multi-Terawtt Femtosecond Cr: LiSAF Laser. *IEEE J Quantum Eletron* 1995; 31: 317–325.

65 Kopf D, Wellingarten KJ, Zhang G, et al. High-power diode-pumped femtosecond CnLiSAF lasers. *Appl Phys B* 1997; 65: 235–243.

66 Lizarelli RFZ, Costa MM, Carvalho-Filho E, Nunes FD, Bagnato VS. Selective ablation of dental enamel and dentin using femtosecond laser pulses. *Laser Phys Lett* 2008; 5: 63–69.

67 Wieger V, Strassl M, Wintner E. Laser dental hard tissue ablation: Comparison Er-lasers and scanned ultra-short pulse laser. *Int J Appl Electromag Mech* 2007; 25: 635–640.

68 Matos AB, Azevedo CS, Ana PA et al. Laser technology for Caries Removal. In: Li M. (ed). *Contemporary Approach of Dental Caries*. Rijeka: In Tech, 2012: 309–330.

CHAPTER 3

Low power lasers: Introduction

Maria Cristina Chavantes,[1] Martha Simões Ribeiro,[2] and Nathali Cordeiro Pinto[3]

[1] Laser Medical Center of the Heart Institute, General Hospital, Medical School, University of São Paulo (USP), São Paulo, SP, Brazil
[2] Center for Lasers and Applications, Institute for Nuclear and Energy Research, IPEN-CNEN/SP, São Paulo, SP, Brazil
[3] Cardiovascular and Thoracic Surgery Department of the Heart Institute, General Hospital, Medical School, University of São Paulo (USP), São Paulo, SP, Brazil

Lasers are among the greatest inventions of the 20th century. According to the National Academy of Sciences, development of the laser ranks among the highest achievements after a century of innovations in the field of engineering. The first medical application by Prof Dr Leon Goldman from the University of Cincinnati, USA, was in patients with dermatological conditions in 1961. The residual or X effect of lasers could not be fully described until the end of the 1980s by Oshiro and Calderhead.

However, in the late 1960s, by virtue of his close observation and diligence, Prof Dr Endre Mester from Semmelweis Medical University, Hungary, established the potential of lasers in cicatricial and analgesic application, later expanding their use to virtually all areas of health sciences. Although at first he did not comprehend the actual mechanisms involved in the biological process, he anticipated the potential impact of lasers in the medical field. Over a decade elapsed before Prof Dr Tiina Karu from the Russian Academy of Laser Sciences unveiled the intricate mechanisms involved in the application of low power lasers and the alterations following their interaction with targeted tissue cells.

In medicine, lasers have been extensively applied over five decades as surgical, diagnostic, and therapeutic tools. Lasers are classified into two broad categories, according to their power: high power lasers and low power lasers.[1]

High power lasers, also known as surgical lasers, can achieve high energy levels and temperatures in a matter of milliseconds to nanoseconds in targeted tissues. They are commonly employed to cut, vaporize different tissues or resect tumors, with a specific action on biological targets. On the other hand, low power lasers can produce photophysical–chemical effects.

Laser treatment requires a good understanding of how they function and how they should be safely handled. Regarding low level laser therapy (LLLT) of tissue/cells, the temperature of the targeted area should not exceed 1 °C, implying a power range of 1–500 mW. The light is typically utilized with a power density between 1 and 5 W/cm² and applied to the injured site for a minute or so, possibly a few times a week for several weeks, depending on the patient's status. Therefore, treatment is non-thermal, based neither on heating nor tissue damage, but on an accumulation of effects depending on the dosage used.

The photophysical–chemical properties of LLLT refer to its effect on molecules and organelle receptors, which in turn assist in the course of biophysical processes and subsequent biochemical responses. The absorption of low levels of red and near infrared laser radiation by the respiratory chain results in a cascade of intracellular biochemical reactions involving a number of cellular components, notably cytochromes (see chapter 4 for more information).

Cytochromes are the primary photoacceptors, being able to absorb low power red and near infrared light irradiated at appropriate wavelengths. This absorption activates the respiratory chain in the mitochondria, resulting in a redox state and enhancing ATP synthesis. Simultaneously, membrane ions carriers (e.g. Na^+, K^+, Ca^{2+}) are activated, controlling cell proliferation as well as metabolism.[2] An intracellular biochemical chain of reactions, which produces a local and systemic response, follows these physical and chemical alterations in photoreceptor molecules. In life sciences, this action is crucial in order to control the process and achieve an antiedematous, anti-inflammatory, angiogenic, healing, and, consequently, analgesic response. As a result, lasers are useful in dentistry, physical therapy, and several medical specialties, such as dermatology, rheumatology, surgery, etc. Furthermore, the effects of LLLT on the immune system and its hemorrheological properties suggest potential for wider application in the health sciences.

In the interest of better understanding of the action of lasers, their photophysical–chemical effects can be divided according to whether their main action is on endogenous or exogenous photoacceptors: (1) photobiomodulation (known as laser therapy or LLLT) and (2) photodynamic therapy (PDT), which depends on the interaction of the laser light with a photosensitizer that produces reactive oxygen species (ROS) upon irradiation with light, leading to microbial reduction (in this case, named Antimicrobial Photodynamic Therapy – aPDT) or cell death. It is important to highlight that in PDT most of the laser light is absorbed by the photosensitizer and biomodulation effects are minimal.

Lasers in Dentistry: Guide for Clinical Practice, First Edition. Edited by Patrícia M. de Freitas and Alyne Simões.
© 2015 John Wiley & Sons, Inc. Published 2015 by John Wiley & Sons, Inc.

Low level laser therapy

When lasers illuminate biological tissues, energy is delivered to the living system and must be absorbed for effective results. Relevant to the process of absorption are laser parameters, such as wavelength and output power, as well as factors of the biological tissue (anatomy, physiology, pathology, and tissue optics). Laser fluence, or energy density (ED), is still considered to be the most important variable in laser therapy when determining maximum and minimum limits. Recent papers have suggested that dosimetry is best described in terms of both (1) irradiation parameters ("the medicine" – wavelength, power density [irradiance or fluence rate], pulse structure, coherence, and polarization) and (2) time/energy/fluence delivered ("the dose" – energy, energy density, irradiation time, and treatment interval)[3,4] (see Chapter 8 for details).

It is well known that if the power density (irradiance or fluence rate) of the applied laser light is not high enough, or exposure time is too short, there is no biological effect. On the other hand, if the power density is too high and irradiation time is too long, the cell/tissue response could be inhibited. Therefore, the optimal combination of power density and exposure time is necessary for stimulation effects. This dose–response effect is related to the biphasic response, known as "Arndt–Schulz's law".[4] Briefly, weak stimuli hasten activity while stronger stimuli increase it further until a peak is reached, and even stronger stimuli suppress activity (see Chapter 8 for details).

Red and near infrared wavelengths are the most commonly used because they have low absorption by blood and water, which are the major chromophores in tissues. In addition, some cellular organelles are particularly responsive to some wavelengths (see Chapter 4).

Although the primary mechanisms of LLLT are not completely understood, *in vitro* and *in vivo* studies suggest that it can avoid apoptosis and increase cellular proliferation[5,6] and motility.[7] In addition, increased uptake of ATP,[8] increased cell membrane permeability to Ca^{2+},[9] regulation of growth factors and cytokines,[10] stimulation of cellular differentiation and proliferation,[11,12] induced synthesis and remodeling of collagen,[13]

increased tensile strength,[14] angiogenesis,[15] and pain relief,[16] have been reported.

This sum of these cellular events stimulated by LLLT restores homeostasis in injured tissues, that is normalization of their shape and function, leading to repair. Laser therapy for the purpose of tissue repair has been widely applied in the treatment of cicatricial lesions and decubitus ulcers, and in postoperative recovery, as well as in the active prevention and treatment of wound dehiscence (Figs 3.1 and 3.2). Despite a shortage of reported studies on the use of LLLT in newborns, laser therapy is safe and efficient for myelomeningocele treatment in infants post neurosurgery (Fig. 3.3).[17]

LLLT can contain the abnormal granulomatous tissue formation after prolonged endotracheal intubation. Some experimental and clinical studies have reported its ability to decrease or even interrupt the development of subglottic and/or tracheal stenosis (Fig. 3.4).[18] Likewise, laser therapy has achieved effective results in the treatment of thoracic-cardiopulmonary problems.[19] According to experimental studies on acute pulmonary inflammation induced by Gram-negative bacterial lipopolysaccharides,[20] LLLT is efficacious in promoting vascular permeability, modulating pro- and anti-inflammatory cytokines, and restraining bronchial hyperresponsiveness.

Others studies have recorded the benefits of LLLT in treating patients with chronic pain unresponsive to psychoneural drugs, due to the blocking of the nociceptor stimulus. The analgesic efficacy of the therapeutic laser in treating pain of traumatic or neuropathic origin has been confirmed and supported by qualified clinicians in the medical field (Fig. 3.5).

In summary, the biomodulatory effects of lasers on targeted tissues alter anti-inflammatory, edematous, and cicatricial processes, as well as inducing an analgesic response.[17–21] Laser therapy can be employed efficiently in a wide range of biological tissues, including soft tissues like derma, nervous tissue, cartilaginous and osseous tissues, as well the immune system. Experimental and clinical studies of LLLT indicate that it promotes regeneration of the damaged tissue structure and reduces the autoimmune response, especially in patients with chronic thyroiditis and rheumatoid arthritis, by altering tissue

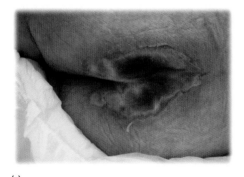
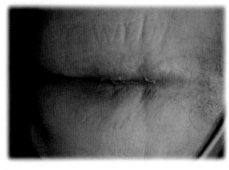

(a)   (b)

Figure 3.1 (a) Decubitus ulcer in a patient who had been bedridden for a prolonged period. (b) Bedsore scar after several LLLT sessions.

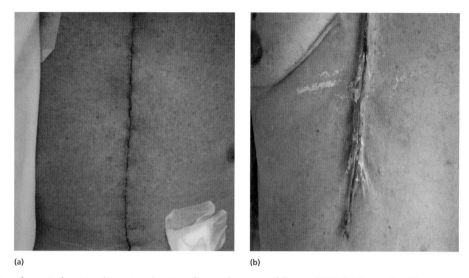

(a) (b)

Figure 3.2 (a) Healing of a surgical incision (sternotomy) post cardiovascular surgery following LLLT. (b) Conventional inpatient treatment of a surgical incision in another patient.

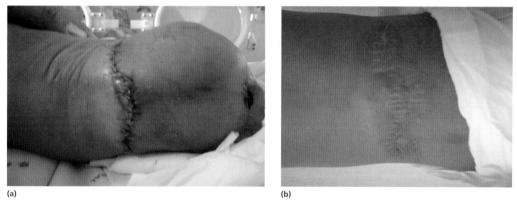

(a) (b)

Figure 3.3 (a) LLLT for healing of a surgical incision following myelomeningocele surgery in a neonate. (b) 10 months later, dehiscence and fistulization of the surgical wound in the medullar area has been successfully avoided.

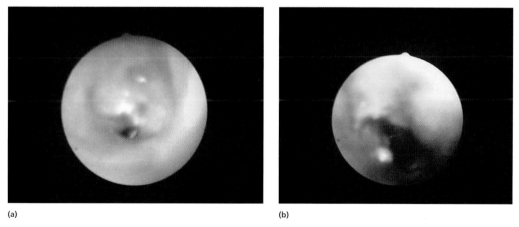

(a) (b)

Figure 3.4 (a) Infraglottis stenosis treated with LLLT in a child. (b) Lumen improvement.

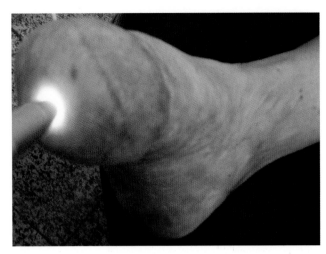

Figure 3.5 LLLT applied to a post-traumatic neuroma on the foot.

conformation and function.[21] Finally, LLLT can be considered a modulator of biological processes in the target tissue area, thus achieving homeostasis. For LLLT to be effective, determination of the most appropriate parameters must be pursued in all medical fields.

Photodynamic therapy

Photodynamic therapy (PDT) has been employed for decades in treating malignant neoplasia. Recent studies have also reported its use in bacterial-induced lesions (periodontitis and endodontic lesions), viral lesions, and fungal infections (see Chapter 7). Three components are involved: molecular oxygen, a photosensitizer, and a light source (e.g. laser or light emitting diode [LED]). More specifically, the photosensitizer must absorb the wavelength of the light source. The photodynamic process is based on the photo-oxidation of organic matter. Following light absorption by the photosensitizer, ROS are generated locally and cause cell death in tumor tissue and/or other diseased tissues and death of infectious agents by oxidative stress.

References

1 Chavantes MC, Tomimura S. Classificação dos lasers. In: Chavantes MC (ed). *Laser em Bio-Medicina*. São Paulo: Atheneu, 2009:41–67.

2 Karu TI. Molecular mechanism of the therapeutic effect of low intensity laser irradiation. *Lasers Life Sci* 1988; 2: 53–74.

3 Huang YY, Chen AC, Carroll JD, Hamblin MR. Biphasic dose response in low level light therapy. *Dose Resp* 2009; 7(4):358–383.

4 Chung H, Dai T, Sharma SK, Huang YY, Carroll JD, Hamblin MR. The nuts and bolts of low-level laser (light) therapy. *Ann Biomed Eng* 2012; 40(2): 516–533.

5 Moore P, Ridgway TD, Higbee RG, Howard EW, Lucroy MD. Effect of wavelength on low-intensity laser irradiation-stimulated cell proliferation in vitro. *Lasers Surg Med* 2005;36(1):8–12.

6 Almeida-Lopes L, Rigau J, Zangaro RA, Guidugli-Neto J, Jaeger MMM. LLLT acts by improving the in vitro fibroblast proliferation – comparison of the low level laser therapy effects on cultured human gingival fibroblasts proliferation using different irradiance and same fluence. *Lasers Surg Med* 2001; 29:179–184.

7 Haas AF, Isseroff RR, Wheeland RG, Rood PA, Graves PJ. Low-energy helium-neon laser irradiation increases the motility of cultured human keratinocytes. *J Invest Dermatol* 1990; 94:822–826.

8 Karu T, Pyatibrat L, Kalendo, G. Irradiation with He-Ne laser increases ATP level in cells cultivated *in vitro*. *J PhotochemPhotobiol B* 1995; 27: 219–233.

9 Lubart R, Friedmann H, Levinshal T, Lavie R, Breitbart H. Effect of light on calcium transport in bull sperm cells. *J PhotochemPhotobiol B* 1992; 15: 337–341.

10 Boschi ES, Leite CE, Saciura VC, et al. Anti-inflammatory effects of low-level laser therapy (660 nm) in the early phase in carrageenan-induced pleurisy in rat. *Lasers Surg Med* 2008; 40: 500–508.

11 Pourreau-Schneider N, Ahmed A, Soudry M, et al. Helium-neon laser treatment transforms fibroblasts into myofibroblasts. *Am J Pathol* 1990; 137:171–178.

12 Stein A, Benayahu D, Maltz L, Oron U. Low-level laser irradiation promotes proliferation and differentiation of human osteoblasts in vitro. *Photomed Laser Surg* 2005; 23: 161–166.

13 De Araújo CE, Ribeiro MS, Favaro R, Zezell DM, Zorn TM. Ultrastructural and autoradiographical analysis shows a faster skin repair in He-Ne laser-treated wounds. *J PhotochemPhotobiol B* 2007; 86:87–96.

14 Vasilenko T, Slezák M, Kovác I, et al. The effect of equal daily dose achieved by different power densities of low-level laser therapy at 635 and 670 nm on wound tensile strength in rats: a short report. *Photomed Laser Surg* 2010; 28:281–283.

15 Melo VA, Anjos DC, Albuquerque Júnior R, Melo DB, Carvalho FU. Effect of low level laser on sutured wound healing in rats. *Acta Cir Bras* 2011; 26: 129–134.

16 Pozza DH, Fregapani PW, Weber JB, et al. Analgesic action of laser therapy (LLLT) in an animal model. *Med Oral Patol Oral Cir Bucal* 2008;13(10): E648–652.

17 PintoNC, Pereira MHC, Stolf NAG, Chavantes, *MC. Low level laser therapy in acute dehiscence saphenectomy: Therapeutic proposal. Rev BrasCirurgiaCardiovasc* 2009; 24(1): 88–91.

18 Pinto FCG, Chavantes MC, Pinto NC, et al. Novel treatment immediately after myelomeningocele repair applying low-level laser therapy in newborns: A pilot study. *PediatrNeurosurg* 2010; 46: 249–254.

19 Chavantes, MC. Pilot study: New treatment applying LLLT in tracheal stenosis using biomodulatedeffect. *JPhotomed Laser Surg* 2005; 23(1): 113.

20 Aimbiri F, Albertini R, Magalhaes RG, et al. Effects of LLLT Ga-Al-As (685 nm) on LPS-induced inflammation of the airway and lung in the rat. *Lasers Med Sci* 2005; 20: 11–20.

21 Hofling DB, Chavantes MC, Juliano AG, et al. Low level laser therapy in chronic autoimmune thyroiditis: Pilot study. *Lasers Surg Med* 2010; 42: 589–596.

CHAPTER 4

Cellular mechanisms of photobiomodulation

Tiina I. Karu

Institute of Laser and Information Technologies of the Russian Academy of Sciences, Troitsk, Moscow Region, Russian Federation

Introduction

Various cellular responses to visible and infrared A (IR-A) radiation have been studied for decades in the context of molecular mechanisms of laser low level light therapy (LLLT) (also called phototherapy or photobiomodulation). LLLT uses monochromatic and quasi-monochromatic light in the optical region of 600–1000 nm to treat in a non-destructive and non-thermal fashion various soft tissue and neurological conditions. Many examples of the successful clinical use of photobiomodulation can be found in other chapters of this book.

Cell response to irradiation

It is well known that practically all types of cells respond to irradiation with monochromatic radiation from laser and non-laser light sources (e.g. LEDs), with changes in their metabolism.[1–3] This consistent character of cell response to irradiation is believed to be due to the universal presence of the photoacceptor, the terminal enzyme of the respiratory chain cytochrome c oxidase, in mitochondria. It is generally accepted that mitochondria are the initial site of light action in cells, and cytochrome c oxidase is the responsible molecule. This event is a starting point for changes in cell metabolism via mitochondrial retrograde signaling.[4] Photoexcitation of certain chromophores in the cytochrome c oxidase molecule influences the redox state of these centers and, consequently, the rate of electron flow in the molecule.[2,4]

At least four types of primary reactions can occur with irradiation[2] (Fig. 4.1). One process possibly involves acceleration of electronic transfer in the respiratory chain due to a change in the redox properties of the carriers following photoexcitation of their electronic states. It is believed that Cu_A and Cu_B, as well as hemes a and a_3, are involved.[3] The action spectrum of stimulation of DNA synthesis and the suggested absorbing chromophores of cytochrome c oxidase are shown in Figure 4.2.

NO hypothesis

The latest developments indicate that under physiological conditions the activity of cytochrome c oxidase is also regulated by nitric oxide (NO).[5] This regulation occurs via reversible inhibition of mitochondrial respiration. It was hypothesized[6,7] that laser irradiation and activation of electron flow in the cytochrome c oxidase molecule could reverse the partial inhibition of the catalytic center by NO and in this way increase the O_2-binding and respiration rate ("NO hypothesis"; Fig. 4.1). This may be a factor leading to the increased concentration of the oxidized form of Cu_B.

Experimental results of the modification of irradiation effects with donors of NO have not excluded this hypothesis,[8,9] as discussed by Lane.[10] Spectroscopic studies of irradiated cellular monolayers showed that the reorganization of two charge-transfer channels, putatively $Cu_{A_{red}}$ and $Cu_{B_{oxid}}$, as well as two reaction channels, putatively connected by d–d transition in $Cu_{B_{red}}$ and $Cu_{A_{oxid}}$ chromophores, is dependent on the presence or absence of NO. It has been suggested that the dissociation of NO (a physiological regulator of cytochrome c oxidase activity) rearranges downstream signaling effects.[6,9] Note also that under pathological conditions the concentration of NO is increased (mainly due to the activation of macrophages producing NO).[11] This circumstance also increases the probability that the respiration activity of various cells will be inhibited by NO. Under these conditions, light activation of cell respiration may have a beneficial effect.

Transient local heating hypothesis

When the electronic states of the photoabsorbing molecule are excited with light, a notable fraction of the excitation energy is inevitably converted to heat, which causes a local transient increase in the temperature of the absorbing chromophores ("transient local heating hypothesis"; Fig. 4.1).[12] Any appreciable time- or space-averaged heating of the sample can be prevented by controlling the irradiation power and dose appropriately. The local transient rise in the temperature of the absorbing

Lasers in Dentistry: Guide for Clinical Practice, First Edition. Edited by Patrícia M. de Freitas and Alyne Simões.
© 2015 John Wiley & Sons, Inc. Published 2015 by John Wiley & Sons, Inc.

biomolecules may cause structural (e.g. conformational) changes and trigger biochemical activity (cellular signaling or secondary dark reactions).[12]

Superoxide anion hypothesis

It was suggested that activation of the respiratory chain by irradiation will also increase the production of superoxide anions ("superoxide anion hypothesis"; Fig. 4.1).[13] It has been shown that the production of $O_2^{\bullet-}$ depends primarily on the metabolic state of the mitochondria.[14]

The belief that only one of the reactions discussed above occurs when a cell is irradiated and excited electronic states are

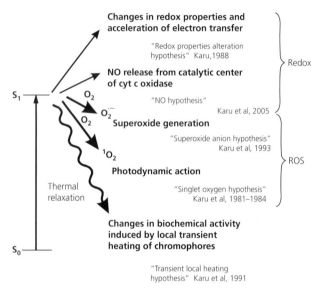

Figure 4.1 Possible primary reactions in the photoacceptor molecule (cytochrome c oxidase) after promotion of excited electronic states. ROS, reactive oxygen species (adapted from Karu 1999. With permission of Elsevier).

produced is groundless. The question is, which mechanism is decisive? It is entirely possible that all the mechanisms discussed above lead to a similar result – a modulation of the redox state of the mitochondria (a shift in the direction of greater oxidation).

Signaling pathways: Role of ATP

The excitation of the photoacceptor molecule by irradiation sets in motion cellular metabolism through cascades of reactions called cellular signaling or retrograde mitochondrial signaling (Fig. 4.3).[4]

Another signaling pathway starting in the mitochondria is connected with ATP. The increased synthesis of ATP in isolated mitochondria and intact cells of various types under irradiation with light of different wavelengths is well documented.[2] ATP is a universal fuel in living cells that drives all biological reactions. It is known that even small changes in the ATP level can significantly alter cellular metabolism. Increasing the amount of ATP may improve the cellular metabolism, especially in suppressed or otherwise ailing cells.[3]

A long series of discoveries has demonstrated that ATP is not only an energy currency inside cells, but is also a critical signaling molecule that allows cells and tissues throughout the body to communicate with one another.[15] This new aspect of ATP as an intercellular signaling molecule allows a broader understanding of the universality phenomenon of LLLT. It is now known that neurons release ATP into muscle, gut, and bladder tissue as a messenger molecule. The specific receptors for ATP as a signaling molecule (P2 family) and for its final breakdown product, adenosine (P1 family), have been identified.[16] This topic is discussed further by Karu.[17,18]

Understanding the multiple roles of ATP in cellular metabolism also provides a better appreciation of the cellular and molecular mechanisms of LLLT. Laboratories worldwide are

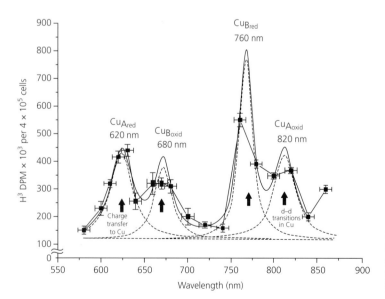

Figure 4.2 Action spectrum for stimulation of DNA synthesis. Suggested absorbing chromophores of the photoacceptor, cytochrome c oxidase, are given (after Karu[17]). Original curve (-■-), curve fitting (■) and Lorentzian fitting (– –) (Karu 2010. Reproduced with permission of Mary Ann Liebert).

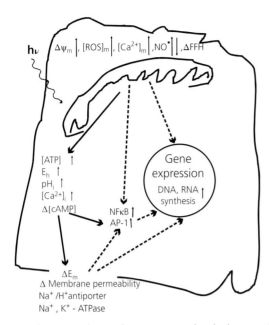

$h\nu$ $\Delta\psi_m\downarrow$, $[ROS]_m\downarrow$, $[Ca^{2+}]_m\downarrow$, $NO^\bullet\downarrow\downarrow$, ΔFFH

[ATP] $\uparrow$
E_h $\uparrow$
pH_i $\uparrow$
$[Ca^{2+}]_i$ $\uparrow$
$\Delta[cAMP]$

Gene
expression

DNA, RNA $\uparrow$
synthesis

$NF\kappa B\uparrow$
$AP\text{-}1\uparrow$

ΔE_m
Δ Membrane permeability
Na^+/H^+ antiporter
Na^+, K^+ - ATPase

Figure 4.3 Schematic explaining the putative mitochondrial retrograde signaling pathways after absorption of visible and infrared A (IR-A) radiation ($h\nu$) by the photoacceptor, cytochrome c oxidase. $\uparrow$ and $\downarrow$, increase or decrease of the values; [], concentration; ΔFFH, changes in mitochondrial fusion–fission homeostasis; AP-1, activator protein-1; NF-κB, nuclear factor kappa B. Experimentally proven ($\rightarrow$) and theoretically suggested (---->) pathways are shown (adapted from Karu 2008, With permission of TI Karu).

racing to turn the data about ATP as a neurotransmitter into therapies.[15] As a neurotransmitter, ATP is directly involved in brain function, sensory reception, and the nervous system control of muscles and organs. When released by non-neuronal cells, it often triggers protective responses, such as bone formation and cell proliferation.[16] Even a very brief look at all the conditions in which ATP is now believed to play a role as a signaling molecule,[16] and comparison of these with the range of clinical actions of LLLT, provides grounds for a new way of thinking. First, chronic and neuropathic pain have been successfully treated with LLLT for many years.[19] ATP signaling is believed to be involved in pain therapy.[16] Second, it is proposed that acupuncture (mechanical deformation of the skin by needles) and application of heat or electrical current lead to release of large amounts of ATP from keratinocytes, fibroblasts, and other cells in the skin.[20] Acupuncture by laser light is a well-known modality[21] (see also Chapter 29).

Respiratory chain enzyme photosensitivity

The photosensitivity of respiratory chain enzymes has not gained researchers' attention, unlike functional photoacceptors, such as chlorophyll and rhodopsin. However, the fragmented knowledge gathered so far forces one to ask whether the photosensitivity of cytochrome c oxidase may have physiological significance in spite of the complete adaptation of living systems to photons as a natural external factor. Let us recall that IR-A radiation penetrates rather deep into the tissues (so-called "optical window" of the skin or "near IR window" into the body). This circumstance also supports the hypothesis of a possible specific biological role of radiation between 600 and 1000 nm and gives new enthusiasm for LLLT clinical methods as well new interest in the biochemical mechanisms at the cellular and molecular levels.

References

1 Karu TI. Photobiology of low-power laser effects. *Health Phys* 1989; 56: 691–704.

2 Karu T. Primary and secondary mechanisms of action of visible-to-near IR radiation on cells. *J. Photochem Photobiol B Biol* 1999; 49: 1–17.

3 Karu T. Ten *Lectures on Basic Science of Laser Phototherapy*. Grängesberg: Prima Books AB, 2007.

4 Karu TI. Mitochondrial signaling in mammalian cells activated by red and near IR radiation. *Photochem Photobiol* 2008; 84: 1091–1099.

5 Brown GC. Nitric oxide and mitochondrial respiration. *Biochem Biophys Acta* 1999; 1411: 351–363.

6 Karu TI, Pyatibrat LV, Afanasyeva NI. A novel mitochondrial signaling pathway activated by visible-to-near infrared radiation. *Photochem Photobiol* 2004; 80: 366–372.

7 Karu TI, Pyatibrat LV, Kalendo GS. Photobiological modulation of cell attachment via cytochrome c oxidase. *Photochem Photobiol Sci* 2004; 3: 211–216.

8 Karu TI, Pyatibrat LV, Kolyakov SF, Afanasyeva NI. Absorption measurements of a cell monolayer relevant to phototherapy: reduction of cytochrome c oxidase under near IR radiation. *J Photochem Photobiol B: Biology* 2005; 81: 98–106.

9 Karu TI, Pyatibrat LV, Afanasyeva NI. Cellular effects of low power laser therapy can be mediated by nitric oxide. *Lasers Surg Med* 2005; 36: 307–314.

10 Lane N. *Power games. Nature* 2006; 443: 901–903.

11 Hothersall JS, Cunha FQ, Neild GH, Norohna-Dutra A. Induction of nitric oxide synthesis in J774 cell lowers intracellular glutathione: effect of oxide modulated glutathione redox status on nitric oxide synthase induction. *Biochem J* 1997; 322: 477–486.

12 Karu TI, Tiphlova OA, Matveyets YuA, Yartsev AP, Letokhov VS. Comparison of the effects of visible femtosecond laser pulses and continuous wave laser radiation of low average intensity on the clonogenicity of Escherichia coli. *J Photochem Photobiol B Biol* 1991; 10: 339–345.

13 Karu T, Andreichuk T, Ryabykh T. Changes in oxidative metabolism of murine spleen following diode laser (660–950nm) irradiation: effect of cellular composition and radiation parameters. *Lasers Surg Med* 1993; 13: 453–462.

14 Forman NJ, Boveris A. Superoxide radical and hydrogen peroxide in mitochondria. In: Pryor A (ed). *Free Radicals in Biology*, Vol. 5. New York: Academic Press, 1982: 65–90.

15 Burnstock G. Purinergic receptors and pain. *Curr Pharm Des* 2009; 15: 1717–1735.

16 Karu TI. Mitochondrial mechanisms of photobiomodulation in context of new data about multiple roles of ATP. *Photomed Laser Surg* 2010; 28: 159–160.

17 Karu TI. Multiple roles of cytochrome c oxidase in mammalian cells under action of red and IR-A radiation. *IUBMB Life* 2010; 62: 607–610.

18 Chow RT, Johnson HI, Lopes-Martins RAB, Bjordal JM. Efficacy of low-level laser therapy in the management of neck pain: a systematic review and meta-analysis of randomised placebo or active-treatment controlled trials. *Lancet* 2009; 374: 1897–1908.

19 Burnstock G. Acupuncture: a novel hypothesis for the involvement of purinergic signaling. *Med Hypoth* 2009; 73: 470–472.

20 Tuner J, Hode L. *Laser Therapy*. Clinical Practice and Scientific Background. Grängesberg: Prima Books, 2002.

21 Karu TI. Molecular mechanism of the therapeutic effect of low-intensity laser radiation. *Lasers Life Sci* 1988; 2: 53–74.

CHAPTER 5

Low level laser therapy – mechanism of action: Inflammatory process

Jan Magnus Bjordal[1], Rodrigo Alvaro Brandão Lopes-Martins[2], and Lucio Frigo[3]

[1]Physiotherapy Research Group, Department of Global and Public Health, University of Bergen, Bergen, Norway
[2]Institute of Biomedical Sciences, Pharmacology Department, University of São Paulo (USP), São Paulo, SP, Brazil
[3]Laser in Dentistry Program, Cruzeiro do Sul University, São Paulo, SP, Brazil

Background

Low level laser therapy (LLLT) has been used for the treatment of musculoskeletal pain for more than two decades. A more appropriate name for this modality would probably be laser phototherapy, because the mechanisms at play are triggered by the laser light without causing irreversible destructive changes to tissue morphology, as seen with laser surgery. This difference is caused by the lower power of the laser devices used for LLLT, typically class 3B lasers with mean output power ranging from 5 mW to 500 mW. Early clinical use relied largely on empirical evidence, but more recent scientific evidence suggests that LLLT can trigger specific photobiological mechanisms. The earliest LLLT experiments pointed in the direction of a biostimulatory effect where LLLT accelerated wound healing and tissue repair processes. Animal studies provided vague and contradictory results, although some suggested that LLLT might even modulate the inflammatory process. However, the evidence base for this hypothesis was not thoroughly investigated until the turn of the last century.

During the last decade, interest in LLLT research has picked up and the effect of LLLT in conditions involving inflammatory processes has been under scrutiny. We first reviewed the LLLT literature in acute injuries and postoperative pain in 2006[1] and later expanded on this issue by reviewing both animal laboratory trials[2] and other musculoskeletal pain conditions with inflammatory components treated by LLLT.[3]

In acute or postoperative pain conditions, non-steroidal anti-inflammatory drugs (NSAIDs) have been the gold standard treatment in treatment guidelines and surveys of clinical practice. NSAIDs are the most frequently recommended or given therapy in traumatic injury,[4] postoperative conditions,[5] and neck and lower back disorders.[6] It is surprising that although inflammation is mostly associated with acute conditions, NSAIDs are also the most common treatment for chronic pain patients in Europe.[7] Another common anti-inflammatory therapy is glucocorticoid injections and they are recommended for subacute and chronic tendinopathies[8] and osteoarthritis.[9] Although anti-inflammatory drug treatment dominates current pain management, there are concerns regarding the adverse effects of this treatment.

There is some evidence that pharmacological management of acute injuries can be associated with significantly better outcomes if prescribed with physical therapies.[10] A timely research question has been whether any of the therapies involving physical agents can modulate inflammation in the same way as anti-inflammatory drugs.

Since the 1980s, LLLT has been a controversial modality with conflicting results.[11] Twenty-five years later, early positive results have yet to be translated into consistent and significant results in clinical trials. The first trial of the effects of LLLT in an experimental animal inflammation model was published in 1985,[12] and a few publications followed during the next decade.[13,14] Still, when basic and clinical LLLT research was reviewed 20 years ago, the conclusion was that LLLT had not made the difficult transition from positive laboratory findings to established therapeutic tool.[15] Today, the situation is changing and the PedRo database, which rates clinical studies for methodology quality, now holds more than 100 randomized controlled clinical LLLT trials with acceptable or high method quality (60% or more of method criteria met). Efficacy results are however mixed. Administration of LLLT involves a number of potential pitfalls of a biophysical, photobiological, pathological, and clinical character that may compromise treatment success. Hence, a considerable number of LLLT studies have been published with negative results. However, if we acknowledge the important pitfalls and adhere to the guidelines of the World Association for Laser Therapy (WALT) (www.walt.nu), then it is quite easy to achieve good results with LLLT. The WALT guidelines are evidence based and have been validated for chronic joint disorders like arthritis[16] and tendinopathies.[17] Both of these meta-analyses found that more than 90% of the trials adhering to WALT dosage recommendations achieved significantly positive results.

Lasers in Dentistry: Guide for Clinical Practice, First Edition. Edited by Patrícia M. de Freitas and Alyne Simões.
© 2015 John Wiley & Sons, Inc. Published 2015 by John Wiley & Sons, Inc.

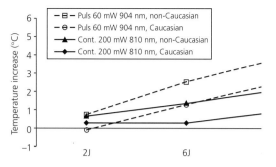

Figure 5.1 Non-significant increase in skin temperature among patients with white and non-white skin after LLLT irradiation with recommended doses of 2 and 6 J from two lasers with continuous wavelengths of 810 nm and superpulsed 904 nm, respectively.

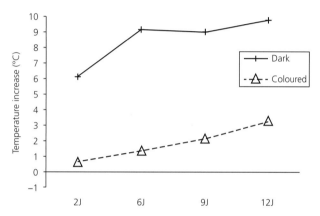

Figure 5.2 Significant increase in dark skin temperature compared to colored skin temperature after LLLT irradiation with recommended doses of 2 and 6 J and higher doses of 9 and 12 J with a continuous 810-nm laser.

How does LLLT work?

LLLT works mostly through non-thermal photobiological mechanisms where laser light is absorbed by chromophores and thereby modulates pathophysiological processes. Typical LLLT doses only induce minor and non-significant changes in human skin temperature in patients with varying levels of skin pigmentation (Fig. 5.1). However, the strong continuous output lasers with wavelengths of 780–860 nm may induce significant thermal effects in patients with dark skin (Fig. 5.2).

Characteristics of some common inflammatory conditions

Inflammation may be present in both acute and chronic musculoskeletal pain disorders. For instance, flares of symptom aggravation in degenerative and systemic arthritis are associated with increased synovial inflammatory activity.[18] For tendon disorders, short-lived flares in disease activity seem to be associated with physical overload, although a definite link between pain aggravation and inflammatory activity is still uncertain.[19]

However, anti-inflammatory treatment with NSAIDs and steroids appears to provide short-term pain relief in acute and subacute tendinopathies.[20] In chronic muscle pain, both the capacity of the muscle cells to withstand fatigue and the vasoactive response to muscle contractions appear to be impaired.[21] More recently, signs of inflammation have also been detected at active myofascial trigger points[22] and one study found significant effects of anti-inflammatory treatment with a topical NSAID patch placed on active myofascial trigger points in neck pain patients.[23] This may also have relevance for temporomandibular disorders, where muscular pain may contribute considerably to the overall pain experience.

Literature review of LLLT effects on inflammatory outcome parameters

In addition to our review from 2006,[1] our literature search has identified one review of cell studies.[24] The latter review focused on the molecular and proliferative effects of LLLT, and inflammation was only superficially covered, with references to a study from our research group[25] and three studies from other research groups.[26-28] It briefly concluded that the expression and secretion of the inflammatory cytokines prostaglandin E_2 (PGE_2), tumor necrosis factor alpha (TNF-α), cyclooxygenase 2 (COX-2), and interleukin 1 beta (IL-1β) can be inhibited by LLLT exposure.[24]

In total we identified 34 potentially eligible studies in cell cultures and 54 eligible studies in animals. Closer examination revealed that 11 cell culture studies and 27 animal studies were relevant. We also included six studies investigating head-to-head comparisons between LLLT and anti-inflammatory drugs and negative drug interactions.

The results of the laboratory studies (cell culture and animal) were consistently in favour of LLLT. All except one study[29] showed anti-inflammatory effects in at least one of the LLLT dose groups studied.

Biochemical markers of inflammation in the initial stage of inflammation

One cell study found no anti-inflammatory effects from LLLT on blood monocytes, vein endothelial cells, and TNF-α.[29] The inflammatory marker PGE_2 was significantly reduced by LLLT in three cell studies.[28,30,31] Three animal studies[32-34] also showed significant reductions in PGE_2 levels after LLLT. In addition, two human studies were performed with microdialysis in symptomatic peritendinous Achilles tissue[3] and in blood serum in patients with rheumatoid arthritis.[35] LLLT inhibition of TNF-α release was reported in three animal studies,[25,36,37] but only in a narrow dose range. Two cell studies demonstrated significant reduction of COX-2 mRNA levels after LLLT exposure.[28,38] COX-2 inhibition was also found in two animal studies,[39,40] but not in animals receiving shorter than 16 seconds of laser irradiation.[40] Five cell studies found that LLLT partially reduced levels of IL-1β[31,41-44] and four animal studies showed the same effect.[45–48] One cell study observed reduced levels of plasminogen activator in stretched periodontal ligament cells.[49]

Inflammatory cell infiltration and formation of edema, hemorrhage, and necrosis in animal studies

Local reduction of inflammatory neutrophil cell infiltration after LLLT was observed in eight animal studies.[37,46,50–55] Four studies in rats and dogs have investigated hemorrhage and myocardial infarct size, and all found significant reductions in size after LLLT as compared to sham-irradiated controls.[37,56–58] In three trials, the necrotic area after snake venom injection was reduced after LLLT.[50,59,60] LLLT showed a significant reduction in edema volume after soft tissue injury in all five animal studies.[13,34,61–63]

Anti-inflammatory effects of LLLT versus non-steroidal anti-inflammatory drugs and glucocorticoid steroids in laboratory trials

In four out of five head-to-head comparisons between LLLT and NSAIDs, human equipotent doses of NSAIDs did not exert significantly different effects from LLLT. The anti-inflammatory effect was measured within the first 3 days after experimental injury, and studies included the NSAIDs indomethacin,[13] meloxicam,[64] celecoxib,[37] and diclofenac.[61] The only study showing a significantly lower effect of LLLT[45] did not report irradiation time, but if the reported parameters are used to calculate irradiation time it may have been as short as 4 seconds. The results of a typical comparison between NSAID and LLLT in edema formation from one of our animal experiments is shown in Figure 5.3.

There are mixed results for the comparison between the anti-inflammatory effect of glucocorticoid steroids (dexamethasone) and LLLT. Dexamethasone anti-inflammatory effects were not significantly different from those of LLLT in two studies,[63,65] but slightly superior to LLLT in three other studies.[55,62,66]

Negative drug interactions with anti-inflammatory effects of LLLT

Four animal studies have reported negative interactions and reduced effect from LLLT with concomitant use of glucocorticoid steroids.[55,67]

Dose–response patterns for LLLT anti-inflammatory effects

Most investigated wavelengths between 632 nm and 904 nm have induced significant anti-inflammatory effects in cell and animal trials. Regarding optimal dosing for these wavelengths, the following lower limits and medians for doses and irradiation times have been reported. The median value for laser mean optical output was 25 mW. Lower limits for anti-inflammatory effects were found to be 0.6 J/cm² in animal studies, and the lower limit for irradiation time was 16 seconds. Median irradiation time was 80 seconds in animal studies, but one study reported significantly better effect when 3 J/cm² was delivered at low power density (5 mW/cm²) over a longer period of time (600 seconds) than at high power density (50 mW/cm²) over a shorter period of time (60 seconds). Two studies reported significantly better anti-inflammatory effects when doses were equal, but they were delivered with longer irradiation times in a model of zymosan-induced arthritis.[65] Upper limits for anti-inflammatory effects remain uncertain for power densities above 135 mW/cm² and doses above 15 J. Both infrared and red lasers were significantly better than LEDs emitting red wavelength in the same experimental model.[62]

Discussion

In our most recent review we found consistent anti-inflammatory effects from LLLT in 43 out of 44 controlled laboratory trials. One may question the clinical relevance of laboratory studies, but

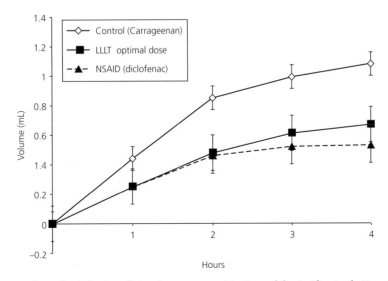

Figure 5.3 Development of rat paw edema after induction of injury by carrageenan injection and the significant reduction of edema formation after LLLT and NSAID (diclofenac) administration. They were equally effective and significantly better than the placebo control.

they form the scientific foundation for the development of pharmaceutical agents and are a compulsory hurdle before marketing approval can be given for drugs. Animal studies are also used to determine optimal doses and administration of anti-inflammatory drugs.[68] It is encouraging that the understanding of the scientific basis for LLLT mechanisms has improved to a level where it can compare and compete well with anti-inflammatory drug treatment. At present there is very limited evidence for the anti-inflammatory effects of other electrophysical agents. A few reports have appeared for shortwave diathermy[69] and high voltage electrical stimulation,[70] but this evidence base is far smaller than that from the 44 studies found for LLLT. The crucial question is whether the evidence for anti-inflammatory effect can translate into effective clinical treatment. There are strong indications that it directly modulates inflammatory marker levels in human studies. One study has shown that LLLT significantly reduces the level of the inflammatory cytokine PGE_2 in the synovial membranes of rheumatoid arthritis patients.[71] Another study in female musculoskeletal pain patients found that decreased PGE_2 blood serum levels were significantly associated with LLLT treatment success.[35] Our research group has also found that LLLT reduced PGE_2 levels measured by microdialysis in activated Achilles tendinitis.[3] We have also found that levels of creatine kinase activity, a cytokine involved in the early phase of muscle damage, and C-reactive protein, a marker of systemic inflammation, could be reduced by LLLT after heavy exercise in animals[72,73] and in humans.[74–76] In the USA, most drugs for acute pain have been approved on the basis of clinical studies in models of minor oral surgery.[77] In our earlier review of human studies,[1] we found that LLLT exhibited a significant dose-dependent anti-inflammatory effect in randomized controlled studies of minor oral surgery. Typically, studies with non-significant effects were underdosed with doses below 0.5 J, while doses ranging from 1 to 6 J typically reported positive effects.

The available evidence can tell us something about the areas where LLLT has clinical potential. LLLT can be used in combination with active exercise or manual therapy to control possible inflammatory responses to loading of joints, muscles, and tendons.[78] New knowledge about the inflammatory manifestations at active myofascial trigger points offers an additional explanation for why LLLT seems to work so well in neck pain patients.[79] Also, LLLT effects at active trigger points have been demonstrated in one animal study.

The anti-inflammatory effects of monochromatic LLLT seem to occur as a class effect irrespective of laser wavelengths if applied with narrow bandwidth in the red or infrared laser light spectra. The difficult transition of LLLT into clinical practice has been hampered by a lack of knowledge about LLLT mechanisms and their dose-dependency. In short, two major factors seem to cause treatment failure in clinical trials. In studies in small animals, most of the inflamed area can be covered even with a small laser spot size and doses are reported in J/cm^2. Extrapolating these results into clinical practice where larger areas need to be irradiated calls for reporting of doses in Joules. Several studies have based their calculation of clinical doses on tiny spot sizes in J/cm^2, leading to insufficient doses in studies of osteoarthritis $(0.18 J)$[80] and carpal tunnel syndrome $(0.9 J)$.[81] Current guidelines state that clinical doses should be given in Joules instead of J/cm^2 (www.walt.nu/dosage-recommendations.html). Secondly, steroids will erase the possible anti-inflammatory effect of LLLT, and several tendinopathy trials have recruited more than 40% of their patients from failures after steroid injection therapy.[82] Possibly the most important contribution from this analysis is the finding that the anti-inflammatory effect occurs locally in the inflamed tissue through inhibition of COX-2 expression. Bearing in mind that the tiny laser beam only penetrates with sufficient energy into $1–4 cm^3$ of human tissue,[83] large pathological tissue volumes need to be irradiated at several points to make a clinical difference.

More research of LLLT in inflammatory experimental models is clearly needed and several aspects of LLLT mechanisms have still to be investigated.

LLLT is still viewed with skepticism by parts of established medicine and it has received very little recommendation in clinical guidelines. During the recent years, much attention has been paid to the side effects of anti-inflammatory drugs[84,85] and the negative long-term effects of steroid injections in tendon disorders.[86] It is agreed that toxicity for LLLT is lower than that for most drugs,[87] and in view of its superior safety, LLLT should be considered as an alternative to pharmaceutical agents.

Clinical aspects for evidence-based use of LLLT in dentistry

There is strong evidence that red and infrared LLLT exhibits a dose-dependent anti-inflammatory effect in cell and animal studies. The effect can be compromised if LLLT is combined with glucocorticoid steroids, which have a negative interaction with LLLT. Most red and infrared LLLT is administered with mean laser outputs ranging from 10 to100 mW and irradiation times from 20 to 60 seconds, and doses between 0.6 and 9.6 J, reduce inflammation significantly and are as effective as NSAIDs in cell and animal studies.[88] However, for the clinician, it may be useful to differentiate between laser types. Technically speaking, one can achieve significant effects with all laser types, but some types have been more extensively investigated and are possibly slightly more effective than others for certain conditions.[88–90]

When one the laser ouput is known, LLLT doses can be easily calculated using the formula:

$$\frac{\text{Mean output (mW)} \times \text{irradiation time (s)}}{1000} = \text{Dose (J)}$$

An angled adapter for the laser probe tip should be considered when performing some intraoral procedures. Several LLLT devices have this option (Fig. 5.4).

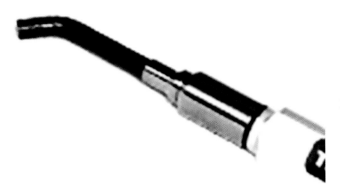

Figure 5.4 Angled LLLT probe tip for intraoral use.

The practical use of LLLT is easy once the optimal dose and target points have been determined. LLLT could even be applied by a properly trained dental assistant. It is important to remember that most of the literature has been performed with the laser probe in a fixed position during treatment. As a rule of thumb, each irradiated point will cover about 1–2 cm^3 of the pathology, so one should assure that a sufficient number of points are selected to cover the entire pathology.

If LLLT is used as recommended in WALT guidelines, then it is an effective and safe therapy.

References

1 Bjordal JM, Johnson MI, Iversen V, Aimbire F, Lopes-Martins RA. Low Level Laser Therapy in acute pain: a systematic review of possible mechanisms of action and clinical effects in randomized placebo-controlled trials. *Photomed Laser Surg* 2006; 24: 158–168.

2 Ramos L, Leal Junior EC, Pallotta RC, et al. Infrared (810 nm) low-level laser therapy in experimental model of strain-induced skeletal muscle injury in rats: effects on functional outcomes. *Photochem Photobiol* 2012; 88: 154–160.

3 Bjordal JM, Lopes-Martins RA, Iversen VV. A randomised, placebo controlled trial of low level laser therapy for activated Achilles tendinitis with microdialysis measurement of peritendinous prostaglandin E2 concentrations. *Br J Sports Med* 2006; 40: 76–80.

4 Bleakley CM, McDonough SM, MacAuley DC. Some conservative strategies are effective when added to controlled mobilisation with external support after acute ankle sprain: a systematic review. *Aust J Physiother* 2008; 54: 7–20.

5 Derry P, Derry S, Moore RA, McQuay HJ. Single dose oral diclofenac for acute postoperative pain in adults. *Cochrane Database Syst Rev* 2009: CD004768.

6 Chou R, Qaseem A, Snow V, et al. Diagnosis and treatment of low back pain: a joint clinical practice guideline from the American College of Physicians and the American Pain Society. *Ann Intern Med* 2007; 147: 478–491.

7 Breivik H, Collett B, Ventafridda V, Cohen R, Gallacher D. Survey of chronic pain in Europe: prevalence, impact on daily life, and treatment. *Eur J Pain* 2006; 10: 287–333.

8 Gaujoux-Viala C, Dougados M, Gossec L. Efficacy and safety of steroid injections for shoulder and elbow tendonitis: a meta-analysis

of randomised controlled trials. *Ann Rheum Dis* 2009; 68: 1843–1849.

9 Bjordal JM, Klovning A, Ljunggren AE, Slordal L. Short-term efficacy of pharmacotherapeutic interventions in osteoarthritic knee pain: A meta-analysis of randomised placebo-controlled trials. *Eur J Pain* 2007; 11: 125–138.

10 Castillo RC, MacKenzie EJ, Archer KR, Bosse MJ, Webb LX. Evidence of beneficial effect of physical therapy after lower-extremity trauma. *Arch Phys Med Rehabil* 2008; 89: 1873–1879.

11 Devor M. What`s in a laser beam for pain therapy? *Pain* 1990; 43: 139.

12 Bagnasco G. Mid-laser treatment of inflammation experimentally induced with formaldehyde. *Med Laser Rep* 1985; 3: 19–22.

13 Honmura A, Yanase M, Obata J, Haruki E. Therapeutic effect of Ga-Al-As diode laser irradiation on experimentally induced inflammation in rats. *Lasers Surg Med* 1992; 12: 441–449.

14 Xu, Yong-Qing. Experimental study of the effects of helium-neon laser radiation on repair of injured tendon. *In: Proc SPIE* 1993; 1616: 598–604.

15 Basford JR. Low intensity laser therapy: still not an established clinical tool. *Lasers Surg Med* 1995; 16: 331–342.

16 Jang H, Lee H. Meta-analysis of pain relief effects by laser irradiation on joint areas. *Photomed Laser Surg* 2012; 30: 405–417.

17 Tumilty S, Munn J, McDonough S, Hurley DA, Basford JR, Baxter GD. Low level laser treatment of tendinopathy: A systematic review with meta-analysis. *Photomed Laser Surg* 2010; 28: 3–16.

18 Felson DT. An update on the pathogenesis and epidemiology of osteoarthritis. *Radiol Clin North Am* 2004; 42: 1–9, v.

19 Alfredson H, Lorentzon R. Chronic tendon pain: no signs of chemical inflammation but high concentrations of the neurotransmitter glutamate. Implications for treatment? *Curr Drug Targets* 2002; 3: 43–54.

20 Smidt N, van der Windt DA. Tennis elbow in primary care. *BMJ* 2006; 333: 927–928.

21 Larsson R, Oberg PA, Larsson SE. Changes of trapezius muscle blood flow and electromyography in chronic neck pain due to trapezius myalgia. *Pain* 1999; 79: 45–50.

22 Shah JP, Danoff JV, Desai MJ,et al. Biochemicals associated with pain and inflammation are elevated in sites near to and remote from active myofascial trigger points. *Arch Phys Med Rehabil* 2008; 89: 16–23.

23 Hsieh LF, Hong CZ, Chern SH, Chen CC. Efficacy and side effects of diclofenac patch in treatment of patients with myofascial pain syndrome of the upper trapezius. *J Pain Symptom Management* 2010; 39: 116–125.

24 Gao X, Xing D. Molecular mechanisms of cell proliferation induced by low power laser irradiation. *J Biomed Sci* 2009; 16: 4.

25 Aimbire F, Albertini R, Pacheco MT, et al. Low-level laser therapy induces dose-dependent reduction of TNFalpha levels in acute inflammation. *Photomed Laser Surg* 2006; 24: 33–37.

26 Gavish L, Perez L, Gertz SD. Low-level laser irradiation modulates matrix metalloproteinase activity and gene expression in porcine aortic smooth muscle cells. *Lasers Surg Med* 2006; 38: 779–786

27 Gavish L, Asher Y, Becker Y, Kleinman Y. Low level laser irradiation stimulates mitochondrial membrane potential and disperses subnuclear promyelocytic leukemia protein. *Lasers Surg Med* 2004; 35: 369–376.

28 Sakurai Y, Yamaguchi M, Abiko Y. Inhibitory effect of low-level laser irradiation on LPS-stimulated prostaglandin E2 production

and cyclooxygenase-2 in human gingival fibroblasts. *Eur J Oral Sci* 2000; 108: 29–34.

29 Bouma MG, Buurman WA, van den Wildenberg FA. Low energy laser irradiation fails to modulate the inflammatory function of human monocytes and endothelial cells. *Lasers Surg Med* 1996; 19: 207–215.

30 Barberis G, Gamron S, Acevedo G, et al. In vitro synthesis of prostaglandin E2 by synovial tissue after helium-neon laser radiation in rheumatoid arthritis. *J Clin Laser Med Surg* 1996; 14: 175–177.

31 Shimizu N, Yamaguchi M, Goseki T, et al. Inhibition of prostaglandin E2 and interleukin 1-beta production by low-power laser irradiation in stretched human periodontal ligament cells. *J Dent Res* 1995; 74: 1382–1388.

32 Campana V, Catsel A, Vidal AE, Juri H, Palma JA. Prostaglandin E2 in experimental arthritis of rats irradiated with HeNe laser. *J Clin Laser Med Surg* 1993; 11: 79–81.

33 Iwatsuki K, Yoshimine T, Sasaki M, Yasuda K, Akiyama C, Nakahira R. The effect of laser irradiation for nucleus pulposus: an experimental study. *Neurol Res* 2005; 27: 319–323.

34 Ferreira DM, Zangaro RA, Villaverde AB, et al. Analgesic Effect of He-Ne (632.8 nm) Low-level laser therapy on acute inflammatory pain. *Photomed Laser Surg* 2005; 23: 177–181.

35 Mizutani K, Musya Y, Wakae K, et al. A clinical study on serum prostaglandin E2 with low-level laser therapy. *Photomed Laser Surg* 2004; 22: 537–539.

36 Campana V, Moya M, Gavotto A, et al. He-Ne laser on microcrystalline arthropathies. *J Clin Laser Med Surg* 2003; 21: 99–103.

37 Aimbire F, Albertine R, Magalhaes RG, et al. Effect of LLLT Ga-Al-As (685 nm) on LPS-induced inflammation of the airway and lung in the rat. *Lasers Med Sci* 2005; 20: 11–20.

38 Pourzarandian A, Watanabe H, Ruwanpura SM, Aoki A, Noguchi K, Ishikawa I. Er:YAG laser irradiation increases prostaglandin E production via the induction of cyclooxygenase-2 mRNA in human gingival fibroblasts. *J Periodontal Res* 2005; 40: 182–186.

39 Albertini R, Aimbire F, Villaverde AB, Silva JA, Jr., Costa MS. COX-2 mRNA expression decreases in the subplantar muscle of rat paw subjected to carrageenan-induced inflammation after low level laser therapy. *Inflamm Res* 2007; 56: 228–229.

40 Lopes NN, Plapler H, Chavantes MC, Lalla RV, Yoshimura EM, Alves MT. Cyclooxygenase-2 and vascular endothelial growth factor expression in 5-fluorouracil-induced oral mucositis in hamsters: evaluation of two low-intensity laser protocols. *Support Care Cancer* 2009; 17: 1409–1415.

41 Sattayut S, Hughes F, Bradley P. 820 nm Gallium aluminium arsenide laser modulation of prostaglandin E2 production in interleukin-1 stimulated myofibroblasts. *Laser Ther* 1999; 11: 88–95.

42 Gavish L, Perez LS, Reissman P, Gertz SD. Irradiation with 780 nm diode laser attenuates inflammatory cytokines but upregulates nitric oxide in lipopolysaccharide-stimulated macrophages: implications for the prevention of aneurysm progression. *Lasers Surg Med* 2008; 40: 371–378.

43 Nomura K, Yamaguchi M, Abiko Y. Inhibition of interleukin-1beta production and gene expression in human gingival fibroblasts by low-energy laser irradiation. *Lasers Med Sci* 2001; 16: 218–223.

44 Yamaura M, Yao M, Yaroslavsky I, Cohen R, Smotrich M, Kochevar IE. Low level light effects on inflammatory cytokine production by rheumatoid arthritis synoviocytes. *Lasers Surg Med* 2009; 41: 282–290.

45 Viegas VN, Abreu ME, Viezzer C, et al. Effect of low-level laser therapy on inflammatory reactions during wound healing: comparison with meloxicam. *Photomed Laser Surg* 2007; 25: 467–473.

46 Aimbire F, Ligeiro de Oliveira AP, Albertini R, et al. Low level laser therapy (LLLT) decreases pulmonary microvascular leakage, neutrophil influx and IL-1beta levels in airway and lung from rat subjected to LPS-induced inflammation. *Inflammation* 2008; 31: 189–197.

47 Safavi SM, Kazemi B, Esmaeili M, Fallah A, Modarresi A, Mir M. Effects of low-level He-Ne laser irradiation on the gene expression of IL-1beta, TNF-alpha, IFN-gamma, TGF-beta, bFGF, and PDGF in rat's gingiva. *Lasers Med Sci* 2008; 23: 331–335.

48 Ferreira MC, Gameiro J, Nagib PR, Brito VN, Vasconcellos Eda C, Verinaud L. Effect of low intensity helium-neon (HeNe) laser irradiation on experimental paracoccidioidomycotic wound healing dynamics. *Photochem Photobiol* 2009; 85: 227–233.

49 Ozawa Y, Shimizu N, Abiko Y. Low-energy diode laser irradiation reduced plasminogen activator activity in human periodontal ligament cells. *Lasers Surg Med* 1997; 21: 456–463.

50 Barbosa AM, Villaverde AB, Guimaraes-Souza L, Ribeiro W, Cogo JC, Zamuner SR. Effect of low-level laser therapy in the inflammatory response induced by Bothrops jararacussu snake venom. *Toxicon* 2008; 51: 1236–1244.

51 Boschi ES, Leite CE, Saciura VC, et al. Anti-Inflammatory effects of low-level laser therapy (660 nm) in the early phase in carrageenan-induced pleurisy in rat. *Lasers Surg Med* 2008; 40: 500–508.

52 Correa F, Martins RA, Correa JC, Iversen VV, Joenson J, Bjordal JM. Low-level laser therapy (GaAs lambda = 904 nm) reduces inflammatory cell migration in mice with lipopolysaccharide-induced peritonitis. *Photomed Laser Surg* 2007; 25: 245–249.

53 Lopes-Martins RA, Albertini R, Martins PS, Bjordal JM, Faria Neto HC. Spontaneous effects of low-level laser therapy (650 nm) in acute inflammatory mouse pleurisy induced by Carrageenan. *Photomed Laser Surg* 2005; 23: 377–381.

54 Aimbire F, Santos FV, Albertini R, Castro-Faria-Neto HC, Mittmann J, Pacheco-Soares C. Low-level laser therapy decreases levels of lung neutrophils anti-apoptotic factors by a NF-kappaB dependent mechanism. *Int Immunopharmacol* 2008; 8: 603–605.

55 Pessoa ES, Melhado RM, Theodoro LH, Garcia VG. A histologic assessment of the influence of low-intensity laser therapy on wound healing in steroid-treated animals. *Photomed Laser Surg* 2004; 22: 199–204.

56 Ad N, Oron U. Impact of low level laser irradiation on infarct size in the rat following myocardial infarction. *Int J Cardiol* 2001; 80: 109–116.

57 Oron U, Yaakobi T, Oron A, et al. Attenuation of infarct size in rats and dogs after myocardial infarction by low-energy laser irradiation. *Lasers Surg Med* 2001; 28: 204–211.

58 Oron U, Yaakobi T, Oron A, et al. Low-energy laser irradiation reduces formation of scar tissue after myocardial infarction in rats and dogs. *Circulation* 2001;103: 296–301.

59 Barbosa AM, Villaverde AB, Sousa LG, et al. Effect of low-level laser therapy in the myonecrosis induced by Bothrops jararacussu snake venom. *Photomed Laser Surg* 2009; 27: 591–597.

60 Dourado DM, Favero S, Baranauskas V, da Cruz-Hofling MA. Effects of the Ga-As laser irradiation on myonecrosis caused by Bothrops Moojeni snake venom. *Lasers Surg Med* 2003; 33: 352–357.

61 Albertini R, Aimbire FS, Correa FI, et al. Effects of different protocol doses of low power gallium-aluminum-arsenate (Ga-Al-As) laser radiation (650 nm) on carrageenan induced rat paw ooedema. *J Photochem Photobiol B* 2004; 74: 101–107.

62 de Morais NC, Barbosa AM, Vale ML, et al. Anti-Inflammatory Effect of Low-Level Laser and Light-Emitting Diode in Zymosan-Induced Arthritis. *Photomed Laser Surg* 2010; 28: 227–232.

63 Reis SR, Medrado AP, Marchionni AM, Figueira C, Fracassi LD, Knop LA. Effect of 670-nm laser therapy and dexamethasone on tissue repair: a histological and ultrastructural study. *Photomed Laser Surg* 2008; 26: 307–313.

64 Campana VR, Moya M, Gavotto A, et al. The relative effects of HeNe laser and meloxicam on experimentally induced inflammation. *Laser Ther* 1999; 11: 36–41.

65 Castano AP, Dai T, Yaroslavsky I, et al. Low-level laser therapy for zymosan-induced arthritis in rats: Importance of illumination time. *Lasers Surg Med* 2007; 39: 543–550.

66 Aimbire F, Lopes-Martins RA, Albertini R, et al. Effect of low-level laser therapy on hemorrhagic lesions induced by immune complex in rat lungs. *Photomed Laser Surg* 2007; 25: 112–117.

67 Gal P, Mokry M, Vidinsky B, et al. Effect of equal daily doses achieved by different power densities of low-level laser therapy at 635 nm on open skin wound healing in normal and corticosteroid-treated rats. *Lasers Med Sci* 2009; 24: 539–547.

68 Czock D, Keller F, Rasche FM, Haussler U. Pharmacokinetics and pharmacodynamics of systemically administered glucocorticoids. *Clin Pharmacokinet* 2005; 44: 61–98.

69 Ogilvie-Harris DJ, Gilbart M. Treatment modalities for soft tissue injuries of the ankle: A critical review. *Clin J Sports Med* 1995; 5: 175–186.

70 Dolan MG, Graves P, Nakazawa C, Delano T, Hutson A, Mendel FC. Effects of ibuprofen and high-voltage electric stimulation on acute edema formation after blunt trauma to limbs of rats. *J Athl Train* 2005; 40: 111–115.

71 Amano A, Miyagi K, Azuma T, et al.. Histological studies on the rheumatoid synovial membrane irradiated with a low energy laser. *Lasers Surg Med* 1994; 15: 290–294.

72 Leal Junior EC, Lopes-Martins RA, de Almeida P, Ramos L, Iversen VV, Bjordal JM. Effect of low-level laser therapy (GaAs 904 nm) in skeletal muscle fatigue and biochemical markers of muscle damage in rats. *Eur J Appl Physiol* 2010; 108: 1083–1088.

73 Lopes-Martins RA, Marcos RL, Leonardo PS, et al. Effect of low-level laser (Ga-Al-As 655 nm) on skeletal muscle fatigue induced by electrical stimulation in rats. *J Appl Physiol* 2006; 101: 283–288.

74 Junior EC, Lopes-Martins RA, Baroni BM, et al. Comparison between single-diode Low-Level Laser Therapy (LLLT) and LED multi-diode (cluster) therapy (LEDT) applications before high-intensity exercise. *Photomed Laser Surg* 2009; 41: 572–577.

75 Leal Junior EC, Lopes-Martins RA, Baroni BM, et al. Effect of 830 nm low-level laser therapy applied before high-intensity exercises on skeletal muscle recovery in athletes. *Lasers Med Sci* 2009; 24: 857–863.

76 Leal Junior EC, Lopes-Martins RA, Rossi RP, et al. Effect of cluster multi-diode light emitting diode therapy (LEDT) on exercise-induced skeletal muscle fatigue and skeletal muscle recovery in humans. *Lasers Surg Med* 2009; 41: 572–577.

77 Ridgway D. Analgesics for acute pain: Meeting the United States Food and Drug Administration's requirements for proof of efficacy. *Clin J Pain* 2004; 20: 123–132.

78 Stergioulas A, Stergioula M, Aarskog R, Lopes-Martins RA, Bjordal JM. Effects of low-level laser therapy and eccentric exercises in the treatment of recreational athletes with chronic achilles tendinopathy. *Am J Sports Med* 2008; 36: 881–887.

79 Chow RT, Johnson MI, Lopes-Martins RA, Bjordal JM. Efficacy of low-level laser therapy in the management of neck pain: a systematic review and meta-analysis of randomised placebo or active-treatment controlled trials. *Lancet* 2009; 374: 1897–1908.

80 Brosseau L, Wells G, Marchand S, et al. Randomized controlled trial on low level laser therapy (LLLT) in the treatment of osteoarthritis (OA) of the hand. *Lasers Surg Med* 2005; 36: 210–219.

81 Irvine J, Chong SL, Amirjani N, Chan KM. Double-blind randomized controlled trial of low-level laser therapy in carpal tunnel syndrome. *Muscle Nerve* 2004; 30: 182–187.

82 Haker E, Lundeberg T. Lateral epicondylalgia (tennis elbow): Report of noneffective midlaser treatment. *Arch Phys Med Rehab* 1991; 72: 984–988.

83 Stolik S, Delgado JA, Perez A, Anasagasti L. Measurement of the penetration depths of red and near infrared light in human "ex vivo" tissues. *J Photochem Photobiol B* 2000; 57: 90–93.

84 Juni P, Nartey L, Reichenbach S, Sterchi R, Dieppe PA, Egger M. Risk of cardiovascular events and rofecoxib: cumulative meta-analysis. *Lancet* 2004; 364: 2021–2029.

85 Helin-Salmivaara A, Virtanen A, Vesalainen R, et al. NSAID use and the risk of hospitalization for first myocardial infarction in the general population: a nationwide case-control study from Finland. *Eur Heart J* 2006; 27: 1657–1663.

86 Smidt N, Lewis M, Van der Windt DA, Hay EM, Bouter LM, Croft P. Lateral epicondylitis in general practice: course and prognostic indicators of outcome. *J Rheumatol* 2006; 33: 2053–2059.

87 Jordan KM, Arden NK, Doherty M, et al. EULAR Recommendations 2003: an evidence based approach to the management of knee osteoarthritis: Report of a Task Force of the Standing Committee for International Clinical Studies Including Therapeutic Trials (ESCISIT). *Ann Rheum Dis* 2003; 62: 1145–1155.

88 Bjordal JM, Lopes-Martins RAB, Joensen J, Iversen VV. The anti-inflammatory mechanism of low level laser therapy and its relevance for clinical use in physiotherapy. *Physical Ther Rev* 2010; 15: 286–293.

89 Bjordal JM, Bensadoun RJ, Tuner J, Frigo L, Gjerde K, Lopes-Martins RA. A systematic review with meta-analysis of the effect of low-level laser therapy (LLLT) in cancer therapy-induced oral mucositis. *Support Care Cancer* 2011; 19: 1069–1077.

90 Bjordal JM. Low Level Laser Therapy (LLLT) and World Association for Laser Therapy (WALT) dosage recommendations. *Photomed Laser Surg* 2012; 30: 61–62.

CHAPTER 6

Low level laser therapy – mechanism of action: Analgesia

Roberta Chow

Nerve Research Foundation, Brain and Mind Institute, The University of Sydney, Camperdown, Australia

History

Research into the analgesic effects of laser applications in dentistry commenced within a decade of the production of the first ruby laser in 1960.[1,2] One of the earliest references to the analgesic effects of laser irradiation in dentistry related to laser acupuncture (LA)[3] and many Japanese laser studies were published during the 1980s.[4] Helium–neon (HeNe) laser devices were used almost exclusively for LA and were characterized by power outputs of less than 10 mW and energy densities (EDs) of less than 4 J/cm². As diode technology developed, the output power of laser devices increased from the early 1-mW devices up to 500 mW. Near and far infrared wavelengths were widely adopted and used for their direct analgesic effects. Pulsed, defocused ablative lasers such as CO_2 and Nd:YAG lasers have more recently been adapted to deliver pain relief in dentistry.

Treated painful conditions

There are a number of dental situations and conditions where the analgesic effects of low level laser therapy (LLLT) are used to good effect. Prior to invasive procedures such as pre-extraction[5] or immediately postoperatively, laser significantly reduces acute pain. For example, a red 632.8-nm laser applied immediately after removal of third molar teeth[6,7] and a 809-nm laser applied prior to endodontic surgery[8] reduced postoperative pain. Other chronic painful conditions such as hypersensitive dentin,[9] temporomandibular joint dysfunction (TMD),[10,11] trigeminal neuralgia,[12,13] and mucosal conditions such as aphthous ulcers[14] and herpes simplex[15,16] represent a range of disparate conditions in which analgesia is central to management. In each of these clinical scenarios there is a complex mix of pathophysiology of inflammation, muscle pain, and peripheral nerve sensitization. Understanding the mechanism of analgesia enables more effective treatment and in each of these conditions laser-induced neural inhibition provides a plausible mechanism for analgesic effects.

Evidence for the inhibitory neural mechanisms

Clinical pain arises from activation of peripheral nerve endings of nociceptors, the thinly myelinated Aδ and unmyelinated, slow conducting C fibers, which lie within the epidermis and mucosa, forming a complex neural network.[17,18] These somatosensory nerve fibers transduce noxious stimuli, such as heat, mechanical force, and the chemical stimuli of inflammatory neuropeptides into action potentials.[19] Blockade of these nerves would therefore lead to reduced transmission of noxious signaling and hence to reduced pain.

Slowing of conduction velocity and decrease in action potential amplitudes reflecting inhibition of electrophysiological activity was demonstrated in a review of laser effects on nerves.[20] Illustrative of these findings is a series of studies which demonstrated conduction block in sensory (somatosensory evoked potentials [SSEPs]) and motor nerves (compound muscle action potentials [CMAPs]) following transcutaneous 808-nm (450 mW, continuous wave) and 650-nm (35 mW, continuous wave) irradiation for 30 seconds to each of four points overlying a rat sciatic nerve.[21] The latter effects are relevant to myofascial pain syndromes, such as TMD dysfunction and treatment of trigger points.[22,23] Neural blockade of up to 30% reduction in amplitude occurred within 10–20 minutes of laser application and was reversed by 24 hours. In a more complex study involving stimulation of the trigeminal nerve, 830-nm (350 mW, continuous wave), 120-second laser irradiation to root pulp blocked evoked electrical activity in the trigeminal nucleus[24] (Figs 6.1 and 6.2). In a similar human model and in line with the findings of Wakabayashi et al.,[24] Nelson and Friedman[25] found that HeNe laser irradiation suppressed somatosensory trigeminal evoked potentials amplitudes (but not latencies) by intraoral irradiation of the maxillary nerve. In contrast to the other studies cited, this study used pulsed HeNe (1.7 mW, 632.5 nm, 50 Hz, 1.73 W/cm²) for 2 minutes. Of particular interest, these effects occurred at 10 and 20 minutes, which is the same time frame reported by Yan et al.[21] for suppression of transcutaneous effects of 650-nm and

Lasers in Dentistry: Guide for Clinical Practice, First Edition. Edited by Patrícia M. de Freitas and Alyne Simões.

© 2015 John Wiley & Sons, Inc. Published 2015 by John Wiley & Sons, Inc.

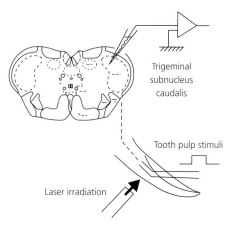

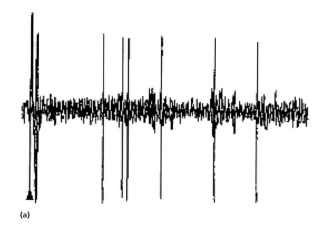

(a)

Figure 6.1 Schematic of the electrophysiological experiment in rats. The pulp of the lower incisor was electrically stimulated and the evoked action potentials were extracellularly recorded in the ipsilateral caudal neurons. The GaAlAs semiconductor laser was irradiated on the cervical surface of the stimulated incisor toward the tooth pulp (Wakabayashi et al. 1993. Reproduced with permission of John Wiley and Sons).

808-nm irradiation on nerve conduction. These findings provide strong evidence that transcutaneous laser can inhibit nerve conduction in underlying nerves. Such inhibitory effects do not provide direct evidence for analgesia; however, Chan and Armati[26] established direct correlation between neural blockade and pain relief. In this study, Nd:YAG laser irradiation (240 seconds) to the buccal sulcus of premolar teeth suppressed neural activity in the pulpo-dental nerve and at the same time significantly reduced pain. Moreover, these analgesic effects were equivalent to the analgesic EMLA. This is strong evidence for the "neural hypothesis" of laser-induced analgesia.

Nociceptor specificity

Of particular relevance to the analgesic effects of laser is the specific suppression of nociceptor activity. As an example, action potentials in nociceptors induced by mechanical and thermal noxious stimuli were blocked by laser irradiation.[27,28] In the first of these studies, 632.8-nm (1 mW, 100 Hz) irradiation applied to the sural nerve blocked pinch stimulation in the rabbit paw, and in the second study, GaAlAs (904 nm, 2 W, 200 ns) blocked noxious heat stimulation in cat tongue nociceptors. Nociceptor specificity was further explored in a study where 830-nm (40 mW), continuous wave laser irradiation to the saphenous nerve blocked pinch, cold, and stimulation heat applied to the rat paw, but not brush stimulation (light touch), which is conveyed by Aβ fibers.[29] Furthermore, a parallel study showed that rats without Aδ and C fibers, having been destroyed at birth by capsaicin, could not respond to painful stimuli or laser irradiation, though brush sensitivity, as in the previous experiment, was unaffected. Other wavelengths, such as 1064 nm (Nd:YAG) used widely in dentistry, have also demonstrated C fiber specificity in peroneal, tibial, and saphenous nerve models.[30,31]

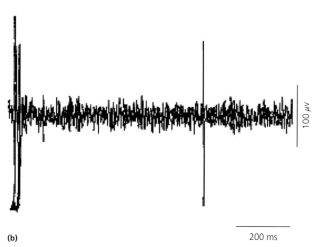

(b)   200 ms

Figure 6.2 Effect of laser irradiation on the evoked responses of a wide dynamic range neuron in the trigeminal subnucleus caudalis. (a) Tooth pulp stimulation (0.4 mA, 0.2 ms) applied to the ipsilateral lower incisor evoked early discharges reflecting temporal convergence A-fiber afferent input and late discharges. (b) When the laser was irradiated on the surface of the lower incisor for 120 seconds, the late discharges were suppressed, whereas the early discharges were not suppressed by the irradiation (Wakabayashi et al. 1993. Reproduced with permission of John Wiley and Sons).

Neural blockade and anti-inflammatory effects

Not only does laser irradiation inhibit neural response to noxious stimuli, but it also blocks action potentials generated by pro-inflammatory stimuli. Specifically, increased electrical activity in sensory nerves was blocked by 830-nm (continuous wave) irradiation when pro-inflammatory substances, such as formalin or turpentine, were injected into the skin of the rat paw.[29,32,33] Injection of bradykinin into the skin of the rat face resulted in increased mitochondrial proliferation in the trigeminal nucleus. The 830-nm (60 mW, continuous wave) laser applied daily for 12 days to the site of injection reduced the extent of proliferation to control levels.[34] Anti-inflammatory effects of LLLT constitute one of the most important of the pain-relieving mechanisms of LLLT and are affected by stimulation of cells which promote the inflammatory cascade, such as neutrophils and macrophages.[35,36] However, in addition to the cellular effects, suppression of neural activity also has the capacity to reduce inflammation, as shown in the previously discussed studies which directly link neural suppression with anti-inflammatory activity. Neurogenic inflammation, in particular, is a specific, sterile inflammatory response caused by the local release of pro-inflammatory neuropeptides, such as substance P, bradykinin, and prostaglandin E_2 (PGE_2) from nerve endings.[37] This response in acute injury causes peripheral nerve sensitization, adding further to the cascade of pain and inflammation. Central sensitization and persistent pain can then follow. Laser-induced neural blockade of nociceptors both pre-emptively or for established pain and inflammation has a strong evidence base with important clinical implications.

Mechanisms for inhibitory effects

The anatomy of individual neurons is very different from that of compact cells such as fibroblasts and may underlie their specific sensitivity to laser irradiation. An axon is the elongated cell body of a neuron, which can be up to 1 m in length (e.g. the sciatic nerve). It extends distally from its cell body which lies within the dorsal root ganglia (DRG) and in proximity to the spinal cord at each spinal level. The trigeminal ganglion is equivalent to the dorsal root ganglion and conveys somatosensory information from the face and teeth via its three branches. Sensory fibers terminate as fine, unmyelinated nerve endings in skin or mucosa, while the proximal, short portion of the neuron enters the dorsal horn.

The elongated structure of the neuron makes it uniquely vulnerable to the effects of laser irradiation. ATP, the source of energy for all cells, is transported in ATP-rich mitochondria via anterograde fast axonal flow (FAF) along the cytoskeleton by molecular motors, kinesins, from the cell body.[38–40] There is no rough endoplasmic reticulum (ER) within the axon so all synthesis of proteins, neurotransmitters, and ATP occurs in the cell body. Retrograde flow of depleted mitochondria occurs by dyneins, another set of molecular motors. When the cytoskeleton is disrupted, FAF and hence transport of mitochondria and other organelles is blocked, leading to the reduction in ATP for nerve function. For example, as the ATP-requiring enzyme Na$^+$K$^+$-ATPase maintains the resting potential of the nerve, decreased activity would therefore have profound effects on the electrophysiology, resulting in depolarization blockade.[41]

Immunohistochemistry demonstrated that 830-nm (300 mW), 808-nm (450 mW, continuous wave), and 650-nm (35 mW, continuous wave) laser irradiation to cultured rat DRG neurons caused the formation of reversible varicosities, or "beading," along axons, in which mitochondria "pile up" where the cytoskeleton is disrupted.[42,43] This is also seen with a 1064-nm Nd:YAG laser in tibial nerves.[44] Live imaging of DRG neurons showed that a 830-nm laser inhibited FAF and decreased mitochondrial membrane potential (MMP) in DRG neurons.

As MMP is a surrogate measure of ATP, it is proposed that decreased MMP will lead to decreased activity in all ATPases.

The relationship between varicosity formation and slowing of conduction velocity has been demonstrated with high dose local anesthetic agents, which also cause varicosities in DRG neurons.[45,46] The authors developed a mathematic model showing how varicosity formation slowed conduction velocity. This suggests that varicosity formation may be a common mechanism for the analgesic effects of laser and local anesthetic agents.

Clinical consequences of nociceptor blockade

Laser-induced neural blockade initiates a cascade of events in the peripheral nerve endings in the skin and dermis with important clinical consequences. The most immediate effect is pain relief, which occurs within a few minutes of LLLT application and is consistent with the experimental findings of the timing of onset of conduction blockade in sensory nerves. The important clinical consequence for the patient is reduced drug intake, improved mobility, and reduced anxiety. A second consequence of local neural blockade is inhibition of peripheral nerve sensitization, which reduces the intensity of local inflammatory response and axon reflexes, limiting vasodilation and swelling in acute injury and inflammation.

These direct effects occur within the penetration depths of laser irradiation of skin and mucosa; however, subsequent central effects occur in the proximal nerve and the dorsal horn as a result of local peripheral nerve inhibition. A consequence of reducing noxious afferent input to the dorsal horn is the down-regulation of synaptic transmission at the spinal cord level, which can limit the progression of acute to chronic pain. This is important in understanding how laser irradiation can modulate the pain matrix[47,48] and prevent persistent pain.[49] A number of studies have demonstrated "central" effects. Illustrative of these is a study where 830-nm laser irradiation to the root pulp blocked electrical activity in the trigeminal nucleus.[24] In a single neuron experiment, bradykinin applied to the axon generated an action potential in the cell body, in a separate chamber.[50] A 830-nm (16.2 mW) laser for 1 minute following bradykinin blocked the action potentials in the cell body. In an *in vivo* model, action potentials generated by electrical stimulation to the sciatic nerve were measured at the L5 dorsal roots.[51] When a 632.8-nm, 1-mW, 100-Hz laser was applied proximal to the site of stimulation in the peripheral nerve, the action potentials generated at the dorsal root were significantly reduced. All these studies, though differing in the experimental models used, demonstrate that laser irradiation applied peripherally has proximal effects. The cascade from peripheral nerve inhibition leads to suppressed synaptic activity in second-order neurons so that cortical areas of the pain matrix are not activated. Importantly, the result of local peripheral nerve blockade has long-term consequences in pain modulation.

Other mechanisms of analgesia

In any clinical situation where laser is transmitted, scattered, and absorbed, many different tissue types will be affected and several mechanisms can act simultaneously, though one may dominate at any one time. In this context, it is relevant to note that not all analgesic effects are related directly to neural inhibition.[52]

Alteration in the release of neurotransmitters that are associated with pain relief has been demonstrated in both animal and human experiments. For example, serotonin levels are increased with treatment of myofascial pain with laser therapy[53,54]; β-endorphin and precursors increase with laser irradiation of trigger points[22]; endorphins in skin are also increased with laser irradiation.[55]

Improving lymphatic flow is also an important component of pain relief as swelling occurs in acute injury and in some chronic conditions.[56,57] Increased motoricity of endothelial cells, which form the pulsatile lymphagion and increase uptake of interstitial fluid by opening up small intercellular spaces, has been demonstrated. In addition, lymphogenesis, in which new lymphatics are formed, increases the capacity to reduce swelling in the long term.

Several lines of evidence also support pain relief by mechanisms which reduce muscle pain and spasm, such as occurs with TMD. Direct laser-induced blockade of amplitude and latencies of CMAPs with 808-nm (450 mW, continuous wave) and 650-nm (35 mW, continuous wave) lasers indicates that laser irradiation can directly inhibit motor nerves. Studies of laser irradiation on the neuromuscular junction end-plate potentials showed reduced amplitude with release of acetylcholine with a 830-nm (86 mW, continuous wave, 12 J/cm²) laser, but not with a 808-nm laser at 4 J/cm²,[58] or with a 655-nm laser at the same EDs.[59] Clinical studies have demonstrated the reduction of tenderness and pain by treatment of trigger points.[23,60–63] A study of particular interest demonstrated that not only did a 904-nm laser significantly reduce tenderness in the treated neck and shoulder girdle trigger points, but also increased the pain threshold in the non-treated contralateral trigger points 15 minutes later.[64] Of note, treatment response occurs within the same time frame as animal studies show conduction block of CMAPs within 10–20 minutes. Moreover, the response on the contralateral side of the body suggests modulation through cross-over of second-order neurons in the spinal cord affecting the same segment. It also suggests that care must be taken when using the contralateral side of the body as a control in randomized controlled studies. Acknowledging the evidence, an International Association for the Study of Pain (IASP) fact sheet now includes LLLT as an evidence-based treatment for myofascial pain.[65]

Future directions for laser use in pain relief

The evidence for LLLT in the treatment of pain and application in dentistry is gaining strength as evidence for its mechanisms accumulates. While neural mechanisms are important in understanding the application of LLLT, it is ultimately the application in practice which will reinforce and assist in progressing the use of LLLT in medicine and dentistry.

References

1 Stern RH, Renger HL, Howell FV. Laser effects on vital dental pulps. *Br Dent J* 1969; 127(1): 26–28.

2 Eichler J, Lenz H. Laser applications in medicine and biology: a bibliography. *Appl Optics* 1977; 16(1): 27.

3 Zhou YC. An advanced clinical trial with laser acupuncture anesthesia for minor operations in the oro-maxillofacial region. *Lasers Surg Med* 1984; 4(3): 297–303.

4 Nagasawa A (ed). Dental and Oral Surgical Aspects of LLLT. International Laser Therapy Association (ILTA) 1990; 1990 October 26–28; Okinawa. Chichester: John Wiley and Sons Ltd, 1991.

5 Chan A, Armati P, Moorthy AP. Pulsed Nd:YAG laser induces pulpal analgesia: a randomized clinical trial. *J Dent Res* 2012; 91(7 Suppl): 79S–84S.

6 Clokie C, Bentley KC, Head TW. The effects of the helium-neon laser on postsurgical discomfort: a pilot study. *J Can Dent Assoc* 1991; 57(7): 584–586.

7 Markovic AB, Todorovic L. Postoperative analgesia after lower third molar surgery: contribution of the use of long-acting local anesthetics, low-power laser, and diclofenac. *Oral Surg Oral Med Oral Pathol Oral Radiol Endodont* 2006; 102(5): e4–8.

8 Kreisler M, Haj H, Noroozi N, Willershausen B. Efficacy of low level laser therapy in reducing postoperative pain after endodontic surgery - a randomized double blind clinical study. *Int J Oral Maxillofac Surg* 2004; 33(1): 38–41.

9 Schwarz F, Arweiler N, Georg T, Reich E. Desensitizing effects of an Er:YAG laser on hypersensitive dentine. *J Clin Periodontol* 2002; 29(3): 211–215.

10 Çetiner S, Kahraman SA, Yucetas S. Evaluation of low-level laser therapy in the treatment of temporomandibular disorders. *Photomed Laser Surg* 2006; 24(5): 637–641.

11 Mazzetto MO, Carrasco TG, Bidinelo EF, de Andrade Pizzo RC, Mazzetto RG. Low intensity laser application in temporomandibular disorders: a phase I double-blind study. *Cranio* 2007; 25(3): 186–192.

12 Walker J, Akhanjee L, Cooney M, Goldstein J, Tamayoshi S, Segal-Gidan F. Laser therapy for pain of trigeminal neuralgia. *Clin J Pain* 1988; 3(4): 183–187.

13 Eckerdal A, Bastian H. Can low reactive level laser therapy be used in the treatment of neurogenic facial pain? A double blind placebo controlled investigation of patients with trigeminal neuralgia. *Laser Ther* 1996; 8(4): 247–251.

14 Colvard M, Kuo P. Managing aphthous ulcers: laser treatment applied. *J Am Dent Assoc* 1991; 122(6): 51–53.

15 Munoz Sanchez PJ, Capote Femenias JL, Diaz Tejeda A, Tuner J. The effect of 670-nm low laser therapy on herpes simplex type 1. *Photomed Laser Surg* 2012; 30(1): 37–40.

16 Schindl A, Neumann R. Low-intensity laser therapy is an effective treatment for recurrent herpes simplex infection. *Results from a randomized double-blind placebo-controlled study. J Invest Dermatol* 1999; 113(2): 221–223.

17 Lauria G. Innervation of the human epidermis. A historical review. *Ital J Neurol Sci* 1999; 20(1): 63–70.

18 Kennedy W, Wendelschafter-Crabb G, Polydefikis M, McArthur J. Pathology and quantitation of cutaneous innervation. In: Dyck P, Thomas P (eds). *Peripheral Neuropathy*, 4 edn. Philadelphia: W.B Saunders, 2005: 873.

19 Siddall PJ, Cousins MJ. Introduction to pain mechanisms - implications for neural blockade. In: Cousins M, Bridenbaugh P ,(eds). *Neural Blockade in Clinical Anesthesia*. Philadelphia: Lippincott-Raven, 1998: 675–713.

20 Chow R, Armati P, Laakso EL, Bjordal JM, Baxter GD. Inhibitory effects of laser irradiation on peripheral mammalian nerves and relevance to analgesic effects: a systematic review. *Photomed Laser Surg* 2011; 29(6): 365–381.

21 Yan W, Chow R, Armati PJ. Inhibitory effects of visible 650-nm and infrared 808-nm laser irradiation on somatosensory and compound muscle action potentials in rat sciatic nerve: implications for laser-induced analgesia. *J Peripher Nerv Syst* 2011; 16(2): 130–135.

22 Laakso E, Cramond T, Richardson C, Galligan J. Plasma ACTH and Beta-endorphin levels in response to low-level laser therapy (LLLT) for myofascial trigger points. *Laser Ther* 1994; 6(3): 133–142.

23 Laakso E, Richardson C, Cramond T. Pain scores and side effects in response to low level laser therapy (LLLT) for myofascial trigger points. *Laser Ther* 1997; 9(2): 67–72.

24 Wakabayashi H, Hamba M, Matsumoto K, Tachibana H. Effect of irradiation by semiconductor laser on responses evoked in trigeminal caudal neurons by tooth pulp stimulation. *Laser Surg Med* 1993; 13(6): 605–610.

25 Nelson A, Friedman M. Somatosensory trigeminal evoked potential amplitudes following low-level laser and sham irradiation over time. *Laser Ther* 2001; 13: 60–64.

26 Chan A, Armati P. Pulsed Nd:YAG laser induces pulpal analgesia: a randomized clinical trial. *J Dent Res* 2012; 91 (7 Suppl): 79S–84S.

27 Kasai S, Kono T, Sakamoto T, Mito M. Effects of low-power laser irradiation on multiple unit discharges induced by noxious stimuli in the anesthetized rabbit. *J Clin Laser Med Surg* 1994; 12(4): 221–224.

28 Mezawa S, Iwata K, Naito K, Kamogawa H. The possible analgesic effect of soft-laser irradiation on heat nociceptors in the cat tongue. *Arch Oral Biol* 1988; 33(9): 693–694.

29 Tsuchiya D, Kawatani M, Takeshige C. Laser irradiation abates neuronal responses to nociceptive stimulation of rat-paw skin. *Brain Res Bull* 1994; 34(4): 369–374.

30 Wesselmann U, Lin S, Rymer W. Effects of Q-switched Nd:YAG laser irradiation on neural impulse propagation: II. *Dorsal Roots and Peripheral Nerves. Physiol Chem Phys Med NMR* 1991; 23: 81–100.

31 Wesselmann U, Kerns J, Rymer W. Laser effects on myelinated and non-myelinated axons in rat peroneal nerve. *Soc Neurosci Abstr* 1992; 18: 134.

32 Sato T, Kawatani M, Takeshige C, Matsumoto I. Ga-Al-As laser irradiation inhibits neuronal activity associated with inflammation. *Acupunct Electrother Res* 1994; 19(2–3): 141–151.

33 Shimoyama N, Iijima K, Shimoyama M, Mizuguchi T. The effects of helium-neon laser on formalin-induced activity of dorsal horn neurons in the rat. *J Clin Laser Med Surg* 1992; 10(2): 91–94.

34 Maeda T. Morphological demonstration of low reactive laser therapeutic pain attenuation effect of the gallium aluminium arsenide diode laser. *Laser Ther* 1989; 1(1): 23–30.

35 Young S, Dyson M, Bolton P. Effect of light on calcium uptake by macrophages. *Laser Ther* 1990; 2: 53–57.

36 Hemvani N, Chitinis DS, Bhagwanai NS. Effect of helium–neon laser on cultured human macrophages. *Laser Ther* 1998; 10(4): 159–164.

37 Richardson JD, Vasko MR. Cellular mechanisms of neurogenic inflammation . *J Pharmacol Exp Ther* 2002; 302(3): 839–845.

38 Hirokawa N, Niwa S, Tanaka Y. Molecular motors in neurons: transport mechanisms and roles in brain function, development, and disease. *Neuron* 2010; 68(4): 610–638.

39 Spudich JA. Biochemistry. Molecular motors, beauty in complexity. *Science* 2011; 331(6021): 1143–1144.

40 Walter WJ, Diez S. Molecular motors: A staggering giant. *Nature* 2012; 482(7383): 44–45.

41 Kudoh C, Inomata K, Okajima K, Motegi M, Ohshiro T. Effects of 830nm Gallium Aluminium Garsenide diode laser radiation on rat saphenous nerve sodium-potassium-adenosine triphosphatase activity: a possible pain attenuation mechanism examined. *Laser Ther* 1989; 1: 63–67.

42 Chow R, David M, Armati P. 830-nm laser irradiation induces varicosity formation, reduces mitochondrial membrane potential and blocks fast axonal flow in small and medium diameter rat dorsal root ganglion neurons: implications for the analgesic effects of 830-nm laser. *J Peripher Nerv Syst* 2007; 12(1): 28–39.

43 Chen M, Shimada K, Fujita K, Ishii J, Hirata T, Fujisawa H. Neurite elongation from cultured dorsal root ganglia is inhibited by Ga-Al-As diode laser irradiation. *Laser Life Sci* 1993; 5(4): 237–242.

44 Wesselmann U, Kerns J, Rymer W. Laser effects in myelinated and nonmyelinated fibres in the rat peroneal nerve: a quantitative ultrastructural analysis. *Exp Neurol* 1994; 129(2): 257–265.

45 Poste G, Papahadjopoulos D, Nicholson G. Local anaesthetics affect transmembrane cytoskeletal control of mobility and distribution of cell surface receptors. *Proc Natl Acad Sci USA* 1975; 72: 4430–4434.

46 Nicolson G, Smith JR, Poste G. Effects of local anaesthetics on cell morphology and membrane-associated cytoskeletal organization in BALB3/3T3. *J Cell Biol* 1976; 68: 395–402.

47 Legrain V, Iannetti GD, Plaghki L, Mouraux A. The pain matrix reloaded: a salience detection system for the body. *Prog Neurobiol* 2011; 93(1): 111–124.

48 Iannetti GD, Mouraux A. From the neuromatrix to the pain matrix (and back). *Exp Brain Res* 2010; 205(1): 1–12.

49 Siddall PJ, Cousins MJ. Persistent pain as a disease entity: implications for clinical management. *Anesth Analg* 2004; 99(2): 510–520.

50 Jimbo K, Noda K, Suzuki H, Yoda K. Suppressive effects of low-power laser irradiation on bradykinin evoked action potentials in cultured murine dorsal root ganglia cells. *Neurosci Lett* 1998; 240(2): 93–96.

51 Kono T, Kasai S, Sakamoto T, Mito M. Cord dorsum potentials suppressed by low power laser irradiation on a peripheral nerve in the cat. *J Clin Laser Med Surg* 1993; 11(3): 115–118.

52 Navratil L, Dylevsky I. Mechanisms of the analgesic effect of therapeutic lasers in vivo. *Laser Ther* 1997; 9(1): 33–39.

53 Walker J. Relief from chronic pain by low power laser irradiation. *Neurosci Lett* 1983; 43(2–3): 339–344.

54 Ceylan Y, Hizmetli S, Silig Y. The effects of infrared laser and medical treatments on pain and serotonin degradation products in patients with myofascial pain syndrome. *A controlled trial. Rheumatol Int* 2004; 24(5): 260–263.

55 Peres e Serra A, Ashmawi HA. Influence of naloxone and methysergide on the analgesic effects of low-level laser in an experimental pain model. *Revista Brasileira Anestesiol* 2010; 60(3): 302–310.

56 Lievens PC. The effect of a combined HeNe and I.R. laser treatment on the regeneration of the lymphatic system during the process of wound healing. *Lasers Med Sci* 1991; 6(193): 193–199.

57 Carati CJ, Anderson SN, Gannon BJ, Piller NB. Treatment of post-mastectomy lymphedema with low-level laser therapy: a double-blind, placebo-controlled trial. *Cancer* 2003; 98(6): 1114–1122.

58 Nicolau R, Martinez M, Rigau J, Tomas J. Neurotransmitter release changes induced by low power 830nm diode laser irradiation on the neuromuscular junction. *Lasers Surg Med* 2004; 35(3): 236–241.

59 Nicolau RA, Martinez MS, Rigau J, Tomas J. Effect of low power 655nm diode laser irradiation on the neuromuscular junctions of the mouse diaphragm. *Lasers Surg Med* 2004; 34(3): 277–284.

60 Snyder-Mackler L, Bork C, Bourbon B. Effects of helium-neon laser on musculoskeletal trigger points. *Physical Ther* 1986; 68: 223–225.

61 Waylonis G, Wilke S, O'Toole D, Waylonis D, Waylonis D. Chronic myofascial pain: management by low-output helium-neon laser therapy. *Arch Physical Med Rehab* 1988; 69: 1017–1020.

62 Snyder-Mackler L, Barry A, Perkins A, Soucek M. Effects of helium-neon laser irradiation on skin resistance and pain with trigger points in the neck and back. *Physical Ther* 1989; 69: 336–341.

63 Carrasco TG, Guerisoli LD, Guerisoli DM, Mazzetto MO. Evaluation of low intensity laser therapy in myofascial pain syndrome. *Cranio* 2009; 27(4): 243–247.

64 Airaksinen O, Rantanen P, Pertti K, Pontinen P. Effects of the infrared laser therapy at treated and non-treated trigger points. *Acupunct Electro-ther Res Int J* 1989; 14: 9–14.

65 International Association for the Study of Pain (IASP). Global Year against Musculoskeletal Pain October 2009 - October 2010 Myofascial Pain. IASP, 2009. Available from: http://www.iasp-pain.org/Content/NavigationMenu/GlobalYearAgainstCancerPain/20092010MusculoskeletalPain/FactSheets/default.htm [accessed 4 April 2010].

CHAPTER 7

Antimicrobial photodynamic therapy in dentistry

Felipe F. Sperandio,[1,2,3] **Caetano P. Sabino,**[3,4] **Daniela Vecchio,**[2,3] **Maria Garcia-Diaz,**[3,5] **Liyi Huang,**[2,3,6] **Ying-Ying Huang,**[2,3,7] **and Michael R. Hamblin**[2,3,8]

[1] Department of Pathology and Parasitology, Institute of Biomedical Sciences, Federal University of Alfenas, Alfenas, MG, Brazil
[2] Department of Dermatology, Harvard Medical School, Boston, MA, USA
[3] Wellman Center for Photomedicine, Massachusetts General Hospital, Boston, MA, USA
[4] Center for Lasers and Applications, IPEN-CNEN/SP, São Paulo, SP, Brazil
[5] Molecular Engineering Group, IQS School of Engineering, University of Ramon Llull, Barcelona, Spain
[6] Department of Infectious Diseases, First Affiliated College & Hospital, Guangxi Medical University, Nanning, China
[7] Aesthetic and Plastic Center of Guangxi Medical University, Nanning, China
[8] Harvard–MIT Division of Health Sciences and Technology, Cambridge, MA, USA

Introduction

Antimicrobial photodynamic therapy (aPDT), also known as photodynamic inactivation (PDI), photoactivated disinfection (PAD) or photodynamic antimicrobial chemotherapy (PACT), involves the administration of a photoactive dye or photosensitizer (PS) that is able to produce reactive oxygen species (ROS) upon irradiation with light of the correct wavelength to be absorbed by the PS. Studies on the use of PDT for treatment of oral and dental infections are increasing in number. The particular features of this non-invasive method and the increased antibiotic resistance amongst many species of pathogenic bacteria suggest PDT as an alternative or an adjunctive treatment to chemical agents in order to eliminate the bacteria in oral infections such as periodontitis and peri-implantitis.

When the PS absorbs a photon, an electron is promoted from the ground state to an electronically-excited singlet state that can transition to a long-lived triplet state that can then undergo electron transfer with oxygen (type I reaction) generating superoxide and hydroxyl radicals; or can transfer energy to molecular oxygen to produce highly cytotoxic singlet oxygen (type II reaction) (Fig. 7.2)[1,2] Both mechanisms can lead to the photooxidation of certain amino acids, pyrimidine and purine bases of DNA/RNA, and unsaturated lipids, leading to DNA damage and/or damage to the cytoplasmic membrane allowing leakage of cellular contents or inactivation of membrane transport systems.[3]

A good PS for antimicrobial PDT should be endowed with specific features in addition to the expected photophysical properties: (1) extensive killing of disease-inducing microbial cells with no damage to the host tissue, (2) prevention of regrowth of pathogens after treatment, and (3) high affinity for the broadest possible range of microbial agents: bacteria, fungi, viruses, and parasites.[3] Moreover, the PS should have a long-lived triplet state, a high quantum yield of ROS generation, and a high extinction coefficient mainly in the red and far red region where light transmission through tissue is maximal.[3,4] Nevertheless, for the treatment of superficial infections, the absorption of blue light (400–420 nm) is useful.

Photosensitizers

The optimal structures of PS for killing various classes of pathogenic microorganisms has been studied in some detail.[5] The structure of the cell walls of different classes of microbial cells is shown in Fig. 7.1.[2] Gram-positive bacteria and fungal cells have a single plasma membrane surrounded by a relatively porous coating composed of peptidoglycan or beta-glucan, respectively. Gram-negative bacteria have a double membrane structure that is a more effective permeability barrier. However, all microorganisms have an overall anionic charge on the cell surface that is more pronounced than that found on host mammalian cells. Therefore, considering the wide range of PS that have commonly been used in antimicrobial PDT, the most important structural feature is the presence of at least one, and preferably more than one, cationic charge.[2] The positive charge on PS allows the molecules to bind to and, when illuminated, inactivate all classes of microorganisms: Gram-positive and Gram-negative bacteria, viruses, fungi, and other parasites, thus exhibiting a broad-spectrum antimicrobial effect. Phenothiazinium dyes,[6–8] phthalocyanines,[9] natural PS such as curcumin,[10] and a conjugate between chlorin e6 and polyethylenimine[11,12] have been used for oral and dental infections (see Fig. 7.3 for chemical structures[2,13–18]). Methylene blue (MB;

Lasers in Dentistry: Guide for Clinical Practice, First Edition. Edited by Patrícia M. de Freitas and Alyne Simões.
© 2015 John Wiley & Sons, Inc. Published 2015 by John Wiley & Sons, Inc.

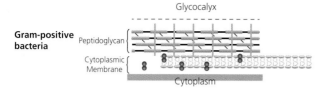

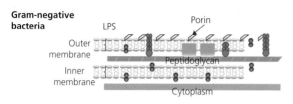

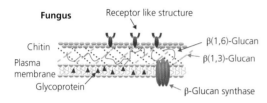

Figure 7.1 Structures of the cell walls of three different classes of microbial pathogens. (a) Gram-positive bacterium showing porous layer of peptidoglycan and single lipid bilayer; (b) Gram-negative bacterium showing double lipid bilayer sandwiching the peptidoglycan layer and an outer layer of lipopolysaccharide; (c) fungal cell with a less porous layer of beta-glucan and chitin surrounding a single lipid bilayer. LPS, lipopolysaccharide (adapted from references[1,2]).

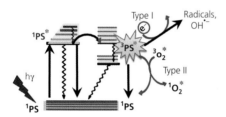

Figure 7.2 Schematic of the mechanism of antimicrobial PDT. Type I and Type II photochemical mechanisms operate from photosensitizer (PS) triplet state producing reactive oxygen species (ROS) that are able to destroy all known microorganisms (adapted from reference[2]).

Ondine Biopharma, Canada) has been approved as a potent PDT drug for local treatment of periodontal diseases because of its relatively low toxicity and high singlet oxygen generation. Toluidine blue O (TBO; (Denfotex, UK and HELBO Photodynamic Systems, Austria) is used as an adjunct in the diagnosis of oral cancer and when photoactivated is also indicated for periodontitis, endodontic infections, and caries.

Periodontitis

The presence of microorganisms on the dental surfaces is one of the predisposing factors for the development of oral diseases. Mechanical removal of biofilm combined with antibiotics is the current standard treatment for periodontitis; however, the

limitations of manual curettage or ultrasound have been shown in areas that are difficult to access, such as bifurcations and concavities. Likewise, the rapid emergence of antibiotic resistance among pathogenic bacteria has led to a growing interest in finding alternatives to antimicrobial therapy.[19]

Treatment of all periodontal diseases involves mechanical cleaning of tooth surfaces to remove mineralized and non-mineralized bacterial deposits (calculus and plaque),[20] and leads to irreversible hard tissue damage[21–24] and gingival recession[25,26] as adverse effects. In addition, hard tissue loss may cause increased sensitivity of treated teeth to evaporative, tactile, thermal, and osmotic stimuli.[27–33]

Therefore, many studies have been performed to evaluate the clinical and antimicrobial effects of PDT and to compare it with conventional therapy in animal and human models of dental infections. Studies on the use of PDT in different models of peri-implantitis demonstrated a decrease in different bacterial strains. A significant reduction of *Aggregatibacter actinomycetemcomitans*, *Porphyromonas gingivalis*, and *Prevotella intermedia* after treatment with TBO-mediated PDT has been reported,[34] Two other studies[35,36] in a dog model for peri-implantitis reported that PDT was able to reduce bacterial counts. In the first, *Prevotella* spp, *Fusobacterium* spp, and *Streptococcus betahaemolyticus* were not 100% destroyed in all samples.[35] Similarly, in the second study a 99.8% reduction of *Prevotella* was shown.[36]

Significant results were obtained also in non-surgical treatment of periodontitis in *in vivo* models[37–40] and many PS have been tested. The use of toluidine blue-mediated PDT showed a significant reduction of *P. gingivalis* in an *in vivo* model.[39] A significant reduction in *P. gingivalis* infected sites was observed using PDT with chlorin e6 in a beagle dog model. In the same study, BLC1010 was shown not to suppress bacteria.[38] Recently, Bottura et al. demonstrated the effect of PDT on reducing bone loss caused by experimental periodontitis in immunosuppressed rats.[41] The results of this study were in agreement with the literature demonstrating the effectiveness of PDT in the treatment of periodontal disease.[42–44] In one further study,[45] the effect of PDT was evaluated on inflammatory cells. These findings demonstrated that the treatment of chronic periodontitis by PDT led to a specific decrease of antigen-presenting cell populations according to the drug delivery system.

The incomplete eradication of biofilm microorganisms observed in periodontal diseases could be due to restricted penetration of the PS in oral biofilms[46] or the ability of bacterial cells to expel PS via multidrug resistance pumps.[47] In a recent study,[48] the effect of PDT on human dental plaque bacteria was investigated *in vitro* using poly(lactic-co-glycolic) (PLGA) nanoparticles as carriers of MB. The results suggested that PLGA nanoparticles have the potential to be used as nanocarriers of MB, to increase diffusion into biofilms, and to help release the encapsulated drug in active form. They showed a greater PDT bacterial killing, but more studies are necessary to define the physical characteristics of the nanoparticles.[48]

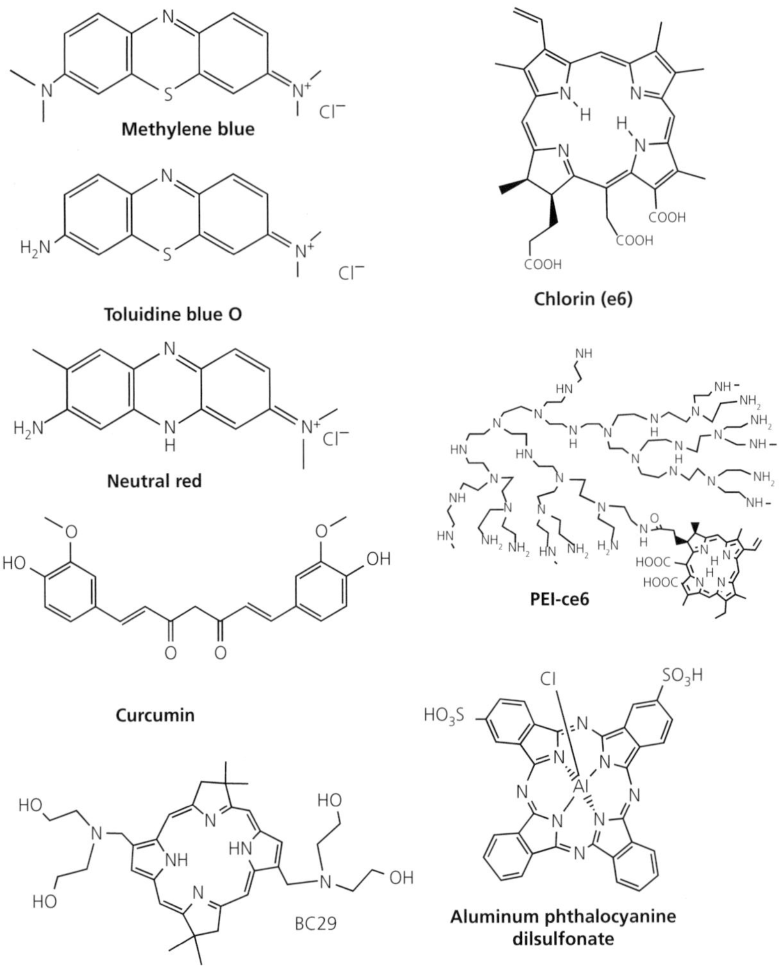

Methylene blue

Toluidine blue O

Neutral red

Curcumin

Chlorin (e6)

PEI-ce6

BC29

Aluminum phthalocyanine dilsulfonate

Figure 7.3 Chemical structures of photosensitizers used in antimicrobial PDT for dental and oral infections. Methylene blue (MB), toluidine blue O (TBO), neutral red, curcumin, chlorin e6, conjugate between polyethylenimine and chlorin e6 (PEI-ce6), chloroaluminum phthalocyanine disulfonate (ClAlPCS2), and basic bacteriochlorin (BC29). (adapted from references[2,13–18]).

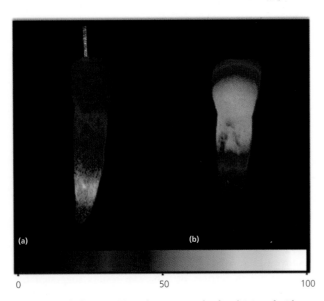

Figure 7.4 Endodontic PDT involves root canals of teeth injected with photosensitizer and then irradiated with fiber. (a) Diffusing tip inserted into root canal. (b) Laser tip at the entrance to the instrumented canal. Normalized scale where 0 is under the charge-coupled device (CCD) threshold and 100 is saturation.

Endodontic therapy

The complex anatomy of the root canal system with isthmuses, anastomoses, re-entrances, and dentin tubules allows micro-organisms to remain in these structures and to compromise the outcome of root canal treatment.[49,50] For endodontic treatment to succeed, intracanal bacterial populations and their products need to be eliminated[49] and PDT has shown encouraging results for significant bacterial reduction in the root canal system.[8,51–53]

The use of PDT to treat endodontic infections caused by bacterial biofilms has been studied in *ex vivo*-extracted teeth as a laboratory model. *Enterococcus faecalis* is the pathogen most commonly associated with current endodontic infections[54] and several studies have been carried out to evaluate the effect of toluidine blue[55,56] and methylene blue[56–58] with PDT in endodontic treatment. As an important aspect, endodontic light delivery is superior when delivered by a diffusing fiber as compared to flat tip fiber being able to produce optimized microbicidal results (Fig. 7.4).[59]

The use of a conjugate between polyethylenimine and chlorin e6 and 660-nm diode laser light delivered into the root canal via a 200 μm fiber was evaluated, both compared with and combined with standard endodontic treatment. In this study, Garcez et al.[60]

used PDT to kill Gram-negative (*Pseudomonas aeruginosa* and *Proteus mirabilis*) bacteria growing as biofilms in root canals of extracted teeth. Gram-negative bacteria are harder to kill than Gram-positive species. The combined therapies reduced the bacterial charge and interestingly, the bacterial regrowth observed 24 hours after treatment was much lower.

Viral lesions

Another possible application of PDT related to oral infections is treatment of recurrent *Herpes labialis* (RHL).[61,62] Better explained in Chapter 35 of this book, RHL is a recurrent herpes simplex virus (HSV-1) infection[63,64] and has a well-known clinical course that begins with prodromal signs or symptoms, such as burning or swelling, leading to the development of vesicles and further ulceration and crusting within 72–96 hours.[65] Although antiviral compounds such as acyclovir or valacyclovir are widely prescribed for the management of RHL, the intermittent administration of acyclovir can promote drug resistance and only provides a good response if applied before the onset of the vesicles.[66–68]

The outcome of the vesicle states of the disease was better for RHL patients who received treatment with PDT combined with low level laser therapy (LLLT) compared to ordinary treatments involving antiviral compounds.[69] Recent studies compared the use of high power laser or MB-mediated PDT in combination with LLLT. The results suggested that both treatments, in combination with LLLT, may be beneficial when treating herpes.[70]

In fact, many clinical studies on infectious diseases have tested PDT to treat herpes simplex lesions. Herpes keratitis was healed by proflavine photodynamic viral inactivation,[71] and the topical application of methylene blue and neutral red eradicated genital herpes but could not prevent its recurrence.[72] In other studies, photoinactivation of herpes virus with neutral red was found to be ineffective.[73,74]

Oral candidiasis and fungal infections

Many PS have been employed to kill fungal cells such as *Candida*. The PS needs to enter the fungal cell to be effective, unlike for bacterial cells where the PS may only need to bind to the cell membrane. Figure 7.5 shows confocal microscopy images of a basic bacteriochlorin (BC29, see Fig. 7.3) emitting red fluorescence inside *Candida albicans* cells whose nucleus has a green autofluorescence.

The effectiveness of PDT has also been evaluated in the inactivation of *C. albicans* in oral candidiasis. Recently, Mima *et al.* evaluated the efficacy of using hematoporphyrin with PDT in an animal model of oral candidiasis.[75] In this study, candidiasis was verified by the presence of white patches or pseudomembranes on the dorsal tongue associated with a significant number of colony forming units (CFU)/mL of *C. albicans*, and PDT significantly reduced the viability of *C. albicans*.

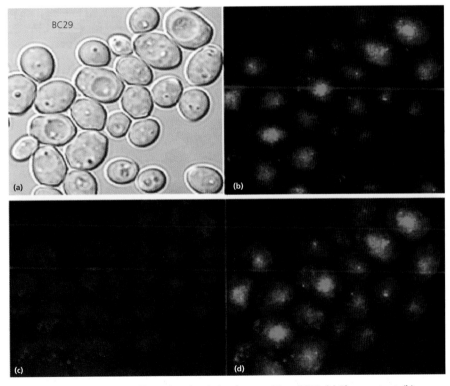

Figure 7.5 Confocal microscopy of *Candida albicans* cells incubated with the photosensitizer, BC29. (a) Phase contrast, (b) green autofluorescence, (c) red BC29 fluorescence, (d) overlay of red and green.

An earlier study described the dose-dependent photoeradication of *C. albicans* in an immunodeficient murine model.[76] In this study, Teichert et al. evaluated the efficacy of using MB-mediated PDT to treat oral candidiasis in an immunosuppressed mouse model, mimicking what is found in human patients. The results indicated a MB-dependent effect of PDT, and complete eradication of bacteria from the oral cavity was achieved when 450–500 μg/mL of MB was used.

Caries

Classified as pandemic by the World Health Organization, caries disease is among the most common pathologies in humans. It is a multifactorial condition resulting from several possible interactions between the host and the oral microflora. A pH imbalance (acid) is generally caused by the fermentation of metabolites of bacterial species (mainly streptococci and lactobacilli) organized as consortiums in a biofilm structure on the tooth surface. This acid production increases the solubility of hydroxyapatite in the tooth dentin, enabling microbial infiltration into the dentin and promoting deeper lesions, further demineralization, and pulpal infection.[77,78]

The change in emphasis towards minimally invasive procedures in modern dentistry places antimicrobial PDT in a promising position. The ability of PDT mediated by phenothiazinum dyes (commonly TBO and MB) to efficiently kill bacteria in cariogenic biofilms[79,80] existing on enamel surfaces and in infected dentin structures,[81–83] even if located in hard to reach regions such as bifurcations and fissures, turns this technique into a unique tool. Furthermore, the possibility of enabling the remineralization of affected tissues through a biological or therapeutic approach is currently a promising strategy in dentistry, reducing drastically the invasiveness of traditional restorative treatments.[78,84,85]

Baptista et al.[81] studied the treatment with MB-mediated PDT of rats with incipient caries induced by feeding them with *S. mutans*-infected food and water enriched with high concentrations of sucrose. Microbiological and optical coherence tomography (OCT) data collected from experimental animals' molars showed effective decrease of microbial burden and arrest of demineralization without any further mechanical or chemical procedures.

Multi-species biofilms cultured on dentin slabs maintained inside the oral cavity of human volunteers for 7 days and irrigated by sucrose solution 10 times a day were studied to determine the effectiveness of PDT on common caries-associated microorganisms.[83] Statistically relevant bacterial reduction was measured for the entire treated microbiota, including all streptococci and lactobacilli species employing TBO solution combined with red LED irradiation.

Antimicrobial PDT has also been employed combined with traditional restorative treatments in order to preserve the pulpal integrity by decreasing the volume of removed dentin once affected tissues are encouraged to remineralize after microbial reduction. Guglielmi et al.[82] demonstrated a general microbial reduction in carious dentin at the pulpal wall after performing PDT for deep carious lesions in molar cavities, suggesting a significant increase in the treatment success rate and decrease in its invasiveness.

Conclusion

The rapid introduction and growing acceptance of antimicrobial PDT for the treatment of periodontitis can be considered a good omen for its application in other dental infections.[86] Part of the problem with introducing new therapies into clinical practice is overcoming the relatively conservative assessment that clinicians frequently adopt towards cutting-edge techniques. Furthermore, PDT may be considered too complicated, requiring both the application of a dye and the use of a separate light source. The growing number of papers on PDT for periodontitis appearing not only in the general dental journals but also in the popular scientific press will bring it to the attention of both dentists and patients alike, and the latter will begin to specifically request the therapy by name.

Acknowledgments

Research in the Hamblin Laboratory is funded by NIH grants (R01A1050875 and R01CA/AI838801to MRH; R01CA137108 to Long Y. Chiang), US Air Force MFEL Program (FA9550-04-1-0079), Center for Integration of Medicine and Innovative Technology (DAMD17-02-2-0006), and CDMRP Program in TBI (W81XWH-09-1-0514). FFS was supported by the CAPES Foundation, Ministry of Education of Brazil, Brasília, DF 70040-020, Brazil and FAPESP Foundation, Brazil.

References

1 Mroz P. *Advances in photodynamic therapy: basic, translational and clinical.* Norwood, MA: Artech House; 2008.

2 Sharma SK, Dai T, Kharkwal GB, et al. Drug discovery of antimicrobial photosensitizers using animal models. *Curr Pharm Des* 2011; 17: 1303–1319.

3 Hamblin MR, Hasan T. Photodynamic therapy: a new antimicrobial approach to infectious disease? *Photochem Photobiol Sci* 2004; 3: 436–450.

4 Jori G, Fabris C, Soncin M, et al. Photodynamic therapy in the treatment of microbial infections: basic principles and perspective applications. *Lasers Surg Med* 2006; 38: 468–481.

5 Sharma SK, Dai T, Kharkwal GB, et al. Drug discovery of antimicrobial photosensitizers using animal models. *Curr Pharm Des* 2011; 17: 1303–1319.

6 Fonseca MB, Junior PO, Pallota RC, et al. Photodynamic therapy for root canals infected with *Enterococcus faecalis*. *Photomed Laser Surg* 2008; 26: 209–213.

7 Schlafer S, Vaeth M, Horsted-Bindslev P, Frandsen EV. Endodontic photoactivated disinfection using a conventional light source: an in vitro and ex vivo study. *Oral Surg Oral Med Oral Pathol Oral Radiol Endod* 2010; 109: 634–641.

8 Soukos NS, Chen PS, Morris JT, et al. Photodynamic therapy for endodontic disinfection. *J Endod* 2006; 32: 979–984.

9 Wilson M, Burns T, Pratten J. Killing of *Streptococcus sanguis* in biofilms using a light-activated antimicrobial agent. *J Antimicrob Chemother* 1996; 37: 377–381.

10 Araujo NC, Fontana CR, Gerbi ME, Bagnato VS. Overall-mouth disinfection by photodynamic therapy using curcumin. *Photomed Laser Surg* 2012; 30: 96–101.

11 Garcez AS, Nunez SC, Hamblin MR, Ribeiro MS. Antimicrobial effects of photodynamic therapy on patients with necrotic pulps and periapical lesion. *J Endod* 2008; 34: 138–142.

12 Huang L, Zhiyentayev T, Xuan Y, Azhibek D, Kharkwal GB, Hamblin MR. Photodynamic inactivation of bacteria using polyethylenimine-chlorin(e6) conjugates: Effect of polymer molecular weight, substitution ratio of chlorin(e6) and pH. *Lasers Surg Med* 2011; 43: 313–323.

13 Alam S, Panda JJ, Chauhan VS. Novel dipeptide nanoparticles for effective curcumin delivery. *Int J Nanomed* 2012; 7: 4207–422.

14 Dai T, Fuchs BB, Coleman JJ, et al. Concepts and principles of photodynamic therapy as an alternative antifungal discovery platform. *Front Microbiol* 2012; 3: 120.

15 Huang L, Huang YY, Mroz P, et al. Stable synthetic cationic bacteriochlorins as selective antimicrobial photosensitizers. *Antimicrob Agents Chemother* 2010; 54: 3834–3841.

16 Li P, Zhou G, Zhu X, et al. Photodynamic therapy with hyperbranched poly(ether-ester) chlorin(e6) nanoparticles on human tongue carcinoma CAL-27 cells. *Photodiagnosis Photodyn Ther* 2012; 9: 76–82.

17 Norum OJ, Selbo PK, Weyergang A, Giercksky KE, Berg K. Photochemical internalization (PCI) in cancer therapy: from bench towards bedside medicine. *J Photochem Photobiol B Biol* 2009; 96: 83–92.

18 Rauf MA, Soliman AA, Khattab M. *Solvent effect on the spectral properties of Neutral Red Chem Cent J* 2008; 2: 19.

19 Harrison JW, Svec TA. The beginning of the end of the antibiotic era? Part II. Proposed solutions to antibiotic abuse. *Quintessence Int* 1998; 29: 223–229.

20 Giannopoulou C, Cappuyns I, Cancela J, Cionca N, Mombelli A. Effect of photodynamic therapy, diode laser and deep scaling on cytokine and acute-phase protein levels in gingival crevicular fluid of residual periodontal pockets. *J Periodontol* 2012; 83: 1018–1027.

21 Kocher T, Fanghanel J, Sawaf H, Litz R. Substance loss caused by scaling with different sonic scaler inserts--an in vitro study. *J Clin Periodontol* 2001; 28: 9–15.

22 Flemmig TF, Petersilka GJ, Mehl A, Hickel R, Klaiber B. The effect of working parameters on root substance removal using a piezoelectric ultrasonic scaler in vitro. *J Clin Periodontol* 1998; 25: 158–163.

23 Ritz L, Hefti AF, Rateitschak KH. An in vitro investigation on the loss of root substance in scaling with various instruments. *J Clin Periodontol* 1991; 18: 643–647.

24 Zappa U, Smith B, Simona C, Graf H, Case D, Kim W. Root substance removal by scaling and root planing. *J Periodontol* 1991; 62: 750–754.

25 Badersten A, Nilveus R, Egelberg J. Effect of nonsurgical periodontal therapy. I. Moderately advanced periodontitis. *J Clin Periodontol* 1981; 8: 57–72.

26 Badersten A, Nilveus R, Egelberg J. Effect of nonsurgical periodontal therapy. II. Severely advanced periodontitis. *J Clin Periodontol* 1984; 11: 63–76.

27 Chabanski MB, Gillam DG. Aetiology, prevalence and clinical features of cervical dentine sensitivity. *J Oral Rehabil* 1997; 24: 15–19.

28 Fischer C, Fischer RG, Wennberg A. Prevalence and distribution of cervical dentine hypersensitivity in a population in Rio de Janeiro, Brazil. *J Dent* 1992; 20: 272–276.

29 Fischer C, Wennberg A, Fischer RG, Attstrom R. Clinical evaluation of pulp and dentine sensitivity after supragingival and subgingival scaling. *Endod Dent Traumatol* 1991; 7: 259–265.

30 Kerns DG, Scheidt MJ, Pashley DH, Horner JA, Strong SL, Van Dyke TE. Dentinal tubule occlusion and root hypersensitivity. *J Periodontol* 1991; 62: 421–428.

31 Orchardson R, Gangarosa LP, Sr., Holland GR, et al. Dentine hypersensitivity-into the 21st century. *Arch Oral Biol* 1994; 39 (Suppl): 113S-119S.

32 Tammaro S, Wennstrom JL, Bergenholtz G. Root-dentin sensitivity following non-surgical periodontal treatment. *J Clin Periodontol* 2000; 27: 690–697.

33 von Troil B, Needleman I, Sanz M. A systematic review of the prevalence of root sensitivity following periodontal therapy. *J Clin Periodontol* 2002; 29 (Suppl 3): 173–177; discussion 95–96.

34 Dortbudak O, Haas R, Bernhart T, Mailath-Pokorny G. Lethal photosensitization for decontamination of implant surfaces in the treatment of peri-implantitis. *Clin Oral Implants Res* 2001; 12: 104–108.

35 Shibli JA, Martins MC, Theodoro LH, Lotufo RF, Garcia VG, Marcantonio EJ. Lethal photosensitization in microbiological treatment of ligature-induced peri-implantitis: a preliminary study in dogs. *J Oral Sci* 2003; 45: 17–23.

36 Hayek RR, Araujo NS, Gioso MA, et al. Comparative study between the effects of photodynamic therapy and conventional therapy on microbial reduction in ligature-induced peri-implantitis in dogs. *J Periodontol* 2005; 76: 1275–1281.

37 de Oliveira RR, Schwartz-Filho HO, Novaes AB, Jr., Taba M, Jr. Antimicrobial photodynamic therapy in the non-surgical treatment of aggressive periodontitis: a preliminary randomized controlled clinical study. *J Periodontol* 2007; 78: 965–973.

38 Sigusch BW, Pfitzner A, Albrecht V, Glockmann E. Efficacy of photodynamic therapy on inflammatory signs and two selected periodontopathogenic species in a beagle dog model. *J Periodontol* 2005; 76: 1100–1105.

39 Komerik N, Nakanishi H, MacRobert AJ, Henderson B, Speight P, Wilson M. In vivo killing of *Porphyromonas gingivalis* by toluidine blue-mediated photosensitization in an animal model. *Antimicrob Agents Chemother* 2003; 47: 932–940.

40 Malik Z, Hanania J, Nitzan Y. Bactericidal effects of photoactivated porphyrins--an alternative approach to antimicrobial drugs. *J Photochem Photobiol B* 1990; 5: 281–293.

41 Bottura PE, Milanezi J, Fernandes LA, et al. Nonsurgical periodontal therapy combined with laser and photodynamic therapies for periodontal disease in immunosuppressed rats. *Transplant Proc* 2011; 43: 2009–2016.

42 Fernandes LA, de Almeida JM, Theodoro LH, et al. Treatment of experimental periodontal disease by photodynamic therapy in immunosuppressed rats. *J Clin Periodontol* 2009; 36: 219–228.

43 de Almeida JM, Theodoro LH, Bosco AF, Nagata MJ, Bonfante S, Garcia VG. Treatment of experimental periodontal disease by

photodynamic therapy in rats with diabetes. *J Periodontol* 2008; 79: 2156–2165.

44 de Almeida JM, Theodoro LH, Bosco AF, Nagata MJ, Oshiiwa M, Garcia VG. Influence of photodynamic therapy on the development of ligature-induced periodontitis in rats. *J Periodontol* 2007; 78: 566–575.

45 Seguier S, Souza SL, Sverzut AC, et al. Impact of photodynamic therapy on inflammatory cells during human chronic periodontitis. *J Photochem Photobiol B* 2010; 101: 348–354.

46 Ogura Y, Ooka T, Asadulghani M, et al. Extensive genomic diversity and selective conservation of virulence-determinants in enterohemorrhagic *Escherichia coli* strains of O157 and non-O157 serotypes. *Genome Biol* 2007; 8: R138.

47 Tegos GP, Masago K, Aziz F, Higginbotham A, Stermitz FR, Hamblin MR. Inhibitors of bacterial multidrug efflux pumps potentiate antimicrobial photoinactivation. *Antimicrob Agents Chemother* 2008; 52: 3202–3209.

48 Klepac-Ceraj V, Patel N, Song X, et al. Photodynamic effects of methylene blue-loaded polymeric nanoparticles on dental plaque bacteria. *Lasers Surg Med* 2011; 43: 600–606.

49 Nunes MR, Mello I, Franco GC, et al. Effectiveness of photodynamic therapy against *Enterococcus faecalis*, with and without the use of an intracanal optical fiber: an in vitro study. *Photomed Laser Surg* 2011; 29: 803–808.

50 Siqueira JF, Jr., Araujo MC, Garcia PF, Fraga RC, Dantas CJ. Histological evaluation of the effectiveness of five instrumentation techniques for cleaning the apical third of root canals. *J Endod* 1997; 23: 499–502.

51 Seal GJ, Ng YL, Spratt D, Bhatti M, Gulabivala K. An in vitro comparison of the bactericidal efficacy of lethal photosensitization or sodium hyphochlorite irrigation on *Streptococcus intermedius* biofilms in root canals. *Int Endod J* 2002; 35: 268–274.

52 Bonsor SJ, Nichol R, Reid TM, Pearson GJ. Microbiological evaluation of photo-activated disinfection in endodontics (an in vivo study). *Br Dent J* 2006; 200: 337–341, discussion 29.

53 Williams JA, Pearson GJ, Colles MJ. Antibacterial action of photo-activated disinfection {PAD} used on endodontic bacteria in planktonic suspension and in artificial and human root canals. *J Dent* 2006; 34: 363–371.

54 Rocas IN, Siqueira JF, Jr., Santos KR. Association of *Enterococcus faecalis* with different forms of periradicular diseases. *J Endod* 2004; 30: 315–320.

55 Fonseca MB, Junior PO, Pallota RC, et al. Photodynamic therapy for root canals infected with *Enterococcus faecalis*. *Photomed Laser Surg* 2008; 26: 209–213.

56 Souza LC, Brito PR, de Oliveira JC, et al. Photodynamic therapy with two different photosensitizers as a supplement to instrumentation/irrigation procedures in promoting intracanal reduction of Enterococcus faecalis. *J Endod* 2010; 36: 292–296.

57 Ng R, Singh F, Papamanou DA, et al. Endodontic photodynamic therapy ex vivo. *J Endod* 2011; 37: 217–222.

58 Soukos NS, Chen PS, Morris JT, et al. Photodynamic therapy for endodontic disinfection. *J Endod* 2006; 32: 979–984.

59 Garcez AS1, Fregnani ER, Rodriguez HM, et al. The use of optical fiber in endodontic photodynamic therapy. Is it really relevant? *Lasers Med Sci* 2013; 28(1): 79–85.

60 Garcez AS, Ribeiro MS, Tegos GP, Nunez SC, Jorge AO, Hamblin MR. Antimicrobial photodynamic therapy combined with conventional endodontic treatment to eliminate root canal biofilm infection. *Lasers Surg Med* 2007; 39: 59–66.

61 Marotti J, Sperandio FF, Fregnani ER, Aranha AC, de Freitas PM, Eduardo Cde P. High-intensity laser and photodynamic therapy as a treatment for recurrent herpes labialis. *Photomed Laser Surg* 2010; 28: 439–444.

62 Sperandio FF, Marotti J, Aranha AC, Eduardo Cde P. Photodynamic therapy for the treatment of recurrent herpes labialis: preliminary results. *Gen Dent* 2009; 57: 415–419.

63 Embil JA, Stephens RG, Manuel FR. Prevalence of recurrent herpes labialis and aphthous ulcers among young adults on six continents. *Can Med Assoc J* 1975; 113: 627–630.

64 Young SK, Rowe NH, Buchanan RA. A clinical study for the control of facial mucocutaneous herpes virus infections. I. Characterization of natural history in a professional school population. *Oral Surg Oral Med Oral Pathol* 1976; 41: 498–507.

65 Woo SB, Challacombe SJ. Management of recurrent oral herpes simplex infections. *Oral Surg Oral Med Oral Pathol Oral Radiol Endod* 2007; 103 (Suppl:S12): e1–8.

66 Raborn GW, Grace MG. Recurrent herpes simplex labialis: selected therapeutic options. *J Can Dent Assoc* 2003; 69: 498–503.

67 Spruance SL, Overall JC, Jr., Kern ER, Krueger GG, Pliam V, Miller W. The natural history of recurrent herpes simplex labialis: implications for antiviral therapy. *N Engl J Med* 1977; 297: 69–75.

68 Spruance SL, Nett R, Marbury T, Wolff R, Johnson J, Spaulding T. Acyclovir cream for treatment of herpes simplex labialis: results of two randomized, double-blind, vehicle-controlled, multicenter clinical trials. *Antimicrob Agents Chemother* 2002; 46: 2238–2243.

69 Sperandio FF, Marotti J, Aranha AC, Eduardo Cde P. Photodynamic therapy for the treatment of recurrent herpes labialis: Preliminary results. *Gen Dent* 2009; 57: 415–419.

70 Marotti J, Sperandio FF, Fregnani ER, Aranha AC, de Freitas PM, Eduardo C de P. High-intensity laser and photodynamic therapy as a treatment for recurrent herpes labialis. *Photomed Laser Surg* 2010; 28: 439–444.

71 Moore C, Wallis C, Melnick JL, Kuns MD. Photodynamic treatment of herpes keratitis. *Infect Immun* 1972; 5: 169171.

72 Chang TW, Fiumara N, Weinstein L. Genital herpes: Treatment with methylene blue and light exposure. *Int J Dermatol* 1975; 14: 69–71.

73 Myers MG, Oxman MN, Clark JE, Arndt KA. Failure of neutral-red photodynamic inactivation in recurrent herpes simplex virus infections. *N Engl J Med* 1975; 293: 945–949.

74 Roome AP, Tinkler AE, Hilton AL, Montefiore DG, Waller D. Neutral red with photoinactivation in the treatment of herpes genitalis. *Br J Vener Dis* 1975; 51: 130–133.

75 Mima EG, Pavarina AC, Dovigo LN, et al. Susceptibility of *Candida albicans* to photodynamic therapy in a murine model of oral candidosis. *Oral Surg Oral Med Oral Pathol Oral Radiol Endod* 2010; 109: 392–401.

76 Teichert MC, Jones JW, Usacheva MN, Biel MA. Treatment of oral candidiasis with methylene blue-mediated photodynamic therapy in an immunodeficient murine model. *Oral Surg Oral Med Oral Pathol Oral Radiol Endod* 2002; 93: 155–160.

77 Takahashi N, Nyvad B. The role of bacteria in the caries process: ecological perspectives. *J Dent Res* 2011; 90: 294–303.

78 Gonzalez-Cabezas C. The chemistry of caries: remineralization and demineralization events with direct clinical relevance. *Dent Clin North Am* 2010; 54: 469–478.

79 Schneider M, Kirfel G, Berthold M, Frentzen M, Krause F, Braun A. The impact of antimicrobial photodynamic therapy in an artificial biofilm model. *Lasers Med Sci* 2012; 27: 615–620 .

80 Zanin IC, Goncalves RB, Junior AB, Hope CK, Pratten J. Susceptibility of *Streptococcus mutans* biofilms to photodynamic therapy: an in vitro study. *J Antimicrob Chemother* 2005; 56: 324–330.

81 Baptista A, Kato IT, Prates RA, et al. Antimicrobial photodynamic therapy as a strategy to arrest enamel demineralization: A short-term study on incipient caries in a rat model. *Photochem Photobiol* 2012; 88: 584–589.

82 Guglielmi C de A, Simionato MR, Ramalho KM, Imparato JC, Pinheiro SL, Luz MA. Clinical use of photodynamic antimicrobial chemotherapy for the treatment of deep carious lesions. *J Biomed Opt* 2011; 16: 088003.

83 Lima JP, Sampaio de Melo MA, Borges FM, et al. Evaluation of the antimicrobial effect of photodynamic antimicrobial therapy in an in situ model of dentine caries. *Eur J Oral Sci* 2009; 117: 568–574.

84 Peters MC. Strategies for noninvasive demineralized tissue repair. *Dent Clin North Am* 2010; 54: 507–525.

85 Rao A, Malhotra N. The role of remineralizing agents in dentistry: a review. *Compend Contin Educ Dent* 2011; 32: 26–33; quiz 4, 6.

86 Kharkwal GB, Sharma SK, Huang YY, Dai T, Hamblin MR. Photodynamic therapy for infections: Clinical applications. *Lasers Surg Med* 2011; 43: 755–767.

CHAPTER 8

Dosimetry

Jan Tunér,[1] Martha Simões Ribeiro,[2] and Alyne Simões[3]

[1]Private Dental Practice, Grängesberg, Sweden
[2]Center for Lasers and Applications, Institute for Nuclear and Energy Research, IPEN-CNEN/SP, São Paulo, SP, Brazil
[3]Department of Biomaterials and Oral Biology, School of Dentistry, University of São Paulo (USP), São Paulo, SP, Brazil

The dosage parameters for dental lasers such as the Nd:YAG and Er:YAG present few problems for the beginner. There are pre-set parameters for most situations and only the advanced operator will feel a need to adjust these settings. Also, it is easy to confirm the accuracy of these parameters as the results can often be seen with the naked eye.

For low power lasers, the situation is quite different. Many parameters have to be taken into consideration and their immediate effects often cannot be seen with the naked eye. Some calculation is required to determine the optimal choice of parameters, as will be described in this chapter. Therefore, the starting point and more difficult aspect is the dosimetry, which is needs to consider the clinician, patient and/or equipment.

Equipment

Basic parameters

First, the *power* of the laser needs to be known. This is stated in the manual in milliWatt (mW). However, it needs to be remembered that diodes degrade with use and age and an initial power of 100 mW can be considerably lower a year later. A power meter is needed to assess the power of a laser at any given time (Fig. 8.1) and many manufacturers supply a simple power meter along with the laser.

The *energy* directed at a spot or during a therapy session can then be calculated using the formula:

$$E\ (J) = P\ (W) \times t\ (s)$$

where P is the power and t the time during which the laser is used. For instance, 100 mW used for 10 seconds delivers 1000 mJ (1 J) of energy. It must be noted that this is the energy, not the dose. *Dose* (also called radiant exposure or energy density) is the amount of energy applied to an area:

$$D\ (J/cm^2) = E\ (J)/cm^2$$

If the area is 1 cm² and the applied energy is 1 J, then the dose is 1 J/cm², and if the irradiated area is 0.5 cm², the calculation is

1 J/0.5 cm² = 2 J/cm². It is clear that the dose increases as the irradiated area decreases. This is easy to understand as photons will be concentrated over a smaller area. So, if the laser probe is thin, the dose increases.

If the laser power (P), the area to be irradiated (A), and the optimum dose (D) for a determined condition are known, the exposure time (t), that is the time the light is turned on during treatment, can be determined:

$$t\ (s) = D\ (J/cm^2) \times A\ (cm^2)/P\ (W)$$

Note that even if the laser power is given in milliWatts (0.001 W), to calculate exposure time milliWatts must be converted to Watts.

It is important to highlight that the calculation of area differs greatly in the literature. Some studies use the area of the laser beam in the calculation (e.g. 0.04 cm²), while others use the area of the "lesion" (e.g. 1 cm²). This is an extremely important point if the amount of energy delivered to the target tissue is to be appreciated.

In others words, there are two ways of calculating the dose (J/cm²). If a laser with an output of 50 mW and an aperture diameter of 1 mm (0.785 mm² = 0.00785 cm²) is used for 15 seconds, the energy delivered is 0.750 J (E = P × T) and the "dose" is 0.750 J/0.00785 cm² = 95.5 J/cm². Depending on how dose is defined, different opinions can be formed as to whether this is the actual dose or not. The cells outside the aperture border will receive laser light due to the scattering in tissue below and around the aperture. Thus, in the area surrounding the 1 cm² circle (a circle with a total diameter of 1.13 cm), the dose is 0.750 J/cm². The method used when calculating the dose must be reported, or alternatively all the relevant parameters so that a qualified reader can determine how it was calculated.

The *power density* (or irradiance) is a third parameter to observe. Most dentists will be familiar with the expression power density, but are not very aware of it. Power density (mW/cm²) is the expression of the intensity of curing lasers. These values are often around 1000 mW/cm². Some curative lasers use "turbo tips," but these light guides do not increase the

Lasers in Dentistry: Guide for Clinical Practice, First Edition. Edited by Patrícia M. de Freitas and Alyne Simões.
© 2015 John Wiley & Sons, Inc. Published 2015 by John Wiley & Sons, Inc.

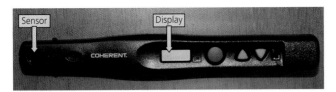

Figure 8.1 The Coherent Lasercheck power meter. Its range is from 400 to 1064 nm and measures up to 1 W.

power of the light; they only concentrate the photons in a smaller area, thus increasing the local intensity. The power density is constant and not related to time.

Dose at target

The above calculations tell us what is happening at the surface. This is appropriate for mucosa and skin, but other targets are deeper inside the body. In order to saturate such tissues with an appropriate amount of energy, we need to know the distance from the surface to the target tissue and what kind of tissue lies between the surface and the target. Much energy is lost immediately after the passage of the light through the skin.[1] Mucosa is rather transparent, bone less transparent, and muscle even less so. Although a small part of the tissue volume, the main absorber of the red and near infrared light is blood, so the vascularization of the area has to be calculated. It is obvious that the initial calculation described above is only a starting point in the calculation of the desired dose at the target.

Another important point is that radiometric quantities and units can quantify only the exposure responsible for the initial event – the optical radiation exposure of the target substance or biological tissue, so dose is the term commonly used in photobiology to express light delivered at the tissue surface.[2] However, it is important to appreciate that there are other concepts that are helpful to describe events within biological tissue: fluence rate (mW/cm²) and fluence (J/cm²). Despite having the same units as power density and dose, respectively, these parameters include backscattered light and are used to modulate the light–tissue interaction.

The quantity intensity, defined as power per solid angle (mW/sr), is commonly misunderstood. This quantity takes into account the light propagation inside biological tissue, which, until now, has been difficult to predict.

In summary, the quantities irradiance and radiant exposure are what instruments measure at the exposed surface. Fluence rate and fluence consider the light interaction with the target and are used to quantify events within a scattering medium, such as biological tissue.[2]

Wavelength

The penetration of light differs from the wavelength. From 200 nm to 400 nm (UV), proteins and DNA are the main chromophores (absorption centers), therefore this region is strongly absorbed by biological tissues, and the influence of scattering is relatively small. Consequently, the radiation does not penetrate deeply into tissues.

From 400 nm to 600 nm (short-wave visible), oxyhemoglobin, hemoglobin, and melanin are the main chromophores, but scattering and absorption occur and the light penetrates approximately 0.5–2.5 mm. From 600 nm to 1500 nm (the end of the visible and near infrared spectrum), scattering predominates over absorption and light penetrates to a depth of 8–10 mm. Above 1500 nm (infrared), water and hydroxyapatite are the main chromophores and the depth of penetration of the radiation is small.

Red light has a low rate of penetration compared to near infrared light. There is greater penetration as the wavelength increases and around 810 nm there is an "optical window" where the light can penetrate several centimeters into tissue. The superpulsed 904-nm laser has the best penetration of all,[1] but this effect is not only related to the wavelength, but also to the extremely short and extremely powerful pulses emitted by this laser.

The eye is a poor "power meter." If a fingertip is irradiated with red laser light, the entire fingertip lights up and it is evident that light has penetrated through the finger. However, if a power meter is used, it shows a loss of 99% of the light. Green light appears to be stronger than red light, but only because our eyes are more sensitive in this region.

How to modify the penetration

It is clear that the wavelength is the most important factor when estimating the penetration of light into tissue (Fig. 8.2). However, there are ways to modify the penetration. By irradiating from a distance, there is more reflection of the light and fewer photons entering the tissue.

By holding the laser in contact with the tissue, the photons are "forced" into the tissue. If pressure is used, the probe will be closer to the target and a less vascularized area will be created with reduced absorption by blood (Fig. 8.3). It is obvious that the therapist can use a range of options to deliver the light to different parts of the body.

Pulsing

There are two types of pulsing. The InGaAlP and GaAlAs lasers can be "chopped." This means that the light is turned on and shut off by a mechanical or electronic device. If the emission is off for 50% of the time, it is called a 50% duty cycle. This also means that it takes twice as long to reach a determined amount of energy, but not that the penetration increases. The 904-nm GaAs lasers, on the other hand, are always pulsed and the strong peak powers do increase the penetration of the photons. Many "chopped" laser manuals suggest different pulse repetition rates for different indications. From *in vitro* studies[3] we know that pulsing is of importance, but in the clinical situation there is no firm evidence on which to base recommendations for pulse repetition rate.

Therapeutic window

The above may seem complicated and indeed takes some consideration to be understood. Fortunately, a fair clinical result is easy to obtain. It is more difficult to obtain the optimal result.[5]

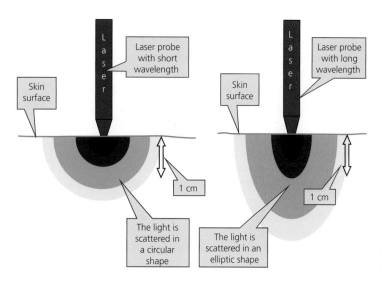

Figure 8.2 Shape of the light profile in illuminated tissue (Tunér 2010. Reproduced with permission of Prima Books).

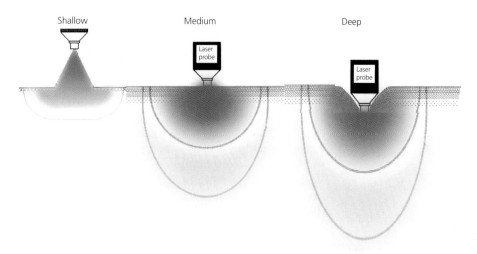

Figure 8.3 Three modes of laser treatment (Tunér 2010. Reproduced with permission of Prima Books).

The dosage follows Arndt–Schultz's law (Fig. 8.4). It is obvious that too low doses have no effect and too high doses likewise have no effect or even a negative effect. However, between those extremes is "the therapeutic window." Getting inside this window is simple, but again, effort is required to approach the optimum.

Some "biostimulation" is actually a matter of inhibition, meaning that the extreme doses are not to be ignored in this discussion. Relief of acute pain requires inhibition of neural activity, and even though the patient feels "stimulated," the pain response has actually been inhibited.[6]

Pitfalls

Energy and dose are related but separate parameters. Both have to be within "the therapeutic window." In many published research papers, only the dose (J/cm^2) is stated. However, as discussed above, it is easy to reach an impressive value for the dose just by

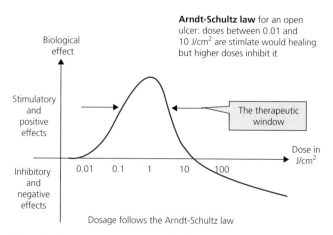

Figure 8.4 Dosage follows Arndt–Schultz's law (Tunér 2010. Reproduced with permission of Prima Books).

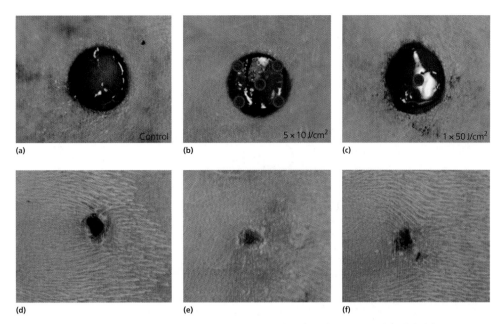

Figure 8.5 (a–c) Wounds were made in a rat's dorsal skin; (d–f) the wounds 10 days later. Rats from group 1 (a and d) did not receive any treatment. The animals from group 2 (b and e) received laser irradiation at five points of 10 J/cm^2 immediately after the completion of the wound and rats from group 3 (c and f) received irradiation at just one point of 50 J/cm^2 (courtesy of Alyne Simões, Luana Campos, and Juliana Rodrigues de Castro).

using a thin probe. The energy needs to be within the window, too! Besides, it is important to note that energy (J) or energy density (J/cm^2) is frequently used to describe low level laser therapy (LLLT) dosage; however, it must not be forgotten that energy has two components: power and time. It has been suggested that these are not necessarily reciprocal components; that is if the power is doubled and the time is halved, then the same energy is delivered but a different biological response could be observed.[7]

The delivery mode of the dose to the tissue is also an important issue, that is the clinical results obtained after irradiation of one point with 50 J/cm^2 are different from those after irradiation performed at five points with 10 J/cm^2 (Fig. 8.5).

A clinical solution

After reading the above, a potential laser user may have second thoughts about adding a therapeutic laser to his/her equipment. There are many different therapeutic lasers on the market, and they differ in power, wavelength, and probe size. The newcomer can apply the "energy per point" method with confidence. This simply means that the energy applied to each point is registered in the medical records: 200 mW applied for 20 seconds = 4 J, and a "point" is about 0.5 cm^2.

This is all very simplistic but will serve as a starting point for the gradual development of clinical experience. For the researcher, of course, every parameter has to be accounted for and justified!

Patient

There are several factors related to the patient that may influence the results of LLLT, and irradiation protocols need to individualized.

Age and bodyweight

Children have a faster metabolism than older people and lower laser energy may be sufficient for them. In LLLT, like for pharmaceuticals, the dose is given according to body weight.

The thickness of the adipose tissue can interfere with the laser penetration and thus can change the effect of irradiation upon the target tissue.

Ethnicity

The tonicity of the patient's skin can influence the absorption of the phototherapy since pigments are chromophores for various types of lasers. Traditional energies directed at skin level may even give a heating sensation in persons with dark skin.[9] Irradiation from a distance will reduce the power density and make LLLT possible.

Availability

Although in some treatment protocols, such as those as for oral mucositis, phototherapy should be given daily, but a patient is often unwilling or unable to go to the dental office every day. In some cases, it would be ideal if the patient could borrow a less expensive home laser device between sessions.

Health status

Laser interacts in a more pronounced way over weakened organs or tissues. Indeed, laser irradiation has the best effect on cells in a reduced redox situation. Healthy cells react very modestly to LLLT.[10]

Tissue

In addition to the laser parameters, tissue optical characteristics should be considered. Different tissues require different modes of laser application as well as different protocols. As stated above, for the wavelengths used in this therapy, mucosa is quite transparent and bone is fairly transparent; skin, even that of

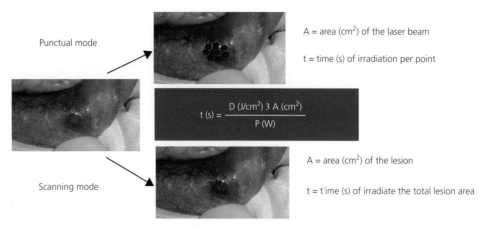

Punctual mode

A = area (cm²) of the laser beam

t = time (s) of irradiation per point

$$t\,(s) = \frac{D\,(J/cm^2)\; 3\; A\,(cm^2)}{P\,(W)}$$

Scanning mode

A = area (cm²) of the lesion

t = t'ime (s) of irradiate the total lesion area

Figure 8.6 Scanning and punctual irradiation modes. "D" is the energy density (J/cm²) and "P" is the power (W).

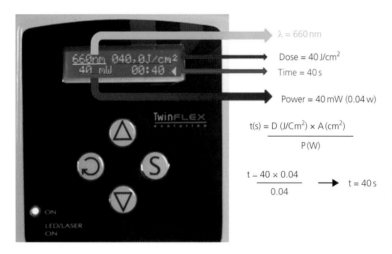

$\lambda = 660\,\text{nm}$

Dose = 40 J/cm²

Time = 40 s

Power = 40 mW (0.04 w)

$$t(s) = \frac{D\,(J/Cm^2) \times A\,(cm^2)}{P\,(W)}$$

$$\frac{t - 40 \times 0.04}{0.04} \longrightarrow t = 40\,s$$

Figure 8.7 Laser equipment display showing wavelength (λ), dose, power, and respective time of irradiation with these laser parameters. The area used in the calculation was the laser beam area (0.04 cm²) and consequently the irradiation mode is punctual. In other words, each point needs to be irradiated for 40 seconds.

persons with a light complexion, is the most important barrier to laser penetration.

Furthermore, it is clear that tissue optics change depending on tissue condition (e.g. healthy and injured tissue) and the latter will influence the protocol.[11] For example, the process of wound healing is dependent upon the coordination of numerous cellular processes. It consists of an inflammatory phase, a proliferative phase, and a remodeling phase. The remodeling phase includes the reorientation and reorganization of the granulation tissue into a scar. It is expected that light penetration in tissue changes during the healing process, suggesting that dosage should be modified during treatment.[12]

Clinician

Equipment

The type of equipment (visible low power laser, infrared low power laser, high power laser, LED) and the clinician's knowledge are directly related to the outcome of the phototherapy. Training is essential for the clinician to be able to offer the best possible therapy for each patient.

Application mode

The clinician's decision between scanning or punctual irradiation mode should be linked to the area of the laser beam or the lesion (Fig. 8.6). It is well established that to calculate the dose, account should be taken of the area to be treated. For example, the optimum dose for healing is suggested to be around 3 J/cm². The area to be irradiated is 1 cm² and the area of the laser beam is 0.04 cm². If the laser output power is 40 mW, exposure time is 100 seconds in an area of 1 cm²; the area can be scanned for 100 seconds or irradiated punctually at 25 points for 4 seconds each to cover the whole lesion area or at 10 standardized spaced points for 10 seconds each.

Commonly, laser equipment displays power and dose on its screen. Once these parameters have been established, exposure time is automatically calculated by the equipment (Fig. 8.7). The dose and consequently the exposure time are then probably calculated based upon 1 cm² or the area of the laser beam. More information from the laser manufacturer on performing this calculation for particular equipment is necessary.

In addition, contact and defocused modes also influence the phototherapy effect, as well as anything that interferes with light absorption by target tissue, such as blood. Open wounds should be irradiated from a distance, but the dermal periphery of the wound should be treated with skin contact.

Diagnosis

A correct diagnosis of the condition is essential for the effectiveness of phototherapy. Pain can have different underlying causes and decreasing the pain intensity with laser treatment may delay a proper diagnosis.

Parameters

Table 8.1 summarizes the key clinical and physical parameters for LLLT. The choice of laser parameters should be made by the clinician according to his/her previous knowledge. Some equipment will already have a protocol recorded in the software and the clinician only has to press a button without further thought. We suggest that clinicians use this tool only if they agree with the proposed protocol.

Dosage recommendations

The World Association for Laser Therapy (WALT) has summarized the present knowledge about dosage (www.walt.nu). These recommendations are based upon a thorough analysis of the literature and are continuously modified when new knowledge becomes available.

Final considerations

Nowadays, there is no doubt that LLLT works. However, there is much controversy and doubt related to dosimetry. For a given patient, what is the best dose, the best mode of application of energy, wavelength, etc.? These concerns are illustrated by considering a Clinical case 8.1.

Table 8.1 Main characteristics and dosimetry associated with LLLT (Silva et al. 2011. Reproduced with permission of Elsevier)

	Synonyms	Units commonly used	Values commonly reported in the literature
Clinical parameters			
Energy density	Dose, radiant exposure, fluence	J/cm²	0.1–1000
Irradiation time (t)	Exposure	Seconds	10–3000
Power density	Intensity, irradiance, fluence rate	mW/cm²	1–1000
Number of irradiated points			1–90
Irradiation method			Contact or non-contact
Mode of application			Punctual, uniform or scanning
Number of treatments			1–14 (or more)
Physical parameters			
Wavelength (λ)		nm	600–1000
Type of emission			Continuous (cw) or pulsing (pw)
Power	Output power	W	10^{-3}–10^{-1}
Repetition rate	Pulse frequency	Hz	0 (cw)–5000
Pulse width		ms	1–500
Beam diameter		mm	
Irradiated area		cm²	
Beam divergence and expansion			
Light source–tissue distance			
Optical tissue properties	Absorption and scattering coefficient	cm⁻¹	

cw (continuous wave).

Clinical case 8.1

A 7-year-old boy diagnosed with Stevens–Johnson syndrome (SJS) was treated with LLLT for his facial and intraoral lesions.[14] On the first day of treatment the clinician was faced with several questions concerning how she would apply the phototherapy to help the patient in the best way.

First, if the clinician is to propose an appropriate treatment for this patient, she should be aware of the syndrome diagnosis and the action mechanism of LLLT. Furthermore, she has to answer some important questions: what were the best wavelength and the best dose? The red lasers are the first choice for healing superficial lesions. In addition, the clinician must be sure not to inhibit wound healing; therefore, a low dose (according to the Arndt–Schultz's law) should be used. The irradiation should be performed in contact mode extraorally and defocused

(non-contact) mode intraorally (the patient was unable to open his mouth widely) and the presence of crusts and blood (on the lips and face) taken into account when considering the laser absorption (Fig. 8.8a–d, g).

Moreover, for extraoral irradiation, a larger laser beam should be used, but for intraoral irradiation a thinner tip should be chosen (Fig. 8.8e, f) to allow the oral cavity to be entered more easily.

It is important to highlight that the patient's age, type of tissue (tongue, buccal mucosa, lip or skin), laser power, etc. should also be considered when determining the best treatment protocol.

The good results observed in this clinical case were only possible thanks to the attention of the clinician to the dosimetry parameters.

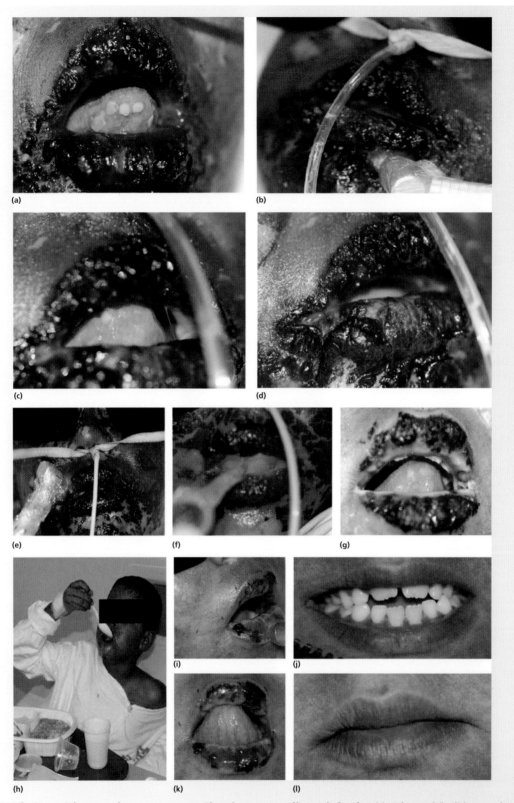

Figure 8.8 LLLT for Steven–Johnson syndrome: a case report. Clinical appearance of lesions before first (a) and second (b–d) laser application. (e) Extraoral and (f) intraoral irradiation with a low power laser. Patient's mouth on fifth (g) and sixth days after the first (h, i, and k) laser irradiation and after complete healing of oral lesions (j and l) (Simões et al. 2011. Reproduced with permission of Mary Ann Liebert).

References

1 Joensen J. *Rat skin penetration during irradiation from 810 nm and 904 nm lasers.* WALT 2010 Congress, Bergen, Norway, September 25–28, Abstract 25G1715.

2 Sliney DH. Radiometric quantities and units used in photobiology and photochemistry: recommendations of the Commission Internationale de L'Eclairage (International Commission on Illumination). *Photochem Photobiol* 2007; 83: 425–432.

3 Karu TI. *Ten lessons on basic science of laser phototherapy.* Grängesberg: Prima Books, 2007: 311–317.

4 Hashmi JT, Huang YY, Sharma SK, et al. Effect of pulsing in low-level light therapy. *Lasers Surg Med* 2010; 42: 450–466.

5 Chung H, Dai T, Sharma SK, et al. The nuts and bolts of low-level laser (light) therapy. *Ann Biomed Eng* 2012; 40: 516–533.

6 Chow R, Armati P, Laakso EL, et al. Inhibitory effects of laser irradiation on peripheral mammalian nerves and relevance to analgesic effects: a systematic review. *Photomed Laser Surg* 2011; 29: 365–381.

7 Huang YY, Chen ACH, Carroll JD, Hamblin MR. Biphasic dose response in low level light therapy. *Dose Response* 2009; 7: 358–383.

8 Guirro RR, Weis LC. Radiant power determination of low-level laser therapy equipment and characterization of its clinical use procedures. *Photomed Laser Surg* 2009; 27: 633–639.

9 Joensen J, Demmink JH, Johnson MI, et al. The thermal effects of therapeutic lasers with 810 and 904 nm wavelengths on human skin. *Photomed Laser Surg* 2011; 29: 145–153.

10 Yamamoto Y, Kono T, Kotani H, et al. Effect of low-power laser irradiation on procollagen synthesis in human fibroblasts. *J Clin Laser Med Surg* 1996; 14: 129–132.

11 Papazoglou ES, Weingarten MS, Zubkov L, Zhu L, Tyagi S, Pourrezaei K. Optical properties of wounds: Diabetic versus healthy tissue. *IEEE T Bio-Med Eng* 2006; 53: 1047–1055.

12 Silva DFT, Ribeiro MS. Light attenuation in rat skin following low level laser therapy on burn healing process. *Progress Biomed Opt Imag* 2010; 11: 77151O1-6.

13 Silva DFT, Almeida-Lopes L, Ribeiro MS. Interação Laser-Tecido Biológico e Princípios de Dosimetria. In: Garcez AS, Ribeiro MS, Núñez SC (eds). *Laser de Baixa Potência: Princípios Básicos e Aplicações Clínicas na Odontologia.* Rio de Janeiro: Elsevier Publishing, 2011: 14–26.

14 Simões A, De Freitas, PM, Bello-Silva, et al. Phototherapy for Stevens-Johnson syndrome: a case report. *Photomed Laser Surg* 2011; 29(1): 67–69.

CHAPTER 9

Risk management and the safe use of laser technology

Rosely Cordon and Dalva Cruz Laganá

Center for Excellence in Prosthesis and Implants (CEPI), School of Dentistry, University of São Paulo (USP), São Paulo, SP, Brazil

This theme, risk management and safety in health care, is studied broadly within the principles of quality management and accreditation in health. Here we focus specifically on the use of laser technology in dentistry, but the principles may well be extended to the use of this technology in health care as a whole, since the risks can be controlled by a range of actions that should be combined in various ways.

Definition of the principles of the quality and implementation of certifiable systems that exist in many countries allows their safe use globally, as long as they are realistic in a given country. Thus, the customer's *safety*, as addressed in Brazil by the National Accreditation Organization (ONA),[1] concerns knowledge, awareness, and selection and implementation of the most appropriate strategies, and addresses the existing regulations, in three levels: structure, processes, and results.

Topics evaluated in a certification process are the availability of control technologies, analysis of costs and benefits, and acceptance of the fact that risks exist and should be minimized by all. This chapter addresses specifically the devices that use laser technology and light emitting diodes (LEDs) in dentistry, as well as the analysis of their impacts on public policy and many other social and political factors.

The World Health Organization (WHO)[2] in its 2010 annual report highlighted the "Ten Facts on Patient Safety," reporting as fact 1: "patient safety is a serious global public health issue. In recent years, countries have increasingly recognized the importance of improving patient safety." Fact 2 states: "Estimates show that in developed countries as many as one in 10 patients is harmed while receiving hospital care. The harm can be caused by a range of errors or adverse events."

This easy access to technologies and information due to the globalized communication that we are now experiencing brings major changes and awareness by all, and its main goal is to improve the quality of health care. Therefore, management has become essential to unifying all aspects of patient care, and technological advances can be seen to be driving constant restructuring in terms of safety and correct use in all healthcare environments. According to the National Health Surveillance Agency (ANVISA), an independent agency under the supervision of the Ministry of Health in Brazil, technology in health care is the set of equipment, medications, materials, and procedures, as well as work procedures, infrastructure, and the organization of health service, all favoring patient safety. One proposed form of technology assessment is a thorough understanding of these technologies with regard to two fundamental aspects. The first concerns the technical dimensions, that is the safety and effectiveness of a technology and its ability to produce the expected result without causing damage when used in normal conditions in healthcare services. The second concerns economic issues, mostly cost-effectiveness, cost-utility or cost-benefit, and the associated economic evaluations. This can be summarized in the formula: cost × effectiveness = expected result/time.

The literature recognizes the existence of different risks to the patient, professional, work environment, and, more recently, global environment, the latter generating a great deal of concern regarding the discarding of technologies. The International Electrotechnical Commission (IEC),[3] a non-profit organization, prepares and publishes with its member countries or affiliates, standards for all electrical, electronic, and related products and is concerned with the adequate use of these devices, especially new technologies in healthcare, such as laser.

The concept of risk is strongly associated with the occurrence of an adverse effect. This risk can be defined as a calculated probability of an adverse or unwanted effect and the severity of the damage that can result from the incorrect use of a technology. Therefore, acceptable risk can be defined for particular situations without compromising safety, as there will never be zero risk when it comes to health care. Thus, it is desirable that institutions manage risk to achieve a high level of safety. The safety culture is a set of values, attitudes, skills, and behaviors that determine the commitment to healthcare management, in a global way, and to safety, reducing failures and guilt and improving attention to care as a whole.

Activities related to the development of consensus and protocols for the use of technologies have been proposed and coordinated both by public officers and by professional associations or even services. These technology assessments, such as "assessment for decision,"[4] aim to promote the use of current scientific knowledge in good practice and to propose recommendations that can support administrators, managers, and clinicians in decision making, as well as providing the necessary information for the patient to give "informed consent," also called "clarified consent," which should wherever possible be individualized for each situation.

Biosafety is defined as "a set of actions aimed at preventing, minimizing or eliminating the risks inherent in research, production, education, technological development, and service delivery, aiming at human and animal health, the preservation of the environment and the quality of the results."[5] Precautions to assure biosafety[6] are recommended by various laws, ordinances, resolutions, and technical standards established by the various international and national agencies. In Brazil, the Ministries of Health and of Labor, and the state and municipal departments, have begun to educate the public in basic concepts through informative campaigns. Such communication is critical to the dissemination of good practices. However, in general, the concepts have not been fully adopted by healthcare professionals. The reasons for this may be related to professional negligence and/or lack of appropriate scientific and technical knowledge, and even a lack of awareness of the population as to their basic rights.

In health services,[7] biosecurity is of utmost importance, as it includes infection control, protection of staff and service users' health, promotion of health awareness, and preservation of the environment through the acquisition, manipulation, and proper disposal of waste. It also includes the care of technologies to assure they are best used to diagnose and treat patients.

ANVISA,[8] through resolution 2/2010, regulates "the management of health technologies used in the provision of health services, to ensure their traceability, quality, efficiency, effectiveness and security, and, where applicable, performance, from their entry into the healthcare facility to their final destination, including the planning of physical, human, and material resources, as well as professionals involved in these proceedings." This resolution covers each stage of management, from planning and entry of the technology into the healthcare facility until its disposal in order to protect workers, and preserve public health, the environment, and patient safety (Fig. 9.1).[9]

Procedures for risk control with laser equipment

The regulations describe procedures for controlling risks directly associated with laser use and also consider the environment in which the laser operates. The regulations for the operation of laser equipment classes 3B and 4 apply to operating rooms or dental procedures where technical control can play the leading role.[10–12]

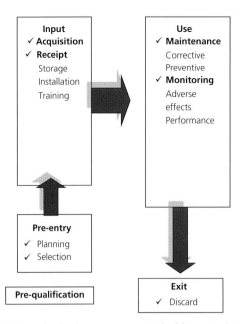

Figure 9.1 Stages of technology management in health services (Garcez et al. 2012. Reproduced with permission of Elsevier).

For *Class 3B* lasers:
- The laser must only be operated within a controlled area;
- Care should be taken to avoid unintentional specular reflections;
- The laser beam optical path must end, whenever possible, in the target area, using a diffuse or absorbing material;
- Eye protection is required if there is any possibility that the beam could be viewed, directly or indirectly, from a distance of less than 13 cm (details in the regulation);
- A standardized warning sign should be fixed at the entrances to the controlled area advising the existence of laser irradiation.

For *Class 4* lasers:
- The beam trajectories must be shielded whenever feasible;
- If practicable, Class 4 lasers must be operated by remote control, thus eliminating the need for the physical presence of people in the environment of the laser;
- Ambient lighting should be increased when eye protection attenuates visible light, using light colored wall surfaces and diffuse lighting, and avoiding specular reflection;
- Whenever possible, the beam and target area should be enclosed in a material opaque to the wavelength of the laser. However, for example, it should be noted that matt metallic surfaces can be highly specular to the wavelength of CO_2 lasers (10 600 nm);
- Whenever practicable, screens should be used to reduce the beam reflection trajectories.

For Class 1M, 2, 2M, and 3R lasers, the regulations only recommend care regarding continuous exposure of the eye to the direct beam. A brief exposure (accidental) of up to 0.25 seconds in the visible spectrum is not considered dangerous. However, the laser beam should not be intentionally targeted at people. It should be noted that the observation of class 1M, 2M, and 3R laser beams with optical devices (e.g. binoculars, microscopes) can be dangerous.

Regulation of safety in the use of laser technology

The IEC[13] is a global organization founded in June 1906 in London but based in Geneva since 1948, with regional centers in Asia Pacific (Singapore), Latin America (São Paulo, Brazil), and North America (Boston, USA). It has 81 member countries and a further 82 countries participate via the National Affiliate Program. Its main goal is to prepare and publish international standards for all electrical and electronic technologies, and their related products. More than 10 000 experts from industry, commerce, government, universities, research laboratories, consumers, and others with interest in the subject, participate in the standardization work.

The IEC[14] is composed of National Committees (NCs), and each NC represents the interests of its nation in the IEC, including those of manufacturers, suppliers and distributors, consumers and users, all levels of governmental agencies, professional organizations and trade associations, and the standards developed by national bodies. NCs are constituted in different ways. Membership of some NCs comes only from the public sector; the membership of others comes from both the public and private sector, or only the private sector. Around 90% of people who prepare IEC standards work in the industry.

IEC regulations have numbers ranging from 60 000 to 79 999 and they are given a standardized named, such as IEC 60417: symbols are for equipment use. The numbers of older regulations were converted in 1997 by the addition of 60 000; for example, the former regulation IEC 27 has become IEC 60027.

The IEC is one of three global partner organizations: the other two are the International Organization for Standardization (ISO) and International Telecommunication Union (ITU), which develop international standards to be applied worldwide. The three cooperate to ensure that the relevant knowledge of experts from related fields is pooled and international standards are complementary.

International standards

The standard is a document established by consensus and approved by a recognized committee that provides, for common and repeated use, rules, guidelines or characteristics for activities or their results in order to obtain the optimum degree of order in a given context.

An international standard (IS) is a standard adopted by an international standards organization and made available to the public. The definition given in all IEC standards is: "A normative document, developed according to consensus procedures, approved by the members of the National Committee of the IEC committee in accordance with Part 1 of ISO and IEC directives."[15]

The IEC is one of the bodies recognized by the World Trade Organization (WTO) and it is entrusted, as part of the WTO technical barriers to trade, to monitor the national and regional organizations agreeing to use its IS as the basis for national or regional principles.

The word "consensus" is important because it indicates a common view of the manufactures, users, consumers, and interested groups. IEC standards are agreed by the international members (IEC NCs). Any member of the IEC may participate in the preparatory work of an IS, and any international organization, governmental and non-governmental, may also participate in this preparation. Another characteristic that gives great credibility to the process of a truly international standard is the fact that it may be subjected to public inquiry in any ISO/IEC member or affiliated country, through democratic consensus and public inquiry.

In Brazil, there is a program of quality control and safety for laser equipment. This control is the responsibility of ANVISA[8] in collaboration with the Institute of National Metrology, Standardization and Industrial Quality (INMETRO),[16] which to this end has adopted the rules of the Brazilian Association of Technical Standards (ABNT); these are based on the IEC 825-1, published in 1998 and replaced by IEC 60825-1 in 2007.

The standards adopted in Brazil for laser technology equipment are NBR IEC 60601.1 and NBR IEC 601.2.22. As set out by the board of resolution (RDC), number 32 in May 2007, ANVISA demands the obligatory registration of all laser equipment; if granted, a certificate of conformity is issued by a laboratory accredited by INMETRO.[16]

Lasers can emit radiation across a wide range of wavelengths, producing an intense, highly focused light beam. The human body is vulnerable to certain lasers; exposure may cause damage to the eyes and skin. Research related to injury to the eyes and skin has been performed in order to understand the biological hazards caused by laser irradiation; the eyes are the most vulnerable and damage to them may be permanent.

For the correct and safe use of lasers it is important to understand the classification of equipment, the dangers involved in their use, and how these can be minimized.[17–20]

The NBR IEC 601.2.22 prescribes minimum safety requirements that must be met by laser equipment. In attempting to regulate the safety of lasers, lasers have been classified according to their wavelength and emitted intensity. The IEC 60.825-1:1993 defines the classes of equipment as 1, 2, 3A, 3B, and 4. More recently the IEC 60.825-1:2007 established a new classification: 1, 1M, 2, 2M, 3R, 3B, and 4, according to a criterion of increasing risk and their potential to cause biological damage.

Lasers classification and safety requirements[21]

All lasers should bear a label giving the class; this is compulsory for Classes 3B and 4 lasers.

Class 1

A Class 1 laser is safe under all conditions of normal use, including when used with magnifying optics (e.g. microscopes, magnifying glasses, binoculars). The optical power output, measured in milliWatts, does not cause damage (e.g. CD player and DVD player). No protective procedures or equipment are required.

Class 1M

Class 1M lasers emit wavelengths between 302.5 nm and 400 nm and are safe in foreseeable operating conditions, but they can be harmful if viewed with an optical instrument that can focus the light in the eye (e.g. presence sensor detectors). They offer low risk of damage to the eyes and no risk to the skin.

Class 2

Class 2 lasers emit visible radiation ranging from 400 nm to 700 nm (e.g. barcode readers, guiding lights, laser pointers). Eye protection is normally achieved by the aversion effect, including the reflex of closing the eyelid. It is expected that the aversion reflex provides adequate protection for reasonably foreseeable operating conditions, including the use of optical magnifying instruments. These lasers have low risk for the eyes and are no risk to the skin.

Class 2M

Class 2M lasers emit visible radiation ranging from 400 nm to 700 nm, where eye protection is normally achieved by the aversion effect, including the reflex of closing the eyelid. However, they can be harmful if viewed with optical instruments. They present low risk to the eyes and no risk to the skin.

Class 3R

Class 3R lasers emit radiation ranging from 302.4 nm to 1 mm (e.g. low power lasers used in physiotherapy, medicine, and dentistry). Beam visualization is potentially dangerous, but the risk is less than that for Class 3B lasers. Manufacturing requirements and control measures are less stringent that those for Class 3B lasers. The access emission limit (AEL) cannot be greater than five times the AEL for Class 2 lasers emitting wavelengths between 400 nm and 700 nm and less than five times the AEL for Class 1 lasers emitting other wavelengths. They present low risk to the eyes and skin.

Class 3B

Class 3B lasers are normally hazardous when their direct beam is viewed within the nominal ocular hazard distance (NOHM). Diffuse reflection viewing is normally safe. They can cause eye damage, but present low risk to the skin. The area of laser operation should be restricted or controlled.

Class 4

Class 4 lasers are capable of causing injuries even through diffuse reflections. They can damage the skin and eyes and are a fire hazard. Their use requires extreme caution. All commercial electrical equipment belonging to laser Classes 3B and 4 in Brazil must comply with the standards. Some of the recommended requirements should be incorporated into the equipment design and others stipulate information that the manufacturer must provide to the user.

Types of tissue damage

The laser can damage biological tissues through four different mechanisms.[22]

Thermal mechanisms

Most of the damage caused by laser irradiation is due to tissue absorption and consequent heating. Heat may dissipate beyond the boundaries of the irradiated target area. Cells within this area show characteristic burns and tissue is damaged by protein denaturation.

Chemical mechanisms

The absorbed radiation can initiate chemical reactions that often result in oxidation and cell death. Usually the damage threshold is low and chemical reactions continue after irradiation ceases.

Photoacoustic mechanisms

When radiation is absorbed and transformed into heat over a short time interval, there can be rapid expansion of the heated volume, generating an acoustic wave that propagates through the tissue and interacts with other tissues in remote regions.

Photoelectric mechanisms

Lasers operating with high power densities, usually with ultrashort pulses, may produce a power density high enough to cause dielectric breakdown of biological tissue.

Adverse health effects

Laser irradiation may be potentially dangerous to eyes and skin. The degree of risk depends on the type of laser beam, frequency, power, beam divergence and intensity, and duration of exposure.

The eye is very vulnerable to the effect of any light, but special care must be taken with laser light. Due to its positioning, the eye can suffer various types of damage. Direct exposure or exposure by reflection of the beam onto the retina may cause burns, resulting in partial or complete blindness. The cornea and lens have the ability to extend and focus radiation onto the retina: thickening of the retinal pigments, dyschromia, photochemical and thermal cataract may occur in the lens, as well as burning of the cornea and lens.

When a member of staff suffers eye exposure, he/she must be checked immediately with an eye exam. Factors that determine the amount of damage to the eye include the reaction of the cornea and the lens, the presence or absence of reflective material between the laser source and the eye, and the distance from the laser source to the retina.

When working with laser equipment, the use of optical devices such as microscopes and binoculars should be avoided (unless the intensity of the beam is so low that their safe use is guaranteed). This rule should be followed for all optical devices that may serve as beam enhancers, thereby increasing the intensity of the beam. Without doubt, the major damage with laser exposure occurs between the visible and infrared spectrum (400–1400 nm) due to the action of focusing on the retina and the eye lens.

The effect of laser irradiation exposure of the skin ranges from redness and mild swelling to blistering and carbonization. The degree of damage depends on the duration of the exposure, radiation wavelength, and the amount of absorbed radiation. Increased pigmentation, burns, erythema, increased sensitivity, and accelerated aging are more related to excessive exposure of the skin to ultraviolet (UV) radiation.

UV radiation is subdivided into three elements: UVC, UVB, and UVA.

- *UVC*: wavelengths below 286 nm are effectively filtered by the ozone layer. Due to the reduction of the atmospheric layer, the absorption value can vary and be reduced near the equator at high altitudes.
- *UVB*: wavelengths between 286 nm and 320 nm are responsible for sunburn and snow blindness. The level of UV rays that affects a person can be substantially enhanced by their reflection from surfaces such as snow, sand, concrete, and water. The cornea absorbs UV radiation below 300 nm, the lower portion of UVB.
- *UVA*: the most dangerous wavelengths may be between 320 nm and 400 nm, causing chronic damage to the eye, particularly if the exposure is at low doses over long periods. UV protection is very important, especially with the thinning of the ozone layer. The tissues of the eye do not develop tolerance to UVA and UVB rays. It is necessary to protect the eyes against the effects of UV radiation. No one is immune to its effects on the eyes.

Staff care

Some lasers operate in the range of invisible light. CO_2 lasers, for instance, operate in the infrared range (wavelength 10 600 nm) with an output power of hundreds of Watts. To avoid accidents, the laser beam is aligned with a low power HeNe laser serving as a "guide." Even a low power laser can be dangerous when directed at the eye for a long time. Laser irradiation can harm the environment as well as people exposed to it. Lesions of the cornea, retina, and skin are potential risks in the environment where the laser is used. There must be a supervisor responsible for the proper and safe use of equipment, keeping track of authorized personnel who will use the device as well as the evaluation of the authorized personnel.

The use of goggles is mandatory in any laser procedure,[23] and the appropriate protection for the wavelength used must be available. All personnel in the controlled area, including the patient, must wear goggles, with the exception of the operator if the equipment does not require protection. Extra pairs of goggles should be available at the entrance to the procedure room to be used by persons entering the room. It must not be forgotten that some laser equipment acts at more than one wavelength, and therefore full protection goggles may be required.

Vacuum/suction devices are also important. When the laser beam vaporizes the tissue it forms smoke which may contain viable particles of DNA or virus that can be deposited in the airways.

Care of the environment

The use of warning signs at the entrances to rooms where the laser is used is crucial. There should be a controlled area and access restricted to designated staff who are familiar with the use of laser and the required safety procedures. Internationally recognized symbols should be used; illuminated signs, such as "laser in use, do not enter," should be placed at every access to the room. The areas in which the laser is operating must be kept clear of flammable and reflective materials. Tissues must not be used to cover reflective surfaces because of the fire hazard. All equipment that will not be used in the procedure should be removed from the room before the start of any procedure. A CO_2 fire extinguisher should be available in the room where the laser is being used.

It is the operator's responsibility to make sure that the device is properly connected, paying special attention to the laser beam direction in relation to doors and windows. The operator should also be concerned with positioning the device in order to achieve easy reading of the control panel and operation of all controls, as well as checking cables and connections since another health hazard is electric shock, especially when working with laser equipment that requires high voltage components.

Management of risk and the systematic and continuous application of procedures, policies, conducts and resource analysis, communications, and control of risks and adverse events that affect the safety of human health, professional integrity, the environment, as well as the profile of the institution, will minimize to an acceptable level any damage to health – this is safety management of technology related to health.

References

1 ONA. Brazilian Accreditation Manual for Organizations Providing Health Services. ONA, 2010.

2 World Health Organization (WHO). Ten facts on patient safety, 2010. Available at http://www.who.int/features/factfiles/patient_safety/patient_safety_facts/en/index4.html [accessed May 24 2011].

3 International Electrotechnical Commission. *Safety of Lasers Products – Part 1: Equipment Classification, Requirements and User's Guide (IEC 60.825-1:2007)*. Geneva: IEC, 2007.

4 Padoveze MC. Interface between the CME, HICC and risk management: determining factor in quality of patient care. Available at http://www.nascecme.com.br/artigos/Artigo%20Maria%20Clara%20Interface%20entre%20a%20CME,%20CCIH%20e%20G.R.pdf [accessed June 2 2011].

5 Teixeira P, Valle S. *Biosecurity: A Multidisciplinary Approach*. Rio de Janeiro: FIOCRUZ, 1996.

6 Carmo MRC, Costa AMDD. Biosafety procedures in dentistry. *JBC* 2001; 5: 116–119.

7 Krieger D, Bueno R, Gabardo MCL. Perspectives on biosafety in dentistry. *Manage Health Magazine* 2010; 1: 1–10.

8 ANVISA (Brazil). National Agency for Sanitary Vigilance. Resolution in the DRC. 2, 25 January 2010. Provides for the management of health technology in healthcare facilities. Available at: www.anvisa.gov.br [accessed June 1 2011].

9 Official Gazette (DOU). Government, of May 30, 2007. Resolution RDC. 32, May 29, 2007. Provides for the compulsory certification of electrical equipment under the regime of Sanitary Surveillance and other measures. Available at http://e-legis.anvisa.gov.br/leisref/public/showAct.php?id=27014&word [accessed June 5 2011]

10 Banta HD, Oortwijn WJ, Van Beekman WT. *The Organization of Health Care Technology Assessment in the Netherlands*. The Hague: Rathenau Institute, 1995

11 Panerai RB, Mohr JP. *Health Technology Assessment Methodologies for Developing Countries*. Washington, DC: PAHO, 1989.

12 Cordon R. *Evaluation of therapeutic lasers for eye protection at low intensity*. MA Thesis. Sao Paulo: Institute of Energy and Nuclear Research, 2003.

13 International Commission of Non-ionizing Radiation Protection (ICNIRP).An Independent Voice in NIR Protection. Available at http://www.icnirp.de/what.htm [accessed June 2 2011].

14 International Commission OF Non-ionizing Radiation Protection. Set guidelines for exposure of the eye to optical radiation from ocular instruments: statement from a group of tasks (ICNIRP). Available at http://www.icnirp.de/PubOptical.htm [accessed June 5 2011].

15 ISO/IEC Directives, Part 1. 9th edn, 2012. Available from http://www.iec.ch/members_experts/refdocs/iec/isoiecdir1%7Bed9.0%7Den.pdf [accessed June 5 2011].

16 IMETRO. Brazilian System of Conformity Assessment (SBAC). Available at http://www.inmetro.gov.br/qualidade/pdf/guia_ingles.pdf [accessed June 2 2011].

17 Garcez AS, Ribeiro MS, Nunes SC. Low Power Laser: Basic Principles and Clinical Applications in Dentistry. *Rio de Janeiro: Elsevier* 2012; 23: 227–240.

18 Maggioni M, Attanasio T, Scarpelli F. Legal and regulatory aspects of safety precautions in laser-assisted dentistry. *I Laser in Odontoiatria* 2009: 333–346.

19 Son DC. *Assessment of security requirements in a diode laser for surgical purposes in accordance with Brazilian law*. MA Thesis. Institute of Energy and Nuclear Research, São Paulo, 2010.

20 Garbin AJ, Garbin CA, Arcieri RM, Crossato M, Ferreira NF. Biosecurity in public and private office. *J Appl Oral Sci* 2005; 13: 163–166.

21 Matthes R, Cain CP, Courant D, et al. Revision of guidelines on limits of exposure to laser radiation of wavelengths between 400 nm and 1.4 μm. *Health Phys* 2000; 79: 431–440.

22 Sliney D, Aron-Rosa D, Delori F, et al. Adjustment of guidelines for exposure of the eye to optical radiation from ocular instruments: Statement from a task group of the International Commission on Non-Ionizing Radiation Protection (ICNIRP). *Appl Opt* 2005; 44: 2162–2176.

23 Salles MR. *Marketing Iris Safety*. Project Millenium, 2007.

SECTION 2

Preventive, esthetic, and restorative dentistry

CHAPTER 10

Selective caries removal, cavity preparation and adhesion to irradiated tissues

Patrícia M. de Freitas,[1] Marcelo Giannini,[2] Junji Tagami,[3] and Simone Gonçalves Moretto[1]

[1]Special Laboratory of Lasers in Dentistry (LELO), Department of Restorative Dentistry, School of Dentistry, University of São Paulo (USP), São Paulo, SP, Brazil
[2]Department of Restorative Dentistry, Piracicaba Dental School, State University of Campinas (UNICAMP), Piracicaba, SP, Brazil
[3]Department of Cariology and Operative Dentistry, Faculty of Dentistry, Tokyo Medical and Dental University, Tokyo, Japan

With technological development, some alternatives to rotary cutting instruments have been introduced for caries removal and cavity preparation.[1,2] High power lasers are now widely used following their introduction for use in dental hard tissues in 1964.[3–5]

Wavelengths close to 3000 nm, such as those emitted by the erbium lasers, are close to the main absorption peak of water and hydroxyapatite, and therefore they have been demonstrated to be effective for cutting soft and hard (enamel, dentin, and alveolar bone) tissues.[6] The erbium lasers are Er:YAG (erbium:yttrium–aluminum–garnet, 2940 nm) and Er,Cr:YSGG (erbium, chromium:yttrium–scandium–gallium–garnet, 2780 nm), and were approved by the US Food and Drug Administration (FDA) for use in dental hard tissues in the late 1990s.*

How do Er:YAG and Er,Cr:YSGG lasers remove dental hard tissue?

The erbium lasers (Er:YAG and Er,Cr:YSGG) remove enamel and dentin through a process called thermomechanical ablation.[7,8] During this process, the infrared laser energy is absorbed by the subsurface water that is confined by the hard tissue matrix, and this quickly leads to "micro-explosions" that remove the mineralized tissue.[9] The greatest part of the energy is absorbed by the ablation process and only a small fraction may heat the adjacent tissues.[10–12] Air/water cooling of laser systems is important to avoid or minimize thermal damage to irradiated tissue and a possible temperature rise in the pulp chamber, thus preserving tooth vitality.[13,14]

The laser irradiation effects on mineralized tissues vary according to the tissue composition and water concentration.[6,10] The high amount of water inside the carious tissues increases the interaction of the laser with the target tissue, leading to a selective removal of carious tissue and resulting in a more conservative cavity design, which follows the principles of minimally invasive dentistry.[15] Regarding the water coming from the laser handpiece, some authors[16] have shown that a thin water layer on the target tissue surface can increase ablation; however, an excessive water layer can negatively affect the light interaction with enamel/dentin, reducing the laser ablation potential.

What are the differences between irradiated and bur-cut treated tooth surfaces?

The irradiated enamel surface is very rough and irregular, with the enamel prisms clearly visible and similar to the pattern resulting from etching with phosphoric acid. There are also conical craters with sharp enamel projections[9] (Fig. 10.1).

Regarding the irradiated dentin, microscopic analysis displays a rough surface, free of a smear layer, with open dentin tubules and protruding peritubular dentin.[17,18] In contrast, the mechanical preparation of dental tissues with rotary cutting instruments produces a thick smear layer that covers the whole surface[17,19] (Fig. 10.2).

Lasers parameters, such as energy density, repetition rate, water/air flow, and pulse duration, can influence both enamel and dentin surface morphology, as has been extensively reported in the literature. Clinically, whether contact or non-contact irradiation mode is used, as well as the angle of incidence of the laser light with the target tissues, are important aspects that can also influence the ablation potential of the laser.[20]

Adhesion to the laser-treated tooth surface

Bonding to irradiated enamel is not as critical as to irradiated dentin. Some studies have suggested that lased enamel does not require acid etching before the adhesive procedure, due to the fact that the laser irradiation can lead to a rough enamel surface. However, studies have shown that the acid-etched lased surface promotes greater bonding to the composite restorative materials.[19]

Regarding adhesion to the dentin surface, controversial results can be found in the literature. Studies have shown that different adhesive systems behave differently on the lased surface.[2]

---

*Even though the CO_2 (9600 nm) lasers are still reported as successful for caries removal and caries preparation, as they are also absorbed by enamel and dentin, they are not widely used in clinical practice and will not be addressed in this chapter.

Lasers in Dentistry: Guide for Clinical Practice, First Edition. Edited by Patrícia M. de Freitas and Alyne Simões.
© 2015 John Wiley & Sons, Inc. Published 2015 by John Wiley & Sons, Inc.

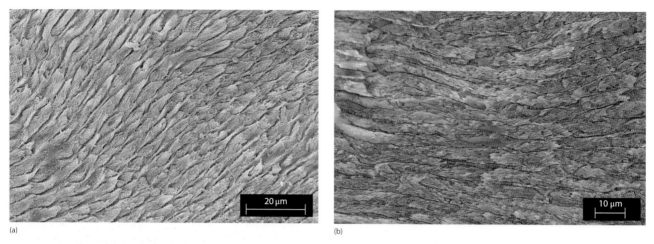

(a)

(b)

Figure 10.1 Enamel after (a) acid etching and (b) Er,Cr:YSGG laser conditioning.

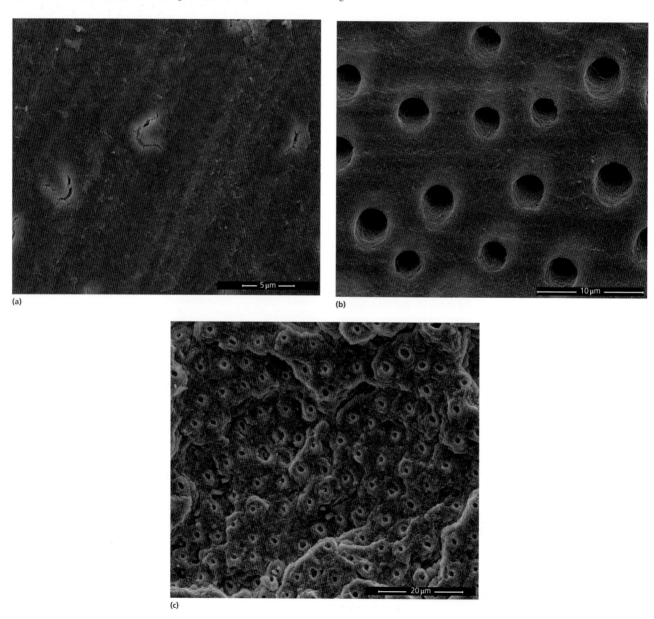

(a)

(b)

(c)

Figure 10.2 (a) Dentin prepared with bur, (b) bur-cut dentin after acid etching, and (c) Er,Cr:YSGG laser-irradiated dentin.

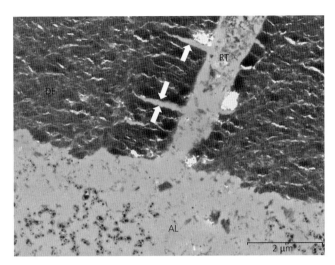

Figure 10.3 Transmission electron micrograph (TEM) of the resin–dentin interface created by a self-etching adhesive system on dentin surface irradiated with the Er:YAG laser (160 mJ/10 Hz). The adhesive is bonded to dentin; however, no infiltration into mineralized dentin was observed at this magnification. Arrows show microcracks in the peritubular dentin (10 000×). DE, dentin; AL, adhesive layer; RT, resin tag. (Vermelho 2011).[55]

Due to the fact that laser irradiation can lead to a smear layer-free surface with a rough pattern, some authors have also suggested that dentin prepared with laser irradiation does not need to be etched.[21] However, later studies demonstrated that laser irradiation does not expose the collagen fibril network to be hybridized with the adhesive system.[12,18,20] When an etch-and-rinse adhesive system is used for cavity restoration, etching the cavity walls remains mandatory in order to expose the collagen fibril network and increase the adhesive monomer infiltration.[19] Selfetching adhesive systems already contain an acidic primer that is able to demineralize the dentin surface, exposing the collagen fibrils and infiltrating the dentin at the same time.

However, depending on the type of bonding agent and laser irradiation parameter of dentin, no adhesive monomer infiltration into mineralized dentin is observed (Fig. 10.3). Some authors have speculated that the lack of adhesive infiltration and mechanical properties of the laser-modified dentin are the main explanation for the lower bond strength of bonding agents to laser-modified dentin when compared to bur-cut surfaces.[22-27]

Although the results of bond strength of the resin composite to the dentin-irradiated surface are mostly similar or lower than those for conventional treatment using a diamond bur, the bond strength values reported in the literature can reach values of higher than 20 MPa, which is considered clinically acceptable. Furthermore, clinical reports support the use of this new technology and its benefits in adhesive restorative procedures,[28-30] microbial reduction,[31-36] selective removal of carious tissue,[37] and other indications.

Even though there is still no consensus in the literature regarding which adhesive should be used, the laser parameters seem to be more important and should effectively remove enamel and/or dentin without causing surface melting (which can negatively affect the resin infiltration into the demineralized tissue), carbonization, and/or pulp tissue damage. It is essential to know the parameters and the laser features in order to use this technology correctly (See clinical case 10.1).

Benefits of using laser irradiation for cavity preparation instead of a high speed drill

The benefits are:

- Effectiveness in selective caries removal and cavity preparation[28,29];
- Great acceptance by the patients due to the absence of noise and vibration, contributing to a less painful/more comfortable treatment[28,38,39];
- In some cases, there is no need for local anesthesia[40,41];
- Bacterial reduction[31-36];
- Effects can be generated in the tissue underlying the tissue being irradiated: these effects are similar to those induced by low power lasers – biomodulation and analgesia.[42]

Limitations to the use of erbium lasers in cavity preparation

The limitations are:

- Should not be used to remove amalgam and ceramic restorations;
- Depending on the location of carious tissue, the use of curettes may be necessary for the complete removal of the caries tissue;
- As the cavity margins are irregular as a consequence of the ablation, resin composite is indicated as the restorative material;
- Extensive theoretical knowledge and practical training are required for the correct use of this technology;
- The working time is two to three times longer than that for the use of burs.[43,44] Strategies to improve the laser ablation (increase of energy density and/or repetition rate) are limited by the temperature increase and discomfort to patients during the clinical procedure[9];
- Cost of the equipment (high power lasers – Er:YAG and Er,Cr:YSGG).

Future perspectives

Erbium lasers (Er:YAG and Er,Cr:YSGG) have long pulse duration (150–400 µs).[9] Studies have demonstrated that long pulse duration can induce high residual heat deposition during laser irradiation,[45] leading to thermal changes in the target tissue,[27] depending on the laser parameters and the cooling (water/air spray) used during the irradiation.

In the early 1990s ultra-short pulsed lasers (USPLs; picosecond [ps; 10^{-12} seconds] and femtosecond [fs; 10^{-15} seconds] were developed. They have been widely tested with the aim of reducing the thermomechanical damage commonly observed as a result of laser irradiation with longer pulsed lasers (nano or microseconds). As the femtosecond pulse duration is so brief, the energy and the laser-generated material dissipate before heat can propagate to the surrounding tissue. As a result, a precise and well-delimited cut can be achieved,[46,47] with no excessive temperature increase or destructive effect on the surrounding matter (Fig. 10.4).[48–50]

This difference in the ablation process with USPLs alters the morphology of the irradiated tissue.[48,51–53] Differently from the pattern described following longer pulsed laser irradiation.[16,18] Figure 10.4 reveals that after USPL irradiation it is possible to verify a well-delimited cavity, without thermal damage to the surrounding tissue, with a rough surface partially covered by a thin layer of debris but with the dentin tubules open. There are still only few studies in the literature evaluating adhesion to

tooth tissue (or dentin) irradiated with USPLs. The available studies indicate very promising results for contemporary adhesive systems bonded to these lased surfaces, with bond strength mean values and hybrid layer formation comparable to those obtained with the conventional cavity preparation (bur-cut)[51,54] even at long-term follow-up.[53]

In contrast to long pulsed lasers, USPLs can interact with different restorative materials, such as composite resin or amalgam.[46] As the ablation threshold fluency to remove the composite resin and amalgam is approximately half the value for enamel, it allows a selective removal of the restorative material while preserving the surrounding tissues.[45]

Nowadays, such lasers are commercially available for ophthalmology and for laboratory use (prototypes),[9] but it is believed that in the near future this new important technology will be used in daily practice in dentistry.

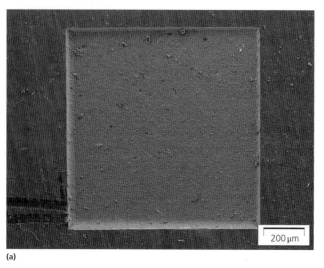
(a)

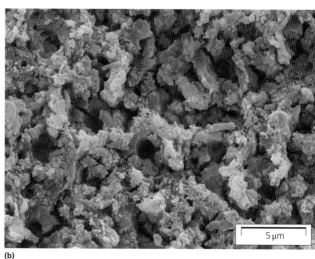
(b)

Figure 10.4 Dentin prepared with the femtosecond laser: (a) 80x and (b) 5000x.

Clinical case 10.1** A 14-year-old female patient attended the clinic of the Special Laboratory of Laser Dentistry (LELO), School of Dentistry, University of São Paulo for a restorative treatment of element 47.

The clinical examination revealed the presence of a temporary restorative material on the occlusal surface of element 47 and, after removal of the material, remaining demineralized dental tissue was observed (Fig. 10.5a,b). The radiographic evaluation revealed the involvement of both enamel and

the dentin structures (Fig. 10.5c) and restorative intervention was required. The patient described little sensitivity to cold and some sweet foods. The treatment of choice was direct composite resin restoration with the use of high and low power lasers (Fig. 10.5d–k).

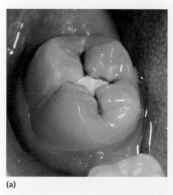
(a)

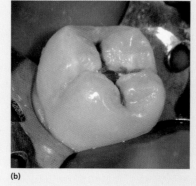
(b)

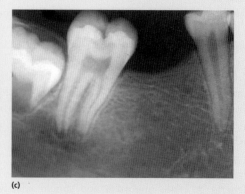
(c)

**Clinical case previously published in Rev Assoc Paul Cir Dent 2011; 65(6): 462–466.

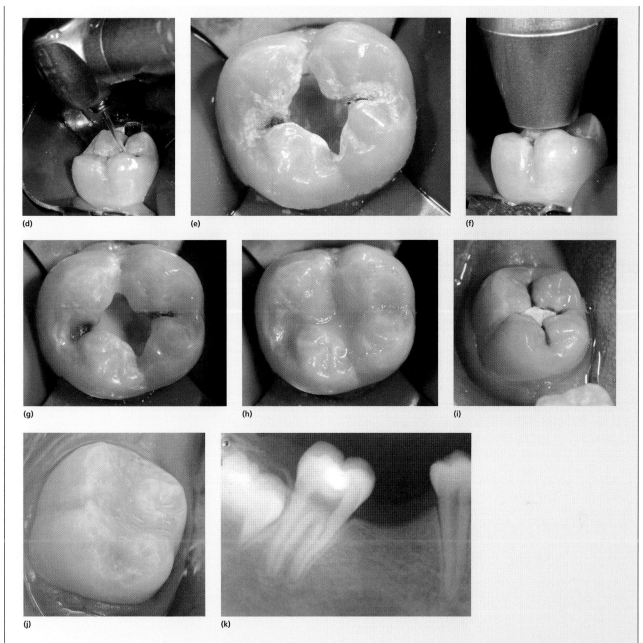

Figure 10.5 (a,b) Initial image of element 47, diagnosed with caries on the occlusal surface, with the presence of temporary restorative material (a) and after removing it (b). (c) Radiographic evaluation of the caries lesion in element 47, with commitment of enamel and dentin structures. (d) Selective removal of carious tissue using a high power laser (Er,Cr: YSGG laser) with water/air cooling (65% air and 55% water). The output power of the laser ranged from 3.5 to 2.0 W; the closer the tissue pulp, the lower the power used. (e) Occlusal view of the cavity after removal of the carious tissue using the high power laser. (f) Irradiation of dentin tissue with a low power laser (660 nm) in order to prevent tooth sensitivity after cavity preparation. (g,h) Occlusal view of the cavity after insertion of a thin layer of a resin-modified glass ionomer liner (g) and completion of the direct composite resin restoration (h). The restoration was performed with an etch-and-rinse adhesive system according to the manufacturer's instructions. (i) Initial image of element 47 and (j) finished direct composite resin restoration. (k) Radiographic image of element 47 after concluding the restorative treatment (2011. Reproduced with permission of Associação Paulista de Cirurgiões Dentistas – APCD).

Conclusion

Erbium lasers (2940 nm and 2780 nm) are interesting alternatives for selective removal of carious tissue and cavity preparation. However, it is important to highlight that the success of this innovative treatment relies not only on the tissue composition and laser settings, but also on the professional's knowledge and experience of working with these wavelengths.

References

1 Oliveira MT, Freitas PM, et al. Influence of diamond sono-abrasion, air-abrasion and Er:YAG laser irradiation on bonding of different adhesive systems to dentin. *Eur J Dent* 2007; 1(3): 158–166.

2 Cardoso MV, Coutinho E, et al. Influence of dentin cavity surface finishing on micro-tensile bond strength of adhesives. *Dent Mater* 2008; 24(4): 492–501.

3 Goldman L, Hornby P, et al. Impact of the laser on dental caries. *Nature* 1964; 203: 417.

4 Stern RH, Sognnaes RF. Laser beam effect on dental hard tissues. *J Dent Res* 1964; 43(5sp): 873.

5 Gordon TE. Some effects of laser impacts on extracted teeth. *J Dent Res* 1966; 45(2): 372–375.

6 Bader C, Krejci I. Indications and limitations of Er:YAG laser applications in dentistry. *Am J Dent* 2006; 19(3): 178–186.

7 Hibst R, Keller U. Experimental studies of the application of the Er:YAG laser on dental hard substances: I. Measurement of the ablation rate. *Lasers Surg Med* 1989; 9(4): 338–344.

8 Altshuler GB, Belikov AV, et al. A laser-abrasive method for the cutting of enamel and dentin. *Lasers Surg Med* 2001; 28(5): 435–444.

9 Matos AB, Azevedo CS, et al. Laser Technology for Caries Removal. Contemporary Approach to Dental Caries. M.-y. Li: *InTech*, 2012: 23.

10 Keller U, Hibst R. Experimental studies of the application of the Er:YAG laser on dental hard substances: II. Light microscopic and SEM investigations. *Lasers Surg Med* 1989; 9(4): 345–351.

11 Ana PA, Bachmann L, et al. Lasers effects on enamel for caries prevention. *Laser Physics* 2006; 16(5): 865–875.

12 Ramos AC, Esteves-Oliveira M, et al. Adhesives bonded to erbium:yttrium-aluminum-garnet laser-irradiated dentin: transmission electron microscopy, scanning electron microscopy and tensile bond strength analyses. *Lasers Med Sci* 2010; 25(2): 181–189.

13 Zach L, Cohen G. Pulp response to externally applied heat. *Oral Surg Oral Med Oral Pathol* 1965; 19: 515–530.

14 Attrill DC, Davies RM, et al. Thermal effects of the Er:YAG laser on a simulated dental pulp: a quantitative evaluation of the effects of a water spray. *J Dent* 2004; 32(1): 35–40.

15 Tyas MJ, Anusavice KJ, et al. Minimal intervention dentistry--a review. FDI Commission Project 1-97. *Int Dent J* 2000; 50(1): 1–12.

16 Freitas PM, Navarro RS, et al. The use of Er:YAG laser for cavity preparation: an SEM evaluation. *Microsc Res Tech* 2007; 70(9): 803–808.

17 Fried D, N. Ashouri, et al. (2002). "Mechanism of water augmentation during IR laser ablation of dental enamel." *Lasers Surg Med* 31(3): 186–193.

18 Moretto SG, Azambuja N, Jr, et al. Análise morfológia de superfícies dentinárias irradiada com os lasers de Er:YAG e Er,Cr:YSGG. *UNOPAR Cient Cienc Biol Saúde* 2012; 12(1): 6.

19 De Munck J, Van Meerbeek B, et al. Micro-tensile bond strength of two adhesives to Erbium:YAG-lased vs. bur-cut enamel and dentin. *Eur J Oral Sci* 2002; 110(4): 322–329.

20 Carvalho RCR, Freitas PM, et al. Influence of Er:YAG laser beam angle, working distance, and energy density on dentin morphology: An SEM investigation. *J Oral Laser Appl* 2005; 5(4): 237–243.

21 Visuri SR, Gilbert JL, et al. Shear strength of composite bonded to Er:YAG laser-prepared dentin. *J Dent Res* 1996; 75(1): 599–605.

22 Kameyama A, Kawada E, et al. Effect of HEMA on bonding of Er:YAG laser-irradiated bovine dentine and 4-META/MMA-TBB resin. *J Oral Rehabil* 2002; 29(8): 749–755.

23 Esteves-Oliveira M, Zezell DM, et al. Bond strength of self-etching primer to bur cut, Er,Cr:YSGG, and Er:YAG lased dental surfaces. *Photomed Laser Surg* 2007; 25(5): 373–380.

24 Lee BS, Lin PY, et al. Tensile bond strength of Er,Cr:YSGG laser-irradiated human dentin and analysis of dentin-resin interface. *Dent Mater* 2007; 23(5): 570–578.

25 de Carvalho RC, de Freitas PM, et al. Micro-shear bond strength of Er:YAG-laser-treated dentin. *Lasers Med Sci* 2008; 23(2): 117–124.

26 de Oliveira MT, Arrais CA, et al. Micromorphology of resin-dentin interfaces using one-bottle etch&rinse and self-etching adhesive systems on laser-treated dentin surfaces: a confocal laser scanning microscope analysis. *Lasers Surg Med* 2010; 42(7): 662–67031.

27 Moretto SG, Azambuja Jr, et al. Effects of ultramorphological changes on adhesion to lased dentin-Scanning electron microscopy and transmission electron microscopy analysis. *Microsc Res Tech* 2011; 74(8): 720–726.

28 Matsumoto K, Hossain M, et al. Clinical assessment of Er,Cr:YSGG laser application for cavity preparation. *J Clin Laser Med Surg* 2002; 20(1): 17–21.

29 Freitas PM, Ramos TM, et al. Benefícios dos lasers de alta e baixa potência no procediemnto restaurador direto: relato de caso." *Rev Assoc Paul Cir Dent* 2011; 65(6): 5.

30 Akin GE, Herguner-Siso S, et al. (2012). Bond strengths of one-step self-etch adhesives to laser-irradiated and bur-cut dentin after water storage and thermocycling. *Photomed Laser Surg* 2012; 30(4): 214–221.

31 Belikov AV, Moroz BT, et al. *Bacterial activity in the products of laser destruction of human dental enamel and dentin Stomatologiia (Mosk)* 1995; 74(6): 32–34.

32 Hibst R, Stock K, et al. Controlled tooth surface heating and sterilisation by Er:YAG laser radiation. *Proc SPIE* 1996; 2922: 119–126.

33 Mehl A, Folwaczny M, et al. Bactericidal effects of 2.94 microns Er:YAG-laser radiation in dental root canals. *J Endod* 1999; 25(7): 490–493.

34 Moritz A, Schoop U, et al. The bactericidal effect of Nd:YAG, Ho:YAG, and Er:YAG laser irradiation in the root canal: an in vitro comparison. *J Clin Laser Med Surg* 1999; 17(4): 161–164.

35 Blay CC. Análise comparativa da redução bacteriana com irradiação do laser de Er:YAG ou ponta montada em alta rotação após remoção de tecido cariado em dentina: estudo in anima nobile. Mestrado Profissionalizante Mestrado Profissionalizante, Instituto de Pesquisas Energéticas e Nucleares/Universidade de São Paulo, 2001.

36 Gordon W, Atabakhsh VA, et al. The antimicrobial efficacy of the erbium, chromium:yttrium-scandium-gallium-garnet laser with radial emitting tips on root canal dentin walls infected with *Enterococcus faecalis. J Am Dent Assoc* 2007; 138(7): 992–1002.

37 Li ZZ, Code JE, et al. Er:YAG laser ablation of enamel and dentin of human teeth: determination of ablation rates at various fluences and pulse repetition rates. *Lasers Surg Med* 1992; 12(6): 625–630.

38 Fried D. *IR laser ablation of dental enamel.* San Jose, CA: SPIE, 2000.

39 Niemz MH. *Laser-tissues interactions - Fundamentals and applications.* Berlin: Springer-Verlag, 2004.

40 Cozean C, Arcoria CJ, et al. Dentistry for the 21st century? Erbium:YAG laser for teeth. *J Am Dent Assoc* 1997; 128(8): 1080–1087.

41 Keller U, Hibst R, et al. Erbium:YAG laser application in caries therapy. Evaluation of patient perception and acceptance. *J Dent* 1998; 26(8): 649–656.

42 Powell GL. Lasers in the limelight: what will the future bring? *J Am Dent Assoc* 1992; 123(2): 71–74.

43 White JM, Goodis HE, et al. Dentin Ablation Rate Using Nd-Yag and Er-Yag Lasers. *J Dent Res* 1994; 73: 318–318.

44 Navarro RS, Gouw-Soares S, et al. The influence of erbium:yttrium-aluminum-garnet laser ablation with variable pulse width on morphology and microleakage of composite restorations. *Lasers Med Sci* 2010; 25(6): 881–889.

45 Fried D, Ragadio J, et al. Residual heat deposition in dental enamel during IR laser ablation at 2.79, 2.94, 9.6, and 10.6 microm. Lasers Surg Med 2001; – (3): 221–229.

46 Freitas AZ, Freschi LR, et al. Determination of ablation threshold for composite resins and amalgam irradiated with femtosecond laser pulses. *Laser Physics Lett* 2010; 7(3): 236–241.

47 Bello-Silva MS, Wehner M, et al. Precise ablation of dental hard tissues with ultra-short pulsed lasers. Preliminary exploratory investigation on adequate laser parameters. *Lasers Med Sci* 2013; 28(1): 171–184.

48 Niemz MH. Cavity preparation with the Nd:YLF picosecond laser. *J Dent Res* 1995; 74(5): 1194–1199.

49 Kim ME, Feit MD, et al. Effects of high repetition rate and beam size on hard tissue damage due to subpicosecond laser pulses. *Appl Phys Lett* 2000; 76(26): 4001–4003.

50 Kim BM, Feit MD, et al. Influence of pulse duration on ultrashort laser pulse ablation of biological tissues. *J Biomed Opt* 2001; 6(3): 332–338.

51 Bello-Silva MS. Análise morfológica e da resistência adesiva dos tecidos dentais duros irradiados com lasers de pulsos ultracurtos. Doctorate Thesis, Dental School from the University of São Paulo, 2010.

52 Ji L, Li L, et al. Ti:sapphire femtosecond laser ablation of dental enamel, dentine, and cementum. *Lasers Med Sci* 2012; 27(1): 197–204.

53 Moretto SG. Estudo longitudinal da resistência e qualidade de união de diferentes sistemas adesivos à dentina irradiada com laser de femtossegundo. Doctorate Thesis, Dental School from the University of São Paulo, 2012.

54 Gerhardt-Szep S, Werelius K, et al. Influence of femtosecond laser treatment on shear bond strength of composite resin bonding to human dentin under simulated pulpal pressure." *J Biomed Mater Res B Appl Biomater* 2012; 100(1): 177–184.

55 Vermelho PM. Avaliação do substrato dentinário irradiado com laser de Er:YAG : resistência de união, padrão de fratura e análise ultramorfológica. Master thesis, Campinas State University.

CHAPTER 11
Management of non-carious cervical lesions

Ana Cecilia Corrêa Aranha,[1] Karen Müller Ramalho,[2] and Marcella Esteves-Oliveira[3]

[1]Special Laboratory of Lasers in Dentistry (LELO), Department of Restorative Dentistry, School of Dentistry, University of São Paulo (USP), São Paulo, SP, Brazil
[2]Biodentistry Master Program, School of Dentistry, Ibirapuera University (UNIB), São Paulo, SP, Brazil
[3]Department of Operative Dentistry, Periodontology and Preventive Dentistry, RWTH Aachen University, Aachen, Germany

Introduction

The substantial and worldwide decrease in the prevalence of dental caries and the improved long-term health of dentition has shifted the attention of both the scientific and clinical communities towards other pathologies that affect dental hard tissues, such as tooth wear.[1-3]

Tooth wear is considered to be a cumulative lifetime process,[1] an universal experience, and a multifactorial condition,[2] which may lead to substantial tooth surface loss. According to Eccles in 1982,[4] tooth surface loss or tooth wear refers to the pathological loss of tooth tissue by a disease process other than dental caries. It is an all-embracing term used to describe the combined processes of erosion, attrition, and abrasion. These processes include the friction of exogenous material (during mastication, tooth brushing, holding tools by the teeth) as it is forced over tooth surfaces (abrasion), the effect of antagonistic teeth (attrition), the chemical dissolution of tooth mineral (erosion), and finally, the impact of tensile and comprehensive forces during tooth flexure (abfraction). Many authors have suggested that the tooth wear observed in an individual will have resulted from a combination of all these processes, even though one may predominate. Examples of non-carious cervical lesions are illustrated in Figure 11.1.

Tooth erosion

The strategies to control tooth erosion include the early diagnosis and evaluation of etiological factors to identify persons at risk.[5] The elimination of the causative factors may be difficult,[6] since they are associated with habits or lifestyle.[7] As erosive lesions frequently require restorative intervention, and currently available fluoride products are not as effective as they are for caries prevention, new preventive treatments are needed to halt lesion progression.[8]

Research has focused on finding new methods for the prevention of dental erosion. The possibility of increasing enamel resistance to demineralization by laser irradiation was

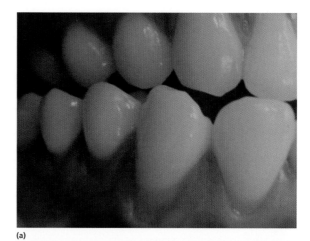
(a)

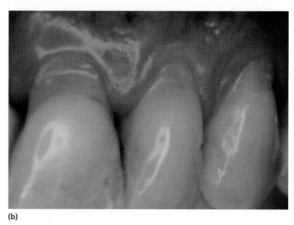
(b)

Figure 11.1 (a,b) Examples of tooth wear in anterior and posterior teeth. The non-carious cervical lesions are easily observed.

first demonstrated with a ruby laser.[9] Over time, due to the strong absorption of the wavelengths between 9000 and 11000 nm by enamel and dentin, the effect of the CO_2 laser in the prevention of demineralization was also tested. Satisfactory results relating to the inhibition of incipient caries were observed (see Chapter 16). However, it was only in the last 5–10 years, with the

Lasers in Dentistry: Guide for Clinical Practice, First Edition. Edited by Patrícia M. de Freitas and Alyne Simões.
© 2015 John Wiley & Sons, Inc. Published 2015 by John Wiley & Sons, Inc.

Table 11.1 Summary of studies testing the role of high power lasers in the prevention of erosion

Authors	Study type	Study description	Results
Vlacic et al. (2007)[10]	*In vitro* study	Different laser wavelengths (argon 488 and 514 nm; KTP 532 nm; diode 633, 670, and 830 nm; Nd:YAG 1064 nm) following previous application of sodium fluoride (1.23%) to increase the resistance of enamel and dentin to acid dissolution (HCl 1 M for 5 minutes). Each wavelength was used at a different power, exposure time, and power density, but fluence was maintained at 15 J/cm^2 for all groups. Vickers hardness number was recorded.	All wavelengths examined had a protective effect against softening.
Magalhaes et al. (2008)[11]	*In vitro* study	Different Nd:YAG laser parameters (35, 52.5, and 70 J/cm^2) combined with acidulated phosphate fluoride (APF) gel or fluoride varnish (FV) were tested in the prevention of dentin erosion (analyzed with profilometry). Samples were stored in artificial saliva for 24 hours and submitted to four erosive 1-minute cycles in Sprite-light®.	Laser irradiation did not reduce dentin erosion. However, fluoride application increased the dentin's resistance to erosion, and APF showed better results than FV.
Rios et al. (2009)[12]	*In vitro* study	As for Magalhaes et al.[11]	The combined used of APF application and laser irradiation seems to be a promising preventive measure against dental erosion.
Sobral et al. (2009)[13]	*In vitro* study	The effect of the Nd:YAG laser (1 W, 100 mJ, 10 Hz; 141.5 J/cm^2, 125 J/cm^2) both combined with and without APF was tested in the prevention of erosion and erosion/abrasion in bovine and human enamel. The teeth were coated with a dark dye (photoabsorber). Microhardness and sample mass were analyzed.	Nd:YAG laser irradiation was more effective when combined with APF (bovine and human enamel) in terms of both increased surface microhardness and reduced wear for both human and bovine enamel.
Wiegand et al. (2010)[14]	*In vitro* study	The effectiveness of the CO$_2$ laser (10 600 nm, 10 μs, 50 Hz) combined with titanium tetrafluoride (TiF$_4$) and amine fluoride (AmF) was tested in protecting enamel and dentin against erosion *in vitro*. Samples were submitted to a 5-day de- and re-mineralization cycle using Sprite Zero® four times daily for 90 seconds. Surface loss was analyzed using profilometry.	AmF decreased enamel and dentin erosion, but CO$_2$ laser irradiation did not improve its efficacy. TiF$_4$ showed only a limited capacity to prevent erosion, but CO$_2$ laser irradiation significantly enhanced its ability to reduce enamel erosion. With the parameters tested, laser alone did not prevent enamel and dentin erosion.
Steiner-Oliveira et al. (2010)[15]	*In vitro* study	The effect of CO$_2$ laser irradiation (10 600 nm, enamel: 1 J/cm^2, 3 W; 5 ms pulse duration, 10 Hz; dentin: 0.6 J/cm^2, 2 W, 5 ms pulse duration, 2 Hz) alone and with previous fluoride gel application on resistance of enamel and dentin to erosion by citric acid (0.3%) was evaluated. Dental surface losses as well as the concentration of calcium, phosphorous, and fluoride in the demineralization solutions were determined after each cycle.	Laser alone did not prevent enamel or dentin surface losses due to erosion. When combined with fluoride, it showed some protective effect, but according to the authors, this was mostly due to the fluoride effect.
Esteves-Oliveira et al. (2011)[16]	*In vitro* study	The effectiveness of CO$_2$ laser irradiation (10 600 nm, 0.3 J/cm^2, 5 μs, 226 Hz) on preventing softening was evaluated in sound and in already softened enamel *in vitro*. Half of the sample was acid softened with citric acid before surface irradiation and the other half after irradiation. Surface microhardness was measured and fluoride uptake in enamel was quantified.	CO$_2$ laser irradiation of dental enamel not only significantly decreased erosive mineral loss (97%), but also rehardened previously softened enamel *in vitro*.
Esteves-Oliveira et al. (2011)[17]	*In vitro* study	The effect of CO$_2$ laser irradiation (10 600 nm, 0.3 J/cm^2, 5 μs, 226 Hz) alone and combined with AmF was tested on the resistance of softened enamel to toothbrushing abrasion (25-day erosive–abrasive cycle in 100 mL of Sprite-light® for 90 seconds; teeth were brushed twice daily with an electric toothbrush). Surface loss was measured with a digital profilometer.	CO$_2$ laser irradiation alone or in combination with AmF gel significantly decreased toothbrushing abrasion of softened enamel.
Ramalho (2011)[18]	*In situ* study	CO$_2$ laser irradiation (10 600 nm, 0.3 J/cm^2, 5 μs, 226 Hz) alone and combined with AmF was evaluated for the prevention of enamel erosion due to citric acid exposure for 20 minutes twice daily for 5 days. Ten volunteers participated in this study. Enamel loss was measured with a digital profilometer.	CO$_2$ laser irradiation at these parameters and combined with AmF decreased enamel surface erosion caused by citric acid. This effect was still observed after 5 days of repeated acid attacks.
Wegehaupt et al. (2011)[19]	*In vitro* study	The protective effect of a cerium solution and a combination of cerium/fluoride solutions was evaluated for the prevention of mineral loss from dentin under erosive conditions. The possible additive effect of concomitant CO$_2$ laser irradiation (10 600 nm, 0.5 W, 20 Hz, 100 ms, 30 s) was tested.	The highest antierosive potential was found for combined cerium chloride and AmF application. Laser irradiation had no adjunctive effect.
Magalhães et al. (2011)[20]	*In vitro* study	The effectiveness of Nd:YAG laser irradiation was tested on the efficacy of TiF$_4$ and NaF varnishes and solutions in the protection of enamel against erosion.	Nd:YAG laser irradiation was not effective in preventing enamel erosion and it did not have any influence on the efficacy of fluoride, except when in TiF$_4$ solution. On the other hand, TiF$_4$ varnish alone protected against enamel erosion.

(Continued)

Table 11.1 (*Continued*)

Authors	Study type	Study description	Results
Altinok et al. (2011)[21]	*In vitro* study	The potential effect of Er:YAG laser irradiation (2940 nm, 1.2 J/cm², 10 Hz, 300 μm) on the prevention of erosive demineralization of human enamel (10 minutes of soft drink immersion) was tested either alone or combined with APF gel (1.23% APF). Microhardness was evaluated.	Er:YAG laser irradiation alone or combined with APF decreased enamel solubility, but combined treatment did not show any significant additional effect.
Ramalho et al. (2012)[22]	*In vitro* study	CO_2 laser irradiation (10 600 nm, 0.3 J/cm², 5 μs, 226 Hz) was evaluated alone and combined with AmF for the prevention of enamel erosion due to citric acid exposure for 20 minutes twice daily for 5 days. After 1, 3, and 5 days, surface loss was measured with a digital profilometer.	On all days there was less enamel loss with both laser irradiation alone and combined with fluoride treatment than in the fluoride and control groups. Laser irradiation could effectively reduce enamel surface loss due to citric acid exposure and the effect was still observed after 5 days of repeated acid exposures.
Esteves-Oliveira et al. (2012)[23]	*In vitro* study	Several CO_2 laser (10 600 nm) parameters were tested on enamel resistance to a continuous flow erosive challenge. The parameters tested varied from 0.1 to 0.9 J/cm², pulse durations from 80 to 400 μs, and repetition rates from 180 to 700 Hz. All samples were eroded by exposure to continuous flow hydrochloric acid (pH 2.6).	The set of CO_2 laser parameters in a new clinical device (200-μs pulse duration) could significantly reduce enamel mineral loss (20%) under *in vitro* erosive conditions. However, this reduction was smaller than that previously observed with an industrial laser and all parameters also caused surface cracking. Therefore, none of the irradiation conditions tested with this new laser equipment is recommended for clinical use.

increase of erosion prevalence, that the first investigations were conducted to translate the efficient CO_2 laser interaction with the dental tissues into a possible positive effect in the prevention of erosion. Table 11.1 describes the published studies testing high power lasers in the prevention of erosion lesions.

As the research methodologies (laser wavelength, fluency, pulse width, erosion challenge, and other variables) used to study high power lasers in the prevention of erosion varies among the studies, it is not possible to compare the effectiveness of the lasers. Some studies showed partial beneficial results with Nd:YAG lasers,[10,12,13] but the studies were not continued and each used different parameters. On the other hand, the preventive effect of CO_2 laser irradiation on erosion has been shown in several studies using the same laser parameters (10 600 nm, 0.3 J/cm², 5 μs, 226 Hz) but different erosion challenges.[16–18,22]

As in *in situ* studies other biological factors present in the oral cavity, such as saliva buffer capacity and contact with soft tissues, are also simulated, this type of research model is recognized as a good predictor of clinical effectiveness of preventive therapies. The single *in situ* study evaluating the impact of CO_2 laser irradiation on increasing enamel resistance to erosion showed a positive result with a special set of parameters (10 600 nm, 0.3 J/cm², 5 μs, 226 Hz), as already had already been observed in caries studies.[18]

Regarding the acid resistance of erbium laser-irradiated enamel, only very few studies have been published. Although irradiation from this laser is relatively well absorbed by tooth tissues, its absorption by hydroxyapatite is lower than that for the CO_2 laser wavelengths. Considering this and the fact that the success rate of wavelengths around 300 nm for increasing enamel caries resistance has not been high and increases are often only observed when combined with fluoride products, there is, at present, no reason to suppose that this irradiation

performs better than that at wavelengths of 9000–11000 nm. However, this should be confirmed in future studies.

In conclusion, based on the current literature, CO_2 laser irradiation at a wavelength of 10 600 nm, low energy density (0.3 J/cm²), and short pulse width (5 μs), seems to be promising in the prevention of tooth erosion. Nevertheless, it is important to point out that this set of parameters is not yet available in any clinical laser equipment.

Dentin hypersensitivity

The growing number of cases of dentin hypersensitivity (DH), whose cause is directly related to the exposure of dentin following removal of enamel (as a result of the processes of tooth wear: erosion, abrasion, and attrition) or loss of periodontal tissue, should be appreciated.[3,24]

DH presents in dentistry as one of the most painful and chronic pathologies. The prevalence is between 4% and 74%; this wide variation is attributed to the different methodologies used and populations studied.[25–29]

According to the Canadian Advisory Board on Dentin Hypersensitivity, DH should be defined as a "short, sharp pain arising from exposed dentin in response to stimuli, typically thermal, evaporative, tactile, osmotic or chemical, and which cannot be ascribed to any other form of dental defect or pathology."[30]

The risk factors for cervical lesions and DH include age, chronic trauma such as from brushing, diet, gastric and esophageal disorders, parafunctional habits, gingival inflammation, and chronic and acute trauma of periodontal surgery.[31,32]

After differential diagnosis, predisposing factors for DH must first be removed or modified, followed by some form of treatment, depending on the severity and extent of the cervical

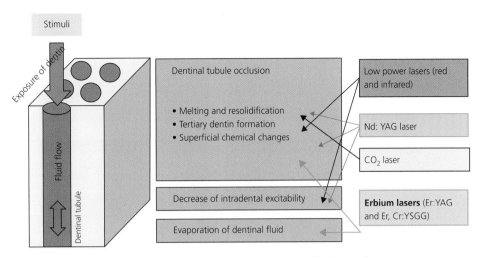

Figure 11.2 Schematic of the mechanisms of treatment of dentin hypersensitivity with low and high power lasers.

lesion.[3] Occlusal adjustment instructions and advice on diet and oral hygiene should be provided to the patient prior to treatment.

As already described, for a diagnosis of DH, exposure of dentinal tubules is a prerequisite. Thus, the treatment should provide a barrier that obliterates all or part of the tubules, preventing the movement of the fluid; this treatment is a logical conclusion from the hydrodynamic theory postulated by Brännström and Aström in the 1960s.[33]

The introduction of laser technology (high and low power lasers) can provide reliable and reproducible therapy for the treatment of DH.[34] Desensitization with laser technology depends on the type of equipment used. Low power lasers, which act by biomodulating cellular responses, will promote a reduction in pain levels by depolarizing nerve fibers and the formation of tertiary dentin.[35] On the other hand, high power lasers block the entrances to the dentinal tubules through thermal and mechanical action (Fig. 11.2).

The low power lasers consist of a crystal of semiconductor diode of gallium arsenide (GaAs) and may include other elements, depending on the desired wavelength; they emit wavelengths in the range of the near infrared part of the spectrum from 780 nm to 900 nm.[34,36]

The proposed mechanisms for the effects of low level power laser therapy (LLLT) require serious considerations and further experiments. It is believed that the low power lasers stimulate nerve cells by interfering with the polarity of the cell membrane by increasing the amplitude of the action potential of the membrane, thereby blocking the transmission of painful stimuli. There is also evidence in the literature that LLLT helps to reduce inflammation and also enhance the formation of reactionary dentin (Fig. 11.2), reducing the repair time of the pulp tissue and, consequently, promoting patient comfort and analgesia.[35,37]

The protocol developed by Groth supports the use of low power lasers in the treatment of DH.[38] The protocol (4 J/cm[2], 15 mW, 10 seconds at four points: mesial, distal, middle and cervical) given in three sessions at intervals of 72 hours showed statistically significant results (Fig. 11.3). Further studies have also shown satisfactory results.[39–41]. Higher dosages have also been tested. Recently, Lopes and Aranha[42] showed the effect of different dosages in a 6-month clinical follow-up trial. The results for the different dosages were distinct, but all were efficient in reducing pain.

The photothermal effects of high power lasers promote melting and recrystallization of the dentin surface and thus partially or completely block the dentinal tubules, supporting the hydrodynamic theory of Brännström and Aström.[33] (Fig. 11.2). It is noteworthy that Nd:YAG laser irradiation melts the dentinal structure, and under refrigeration, these resolidify to form hydroxyapatite crystals larger than those of the initial structures. Investigations into this recrystallized structure have shown a "glazed" non-porous surface with partial or total obliteration of the dentinal tubules.[43–51] Some authors have also suggested that the Nd:YAG laser interferes with the neural cell membrane permeability of the nerve fibers.[52] Figure 11.4 illustrates the high power laser equipment used for DH at the Special Laboratory of Lasers in Dentistry (LELO) at the School of Dentistry of the University of São Paulo, Brazil.

Other high power lasers can be used in the treatment of DH. CO_2 laser irradiation has been shown to narrow the dentinal tubules, reducing dentin permeability.[53,54] When combined with calcium hydroxide paste, it provides satisfactory results, as recently reported by Romano et al.[55] Despite their high water and hydroxyapatite absorption and indication for hard tooth tissue ablation, the erbium lasers (Er:YAG and Er,Cr:YSGG) are suitable for the treatment of DH (Fig. 11.5).[56–61]

Cunha-Cruz et al.[62] recently reviewed the scientific evidence for the use of lasers in DH treatment. Results showed a small clinical advantage over other treatments. However, the authors concluded that larger samples, with assessment of long-term, randomized controlled trials, are needed before definitive conclusions can be made. In another recent systematic review,

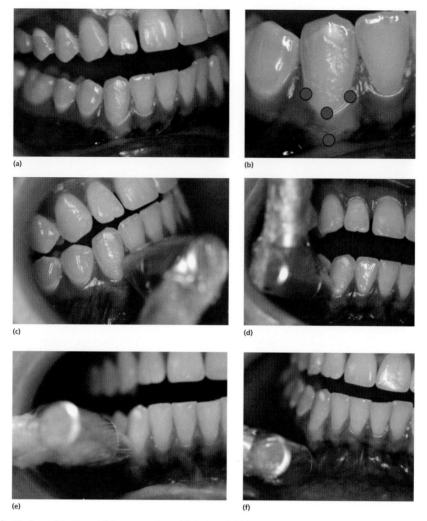

Figure 11.3 Protocol for dentin desensitization with low power laser (Twin Lase/MMOptics: spot size 0.04 cm², 780 nm, 3.8 J/cm², 15 mW, 0.16 J per point, 10 seconds per point). (a) Initial image; (b) four points of irradiation (three cervical: mesial, central and distal; and one apical); (c) irradiation in contact, perpendicular to the surface, in the cervical/mesial part of the tooth; (d) irradiation in the distal portion; (e) irradiation in the central portion of the cervical part; (f) irradiation in the apical part of the tooth. This protocol should be repeated in three sessions with intervals of 72 hours between them. (Clinical case performed at the Special Laboratory of Lasers in Dentistry [LELO] by the postgraduate students at the Discipline of Lasers in Dentistry in the Department of Restorative Dentistry, School of Dentistry, University of São Paulo.)

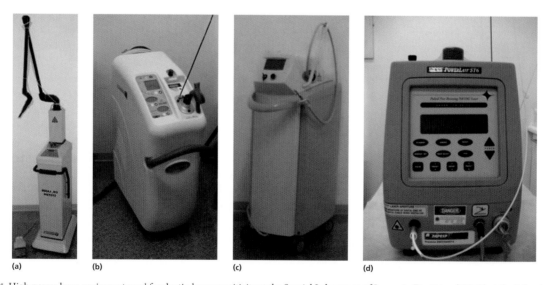

Figure 11.4 High power laser equipment used for dentin hypersensitivity at the Special Laboratory of Lasers in Dentistry (LELO) at the School of Dentistry of University of São Paulo, Brazil. (a) CO_2 laser – Union Medical/10 600 nm; (b) Er,Cr:YSGG laser/Waterlase – Biolase/2780 nm; (c) Er:YAG laser – KaVo/2940 nm; (d) Nd:YAG laser – Lares Research/1094 nm.

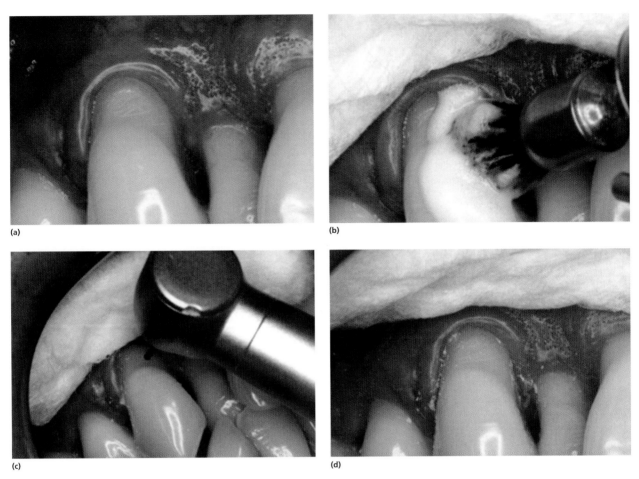

Figure 11.5 Protocol for the irradiation of a non-carious cervical lesion with an Er,Cr:YSGG laser (Waterlase/Biolase). (a) Initial image; (b) oral prophylaxis with pumice; (c) handpiece positioned 2 mm away from the exposed dentin (tip Z6, 600 μm, 0.25 W, 20 Hz); (d) final irradiated surface.

Sgolastra et al.[63] showed that of 18 661 articles published on the subject, only three met the inclusion criteria and a meta-analysis was not possible due to the wide variability of the information reported. The authors showed that although laser irradiation reduced pain, the evidence was not conclusive. Further randomized controlled trials over longer time periods are required to evaluate the effectiveness of lasers in DH.

Consideration of the severity of the DH is necessary prior to the utilization of laser irradiation in order that a correct and safe protocol is used. However, considering its effectiveness and simplicity, laser treatment, both low and high power, is a conservative choice and appropriate for the treatment of DH, provided that correct protocols, based on scientific evidence, are used.

References

1 Lussi A. Erosive tooth wear - a multifactorial condition of growing concern and increasing knowledge. *Monogr Oral Sci* 2006; 20: 1–8.

2 Bartlett D. A new look at erosive tooth wear in elderly people. *J Am Dent Assoc* 2007; 138 (Suppl): 21S–25S.

3 West NX. Dentine hypersensitivity: preventive and therapeutic approaches to treatment. *Periodontol* 2000 2008; 48: 31–41.

4 Eccles JD. Tooth surface loss from abrasion, attrition and erosion. *Dent Update* 1982; 9(7): 373–374, 376–378, 380–381.

5 Lussi A, Hellwig E. Risk assessment and preventive measures. *Monogr Oral Sci* 2006; 20: 190–199.

6 Amaechi BT, Higham SM. *In vitro* remineralization of eroded enamel lesions by saliva. *J Dent* 2001; 29(5): 371–376.

7 Serra MC, Messias DC, Turssi CP. Control of erosive tooth wear: possibilities and rationale. *Braz Oral Res* 2009; 23 (Suppl 1): 49–55.

8 Young A, Amaechi BT, Dugmore C, et al. Current erosion indices-flawed or valid? *Summary. Clin Oral Invest* 2008; 12 (Suppl 1): S59–63.

9 Stern RH, Sognnaes RF. Laser inhibition of dental caries suggested by first tests in vivo. *J Am Dent Assoc* 1972; 85(5): 1087–1090.

10 Vlacic J, Meyers IA, Walsh LJ. Laser-activated fluoride treatment of enamel as prevention against erosion. *Aust Dent J* 2007; 52(3): 175–180.

11 Magalhães AC, Rios D, Machado MA, et al. Effect of Nd:YAG irradiation and fluoride application on dentine resistance to erosion *in vitro*. *Photomed Laser Surg* 2008; 26(6): 559–563.

12 Rios D, Magalhães AC, Machado MA, et al. *In vitro* evaluation of enamel erosion after Nd:YAG laser irradiation and fluoride application. *Photomed Laser Surg* 2009; 27(5): 743–747.

13 Sobral MA, Lachowski KM, de Rossi W, Braga SR, Ramalho KM. Effect of Nd:YAG laser and acidulated phosphate fluoride on bovine

and human enamel submitted to erosion/abrasion or erosion only: an *in vitro* preliminary study. *Photomed Laser Surg* 2009; 27(5): 709–713.

14 Wiegand A, Magalhães AC, Navarro RS, et al. Effect of titanium tetrafluoride and amine fluoride treatment combined with carbon dioxide laser irradiation on enamel and dentin erosion. *Photomed Laser Surg* 2010; 28(2): 219–226.

15 Steiner-Oliveira C, Nobre-dos-Santos M, Zero DT, Eckert G, Hara AT. Effect of a pulsed CO_2 laser and fluoride on the prevention of enamel and dentine erosion. *Arch Oral Biol* 2010; 55(2): 127–133.

16 Esteves-Oliveira M, Pasaporti C, Heussen N, Eduardo CP, Lampert F, Apel C. Rehardening of acid-softened enamel and prevention of enamel softening through CO_2 laser irradiation. *J Dent* 2011; 39(6): 414–421.

17 Esteves-Oliveira M, Pasaporti C, Heussen N, Eduardo CP, Lampert F, Apel C. Prevention of toothbrushing abrasion of acid-softened enamel by CO_2 laser irradiation. *J Dent* 2011; 39(9): 604–611.

18 Ramalho KM. Prevention of enamel erosion through CO_2 laser irradiation. An *in situ* study. PhD Thesis. Universitiy of São Paulo, Brazil and RWTH Aachen Germany, 2011.

19 Wegehaupt FJ, Sener B, Attin T, Schmidlin PR. Anti-erosive potential of amine fluoride, cerium chloride and laser irradiation application on dentine. *Arch Oral Biol* 2011; 56(12): 1541–1547.

20 Magalhães AC, Romanelli AC, Rios D, et al. Effect of a single application of TiF4 and NaF varnishes and solutions combined with Nd:YAG laser irradiation on enamel erosion *in vitro*. *Photomed Laser Surg* 2011; 29(8): 537–544.

21 Altinok B, Tanboga I, Peker S, Eren F, Bakkal M, Peker F. The effect of laser-activated acidulated phosphate fluoride on enamel submitted to erosive solution only: an *in vitro* preliminary evaluation. *Eur J Paediatr Dent* 2011; 12(1): 13–16.

22 Ramalho KM, de Paula Eduardo C, Heussen N, et al. Protective effect of CO_2 laser (10.6 µm) and fluoride on enamel erosion *in vitro*. *Lasers Med Sci* 2013; 28: 71–78.

23 Esteves-Oliveira M, Yu H, Eduardo CD, et al. Screening of CO_2 laser (10.6 µm) parameters for prevention of enamel erosion. *Photomed Laser Surg* 2012; 30.

24 West NX. Dentine hypersensitivity. *Monogr Oral Sci.* 2006; 20: 173–189.

25 Rees JS, Jin LJ, Lam S, Kudanowska I, Vowles R. The prevalence of dentine hypersensitivity in a hospital clinic population in Hong Kong. *J Dent* 2003; 31(7): 453–461.

26 Flynn J, Galloway R, Orchardson R. The incidence of 'hypersensitive' teeth in the West of Scotland. *J Dent* 1985; 13(3): 230–236.

27 Fischer C, Fischer RG, Wennberg A. Prevalence and distribution of cervical dentine hypersensitivity in a population in Rio de Janeiro, Brazil. *J Dent* 1992; 20(5): 272–276.

28 Irwin CR, McCusker P. Prevalence of dentine hypersensitivity in a general dental population. *J Ir Dent Assoc* 1997; 43(1): 7–9.

29 Taani DQ, Awartani F. Prevalence and distribution of dentin hypersensitivity and plaque in a dental hospital population. *Quintessence Int* 2001; 32(5): 372–376.

30 Canadian Advisory Board on Dentin Hypersensitivity. Consensus-based recommendations for the diagnosis and management of dentin hypersensitivity. *J Can Dent Assoc* 2003; 69(4): 221–228.

31 Addy M, Urquhat E. Dentine hypersensitivity: Its prevalence, aetiology and clinical management. *Dent Update* 1992; 19(10): 407–408, 410–412.

32 Jacobsen PL, Bruce G. Clinical dentin hypersensitivity: understanding the causes and prescribing a treatment. *J Contemp Dent Pract* 2001; 2(1): 1–12.

33 Brännström M, Aström A. The hydrodynamics of the dentine; its possible relationship to dentinal pain. *Int Dent J* 1972; 22(2): 219–227.

34 Kimura Y, et al. Treatment of dentine hypersensitivity by lasers: a review. *J Clin Periodontol* 2000; 27(10): 715–721.

35 Ferreira AN, Silveira L, Genovese WJ, et al. Effect of GaAIAs laser on reactional dentinogenesis induction in human teeth. *Photomed Laser Surg* 2006; 24(3): 358–365.

36 Benetti AR, Franco EB, Franco EJ, Pereira JC. Laser therapy for dentin hypersensitivity: A critical appraisal. *J Oral Laser Appl* 2004; 4: 271–278.

37 Matsui S, Tsujimoto Y, Matsushima K. Stimulatory effects of hydroxyl radical generation by Ga-Al-As laser irradiation on mineralization ability of human dental pulp cells. *Biol Pharm Bull* 2007; 30(1): 27–31.

38 Groth EB. *Scientific contribution to the treatment of dentin hypersensitivity with low power laser of Ga-Al-As. (Dissertation).* Sao Paulo. School of Dentistry of University of São Paulo, 1993.

39 Tengrungsun T, Sangkla W. Comparative study in desensitizing efficacy using the GaAlAs laser and dentin bonding agent. *J Dent* 2008; 36(6): 392–395.

40 Aranha AC, Pimenta LA, Marchi GM. Clinical evaluation of desensitizing treatments for cervical dentin hypersensitivity. *Braz Oral Res* 2009; 23(3): 333–339.

41 Orhan K, Aksoy U, Can-Karabulut DC, Kalender A. Low-level laser therapy of dentin hypersensitivity: a short-term clinical trial. *Lasers Med Sci* 2011; 26(5): 591–598.

42 Lopes AO, Aranha ACC. Clinical evaluation of different protocols on cervical dentin hypersensitivity treatment. Medicina Oral, Patologia Oral Y Cirurgia Bucal. 13th Congress of WFLD, Barcelona, 2012.

43 Liu HC, Lin CP, Lan WH. Sealing depth of Nd:YAG laser on human dentinal tubules. *J Endod* 1997; 23(11): 691–693.

44 Lan WH, Liu HC, Lin CP. The combined occluding effect of sodium fluoride varnish and Nd:YAG laser irradiation on human dentinal tubules. *J Endod* 1999; 25(6): 424–426.

45 Lier BB, Rosing CK, Aass AM, Gjermo P. Treatment of dentin hypersensitivity by Nd:YAG laser. *J Clin Periodontol* 2002; 29(6): 501–506.

46 Ciaramicoli MT, Carvalho RC, Eduardo CP. Treatment of cervical dentin hypersensitivity using neodymium: Yttrium-aluminum-garnet laser. *Clinical evaluation. Lasers Surg Med* 2003; 33(5): 358–362.

47 Aranha AC, Domingues FB, Franco VO, Gutknecht N, Eduardo CP. Effects of Er:YAG and Nd:YAG lasers on dentin permeability in root surfaces: a preliminary *in vitro* study. *Photomed Laser Surg* 2005; 23(5): 504–508.

48 Naylor F, Aranha AC, Eduardo Cde P, Arana-Chavez VE, Sobral MA. Micromorphological analysis of dentinal structure after irradiation with Nd:YAG laser and immersion in acidic beverages. *Photomed Laser Surg* 2006; 24(6): 745–752.

49 Birang R, Poursamimi J, Gutknecht N, Lampert F, Mir M. Comparative evaluation of the effects of Nd:YAG and Er:YAG laser in dentine hypersensitivity treatment. *Lasers Med Sci* 2007; 22(1): 21–24.

50 Dilsiz A, Aydin T, Canakci V, Gungormus M. Clinical evaluation of Er:YAG, Nd:YAG, and diode laser therapy for desensitization of teeth with gingival recession. *Photomed Laser Surg* 2010; 28 (Suppl 2): S11–17.

51 Al-Saud L, Al-Nahedh H. Occluding effect of Nd:YAG laser and different dentin desensitizing agents on human dentinal tubules *in vitro*: A scanning electron Microscopy Investigation. *Oper Dent* 2012 Feb 7.

52 Yonaga K, Kimura Y, Matsumoto K. Treatment of cervical dentin hypersensitivity by various methods using pulsed Nd:YAG laser. *J Clin Laser Med Surg* 1999; 17(5): 205–210.

53 Moritz A, Schoop U, Goharkhay K, et al. Long-term effects of CO2 laser irradiation on treatment of hypersensitive dental necks: results of an in vivo study. *J Clin Laser Med Surg* 1998; 16(4): 211–215.

54 Gholami GA, Fekrazad R, Esmaiel-Nejad A, Kalhori KA. An evaluation of the occluding effects of Er;Cr:YSGG, Nd:YAG, CO_2 and diode lasers on dentineal tubules: a scanning electron microscope *in vitro* study. *Photomed Laser Surg* 2011; 29(2): 115–121.

55 Romano AC, Aranha AC, Lopes da Silveira B, Baldochi SL, Eduardo CP. Evaluation of carbon dioxide laser irradiation associated with calcium hydroxide in the treatment of dentineal hypersensitivity. A preliminary study. *Lasers Med Sci* 2011; 26(1): 35–42.

56 Schwarz F, Arweiler N, Georg T, Reich E. Desensitizing effects of an Er:YAG laser on hypersensitive dentine. *J Clin Periodontol* 2002; 29(3): 211–215.

57 Badran Z, Boutigny H, Struillou X, Baroth S, Laboux O, Soueidan A. Tooth desensitization with an Er:YAG laser: *in vitro* microscopical observation and a case report. *Lasers Med Sci* 2011; 26(1): 139–142.

58 Aranha AC, de Paula Eduardo C. Effects of Er:YAG and Er,Cr:YSGG lasers on dentine hypersensitivity. Short-term clinical evaluation. Lasers Med Sci 2011.

59 Aranha AC, de Paula Eduardo C. *In vitro* effects of Er,Cr:YSGG laser on dentine hypersensitivity. Dentine permeability and scanning electron microscopy analysis. Lasers Med Sci 2011.

60 Yilmaz HG, Kurtulmus-Yilmaz S, Cengiz E, Bayindir H, Aykac Y. Clinical evaluation of Er,Cr:YSGG and GaAlAs laser therapy for treating dentine hypersensitivity: A randomized controlled clinical trial. *J Dent.* 2011 Mar; 39(3): 249–54.

61 Yilmaz HG, Cengiz E, Kurtulmus-Yilmaz S, Leblebicioglu B. Effectiveness of Er,Cr:YSGG laser on dentine hypersensitivity: a controlled clinical trial. *J Clin Periodontol.* 2011 Apr; 38(4): 341–6.

62 Cunha-Cruz J, Wataha JC, Zhou L, et al. Treating dentin hypersensitivity: therapeutic choices made by dentists of the northwest PRECEDENT network. *J Am Dent Assoc* 2010; 141(9): 1097–1105.

63 Sgolastra F, Petrucci A, Gatto R, Monaco A. Effectiveness of laser in dentinal hypersensitivity treatment: a systematic review. *J Endod* 2011; 37(3): 297–303.

CHAPTER 12

Antimicrobial photodynamic therapy for carious tissue

Giselle Rodrigues de Sant'Anna and Danilo Antônio Duarte

Pediatric Dentistry, University Cruzeiro do Sul (UNICSUL), São Paulo, SP, Brazil

Minimal invasive dentistry (MID) is a relatively new philosophy that changes the paradigms regarding the restorative treatment of dental caries. The most significant change involves the principle of the maximum preservation of both healthy dental structures and structures capable of remineralization, which is contextualized in atraumatic restorative treatment and conservative dental surgery. Photodynamic therapy (PDT) is a component of two aspects of the minimal intervention protocol for dental caries treatment (i.e. prevention and cure) because the interaction of a specific wavelengths of light with a non-toxic compound (the photosensitizer [PS]) and oxygen can result in the production of reactive species, which are capable of inducing the death of bacterial cells in dental biofilms.

Traditional surgical methods have been shown to be ineffective in MID, and consequently, alternative methods have replaced the surgical procedure proposed by Black, including biological therapies that favor a less invasive treatment of carious lesions.[1] The success of these biological therapies relies on their more selective removal of carious tissue,[2–5] based on the biological principle that the carious lesion is composed of two layers: infected and affected. The first layer is highly infected, necrotic, and irreversibly disorganized, whereas the second layer is less infected and potentially remineralizable.[6,7] The methods for minimally invasive cavity preparation (MICP) reduce or eliminate the amount of bacteria inside the cavity without removing the carious tissue that is capable of remineralization (i.e. the affected dentin).[8] Importantly, the use of less invasive methods, which involve the partial removal of the carious lesion, and of MID have become more prevalent.

The partial removal of carious dentin and the subsequent sealing of the cavity is a treatment that remains under debate. Studies have shown that even the clinical criteria normally used for achieving the complete removal of carious tissue, including dentin staining and the degree of hardness, are not capable of ensuring dentin sterility[9] and cannot be trusted because they are empirical and subject to individual variations.[10] The microorganisms that are not removed are unable to cause further dental destruction under temporary restorations because

sealing prevents them from accessing the substrates that provide nutrients for survival. However, after a certain time has elapsed, some microorganism appear to survive, presumably using pulp fluid as a source of nutrients and the degradation of collagen as substrate and continue to destroy the dentin.[11] Given all of these uncertainties, the partial removal of carious dentin and the subsequent sealing of the cavity is still questionable and a risky strategy for clinicians in routine practice. Indeed, studies have not clearly demonstrated what happens to the bacteria that remain in the dentin after cavity preparation. In addition, there is no consensus about how much of the infected tissue should be removed and the level of residual infection considered to be acceptable for disease control. Therefore, dentin disinfection maneuvers prior to restorative procedures are considered to be salutary protocol measures in minimally invasive approaches.

Antimicrobial photodynamic therapy (aPDT) is a very promising method[12] (see Case studies 12.1 and 12.2) for dentin disinfection prior to restorative procedures because, in the presence of the oxygen found in cells, the light-activated PS is capable of reacting with surrounding molecules by electron or hydrogen transfer to produce free radicals (Type I reaction). Alternatively, energy transfer to oxygen (Type II reaction) can lead to the production of singlet oxygen. These reactions will cause microbial death.[13] One of the advantages of aPDT is that the development of resistance to it by microorganisms appears to be unlikely because singlet oxygen and free radicals interact with several different cell structures and metabolic pathways of microbial cells. aPDT is equally effective against antimicrobial-resistant bacteria and antimicrobial-susceptible bacteria, and repeated photosensitization has not been shown to induce the selection of resistant strains.[14]

The aPDT activity against Gram-positive/Gram-negative cariogenic bacteria (in homogeneous and mixed forms), planktonic cells, and biofilm cells has been reported for a series of PS and dosimetry parameters (Table 12.1).[15–35]

Bacterial variability in a carious lesion (anaerobic Gram-positive cocci in the sub-superficial portion and Gram-positive

Lasers in Dentistry: Guide for Clinical Practice, First Edition. Edited by Patrícia M. de Freitas and Alyne Simões.
© 2015 John Wiley & Sons, Inc. Published 2015 by John Wiley & Sons, Inc.

Table 12.1 Scientific studies on cariogenic bacteria and photodynamic therapy (PDT).

Authors (year)	Type of study	Mineralized hard tissues	Photosensitizer(s) (PS)	Light source	Dosimetry	Bacteria	Results
Okamoto et al.[15] (1992)	In vitro	–	Varied	HeNe laser 632.8 nm	$5\,J/cm^2$ $7\,J/cm^2$ $14.3\,J/cm^2$ $28.6\,J/cm^2$	Streptococcus mutans, Streptococcus rattus, Streptococcus cricetus, Streptococcus sobrinus, planktonic	Cariogenic bacteria were killed by HeNe irradiation and dyes, including toluidine blue, crystal violet, and cresyl blue
Burns et al.[16] (1992)	In vitro	–	Toluidine blue (0.005%) Disulfonated aluminum phthalocyanine	HeNe laser 632 nm and GaAlAs laser 660 nm		Streptococcus mutans, Streptococcus sobrinus, Actinomyces viscosus, Lactobacillus casei, Lactobacillus fermentum	Both PS and lasers led to bacterial death. S. sobrinus was more susceptible than Streptococcus mutans
Sarkar et al.[17] (1993)	In vitro	–	Toluidine blue (50 µg/mL)	HeNe laser 632 nm	–	Streptococcus spp.	94.2% reduction in viability
Burns et al.[18] (1993)	In vitro	–	Toluidine blue (from 0.1 to 1000 µg/mL)	HeNe laser 632.8 nm		Streptococcus mutans, Streptococcus sobrinus, Actinomyces viscosus, Lactobacillus casei	Up to 66% reduction in viable S. mutans, up to 99% in L. casei, up to 62% in S. sobrinus and up to 82% in A. viscosus. A statistically significant reduction in viability was observed with 1 µg/mL
Wilson et al.[19] (1995)	In vitro	–	Toluidine blue Disulfonated aluminum phthalocyanine	HeNe laser 632 nm and GaAlAs laser 660 nm	1.31 J	Streptococcus spp, Actinomyces spp	HeNe and toluidine blue were more effective with $\log_{10}$ reductions of 5.40 for Streptococcus spp and 3.34 for Actinomyces spp.
Burns et al.[20] (1995)	In vitro	Dentin	Toluidine blue	HeNe laser 632 nm	$67.2\,J/cm^2$ $134.4\,J/cm^2$ $268.8\,J/cm^2$	Streptococcus mutans, planktonic	Higher energy densities caused greater reduction in S. mutans viability in dentin
Wilson et al.[21] (1996)	In vitro	Hydroxyapatite	Disulfonated aluminum phthalocyanine	GaAlAs laser 660 nm	$61.2\,J/cm^2$ 12.2 J	Streptococcus sanguinis, biofilm	Significantly reduced viable bacterial counts
Wood et al.[22] (1999)	In situ	–	Pyridinium zinc phthalocyanine (20 µg/mL)	Tungsten light 600–700 nm	$22.5\,mW/cm^2$	Mixed biofilm	Biofilm with less evidence of channels and a less dense biomass. Bacteria under the effect of PDT suffered considerable damage (i.e. cytoplasmic vacuolization and membrane damage)
De Sant'Anna[23] (2001)	In vivo	Dentin	Toluidine blue (50 µg/mL)	Laser 650 nm	$29–100/cm^2$	Total bacteria	Reduction of viable bacteria by an average of 97% after PDT
O'Neill et al.[24] (2002)	In vitro	–	Toluidine blue	HeNe laser 632 nm	$31.5\,J/cm^2$	Mixed biofilm	97.4% level of bacteria death
Zanin et al.[25] (2005)	In vitro	Hydroxyapatite	Toluidine blue	HeNe laser 632 nm and LED 638 nm	$49\,J/cm^2$ $147\,J/cm^2$ $294\,J/cm^2$	Biofilm, Streptococcus mutans	Reduction in viability by 99.9% Older biofilms were less susceptible to aPDT
Wood et al.[26] (2006)	In vitro	–	Erythrosine, methylene blue and Photofrin®	White light	15 min	Biofilm, Streptococcus mutans	Erythrosine was 1–2 $\log_{10}$ more effective than Photofrin in killing bacteria and 0.5–1 $\log_{10}$ more effective than methylene blue Photodynamic activity increased as biofilm age increased

(Continued)

Table 12.1 (Continued)

Authors (year)	Type of study	Mineralized hard tissues	Photosensitizer(s) (PS)	Light source	Dosimetry	Bacteria	Results
Zanin et al.[27] (2006)	In vitro	Enamel	Toluidine blue	LED	$85.7\,J/cm^2$	Biofilm, Streptococcus sobrinus, Streptococcus mutans, Streptococcus sanguinis	Significant reductions of 95% were observed for S. mutans and S. sobrinus and 99.9% for S. sanguinis
Metcalf et al.[28] (2006)	In vitro	–	Erythrosine	White light	Irradiation time 5 min and fractionation	Biofilm, Streptococcus mutans	A 2 $\log_{10}$ reduction in bacterial viability after 5 min. The fractionation of 10 × 30s had the best 3.7 $\log_{10}$ reduction
Müller et al.[29] (2007)	In vitro	Enamel	Methylene blue	Laser 665 nm	Irradiation time 60 s	Biofilm, S. sobrinus, Streptococcus oralis	Bacterial reduction obtained was smaller than one order of magnitude
Giusti et al.[30] (2008)	In vitro	Dentin	Photogem® (hematoporphyrin) (1, 2, and 3 mg/mL) Toluidine blue (0.0025 and 0.1 mg/mL)	LED 630 ± 10 nm	$24\,J/cm^2$ $48\,J/cm^2$	Lactobacillus acidophilus, Streptococcus mutans	Both PS combined with light resulted in a reduction in the number of bacteria; however, toluidine blue was more effective at a concentration of 0.1 mg/mL and $48\,J/cm^2$
Lima et al.[31] (2009)	In situ	Dentin	Toluidine blue (100 μg/mL)	LED	$47\,J/cm^2$ $94\,J/cm^2$	Mixed cultures, Streptococcus mutans, total microorganisms	Both energy densities combined with toluidine blue led to bacterial reduction; the most significant reduction was observed at $94\,J/cm^2$
Longo et al.[32] (2010)	In vitro	Dentin	Methylene blue (25 and 50 μg/mL)	Laser 660 nm	$6.8\,J/cm^2$ $20.55\,J/cm^2$ $61.65\,J/cm^2$	Mixed cultures arising from carious dentin	The energy densities of 20.5 and 61.65 J/cm² were both effective in bacterial reduction, but the latter is more suitable for aPDT
Longo et al.[33] (2012)	In vitro and in vivo	Dentin	Aluminum chloride–phthalocyanine in liposomes	Laser 660 nm	$6.8\,J/cm^2$ $20.55\,J/cm^2$ $61.65\,J/cm^2$ $180\,J/cm^2$ in vivo	Mixed cultures arising from and on carious dentin	82% reduction in total bacteria
Guglielmi et al.[34] (2011)	In vivo	Dentin	Methylene blue (0.01% 100 mg/L)	Laser 660 nm	$320\,J/cm^2$	Streptococcus mutans, Lactobacillus ssp. and total bacteria	A 1.38 $\log_{10}$ reduction for Streptococcus mutans, 0.93 $\log_{10}$ reduction for Lactobacillus ssp. and 0.91 for total bacteria.
Vahabi et al.[35] (2011)	In vitro	–	Toluidine blue (0.1%) Radachlorin® (0.1%)	Laser 662 nm 633 nm	$3\,J/cm^2$ $12\,J/cm^2$	Streptococcus mutans, planktonic	Potential bacterial reduction was only observed with toluidine blue and 3 J/cm²

LED, light emitting diode.

rods and Gram-negative bacteria in the deeper portion) requires the appropriate selection of a PS. The use of a cationic dye, due to the interaction of this type of substance with bacterial characteristics, or a nanostructured PS, such as those found in cationic liposomes, is recommended for the treatment of carious lesions.[33] Cationic dyes can increase the efficiency of the photoinactivation process in Gram-negative bacteria because the positive charges of the PS appear to promote an electrostatic interaction with negatively charged areas on the external surfaces of the bacterial cells.[36] Toluidine blue and methylene blue, which cause bacterial death through lipid photoperoxidation, are attractive choices for the treatment of bacterial infection in carious lesions because of their affinity for bacterial membranes.

One consideration in the practice of dentin disinfection with aPDT is that the depth to which the PS is able to penetrate in the carious dentin is unclear. Lethal photosensitization occurs predominantly in the most external layers of the biofilm and carious tissue,[24] which are believed to be responsible for the inability of the PS to diffuse to inner layers. In addition, the light may not be completely transmitted because the interaction of the demineralized dentin with the light beam is complex. This interaction likely involves the refraction and reflection of the beam on the surface of hydroxyapatite crystals in the peri- and inter-tubular dentin, which results in the dissipation of the energy delivered by the laser source.

In addition to the need for an actual interaction time for the bacteria to be sensitized by the photodynamic agent, the pre-irradiation exposure time is an important factor for the diffusion of PS through the tissue (see Clinical cases 12.1 and 12.2). An interval of 1–5 minutes[37,38] is ideal for the maximum uptake of the PS. A time interval of 3–5 minutes is recommended for dentin disinfection because the microorganisms are both superficial and deep in the dentinal tubules.

The concentration of the PS is another factor that needs to be considered because high concentrations of dyes may induce a "self-quenching" phenomenon, which would decrease the amount of light that actually reaches the bacteria and reduce the generation of reactive oxygen species (ROS). Concentrations of 10–100 µg/mL have been reported to effectively kill cariogenic bacteria[15–35] (see Table 12.1); however, the most frequently recommended concentrations are 25 and 50 µg/mL because of the complexity of the substrates. Nevertheless, it is worth noting that the degree of photodamage depends on the concentration of the dye and the intensity and the wavelength of the light.

There has been a high degree of variability with regards to the power, type of emitter, and energy density of the lasers used for PDT directed at oral microorganisms (see Table 12.1). The efficiency of energy densities is related to the amount of direct radiation that reaches the bacteria, and the interposition of demineralized tissues should be considered because the extent and effect of the light can be reduced by the thickness of the

interposing tissue and by the microscopic characteristics of the structure.[20] In dentin disinfection, the restriction of PS penetration and light transmission through the dentin substrate imposes a requirement for higher energy densities to overcome penetration and transmission obstacles.

Another variable that needs to be considered is the clinical time interval for surgical procedures. Indeed, a short light exposure time is desirable, even for high energy densities such as those recommended for carious dentin (100–300 J/cm²); therefore, the selection of a high power transmitting unit may constitute an advantage.

Many studies[15–35] have shown that different light sources and PS can be combined to promote a bactericidal effect (see Table 12.1). Because longer wavelengths allow for greater light penetration into the tissue, which is necessary with the use of aPDT on dentin, the combination of a blue PS and a red laser source is favorable from an antimicrobial and therapeutic point of view.

Interestingly, laser therapy combined with aPDT leads to cell induction and biomodulation (i.e. a state of normalization in the affected region, which, in the case of dentin, is the pulp cells). When a cell is irradiated with a low energy power that respects the cell's survival threshold, the energy provided will stimulate the cell's membrane or mitochondria.[39,40] For example, De Sant'Anna demonstrated the production of newly formed secondary dentin after the use of aPDT (Figs 12.1, 12.2, and 12.3) with laser on deciduous teeth *in vivo*, which, in turn, led to the obliteration of dentinal tubules[23] (Fig. 12.3). Therefore, the use of laser therapy with aPDT for carious dentin, which offers both disinfection and a biological stimulation for odontoblasts, results in a dentinal tissue response that works toward the control of disease progression and increases the chances of success of minimally invasive approaches.

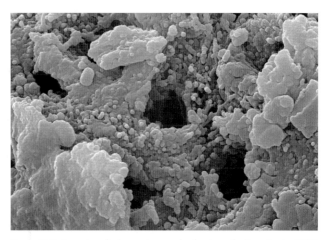

Figure 12.1 Scanning electron micrograph of carious dentin prior to aPDT. There are areas of great bacterial invasion without disruption to dentin, as well as dentinal tubules invaded by bacteria showing tubule disorganization (10 000×).

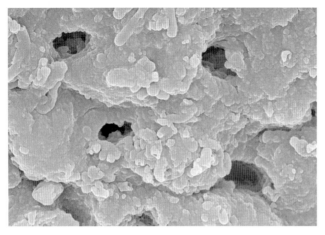

Figure 12.2 Scanning electron micrograph of the dentin surface immediately after aPDT, showing amorphous masses suggestive of bacterial death and an evident reduction in the bacterial population (20000×).

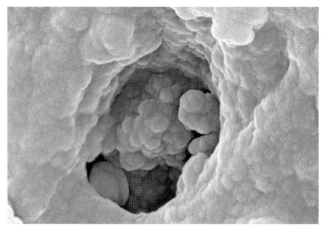

Figure 12.3 Tubular sclerosis or obliteration 90 days after aPDT therapy with lethal photosensitization in carious dentin.

Clinical case 12.1 Early childhood caries

A 4-year-old male child presented with early childhood caries. Some of his teeth presented with major coronary destructions, including teeth 54, 51, 61, 64, 74, and 84. For tooth 64, treatment with dental caries removal by aPDT and restoration with resin glass ionomer cement was chosen. Figure 12.4 shows the treatment step by step.

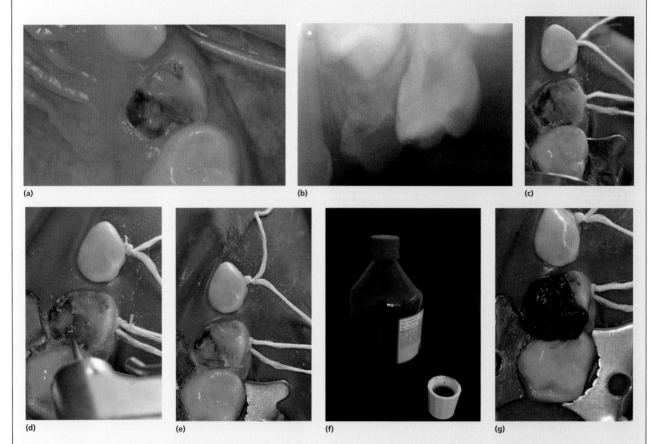

Figure 12.4 (a) Clinical view of carious lesion; (b) radiographic view of carious lesion; (c) necrotic dentin must be removed; (d) removal of necrotic dentin using a low speed rotation instrument; (e) affected and remineralizable dentin; (f) aqueous solution of methylene blue (50 μg/mL); (g) application of photosensitizer for 3 minutes; (h) stained affected dentin; (i) low power laser irradiation (665 nm; 100 J/cm²); (j) dentin after aPDT; (k) cleaning of the cavity with cotton dressing and water; (l) cleaned cavity; (m) resin glass ionomer cement tooth restoration; (n) tooth restoration using aPDT.

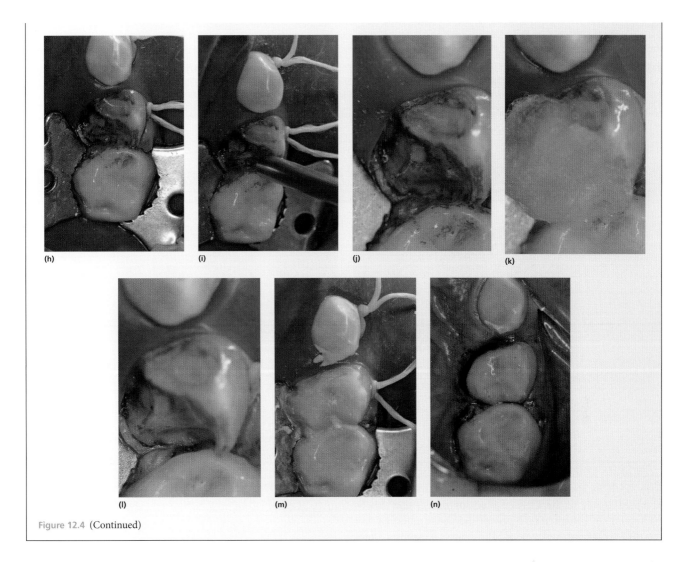

Figure 12.4 (Continued)

A 5-year-old male child attended the pediatric dentistry clinic following dental trauma with the intrusion of teeth 51 and 61. The child also had dental caries in teeth 75 and 85. The chosen treatment for tooth 85 was atraumatic restorative treatment combined with aPDT. Figure 12.5 shows the treatment step by step.

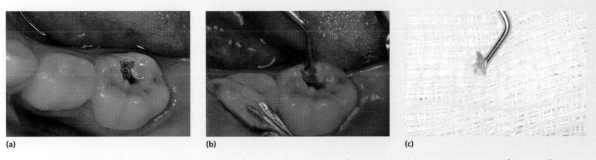

Figure 12.5 (a) Clinical view of carious lesion; (b) removal of necrotic dentin using a dentin curette; (c) macroscopic aspect of necrotic dentin; (d) affected and remineralizable dentin; (e) application of methylene blue (50 μg/mL) for 3 minutes; (f) stained affected dentin; (g) low power laser irradiation (665 nm; 100 J/cm^2); (h) atraumatic restorative treatment using glass ionomer combined with aPDT.

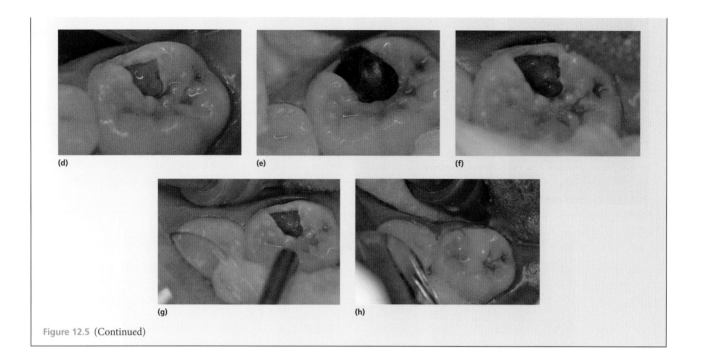

Figure 12.5 (Continued)

Conclusion

Consistent with the philosophy of MID, the use of laser therapy with aPDT for the treatment of dentinal lesions appears to be accepted as one of the least invasive approaches and can be chosen for any patient in both private and public practice.

aPDT with laser therapy as a MID approach assumes a preventive, curative characteristic, eliminates the aggressive nature of traditional clinical procedures, strengthens the natural defense mechanism of the pulp–dentin complex, and suppresses the lesions in a biological and conservative manner.

References

1 Barata TJE, Bresciani E, Mattos MCR, et al. Comparasion of two minimally invasive methods on the longevity of glass ionomer cement restorations: short-term results of a pilot study. *J Appl Oral Sci* 2008; 16: 155–160.

2 Banerjee A, Kidd EA, Watson TF. *In vitro* evaluation of five alternative methods of carious dentin excavation. *Caries Res* 2000; 34: 144–150

3 Banerjee A, Watson TF, Kidd EA. Dentine caries: Take it or leave it? *SADJ* 2001; 56: 186–192

4 Banerjee A, Kidd EA, Watson TF. *In vitro* validation of carious dentin removed using different excavation criteria. *Am J Dent* 2003; 16: 228–230.

5 Kidd EA How clean must a cavity be before restoration? *Caries Res* 2004; 38: 305–313

6 Fusayama T. Two layers of carious dentin; diagnosis and treatment. *Oper Dent* 1979; 4: 63–70.

7 Massler M. Pulpal reactions to dental caries. *Int Dent J* 1967; 17: 441–460.

8 Ericson D. What is minimally invasive dentistry? *Oral Health Prev Dent* 2003; 1: 59–72.

9 Nevesa AA, Coutinho E; Cardoso MV, et al. Current concepts and techniques for caries excavation and adhesion to residual dentin. *J Adhes Dent* 2011; 13: 7–22.

10 Maltz M, Henz S, Oliveira EF. A microbiological study of conventional and incomplete dentine caries removal. *Caries Res* 2004; 38: 367.

11 Mertz-Fairhurst EJ, Curtis JW, Ergle JW, et al. Ultraconservative and cariostatic sealed restorations: results at year 10. *J Am Dent Assoc* 1998; 129: 55–66.

12 Noack MJ, Wicht MJ, Haak R. Lesion orientated caries treatment–a classification of carious dentin treatment procedures. *Oral Health Prev Dent* 2004; 2: 301–306 .

13 Wainwright, M. Photodynamic antimicrobial chemotherapy (PACT). *J Antimicrob Chemother* 1998; 42: 13–28.

14 Wainwright M, Crossley KB. Photosensitizing agents—circumventing resistance and breaking down biofilms: a review. *Int Biodeterior Biodegrad* 2004; 53: 119–126.

15 Okamoto H, Iwase T, Morioka T. Dye-mediated bactericidal effect of He-Ne laser irradiation on oral microorganisms. *Lasers Surg Med* 1992; 12: 450–458.

16 Burns T, Wilson M, Pearson GJ. Laser-induced killing of photosensitized cariogenic bacteria. *J Dent Res* 1992; 71: 675.

17 Sarkar S, Wilson M. Lethal photosensitization of bacteria in subgingival plaque from patients with chronic periodontitis. *J Periodontal Res* 1993; 28: 204–221.

18 Burns T, Wilson M, Pearson GJ. Sensitization of cariogenic bacteria to killing by light from a helium-neon laser. *J Med Microbiol* 1993; 38: 401–405.

19 Wilson M, Burns T, Pratten J, et al. Bacteria in supragingival plaque samples can be killed by low-power laser light in the presence of a photosensitizer. *J Appl Bacteriol* 1995; 78: 569–557.

20 Burns T, Wilson M, Pearson GJ. Effect of dentin and collagen on the lethal photosensitization of *Streptococcus mutans*. *Caries Res* 1995; 29: 192–197.

21 Wilson M, Burns T, Pratten,J. Killing of *Streptococcus sanguis* in biofilms using a light-activated antimicrobial agent. *J Antimicrob Chem* 1996; 37: 377–381.

22 Wood S, Nattress B, Kirkham J, *et al.* An *in vitro* study of the use of photodynamic therapy for the treatment of natural oral plaque biofilms formed in vivo. *J Photochem Photobiol B* 1999; 50: 1–7.

23 De Sant'Anna GR. *In vivo study of photodynamic therapy effect on decidupus dentin: microbiologic and SEM analysis.* Dissertation presented to Sao Paulo University. São Paulo, 2001.

24 O'Neill JF, Hope CK, Wilson M. Oral bacteria in multi-species biofilms can be killed by red light in the presence of toluidine blue. *Lasers Surg Med* 2002; 31: 86–90.

25 Zanin ICJ, Gonçalves RB, Brugnera Junior A, et al. Susceptibility of Streptococcus mutans biofilms to photodynamic therapy: an *invitro* study. *J Antimicrob Chemother* 2005, 56: 324–330.

26 Wood S, Metcalf D, Devine D, et al. Erythrosine is a potential photosensitizer for the photodynamic therapy of oral plaque biofilms. *J Antimicrob Chemother* 2006; 57: 680–684.

27 Zanin IC, Lobo MM, Rodrigues LK. Photosensitization of *in vitro* biofilms by toluidine blue O combined with light-emitting diode. *Eur J Oral Sci* 2006; 114: 64–69.

28 Metcalf D, Robinson C, Devine D, et al. Enhancement of erythrosine-mediated photodynamic therapy of *Streptococcus mutans* biofilms by light fractions. *J Antimicrob Chemother* 2006; 58: 190–192.

29 Müller P, Guggenheim B, Schmidlin PR. Efficacy of gasiform ozone and photodynamic therapy on a multispecies oral biofilm *in vitro*. *Eur J Oral Sci* 2007; 115: 77–80.

30 Giusti JSM, Pinto-Santos L, Pizzolito AC, et al. Antimicrobial photodynamic action on dentin using a light-emitting diode light source. *Photomed Laser Surg* 2008; 26: 281–287.

31 Lima JMP, Melo MAS, Borges FMC, et al. Evaluation of the antimicrobial effect of photodynamic therapy in an in situ model of dentine caries. *Eur J Oral Sci* 2009; 117: 1–7.

32 Longo JPF, de Azevedo RB. Effect of photodynamic therapy mediated by methylene blue in cariogenic bacteria. *Rev Clin Pesq Odontol* 2010; 6: 249–257.

33 Longo JPF, Leal SC, Simioni AR, et al. Photodynamic therapy disinfection of carious tissue mediated by aluminum-chloride-phthalocyanine entrapped in cationic liposomes: an *in vitro* and clinical study. *Lasers Med Sci* 2012; 27: 575–584..

34 Guglielmi CAB, Simionato, MRL, Ramalho KM, et al. Clinical use of photodynamic antimicrobial chemotherapy for the treatment of deep carious lesions. *J Biomed Opt* 2011;16: 088003.

35 Vahabi S, Fekrazad R, Ayremlou S, et al. The effect of antimicrobial photodynamic therapy with radachlorin and toluidine blue on Streptococcus mutans: An *in vitro* study. *J Dent* 2011; 8: 48–54.

36 Bhatti M, Mac Robert A, Meghji S, et al. Uptake and cellular distribution of a light-activated antimicrobial agent by *Porphyromonas gingivalis*. *J Dent Res* 1997; 76: 1035.

37 Bhatti M, Mac Robert A, Meghji S, et al. Effect of dosimetric and physiological factors on the lethal photosensitization of *Porphyromonas gingivalis* in vitro. *Photochem Photobiol* 1997; 65: 1026–1031.

38 Wilson M, Mia, N. Effect of environmental factors on the lethal photosensitization of *Candida albicans in vitro*. *Lasers Med Sci* 1994; 9: 105–109.

39 Ferreira AN, Silveira L, Genovese WJ, et al. Effect of GaAIAs laser on reactional dentinogenesis induction in human teeth. *Photomed Laser Surg* 2006; 24: 358–365.

40 Godoy BM, Arana-Chavez VE, Núñez SC, et al. Effects of low-power red laser on dentine-pulp interface after cavity preparation. An ultrastructural study. *Arch Oral Biol* 2007; 52: 899–903.

CHAPTER 13

Treatment of internal ceramic surfaces

Carlos de Paula Eduardo,[1] Marina Stella Bello-Silva,[2] and Paulo Francisco Cesar[3]

[1]Special Laboratory of Lasers in Dentistry (LELO), Department of Restorative Dentistry, School of Dentistry, University of São Paulo (USP), São Paulo, SP, Brazil
[2]Center for Research and Innovation in Laser, University Nove de Julho, São Paulo, SP, Brazil
[3]Department of Biomaterials and Oral Biology, School of Dentistry, University of São Paulo (USP), São Paulo, SP, Brazil

Introduction

The development of restorative dentistry following the introduction of high technology equipment and innovative techniques has facilitated the achievement of more predictable clinical outcomes, with dental restorations that fulfil functional and esthetic requirements. The evolution of esthetic restorative materials has led to the production of ceramic systems that are capable of withstanding higher levels of masticatory load, enabling the production of metal-free ceramic restorations.[1]

Polycrystalline ceramics and ceramic composites have a microstructure with higher crystalline content compared to porcelains and glass–ceramics. This feature is responsible for their increased strength and better clinical performance compared to other dental ceramics.[2] The higher crystal content and smaller amount of glass hinder crack propagation in these materials, therefore increasing their clinical lifetime.[3]

Ceramic composites are composed of an alumina or alumina–zirconia scaffold that is infiltrated by a lanthanum glass, making it suitable for building crown infrastructures and three element fixed partial dentures, depending on the composition of the material's crystalline phase.[4] Examples of ceramic composites are InCeram System (Vita), Glass-Ceram System (Angelus), and Alglass System (GDS). Unlike ceramic composites, polycrystalline ceramics have a purely crystalline structure, without a glassy phase, and are represented by alumina polycrystal and Y-TZP (yttrium oxide partially-stabilized tetragonal zirconia polycrystals; IPS e.max ZirCAD, Ivoclar; Lava, 3 M; In-Ceram YZ and AL, Vita; Cercon, Dentsply).

Despite its improved mechanical strength, the cementation of highly crystalline ceramic restorations still represents a challenge for clinicians. Although luting can still be carried out with traditional materials, such as zinc phosphate cement or glass ionomer cement, the esthetic demands of these restorations and the excessive propensity of some of these preparations to be expelled may require the use of adhesive cements.[5] Adhesive cementation has the advantage of filling gaps between the tooth and the restoration, as well as providing an optimized esthetic outcome. Bonding the restoration to the dental substrate improves stress distribution, which increases the resistance of the tooth–restoration complex.

Conditioning the ceramic inner surface

In order to obtain a good adhesive cementation of highly crystalline ceramics, it is mandatory that both the tooth surface and ceramic inner surface are adequately conditioned so as to promote an effective and simultaneous bonding of resin cement to tooth and ceramic.[6,7] Conditioning the ceramic inner surface is difficult due to its high crystalline content, and this problem may result in clinical failure of this restoration, because of insufficient bonding promoted by the resin cement.[8–10] Bonding between resin cement and ceramics may be achieved by means of micromechanical retention after conditioning the inner surface of the prosthetic piece.[11–13] Other bonding techniques are based on chemical bonds formed with the use of a silane agent that improves the wettability of the resin cement and bonds chemically and simultaneously to the inorganic portion of the ceramic and the organic portion of the resin cement.[14] Because of their high crystalline content and low amount of glass, polycrystalline ceramics and ceramic composites do not undergo significant morphological changes when hydrofluoric acid is used.[7,15–17]

Therefore, other forms of surface treatment have been used in order to improve the bond strength between cement and ceramic, such as the tribochemical silica coating. This method has proven efficient in terms of adhesion values, since it results in the impregnation of the ceramic surface with silica particles, facilitating the bonding of the former to the silane agent and the adhesive cement.[11,18,19] However, this method still has limitations when used for the surface treatment of Y-TZP polycrystalline ceramic.[20–22]

More recently, high power lasers have been studied for the conditioning of ceramic inner surfaces, and consequently, for the improvement of bonding between ceramic and resin cement. The irradiation of the ceramic substrate with erbium lasers leads to ablation of the structure through a thermomechanical process, in which the water in the tissue or on the surface (from

Case study 13.1

Figure 13.1 shows a case of laser conditioning of the internal surface of teeth prior to restoration.

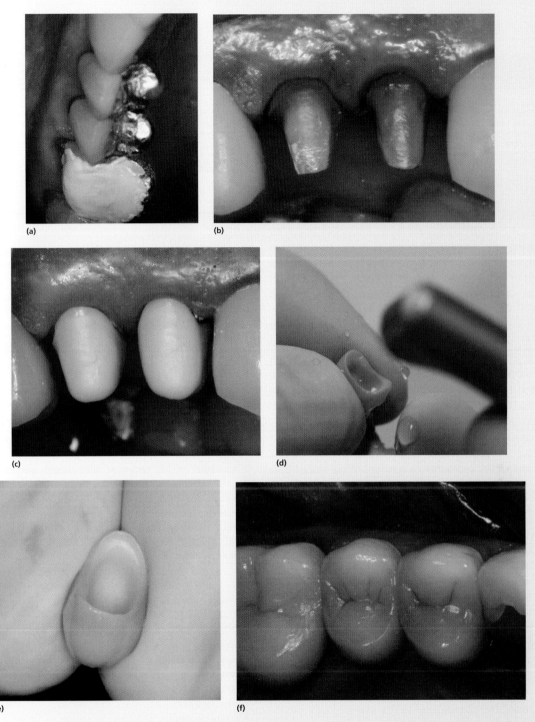

Figure 13.1 (a) Occlusal view of the restorations of teeth 14 and 15 that need replacement. Inflammation and retraction of the buccal gingival tissue can be seen. Metal-free indirect restorations were indicated to enhance the esthetic outcome. (b) After the removal of the crowns, the teeth were prepared in a manner that preserved adjacent periodontal tissue and maintained vitality of both teeth. Particular attention was given to the distance between antagonists, which should be such as to enable the fabrication of restorations with enough body to provide increased resistance and esthetics. (c) Proof of ceramic copings, before the conditioning of the internal surface. (d) Conditioning of the internal surface of the crown with Er:YAG laser irradiation, immediately before cementation. (e) After irradiation with the Er:YAG laser, the inner surface presents an opaque aspect, in contrast to the smooth and shiny surface observed prior to conditioning. (f) Metal-free indirect restoration after final luting: occlusal view. (g) Buccal view. (Eduardo et al.[30] Reproduced with permission of Editora Santos).

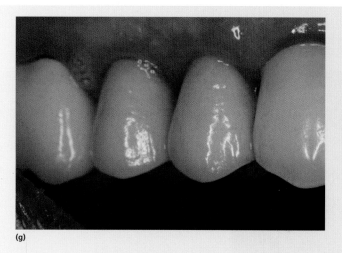

(g)

Figure 13.1 (Continued)

the cooling system) absorbs the energy of the incident photons and vaporizes rapidly, causing micro-explosions that eject adjacent structures.[23] Likewise, neodymium lasers may be used for ceramic conditioning by interacting with the surface so as to melt the material in this region, producing a micro-retentive morphology that favors the adhesion of the cement.[7] In other words, when used properly, high power lasers can cause micro-retentions by ablating or melting the ceramic surface, resulting in better adhesion values between resin cements and ceramic materials. It is important to emphasize that the laser effects on ceramic surfaces depend on the wavelength used, as well as on the chemical composition and microstructure of the ceramic irradiated.

The Nd:YAG laser (1064 nm) has proven to be effective in promoting higher bond strength values between alumina-based ceramic composites and adhesive cements. These values were equivalent to those obtained with tribochemical silica coating.[7,24] For Y-TZP, the Nd:YAG laser significantly increased adhesion in the presence of metal primers, either with or without association with the silica coating.[25] In the same study, the CO_2 laser was not efficient in conditioning Y-TZP surfaces. For ceramic composite, conversely, this laser seemed to favor adhesion to the resin cement.[26] Recent studies also have shown that the Er,Cr:YSGG laser (2780 nm) promotes bonding values similar to those achieved with silicatization in alumina-based ceramic composites.[27] Few studies have assessed the effects of the Er:YAG laser (2940 nm) on the bond strength between ceramic and resin cement. To date, the use of the Er:YAG laser in the conditioning of polycrystalline ceramics, using the parameters tested in the literature, has provided similar adhesion to that achieved with silicatization[28,29] (see Clinical case 13.1[30]).

In summary, one can conclude that each type of ceramic behaves differently when high power lasers are used for surface conditioning prior to cementation.

Many studies have been conducted to establish effective methods for conditioning the inner surface of ceramic restorations. The main objective is to improve adhesion to the resin

cement and thereby optimize clinical performance. The use of metal primers for this purpose has also been advocated.[25,28] The clinician must know the chemical composition and microstructure of the dental ceramic chosen for a determined treatment; this information will allow the professional to choose among different surface treatments, primers, and luting agents in order to provide the patients with a more predictable treatment that will have a better prognosis.

References

1 Anusavice KJ. Recent developments in restorative dental ceramics. *J Am Dent Assoc* 1993; 124(2): 72–74, 76–78, 80–74.

2 Hondrum SO. A review of the strength properties of dental ceramics. *J Prosthet Dent* 1992; 67(6): 859–865.

3 Bottino MA, Valandro LF, Buso L (eds). *Prótese metal-free: tratamento da superfície cerâmica pré-cimentação*. Atualização Clínica em Odontologia, 2004.

4 McLean JW. New dental ceramics and esthetics. *J Esthet Dent* 1995; 7(4): 141–149.

5 Kiyan VH, Saraceni CH, da Silveira BL, et al. The influence of internal surface treatments on tensile bond strength for two ceramic systems. *Oper Dent* 2007; 32(5): 457–465.

6 Madani M, Chu FC, McDonald AV, et al. Effects of surface treatments on shear bond strengths between a resin cement and an alumina core. *J Prosthet Dent* 2000; 83(6): 644–647.

7 da Silveira BL, Paglia A, Burnett LH, et al. Micro-tensile bond strength between a resin cement and an aluminous ceramic treated with Nd:YAG laser, Rocatec System, or aluminum oxide sandblasting. *Photomed Laser Surg* 2005; 23(6): 543–548.

8 Strub JR, Stiffler S, Scharer P. Causes of failure following oral rehabilitation: biological versus technical factors. *Quintessence Int* 1988; 19(3): 215–222.

9 Libby G, Arcuri MR, LaVelle WE, et al. Longevity of fixed partial dentures. *J Prosthet Dent* 1997; 78(2): 127–131.

10 Sorensen JA, Kang SK, Torres TJ, et al. In-Ceram fixed partial dentures: three-year clinical trial results. *J Calif Dent Assoc* 1998; 26(3): 207–214.

11 Kern M, Thompson VP. Sandblasting and silica coating of a glass-infiltrated alumina ceramic: volume loss, morphology, and changes in the surface composition. *J Prosthet Dent* 1994; 71(5): 453–461.

12 Sorensen JA, Engelman MJ, Torres TJ, et al. Shear bond strength of composite resin to porcelain. *Int J Prosthodont* 1991; 4(1): 17–23.

13 Sen D, Poyrazoglu E, Tuncelli B, et al. Shear bond strength of resin luting cement to glass-infiltrated porous aluminum oxide cores. *J Prosthet Dent* 2000; 83(2): 210–215.

14 Jedynakiewicz NM, Martin N. The effect of surface coating on the bond strength of machinable ceramics. *Biomaterials* 2001; 22(7): 749–752.

15 Kim BK, Bae HE, Shim JS, et al. The influence of ceramic surface treatments on the tensile bond strength of composite resin to all-ceramic coping materials. *J Prosthet Dent* 2005; 94(4): 357–362.

16 Della Bona A, Anusavice KJ. Microstructure, composition, and etching topography of dental ceramics. *Int J Prosthodont* 2002; 15(2): 159–167.

17 Wood DJ, Bubb NL, Millar BJ, et al. Preliminary investigation of a novel retentive system for hydrofluoric acid etch-resistant dental ceramics. *J Prosthet Dent* 1997; 78(3): 275–280.

18 Kern M, Strub JR. Bonding to alumina ceramic in restorative dentistry: clinical results over up to 5 years. *J Dent* 1998; 26(3): 245–249.

19 Della Bona A, Donassollo TA, Demarco FF, et al. Characterization and surface treatment effects on topography of a glass-infiltrated alumina/zirconia-reinforced ceramic. *Dent Mater* 2007; 23(6): 769–775.

20 Kern M, Wegner SM. Bonding to zirconia ceramic: adhesion methods and their durability. *Dent Mater* 1998; 14(1): 64–71.

21 Friederich R, Kern M. Resin bond strength to densely sintered alumina ceramic. *Int J Prosthodont* 2002; 15(4): 333–338.

22 Re D, Augusti D, Sailer I, et al. The effect of surface treatment on the adhesion of resin cements to Y-TZP. *Eur J Esthet Dent* 2008; 3(2): 186–196.

23 Fried D. IR laser ablation of dental enamel. *Proc SPIE* 2000; 3910: 136–148.

24 Spohr AM, Borges GA, Junior LH, et al. Surface modification of In-Ceram Zirconia ceramic by Nd:YAG laser, Rocatec system, or aluminum oxide sandblasting and its bond strength to a resin cement. *Photomed Laser Surg* 2008; 26(3): 203–208.

25 Paranhos MP, Burnett LH, Jr., Magne P. Effect Of Nd:YAG laser and CO_2 laser treatment on the resin bond strength to zirconia ceramic. *Quintessence Int* 2011; 42(1): 79–89.

26 Ural C, Kulunk T, Kulunk S, et al. The effect of laser treatment on bonding between zirconia ceramic surface and resin cement. *Acta Odontol Scand* 2010; 68(6): 354–359.

27 Eduardo CdeP, Bello-Silva MS, Moretto SG, et al. Microtensile bond strength of composite resin to glass-infiltrated alumina composite conditioned with Er,Cr:YSGG laser. *Lasers Med Sci* 2012; 27(10): 7–14.

28 Foxton RM, Cavalcanti AN, Nakajima M, et al. Durability of resin cement bond to aluminium oxide and zirconia ceramics after air abrasion and laser treatment. *J Prosthodont* 2011; 20(2): 84–92.

29 Cavalcanti AN, Foxton RM, Watson TF, et al. Bond strength of resin cements to a zirconia ceramic with different surface treatments. *Oper Dent* 2009; 34(3): 280–287.

30 Eduardo CP, Ramalho KM, Bezinelli LM, et al. Laser in contempory clinical dentistry. In: Fernandes CP (ed). *A World Class Dentistry - fdi 2010 Brasil*. Rio de Janeiro: Editora Santos, 2010: 237–263.

CHAPTER 14

Dental bleaching with LEDs and lasers

Fátima Zanin,[1-3] Aldo Brugnera Jr,[1-4] and Mateus Cóstola Windlin[3]

[1] Federal University of Rio de Janeiro (UFRJ), Rio de Janeiro, RJ, Brazil
[2] Master and PhD course at Federal University of Bahia (UFBA), Salvador, BA, Brazil
[3] Private Dental Practice – Brugnera & Zanin Institute, São Paulo, SP, Brazil
[4] Masters and Doctoral Courses of Biomedical Engineering, University of Camilo Castelo Branco – Technological Park, São José dos Campos, SP, Brazil

Introduction

Dental surgeons are concerned with assuring comfort and safety for patients when introducing procedures into their clinical practice, such as esthetic dental bleaching. Dental bleaching, a non-invasive technique, is currently part of the overall dental treatment to fulfil the patient's expectations.

Dental bleaching has been associated with esthetic procedures for decades and has developed much since 1989, when Haywood and Heymann[1] proposed the home bleaching system Nightguard. Since then, many techniques have emerged to improve patient comfort and reduce time of application; these techniques achieve similar outcomes as all are based on the use of hydrogen peroxide (H_2O_2).

Activation of the bleaching gel was first done using a heat source: heated spatulas and high intensity lamps (Photoflood, Photopolymerizer). However, the high penetration of H_2O_2 at increased temperature resulted in increased sensitivity. Since then, techniques have tried to decrease heat generation, thus decreasing sensitivity during the treatment. In photoassisted bleaching there is interaction of a light source with the bleaching gel and some aspects are decisive:

- Type of light used: laser, light emitting diodes (LEDs), xenon, halogen;
- Characteristics of the equipment, such as filters, diameter of tip collimators, and distance at which these tips should be positioned;
- Characteristics of the gel: color, absorption band, thickness, pH;
- Morphology of the enamel and dentin structure;
- Adequate parameters for the equipment used: power density (P/A), energy density (which relates time to power density), application distance.

Activation sources: Laser and LEDs

The bleaching technique increases dentin permeability, thus also increasing dental sensitivity, especially when the temperature increases. The amount of heat generated by the activation source for the bleaching system is directly related to the sensitivity felt by the patient. New bleaching techniques should be developed that require lower light irradiance to photochemically activate the bleaching gel. In addition, infrared therapeutic lasers at low power density do not generate heat and minimize dental sensitivity during the procedure.

Approval of the use of the argon laser in photoassisted bleaching techniques by the Ion Laser Technology (ILT) in 1996, changed the view that activation of the bleaching reaction in the office should be achieved with thermal sources.

The photopolymerizer's halogen light emits blue and infrared light, which heat their target. Although the xenon light/plasma arch has a more efficient optical filter, it still emits infrared wavelengths together with the blue light.

Blue LEDs are used in dental bleaching (Fig. 14.1) because their emission spectrum is similar to that of argon lasers. Their use in composite photopolymerization was proposed by Mills in 1995. This system does not emit wavelengths in the infrared range, but does induce a photochemical interaction.

However, when the blue light emitted by LEDs is combined with the infrared wavelengths of diode lasers at higher power densities, there will be the same undesirable thermal effects of infrared wavelengths associated with the photopolymerizer's blue light.

Argon laser

The argon laser used to activate dental bleaching has a wavelength of 488 nm, emits a bluish–greenish light in the visible part of the electromagnetic spectrum, and is absorbed by dark colors. It seems to be the perfect instrument for dental bleaching when used with 35% H_2O_2 and a dye whose absorption coefficient is appropriate for the light–H_2O_2 interaction, as heat production is minimal.[2,3] The argon laser (LaserMed; Fig. 14.2), with an optical power of up to 200 mW can activate the reaction of the bleaching gel photochemically, because its narrow emission band confers a spectral purity around 488 nm (Fig. 14.3) without emitting infrared rays (which generate heat). The advantage of photochemical activation is that the light acts on the product and does not heat up the dental structure. When using the argon laser, it is important to know that it emits wavelengths in two different bands of the electromagnetic

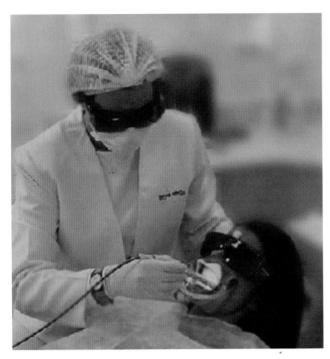

Figure 14.1 Dental bleaching with the blue LED system (reproduced with permission of Livraria Santos Editor).

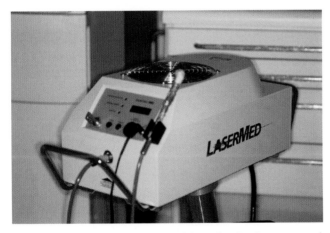

Figure 14.2 Argon laser (LaserMed, USA) (reproduced with permission of Livraria Santos Editor).

spectrum: one in the blue spectrum at 488 nm, which can be used in dental bleaching and composite polymerization, and another in the green spectrum ranging from 512 nm to 540 nm. The KTP laser (532 nm) emits in this latter band. This laser is used in dental bleaching as well as in soft tissue surgeries.[4,5]

In order to accomplish bleaching, the laser energy must be absorbed by the target tissues or materials (Fig. 14.4). The argon laser (488 nm) as well as the KTP laser (532 nm) may be used with a gel that absorbs the wavelength of the blue and green spectra. The red bleaching gel is used with the blue argon laser (488 nm), green argon laser (514 nm), and KTP laser (532 nm). For argon lasers, protection goggles should be orange.

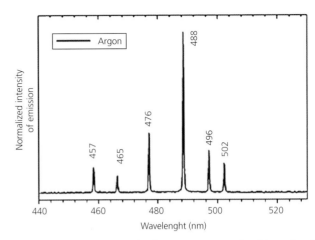

Figure 14.3 Argon laser normalized emission at 488 nm band (reproduced with permission of Livraria Santos Editor).

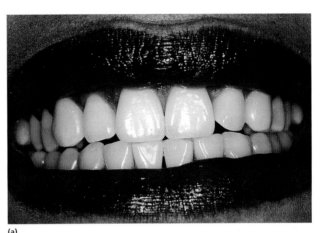

(a)

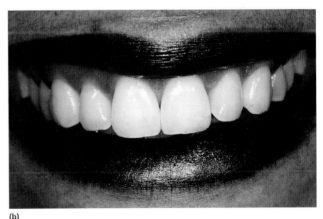

(b)

Figure 14.4 (a) Before and (b) after dental bleaching with the argon laser (reproduced with permission of Livraria Santos Editor).

Diode laser

The diode laser is used in soft tissue surgeries and it emits wavelengths ranging from 810 to 830 nm. It has a power output of 1–10 W and is absorbed by dark substances such as hemoglobin and melanin. It provokes coagulation, vaporization, decontamination, and cutting of soft tissues. In order to decrease its thermal effects in the bleaching process, it should be used at minimum power and with lenses that will blur the ray. The manufacturers' recommendations should be followed, since the correct parameters are crucial to the success of this therapy,[6] as it is an infrared laser that emits in the thermal band. To decrease the thermal effects, it is important to use an appropriate gel, which should absorb the infrared wavelengths, acting like an absorption "filter" that protects the pulp from the penetration of infrared wavelengths.[7] Currently, the gels available on the market for the phototonic interaction with the infrared diode laser are blue.

Blue LEDs

LEDs were developed in the 1950s and emit in the infrared band. The yellow and green LEDs were introduced in 1970, followed by white LEDs. In 1990, blue and ultraviolet LEDs were introduced. LEDs use semiconductor connections to generate light instead of the hot filaments used in halogen lamp bulbs.[8] LEDs do not need filters to produce blue light, are resistant to shocks and vibrations, and consume little energy in their operation. The InGaN (indium–gallium–nitrogen) LED emits a narrow light spectrum of 400–500 nm, which is close to the band absorbed by canforoquinone and makes them efficient in the photopolymerization technique of composites.[8,9]

The use of LEDs in dental bleaching started after Mills[10] proposed using blue LEDs in composite photopolymerization.[11] Since LEDs do not emit wavelengths in the infrared range, they do not heat the target tissue and just induce a photochemical interaction. The first generation of equipment using LEDs produced a 50–300 mW/cm^2 power density, and the ultraLEDs could reach 1200 mW/cm^2. The light produced by blue LEDs emits in a narrow band with a peak close to 470 nm. Therefore, even at low power density, all the light emitted is within the maximum absorption spectrum of canforoquinone (468 nm), which is the photoinitiator generally found in most resinous materials.[9,12–15]

The advantages of blue LEDs presents make them very attractive to dental surgeons, both for dental bleaching and in the polymerization of composite. The basic difference between LEDs and lasers is the type of emission. In LEDs, spontaneous radiation emission prevails, while in lasers there is a predominance of stimulated light emission. Generation of laser light consumes a great amount of energy, while LEDs need little energy to generate light. This has a direct impact on the amount energy that is expended.[16] The emission of light by LEDs does not alter over their lifespan of 100 000 hours as they do not contain filters that can be damaged.[13,17]

As their wavelength compares with that of argon lasers,[18] blue LEDs have become a feasible option for dental bleaching and composite photopolymerization, with similar results and minimal heat generation.

The blue LED dental bleaching system (470 nm) proposed by Zanin et al.,[19] is the Bright Max (MM Optics, São Carlos, Brazil), which is composed of five LEDs, each with a power output of 50 mW (Fig. 14.5).

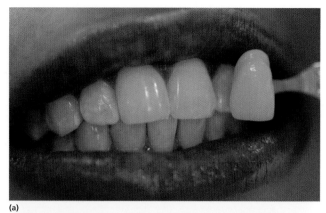
(a)

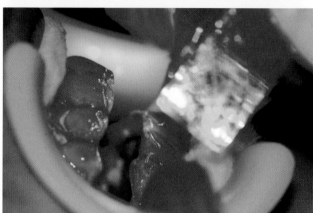
(b)

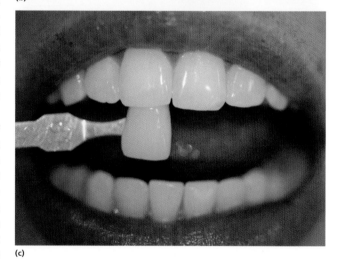
(c)

Figure 14.5 Dental bleaching with the blue LED system (Bright Max; MM Optics, São Paulo, Brazil). (a) Initial image (b) system activation (c) dental bleaching with blue LED system (courtesy of Fátima Zanin).

Bleaching agents

It is important to emphasize that the different sources of activation are not responsible for the bleaching of a dental element; this is achieved by the bleaching gel, which is made more effective by the activation.

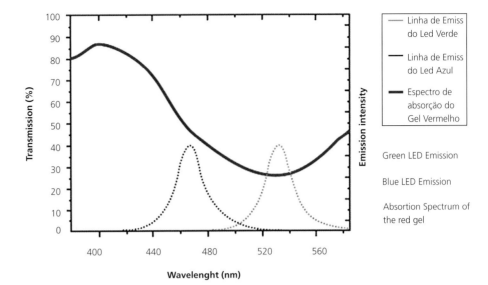

Figure 14.6 Interaction of the green LED and the red gel (reproduced with permission of Livraria Santos Editor).

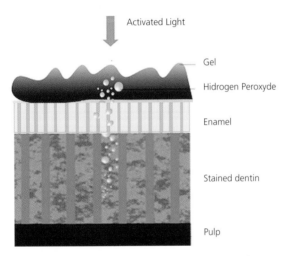

Figure 14.7 Diffusion of hydrogen peroxide through the dental structure (reproduced with permission of Livraria Santos Editor).

Absorption spectrum

In the bleaching process, interaction of the bleaching agent with an energy source increases the former's bleaching potential (photochemical activation). In order to achieve good results, it is best to use an energy source that emits wavelengths close to the absorption peak of the dye in the bleaching gel. It is thus important to investigate the amount of energy absorbed by the bleaching gels when activated by lasers and LEDs. When analyzing the absorption spectrum of the red bleaching gel (Whiteform Perox Red; Fórmula e Ação, São Paulo, Brazil), it was observed to interact well with green LED light, absorbing it in a photochemical process (Fig. 14.6).[7]

Action mechanism

H_2O_2 is the bleaching agent used in all techniques, and diffuses throughout the organic matrix of the enamel during bleaching (Fig. 14.7). During this process, the oxidizing agent reacts with

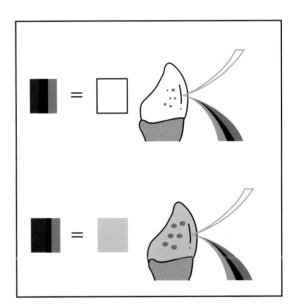

Figure 14.8 The bleaching effect decreases the intensity of the color (reproduced with permission of Livraria Santos Editor).

the organic material in the spaces between the crystals of the enamel and acts on the organic part of the dentin.[20]

LEDs generate minimum temperature increase without damaging the pulpal tissue, as they activate the bleaching gel and not the dental structure.[21] Bleaching breaks down the giant molecules of the pigment that absorb light and thus darken teeth. As a result, smaller molecules are formed, which reflect light and have a bleaching effect, decreasing the intensity of the color[22-25] (Fig. 14.8).

Other products such as carbamide peroxide (used in the home technique) and sodium perborate release H_2O_2 at a low concentration (3–7% for carbamide peroxide, which breaks down into CO_2, urea, ammonia, and H_2O_2),[24] and demand a higher number of sessions when using the conventional bleaching technique.

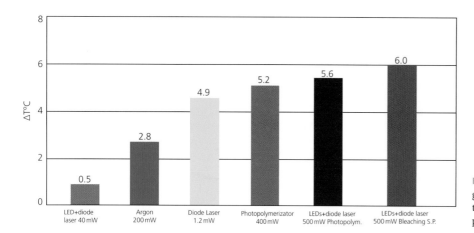

Figure 14.9 Intrapulpar temperature generated by different sources of light during the dental bleaching.[31] (reproduced with permission of Livraria Santos Editor).

The advantage of in-office bleaching is the short time the tooth is in contact with the product (1.5 hours), while in the home technique contact lasts from 7 to 15 days. If there is any sensitivity, it will be milder and more easily controlled. The decrease in application time is due to the potentiation of the reaction.[16]

In-office bleaching is done with 35% H_2O_2, an oxidizing agent that produces free radicals and breaks down into water (H_2O) and a free oxygen radical. The staining undergoes an oxyreduction process (redox), in which organic material (colored) is converted into carbon dioxide and water (colorless).[24,26]

Dental bleaching products may be activated either by heat (photothermal) or by light (photochemical effects). In photothermal activation, heat spreads throughout the dental structure, while in photochemical activation the light acts on the gel layer only.

Thermal effects

Like all living biological tissues, the pulp has a capacity to withstand stimuli. We know from the classic work by Zack and Cohen[27] that to maintain pulpal vitality, temperature increase should not exceed 5.6 °C.

The use of argon laser for dental bleaching, as well as for polymerization of composites, does not cause thermal damage to the dental pulp (≤ 2 °C), which is within the tolerated histopathological limit.[28] Several authors have verified that the argon laser causes significantly less thermal alterations than those obtained with conventional visible light.[29,30]

When correctly used, the dental bleaching technique with the diode laser (810 and 830 nm) is also efficient. However, as it is a high power laser, it should be used with low power densities to avoid thermal damage to tissues.

In the bleaching technique, activation with xenon and halogen lights may generate more thermal energy than activation with lasers and LEDs.

When heat is associated with a highly concentrated product such as 35% H_2O_2, there is higher penetration, which may increase pain and cause pulpal injuries. Depending on the pulpal response, an inflammatory process may evolve. Calmon[31] carried out a study *in vitro* to measure intrapulpal temperatures of samples of extracted human teeth subjected to bleaching using different activation sources (Fig. 14.9). The author used the following equipment: a 400-mW photopolymerizator, wavelength 380–500 nm; a 200-mW argon laser, wavelength 488 nm, a 1.2-W high power diode laser, wavelength 798–805 nm; and two pieces of equipment that conjugated LEDs with infrared laser of different trademarks and power outputs, each used according to its individual protocol.

The blue LEDs system and the argon laser produce a minimal increase in temperature, and thus can be used safely.[31]

Diagnosis and procedure clarification

The first contact with the patient and the clinical exam are of fundamental importance in all odontological specialties. As there is a wide range of new techniques and materials available, it is of utmost importance that the dental surgeon is able to diagnose the causes of color, shape, and dental structure alterations, and recommend the most appropriate procedure, or even combination of procedures, for each case.[32]

The patient's worries and expectations are discussed during the first appointment. The professional should remain very objective when describing the results of dental bleaching, which may not meet the patient's expectations. The patient should sign a dated consent form, which should include a description of the expected results of dental bleaching, as well as an explanation of the bleaching technique to be employed, the product used, the activation sources, approximate duration of procedure, degree of protection needed, and the risks, benefits, and limitations of the technique.

The degree of bleaching will vary from patient to patient. Yellowish or light brown teeth that are monochromatically darkened with external stains are more easily bleached. Bluish teeth or teeth with dark gray stripes caused by antibiotics (tetracycline) and those with irregular staining are more difficult to bleach. Complementary bleaching of the dark stripes can be performed.

With aging, teeth expose a reactional dentin which is of a darker color and makes the bleaching more difficult due to the increase of dentinal calcification. The larger the dentinal mass, the more difficult it is for the gel to penetrate.

Dental trauma or forceful orthodontic movements can also induce dental darkening and obliteration of dental tubules, making bleaching difficult. The presence of white stains may indicate congenital defects with smooth and shiny or initial carious lesions (which should be inactivated), fluorosis or hypoplastic stains of congenital origin. Dental bleaching cannot bleach the tooth until it reaches the white hue. However, there is a lessening of the difference between the hues.[16]

Before starting the dental bleaching process, periodontal health should be assessed and carious lesions temporarily luted with glass ionomer. These lesions should only be definitively restored after bleaching, to match the new hue. Infiltrated restorations and enamel cracks should also be looked for. H_2O_2 penetration favors the dentinal tissue, provoking temporary dentinal hypersensitivity. To avoid patient discomfort, rubber dams should be applied to lute these sites. The composite restorations are not bleached. They should be changed after 1 week to enable dental rehydration and avoid interference with adhesiveness.[33,34]

Evaluation criteria of the dental structure

The evaluation criteria for the dental structure can be used to indicate the required bleaching intensity. The oxyreduction mechanism of the bleaching techniques results in a change of two to three hues on the color scale. Bleaching is not whitening. Therefore, the limitations of bleaching should be explained to the patient for a predictable and satisfactory result.

It is possible to identify the level of dental calcification from laser fluorescence.[35,36] This new detection method measures the amount of fluorescent light irradiated from the tooth demineralization.[37] Fluorescence happens in the organic part of tissues, and the larger the demineralized area, the higher the number shown on the equipment's visor.[38,39] Thus, it is possible to check the degree of dental mineralization before and after bleaching using DIAGNOdent® (KaVo, Biberach, Germany) (Fig. 14.10): Both home and in-office bleaching do not alter the degree of calcification of dentin and enamel.

Photoassisted bleaching technique

In-office dental bleaching allows the dental surgeon to keep control over all the phases of the procedure and if necessary to customize them. Protocols for bleaching techniques using lasers or LEDs must be devised according to the equipment instructions regarding application time of light and intervals between applications. The duration of the applications should

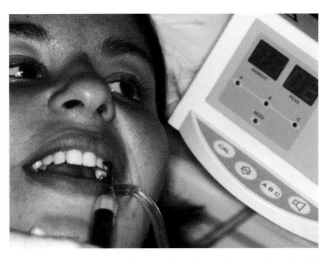

Figure 14.10 Measurement of tooth surface demineralization (reproduced with permission of Livraria Santos Editor).

be of the order of 15–20 minutes, since this is the amount of time it takes the bleaching agent to penetrate to dentin's deepest layers, where pigmentation is more intense.

Protocol proposed for the blue LEDs system (Fig. 14.11)

- Clinical evaluation and consent signed by the patient;
- Prophylaxis with pumice stone and water;
- Picture and color analysis at beginning of treatment;
- Measurement of dental demineralization at beginning of treatment with DIAGNOdent® (optional technique to show the patient that dental bleaching does not cause decalcification);
- Use of the lip and cheek mouth opener with the tongue protection;
- Relative isolation and protection of areas with exposed dentin using a gingival barrier;
- Application of a 2–3-mm layer of *orange* bleaching gel to the vestibular tooth surface;
- Positioning of the equipment in a way that will illuminate the surfaces of all teeth, from premolar to premolar, and activate the LED. The duration of the applications should be of the order of 15 minutes (10 minutes with light on and 5 minutes with light off);
  ○ Repeat the process of gel application and activation twice more;
- Apply colorless fluoride;
- Measure the final dental calcification with DIAGNOdent®;
- Color analysis at end of treatment;
- Final picture;
- Orientation about postoperative care.

Protection of dental and buccal tissues

As part of the safety rules, specific protection goggles for each kind of light should be worn by the patient, dental surgeon, and assistant.

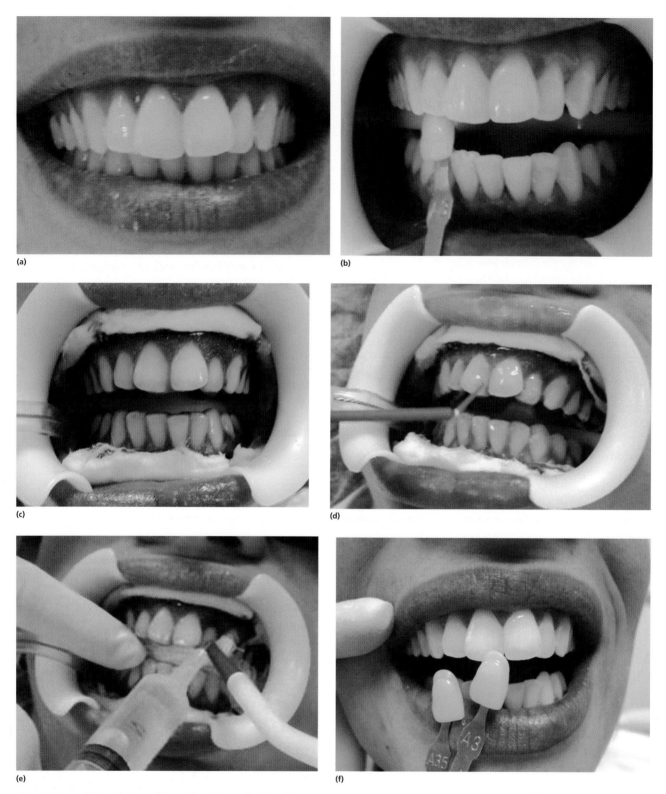

Figure 14.11 11 (a) Initial image; (b) A3 color VITA Scale; (c) application of the gingival barrier – protection of the exposed dentin and gum; (d) orange gel has the ideal color to absorb the blue light of the LEDs; (e) after dental irradiation with blue LED, the gel is vacuumed and then the mouth rinsed first with sodium hypochlorite 3% and then with water; (f) difference between initial and final color following single session dental bleaching; (g) final color B1 VITA Scale (courtesy of Fátima Zanin).

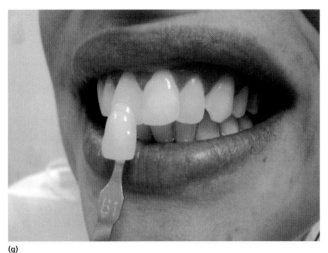

(g)

Figure 14.11 (Continued)

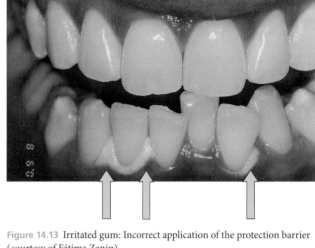

Figure 14.13 Irritated gum: Incorrect application of the protection barrier (courtesy of Fátima Zanin).

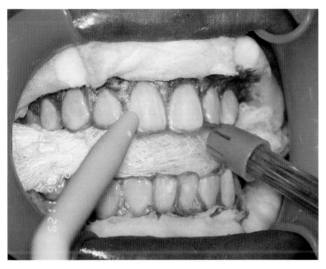

Figure 14.12 Protection of the oral tissues (courtesy of Fátima Zanin).

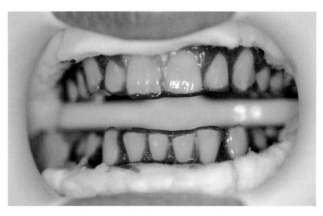

Figure 14.14 Another example of the protection of the dental and mucosal tissues (courtesy of Fátima Zanin).

Relative isolation can be achieved by using a gingival barrier, which is a fluid photopolymerized composite that acts like an artificial gingiva, luting the interproximal dental areas to avoid penetration of H_2O_2 into the cracks and exposed dentin (Fig. 14.12). It should be easy to use and remove, enabling the clinician to work safely without worrying about the protection of periodontal and dental tissues (Figs 14.13 and 14.14).

Post bleaching care

In the first 24 hours after bleaching, patients are advised to:
- Avoid eating foods containing dyes;
- Avoid acidic foods;
- Avoid smoking;
- Rinse the mouth with fluoride substances several times a day to rehydrate enamel and dentin.

Repetition of bleaching

The follow-up of bleaching cases has shown that if patients comply with the suggested protocol, the color is kept very close to that obtained at the end of treatment for about 2 years. However, it is important to appreciate that results vary from patient to patient. Whereas some obtain intense bleaching after a single application, others may obtain a very small change in color. The dental surgeon has no control over this and in some cases it is necessary to repeat the procedure to maintain the bleaching.

Maintenance with tooth pastes and other agents

Whitening dental creams help maintain the color obtained after bleaching for a longer period of time, as they have cleaning agents that minimize the incorporation of new dark pigments contained in food. Additional agents, such as rinses or bleaching brushes, may be used to improve the results after dental bleaching.

Hypersensitivity in dental bleaching

One complaint following dental bleaching can be dental sensitivity. All techniques may occasionally cause some postoperative discomfort. In almost 90% of cases this is a minor and temporary problem. In dental bleaching with the argon laser, about 70% of patients did not experience sensitivity. The other 30% had mild sensitivity during the treatment, which disappeared immediately after its conclusion.

In our analysis of the bleaching technique with the argon laser in 300 patients between 2000 and 2001, 70% did not experience sensitivity and the remaining 30% were treated with therapeutic laser immediately after bleaching. When the latter patients returned the next day for a therapeutic laser session, they no longer experienced any sensitivity.

According to Smigel,[20] dental sensitivity is low, and the temporary sensations that may occur immediately after bleaching disappear after a few hours.

LEDs for therapeutic (red and infrared) purposes are an alternative to the high cost lasers. The use of blue LEDs in composite photopolymerization and the activation of the bleaching process has also made these techniques more affordable to the dental clinic.

Currently, the introduction of LED system into the same tip as the therapeutic laser makes it possible to desensitize the tooth at the same time as bleaching it. This technique increases the patient's comfort as long as the correct parameters of the therapeutic laser are followed. According to most researchers, low irradiation should be emitted.[40-45] Higher or medium power diode lasers conjugated with LEDs heat the gel, and may in turn heat the tooth. Increase in temperature may generate pulpal hyperemia and pain, especially when associated with a high concentration of H_2O_2.[31]

In a clinical study at Instituto Brugnera & Zanin (SP/Brazil), 860 cases of bleaching were carried out with a combined LED and therapeutic laser (power output 40 mW).[45] This equipment had some advantages, especially with regards to decreasing sensitivity during and after the session. Less than 10% of the 860 procedures induced mild and isolated sensitivity in one or two teeth during or after the treatment. These sensations were of short duration and disappeared immediately after the treatment. Clinical results were excellent, demonstrating that the equipment was efficient in the activation of the gel.

Our team has accumulated results from over 800 dental bleaching procedures using argon lasers. These are being compared with the results of procedures using other techniques with lights and lasers. LEDs and the argon laser produce similar results because they work at a very similar emission band with little heat generation, as they do not emit infrared rays. Therapeutic lasers combined with LEDs should have adequate power but should not generate heat and cause pain in the dental biological system. The argon lasers and LEDs as bleaching activators improved results with a minimum increase in temperature (≤2 °C) because they activate the photosensitive gel and not the dental structure.

The application of these new, nevertheless scientifically supported, resources, allied to our clinical knowledge, promotes patient confidence in the quality of the treatment that is delivered to them.

Safety of bleaching agents in vital teeth

Post-bleaching composite restorations

A problem regarding restorative material has been reported. If the application of bleaching agents is immediately followed by a composite restoration procedure, there is an almost immediate decrease of adhesiveness.[46-49] This reduction has been attributed to the presence of residual oxygen in the dental structure, which deters the polymerization of monomers. Due to this, it is recommended that restorative procedures be undertaken 1 week after bleaching.[47,49-53]

Enamel resistance

Researches have shown that the sensible use of laser and LEDs in dental bleaching usually has little or no effect on the enamel, nor causes sensitivity.

When the argon laser is used on sound enamel at low energy fluence, alone or with acidulated phosphate fluoride, there is an increase in the enamel's resistance.[54-56] This also happens when fluoride is given when bleaching with LEDs, as the acid challenge decreases the pH and increases the absorption of fluoride.

Studies carried out by Friedman and Reyto[57] affirm that the enamel's Vickers microhardness is not altered following 120 minutes of continuous laser bleaching, and there was no significant difference in the superficial morphology of the human tooth following up to 2 hours of continuous argon laser/CO_2 irradiation.

Modifications to the enamel surface

The power of bleaching agents may be related to their pH. The 35% H_2O_2 solution has a pH close to 2.0,[26] which is lower than the critical pH of enamel (5.2–5.8) and dentin (6.0–6.8), and therefore may cause demineralization.[58] However, H_2O_2 gels are currently buffered, with a pH close to neutral, and thus are safer. However, it is known that the oxidizing power of bleaching agents leads, albeit mildly, to the degradation of the enamel and dentin's organic matrix, increasing the permeability of the dental structure.[59]

Several studies have demonstrated reductions in microhardness of the enamel and dentin.[57,60-62] Nevertheless, one should question if these reductions are significant from the clinical point of view. According to Haywood et al.,[63] the use of 10% carbamide peroxide for 6 hours has a conditioning effect similar to that from tooth contact with a cola soft drink for 2.5 minutes. Therefore, the demineralizing effects of the bleaching agents are very mild, and may be reversed by the action of the saliva.

With regards to the pulpal tissue, Cooper et al.[64] showed that it takes carbamide peroxide 15 minutes to permeate the enamel and dentin to reach the pulp. However, 35% H_2O_2 has been used on vital teeth for over 30 years and no irreversible damage has been observed.[65] In most studies,[66–69] when an inflammatory pulpal reaction is observed, it promotes transitory and postoperative sensitivity. Usually, sensitivity disappears following completion of bleaching, and the tooth returns to its normal conditions.

As already mentioned, the demineralizing effects of bleaching agents may be reversed by the action of the saliva. Artificial saliva has been used in *in vitro* studies to reproduce the buccal environment to remineralize the teeth.[70–73]

Dental enamels bleached in different ways have shown a considerable fluoride gain after topical application of fluoride solutions.[74]

Level of dental demineralization analysis

In an analysis of laser fluorescence (655 nm, 1 mW, continuous emission) using DIAGNOdent, the level of dental demineralization was observed before and after dental bleaching.[75] A total of 345 teeth from 38 individuals were evaluated. They were divided into two groups according to the bleaching technique: for group A (173 teeth from 19 individuals) dental bleaching was carried out with the Argon laser (488 nm, 200 mW; LaserMed, USA) and group B (172 teeth from 19 individuals) with blue LED (470 nm, 57 mW/cm² combined with a diode laser of 790 nm and 40 mW; Kondortech, Brazil). Identical protocols were followed for both techniques, but their phototonic emissions differed. The degree of demineralization was measured before and after dental bleaching.

The mean degree of demineralization before bleaching in group A was 3.46 and in group B 2.62. Immediately after bleaching, group A presented mean values of 2.93 and group B of 2.13. Differences detected in the degree of demineralization before and after dental bleaching were not statistically significant.

Results obtained by the laser fluorescence technique showed that no mineral loss was detected after dental bleaching using either laser or LED.

Bleaching quality: Time and irradiance of different photonic and chemical action systems

It is the aim that dental bleaching uses the most efficient energy source that avoids any harmful morphological or chemical effect on the enamel. The heat element must be controlled; otherwise it may lead to pulpal reaction.[27,66]

Dostalová et al.[76] compared laser and LED systems with the chemical action of the bleaching gel to analyze the time and quality of the bleaching process as well as to evaluate the modification of the enamel's structure after dental bleaching by scanning electron microscopy (SEM). To activate the bleaching agent, two different systems of laser and LED were used: (1) diode laser, 970 nm, 1 W for 5 minutes and 2 W for 2.5 minutes and (2) diode laser, 790 nm, 40 mW conjugated with eight LEDs, 467 nm, 4000 millicandelas each.

Twenty human, superior, central and lateral higid incisors hydrated in saline solution were analyzed. A 38% H_2O_2, Opalescence Extra Boost (Ultradent Products, South Jordan, UT, USA) was used in the form of a red gel for bleaching with laser and LEDs. The control was 38% H_2O_2 for 15 minutes without light activation.

The color of teeth was visualized using a stereomicroscope (Nikon SMZ 2T, Japan), and pre- and post-operative measurements were taken. The left side of the tooth was used as control and protected with wax before bleaching. The right side was used bleached. The results showed that a minimum of 15 minutes were necessary to achieve adequate bleaching using only chemical activation.

Diode laser (970 nm) and the bleaching agent caused the same effect in a shorter period of time. The enamel's surface was analyzed by SEM JSM 5500 LV (Jeol, Japan). The power had a direct influence on the activation time: power of 1 W, 5 minutes, and of 2 W, 2.5 minutes. The eight blue LEDs (467 nm) conjugated with the infrared diode laser (790 nm, 40 mW) with the bleaching gel, achieved the desired color in 5 minutes.

After bleaching with all techniques, minimal modifications of the enamel's surface were observed by SEM. The procedure with the conjugated system of laser and LEDs left a smooth surface with well-formed hydroxyapatite prisms, and the organic matrix was removed without structural alteration.

This study showed that selective radiation with blue LEDs and therapeutic laser may decrease bleaching time without significant modification of the enamel surface.

Final considerations

Most problems that occur during dental bleaching seem to be associated with lack of technical experience. Therefore, if the steps are correctly followed, the technique becomes faster, easier, and more efficient.

In order to be competent in the technique, hands-on training is essential, and this combined with theoretical knowledge, clinical experience, and a correct diagnosis will produce the expected results.

References

1 Haywood VB, Heymann HO: Nightguard vital bleaching. *Quintessence Int* 20:173–176, 1989.

2 Powell GL, Anderson JR, Blankenau RJ. Laser and curing light induced in vitro pulpal temperature changes. *J Dent Res* 1997; 76: 79 (abstract).

3 Reyto R. Laser tooth whitening. *Dent Clin North Am* 1998; 42(4): 755–762.

4 Walsh LJ, Liu Jackson Y, Verheyen P. Tooth discolouration and its treatment using KTP laser-assisted tooth whitening. *J Oral Laser Appl* 2004; 4(1): 7–21.

5 Goodman JD, Kaufman HW. Effects of an Argon laser on the crystalline properties and rate of dissolution in acid of tooth enamel in the presence of sodium fluoride. *J Dent Res* 1977; 56(10): 1201–1207.

6 Martelli FS, De Leo A, Zinno S. Laser in Odontostomatologia – Applicazioni Cliniche. *Cap*.5. p. 59-72. Milan: Masson S.p.A, 2000.

7 Rocha R. *Interação dos lasers com diferentes agentes clareadores.* Laser Dental Show, Programa Oficial, 2003.

8 Nakamura S, Mukai T, Senoh M. Candelaclass high brightness InGaN/ AlGaN double heterostructure blue-light-emitting diodes. *Appl Phys Lett* 1994; 64: 1687–1689.

9 Stahl F, Ashworth SH, Jandt KD, Mills RW. Light-emitting diode (LED) polymerization of dental composites: flexural properties and polymerization potential. *Biomaterials* 2000; 21: 1379–1385.

10 Mills RW, Jandt KD, Ashworth SH. Dental composite depth of cure with halogen and blue light emitting diode technology. *Br Dent J* 1999; 186: 388–391.

11 Kurachi C, Lizarelli RFZ, Bagnato VS. *Avaliação da microdureza superficial de resina composta curada por LED 468nm.* SBPqO, 1999.

12 Tarle Z, Knezevic A, Meniga A, Sutalo J, Pichler G. Temperature rise in composite samples cured by blue superbright light emitting diodes. *J Dent Res* 1998; 77: 686 (Abstract 433).

13 Mills RW, Jandt KD, Ashworth SH. Dental composite depth of cure with halogen and blue light emitting diode technology. *Br Dent J* 1999; 186: 388–391.

14 Jandt KD, Mills RW, Blackwell GB, Ashworth SH. Depth of cure and compressive strength of dental composites cured with blue light emitting diodes (LED's). *Den Mater* 2000; 16: 41–47.

15 Franco EB, Lopes LG. *Conceitos atuais na polimerização de sistemas restauradores resinosos.* Biodonto Revista Odontológicas 2003; 1(2): 23.

16 Zanin F, Brugnera Jr A. *Clareamento Dental com Luz-laser,* 3rd edn. Sao Paulo: Santos, 2005: 170.

17 Whitters CJ, Mills RW, Carey JJ. Curing of dental composites by use InGaN light-emitting diodes. *Optics Lett* 1999; 24: 67.

18 Frentzen, M.; Viktor, F.; Andreas, B. Photopolymerization of composite resin using LED technology. *J Oral Laser Appl* 2001; 1(3): 189–194.

19 Zanin F, Windlin MC, Brugnera Jr A, Brugnera AP. Photoactivated dental bleaching: bioscience in clinical practice. *Implant News,* 2012; 9(Special Suppl): 30–35.

20 Smigel I. Laser tooth whitening. *Dent Today* 1996; 15(8): 32–36.

21 Tarle Z, Knezevic A, Menija A, Sutalo J, Pichler G. Temperature rise in composite samples cured by blue superbright light emitting diodes. *J Dent Res* 1998; 77: 686(Abstract 433).

22 Haywood VB. Nightguard vital bleaching: Current information and research. *Esthet Dent Update* 1990; 1(2): 20–25.

23 Albers H. Lightening natural teeth. *ADEPT Rep* 1991; 2(1): 1–24.

24 Frysh H, Bowles W, Baker F, Rivera-Hidalgo G, Guillen G. Effect of pH on bleaching efficiency [abstract 2248]. *J Dent Res* 1993; 72: 384.

25 Baratieri LN, Monteiro Jr S, Andrada MAC, Vieira LCC. Clareamento Dental. *Chicago: Quintessence,* 1993: 176.

26 Pécora JD, Sousa Neto MD, Silva RG, et al. Guia de Clareamento Dental. *Sao Paulo: Santos,* 1996: 48.

27 Zach L, Cohen G. Pulp responses to externally applied heat. *Oral Surg Oral Med Oral Pathol* 1965; 19: 515–530.

28 Zanin F. *Avaliação da dureza Vickers e do aumento de temperatura de resinas compostas quando fotopolimerizadas pela luz do laser de argônio 488nm e pelo fotopolimerizadoor de luz halógena.* Tese de mestrado, Universidade do Vale do Paraíba; Instituto de Pesquisa e Desenvolvimento-UNIVAP-IP&D, 2001.

29 Cobb DS, Dederich DN, Gardner TV. In vitro temperature change at the dentin/pulpal interface by using conventional visible light versus argon laser. *Lasers Surg Med* 2000; 26: 386–397.

30 ADA Council on Scientific Affairs. Laser-assisted bleaching Na update. *J Am Dent Assoc* 1998; 129: 1485–1487.

31 Calmon WJ, et al. Estudo do aumento de temperatura intra-pulpar gerado pelo clareamento dental. *RGO* 2004; 52(1): 19–24.

32 Mondelli RFL. Clareamento dental. *Revista de Dentística Restauradora, Bauru* 1998 1(4): 163–215.

33 Ben-Amar A, Liberman R, Gorfil C, Bernstein Y. Effect of mouthguard bleaching on enamel surface. *Am J Dent* 1995; 8(1): 29–32.

34 Haywood VB, Heymann HO. Niteguard vital bleaching: how safe is it? *Quintessence Int* 1991; 22: 515–523.

35 Hibst R, Gall R. Development of a diode laser-based fluorescence caries detector. *Caries Res* 1998; 32: 294.

36 Hibst R, Paulus R. A new approach on fluorescence spectroscopy for caries detection. *Proc SPIE* 1999; 35: 93.

37 Ladalardo TCCGP, Cappellette Jr M, Zanin F, Brugnera Jr A, Pignatari S, Weckx LLM. *Evaluation of the mineralization degree of the vestibular surface of upper central incisors with a 655 nm diode laser in buccal respiring patients.* Lasers in Dentistry IX. Proc SPIE, 2003.

38 Zanin F, Pinheiro A, Campos DHS, Brugnera Jr A, Pécora JD. Caries diagnosis using laser fluorescence. *Lasers in Dentistry VI. Proc SPIE* 2000; 3910: 290–296.

39 Zanin F, Campos DHS, Zanin S, Brugnera Jr A, Harari S. Measurement of fluorescence of restorative dental materials using a diode laser 655 nm. *Lasers in Dentistry VII. Proc SPIE* 2001; 4249: 145–151.

40 Villa RG, Brugnera Jr A, Aun CE. Estudo histológico da atuação do raio laser He:Ne na neoformação dentinária em polpa de ratos. *SBPqO* 1988: 101.

41 Aun CA, Brugnera Jr A, Villa RG. Raio Laser – Hipersensibilidade dentinária. *Rev Assoc Paul Cirur Dent* 1989; 43(2).

42 Matsumoto K, Tomunari H, Bayashi H. Study on the treatment of hypersensitive dentine by laser. *Jpn J Conservat Dent* 1985; 28(4): 208.

43 Tuner J, Hode L. *Laser Therapy in Dentistry and Medicine.* Suécia: Prima Books, 1996.

44 Tuner J; Hode L. *Laser Therapy. Clinical Practice and Scientific Background.* Suécia: Prima Books, 2002: 572.

45 Brugnera Jr A, Zanin F, Pinheiro A, Pécora J, Ladalardo TC, Campos D. *Hypersensitivity: a histologic study and clinical application. 2nd International Nearfield Optical Analysis.* Photobiology Workshop Conference. Houston, TX, USA, May 29–30, 2001.

46 Titlei KC, et al. Adhesion of a resin composite to bleached and unbleached human enamel. *J Endod* 1993; 19(3): 112–115.

47 Spyrides GM. *Resistência adesiva da dentina bovina quando submetida ao peróxido de hidrogênio e de carbamida.* Tese de Doutorado. Faculdade de Odontologia de São José dos Campos, UNESP – São José dos Campos, 1999.

48 Haywood VBE, Barry TG. Natural tooth bleaching. In: Summit JB, Robbins JW, Schwartz RS. *Fundaments of operative dentistry: a contemporary approach,* 2nd edn. Quintessence Cap 2001; 15: 401–426.

49 Borges AB. *A Influência de agentes clareadores na resistência de união de uma resina composta ao esmalte em função do tempo de armazenamento em saliva artificial.* 128p. Tese (Doutorado em

Odontologia, Área de Concentração: Odontologia Restauradora). Faculdade de Odontologia de São José dos Campos, Universidade Estadual Paulista, São José dos Campos, 2003.

50 Haywood VB, Heymann HO. Nightguard vital bleaching: how safe is it? *Quintessence Int* 1991; 22: 515–523.

51 McGuckin RR, Trumond BA, Osovitz S. Enamel shear bond strength after vital bleaching. *Am J Dent* 1992; 5(4): 216–222.

52 Pagani C, Torres RG, Miranda CB. Livro do Ano Clínica Odontológica Brasileira. Cap. 17, Clareamento Dental, Artes Médicas, 2004: 485–487.

53 Sundfeld RH, Briso ALF, Marra de Sá P, Sundefeld MM, Bedran-de-Castro AKB. *Significance of time interval between bleaching and bonding: The effect on Tag formation.* Bull. Tokyo Dental Coll 2005; 46(1–2): 1–6.

54 Flaitz CM, Hicks MJ, Westerman GH, Berg JH, Blankenau RJ. Argon laser irradiation and acidulated phosphate fluoride treatment in caries-like lesion formation in enamel: an *in vitro* study. *Pediatr Dent* 1995; 17(1): 31–35.

55 Haider SM, White GE, Rich A. Combined effects of argon laser irradiation and fluoride treatments in prevention of caries-like lesion formation in enamel: an *in vitro* study. *J Clin Pediatr Dent* 1999; 23(3): 247–257.

56 Namour S. Enamel fluoridation by means of Argon Laser. *Br Dent J* 2004; (15 Special Issue): SI55–156.

57 Friedman G, Reyto R. Laser bleaching: a clinical survey. *Dent Today* 1997; 16(5): 106.

58 Baratieri LN, et al. *Caderno de dentística-clareamento dental.* Sao Paulo: Santos, 2004.

59 Pagani C, Torres RG, Miranda CB. *Livro do ano Cínica Odontológica Brasileira.* Sao Paulo: Artes Médicas, 2004: 485–487.

60 Araújo Jr EM. *Influência do tempo de uso de um gel clareador à base de peróxido de carbamida a 10% na microdureza superficial da dentina de um estudo in situ.* 109p. Dissertação (Mestrado em Odontologia – opção dentística) – Programa de Pós-graduação em odontologia, Universidade Federal de Santa Catarina, Florianópolis, 2002.

61 Arcari GM. *Influência de tempo de uso de um gel clareador a base de peróxido de carbamida a 10% na microdureza superficial da dentina. Um estudo in situ.* 109p. Dissertação (Mestrado em Odontologia – Opção Dentística) – Programa de Pós graduação em Odontologia, Universidade Federal de Santa Catarina, Florianópolis, 2002.

62 Miranda CB. *Avaliação da microdureza e tenacidade do esmalte dental humano submetido ao tratamento clareador.* 321p. Dissertação (Mestrado em Odontologia Restauradora) – Faculdade de Odontologia de São José dos Campos, Universidade estadual Paulista. São José dos campos, 2003.

63 Haywood VB. Nightguard vital bleaching: current information and research. *Esthet. Dent. Update* 1990; 1(2): 20–25.

64 Cooper JS, Bokmeyer TJ, Bowles WH. Penetration of the pulp chamber by carbamide peroxide bleaching agents. *J Endod* 1992; 18: 315–317.

65 Haywood VB, Barry TG. Natural tooth bleaching. In: Summit JB, Robbins JW, Schwartz RS, eds. *Fundamentals of operative dentistry: a contemporary approach*, 2nd edn. Quintessence Int 1991; 22: 515–523.

66 Cohen SC. Human pulpar response to bleaching procedures on vital teeth. *J Endod* 1979; 5: 138–147.

67 Robertson WD, Melfi RC. Pulpal response to vital bleaching procedures. *J Endod* 1980; 6(7): 645–649.

68 Seale NS, et al. Pulpal reaction to bleaching of teeth in dogs. *J Dent Res* 1981; 60: 948–953.

69 Seale NS, Wilson CFG. Pulpal response to bleaching of teeth in dogs. *Pediatr Dent* 1985; 7(3): 209–214.

70 Josey AL, Meyers IA, Romaniuk K, Symons AL. The effect of a vital bleaching technique on enamel. *J Oral Rehabil* 1996; 23: 244–250.

71 Junqueira JC, Colombo CED, Martins CAde P, et al. Efeito da técnica de clareamento, utilizando peróxido de carbamida a 35%, sobre o esmalte dental – avaliação por microscopia de luz polarizada e microscopia eletrônica de varredura. *JBC* 2000; 4(24): 61–65.

72 Rodrigues JA, Basting RT, Serra MC, Rodrígues Jr AL. Effects of 10% carbamide peroxide bleaching materials on enamel microhardness. *Am J Dent* 2001; 14(2): 67–71.

73 Freitas PM, Basting RT, Rodrigues Jr AL, Serra MC. Effects of two 10% peroxide carbamide bleaching agents on dentin microhardness at different time intervals. *Quintessence Int* 2002; 33(5): 370–375.

74 Attin T, Kielbassa AM, Schwanenberg M, Hellwing E. Effect of fluoride treatment on remineralization of bleached enamel. *J Oral Rehabil* 1997; 24: 282–286.

75 Vendramini et al 2004

76 Dostalová T, et al. Diode laser-activated bleaching. *Braz Dent J* 2004; 15: 3–8.

CHAPTER 15

Caries diagnosis

Mariana Minatel Braga,[1] Thais Gimenez,[1] Fausto Medeiros Mendes,[1] Christopher Deery,[2] and David N. J. Ricketts[3]

[1] Department of Pediatric Dentistry, School of Dentistry, University of São Paulo (USP), São Paulo, SP, Brazil
[2] School of Clinical Dentistry, University of Sheffield, Sheffield, UK
[3] Dundee Dental Hospital and School, University of Dundee, Dundee, UK

Contemporary concepts

Caries detection is a key step in the gathering and synthesis of information that makes up the caries diagnostic process.[1,2] Detection is dependent on the identification of signs of dental caries on tooth surfaces. These signs reflect the actual status or severity of dental caries in the oral cavity and consequently aid in the clinical decision-making process that constitutes diagnosis and treatment planning.[2] This is particularly important because patients do not usually report symptoms related to caries lesions, especially in the initial stages. Consequently, it is the clinician who will identify any disease present.[3]

Caries can be detected and diagnosed at different thresholds. Historically, cavitation (presence of a frank hole) has been used; however, such lesions are deep, often involve the dental pulp, and are at the extreme end of the lesion severity spectrum. The D_3 (caries into dentine) threshold has also been used, but there is increasing interest in the D_1 (caries into enamel – the initial stage lesion) threshold as this promotes a preventive approach to oral health care, as early lesion progression can be arrested and lesion remineralization is possible.[4,5] Varying the diagnostic threshold can significantly alter the reporting of epidemiological data collected in population surveys.[6–8]

There are a number of diagnostic systems available to assist in caries detection and assessment; each, whether visual or electronic, has advantages and disadvantages in terms of diagnostic threshold and technique accuracy.[4,5] Therefore, choosing the appropriate caries detection method and threshold is intimately related to the outcome that is hoped for from the method used.[9]

Caries surveys using the World Health Organization criteria have been based on the detection of cavitated dentinal caries lesions.[10]. These lesions are in fact quite advanced D_3 lesions. This level has been chosen because it is the point where operative intervention is unquestioningly indicated (Fig. 15.1a). It has also been erroneously believed that diagnosis at this threshold yields superior validity and reproducibility for diagnosis at less advanced stages of the disease. It has also been argued that detection of lesions prior to cavitation is less cost-effective in the short term and is a measure indicated only for individuals with high caries risk.[11] On the other hand, some authors have criticized caries decision-making based only on the need for operative treatment or presence of cavities, since other important factors can play an important role in prognosis of caries lesions and the opportunity for prevention is lost[3,9] Diagnosis of lesions prior to cavitation may be less cost-effective in the short term, but clinically avoids biological cost in terms of lost tooth tissue.

Increasingly, clinicians, educators, and researchers are seeing the value in diagnosing caries at as early a stage as possible.[4,5,12] Detection of caries lesions at an early stage can give a more realistic picture of the prevalence of dental caries in different populations,[13,14] including its different levels of severity (Fig. 15.1a,b). In addition, these lesions can be managed more efficiently, reducing costs related to operative treatment in short- and long-term analysis.[6,7,15–20] Arguments for early detection in terms of tooth survival, associated benefit to the patient, and reduced costs to the healthcare system have been made. For the researchers, registering initial caries lesions in clinical trials may be important in minimizing costs and study duration.[12]

Although the diagnostic threshold is clearly important to clinical decision-making, caries diagnosis cannot be dissociated from caries activity assessment, if a truly valid prognosis for the lesion is to be reached. Caries activity is an extremely important parameter in the estimation of caries progression and consequently allows the best therapy in each situation to be established,[1,5,21–23] since recent and past signs of dental caries can be distinguished[5] and patients who need some form of intervention to arrest caries lesions can be effectively differentiated from those who do not[1,22] (Fig. 15.1b,c). Therefore, uniting caries detection and activity assessment is an important step in deciding the optimal treatment for a patient.[24]

Lasers in Dentistry: Guide for Clinical Practice, First Edition. Edited by Patrícia M. de Freitas and Alyne Simões.
© 2015 John Wiley & Sons, Inc. Published 2015 by John Wiley & Sons, Inc.

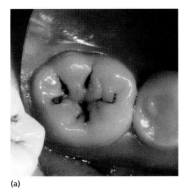
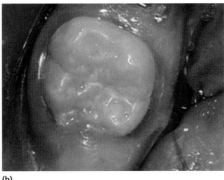
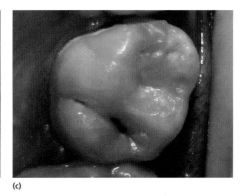

(a) (b) (c)

Figure 15.1 Different stages and prognosis of caries lesions: (a) cavitated caries lesion – more prone to cause pulpal damages and to progress (b) initial active caries lesions: sign of dental caries present – need intervention to be arrested (c) initial inactive caries lesions: past sign of dental caries – do not need intervention to be arrested.

Use of laser fluorescence in caries detection

Fluorescence is the result of an interaction between electromagnetic waves and specific molecules. These molecules are first excited and, when they return to their original state, they fluoresce. In other words, when this process is complete, previously excited molecules emit light across the visible or non-visible light spectra.

Emission of fluorescence from dental structures has been studied for a long time.[25–27] After excitation by ultraviolet light, different spectra of visible fluorescence were found to be emitted from sound and carious dentin.[26] Further, this trend was confirmed using yellow–green light in visible luminescent spectroscopy.[25] Different wavelengths of laser light spectra were then tested in order to distinguish sound from carious areas.[27] The argon laser (488 nm) provided the most suitable wavelength for the detection of caries lesions using fluorescence.[27] Its effectiveness in distinguishing caries lesions from sound areas was related to the higher absorption of argon laser light by carious tissues, thereby resulting in less fluorescence being emitted by them compared to sound tissues.[27]

The HeNe laser (633 nm) did not succeed in differentiating sound areas from caries lesions.[27] However, the diode laser (AsGaIP), which emits a similar wavelength (655 nm), has proved effective. At this wavelength, the distinction between caries lesions and sound surfaces was more evident than had previously been obtained, even though the fluorescence levels were lower when the argon laser was used.[28] The wavelength produced by the diode laser can penetrate dental surfaces,[28,29] which may explain why it has succeeded where other devices have failed.

The fluorescence emitted from dental tissues excited by a diode laser is derived especially from porphyrins (bacterial byproducts) and not directly from the demineralization process.[28–32] Fluorescence tends to be greater from teeth presenting with high concentrations of these bacterial metabolites and also darker teeth.[28,29] Therefore, the basal fluorescence observed in dental tissues is probably the combined fluorescence from

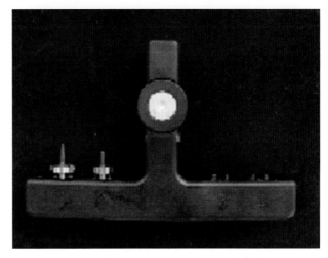

Figure 15.2 Ceramic whose fluorescence is known and used for initial standard calibration of the LFpen.

inorganic components associated with low concentrations of bacterial metabolic components. On the other hand, fluorescence from caries lesions is the result of an association between an increase in porphyrin concentration caused by caries progression and disintegration of the inorganic structure of the tooth.[29]

In order to compensate for variation between and within diode devices, calibration of the device with a ceramic standard is necessary before its use.[29] This inherent fluorescence of a ceramic standard is known and it can therefore be used as a reference against which to check the readings for the device (Fig. 15.2). This is necessary to ensure consistency and to allow comparisons of laser fluorescence measurements over time. As laser fluorescence measurements will also vary according to variation in tooth color from one person to another, an individual calibration should also be done for each patient, to set a baseline fluorescence for that dentition. This second calibration of the device is carried out by measuring the fluorescence of a sound region on the smooth surface of the tooth. This provides the baseline fluorescence value

(Fig. 15.3), which is then subtracted electronically from the fluorescence of the sites subsequently investigated.

It is also possible for the color and baseline fluorescence to vary between different teeth within the same dentition. However, in daily clinical practice, individual calibration (IC) for each and every tooth, prior to each reading, would be extremely time-consuming and unrealistic.[33,34] In order to investigate the

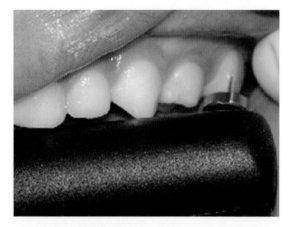

Figure 15.3 Individual calibration of the LFpen on a sound tooth surface.

impact of not calibrating a device on an individual patient and tooth basis, a recent *in vivo* study compared laser fluorescence (LF) readings without any IC with readings taken when the device was calibrated on a sound surface of a permanent incisor or deciduous first or second molar tooth for each patient. When no IC was carried out, the LF readings were higher than when any form of IC was used. LF readings taken following any form of IC were statistically the same, indicating that calibration on only one sound surface is needed to achieve clinically consistent results.[35,36] That said, it has been suggested that if caries lesion progression is to be monitored over a period of time, the method of IC should be standardized.[35,37] Further studies in this field should be encouraged. Certainly, a simplification of the calibration process could contribute to easier utilization of this method in clinical practice.

Based on the use of the diode laser and the principles described above, the first commercially available device based on laser fluorescence was developed, DIAGNOdent (LF; KaVo, Biberach, Germany) (Fig. 15.4a). More recently, a new version of this device has become available – the DIAGNOdent pen (LFpen; KaVo) (Fig. 15.4b). This new version uses similar principles to the original in differentiating fluorescence between sound and caries tissues[29] (Fig 15.5).

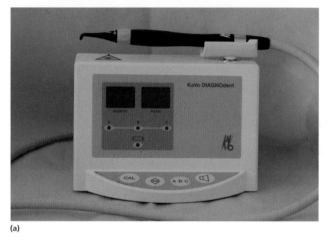

(a)

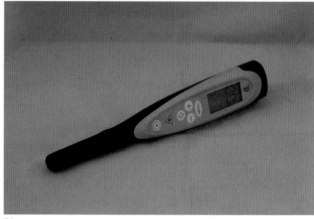

(b)

Figure 15.4 Laser fluorescence devices: (a) LF – DIAGNOdent(b) LFpen – DIAGNOdent pen.

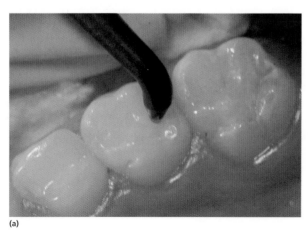

(a)

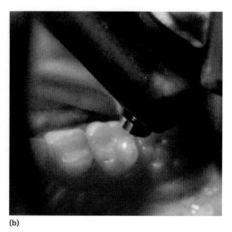

(b)

Figure 15.5 Utilization of (a) LF and (b) LFpen.

The LFpen has an additional function compared to the older LF device, in that it has an attachment which permits application to and the detection of approximal caries lesions in addition to occlusal lesions[38] (Fig 15.6). Another significant difference between the two devices relates to the tips (Fig. 15.7). In the LFpen device, the same solid single sapphire fiber tip is used both for delivery of the excitation and for collection of the fluorescent light. In contrast, the older LF device delivered the light to the angled tip within a central excitation fiber and collected the fluorescent light from dental tissue via additional fibers which were concentrically arranged around the central fiber.[38]

The tip of both the LF and LFpen should be placed on the site under investigation and rotated around a vertical axis. While the tip is in contact with the surface, real time (individual moment) values of fluorescence are read by the device. The highest value read during the evaluation of a single surface is also registered in a specific display (Fig. 15.8a,b).

Since their launch, the LF and LFpen have been extensively studied. The use of these devices as an objective method has been demonstrated.[39] Nevertheless, data about LF/LFpen accuracy have shown different trends in different studies. In addition, several factors that could influence or affect their performance have been investigated and identified (e.g. staining). In order to compile and synthesize the results of different studies in a structured and unbiased way to better evaluate the effectiveness of this method in detecting caries, we undertook a systematic review of the literature.

Performance of laser fluorescence in caries detection: A systematic review

Systematic reviews are scientific studies that summarize the results of individual studies through well-defined steps and strategies that limit bias and random errors.[40,41]

Location and identification of studies
Reviewers
Two reviewers independently performed the search and selection of articles. A researcher with experience in caries diagnosis resolved any cases of conflict or doubt.

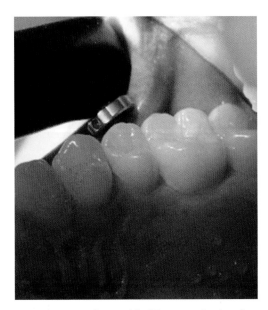

Figure 15.6 Innovation in the use of the LFpen: examination of approximal surfaces.

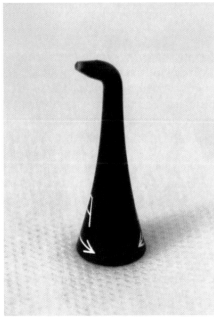
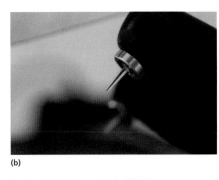
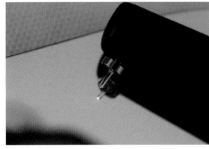

Figure 15.7 Different tips: (a) LF tip; (b) LFpen conical tip; (c) LFpen cylindrical tip.

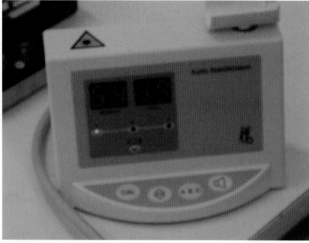

(a)

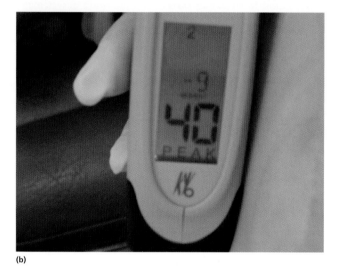

(b)

Figure 15.8 Display of (a) LF and (b) LFpen. Note the moment and peak values registered during examination.

Sources of studies

PubMed is the most frequently used resource for information in the biomedical field. Moreover, it is a very accessible, quick, and easy to use database.[42] Regarding language, some recent studies have shown that the exclusion of published articles that are not in English does not seem to bias the review of conventional medicine,[43,44] but does bias reviews of complementary and alternative medicine.[45]

Thus, we performed a systematic search of the PubMed electronic database for articles published in English until March 1st, 2012. The references of the included articles were checked for verification of possible items not covered by the search.

Search strategy

The search strategy was divided into two parts. The first part corresponded to the optimal search strategy for diagnostic studies[46] and the clinical situation studied. The other part concerned the

Table 15.1 Search strategy for electronic database concerning the diagnostic outcome and clinical situation studied.

Strategy related to the outcome of the diagnostic method	(((((((((((((((((((sensitive and specificity) OR sensitivity and specificity/standards) OR specificity) OR screening) OR false positive) OR false negative) OR accuracy) OR predictive value of tests) OR predictive value) OR predictive value of tests/standards) OR predictive values of tests) OR predictive values) OR reference value) OR reference values) OR reference values/standards)) OR (((((((((((roc) OR roc analyses) OR roc analysis) OR roc and) OR roc area) OR roc auc) OR roc characteristics) OR roc curve) OR roc curve method) OR roc curves) OR roc estimated) OR roc evaluation) OR likelihood ratio)))[46]
Clinical situation	(dental caries[MeSH Terms] OR caries OR carious)

Table 15.2 Search strategy for electronic database related to the method.

Laser fluorescence method	((((lasers[MeSH Terms]) AND fluorescence[MeSH Terms])) OR ((((laser fluorescence) OR DIAGNOdent) OR infrared) OR diode laser fluorescence))

method studied (Tables 15.1 and 15.2)[47]. The strategies were linked using the Boolean tool "AND" in the method evaluated.

Selection of studies

Inclusion criteria

After locating the studies, their titles and abstracts were inspected to determine if they fulfilled the inclusion criteria.

Articles were considered for inclusion if:
- They were related to the performance of the LF or LFpen method;
- They had any type of test as a reference standard;
- They were performed in human teeth, including *in vitro* studies;
- The disease under investigation was dental caries.

Exclusion criteria

The articles that fulfilled the inclusion criteria had their full text evaluated to see if the sample size was reported and whether there were sufficient data related to the prevalence of dental caries and performance of the method (sensitivity and specificity) or sufficient data to calculate this information. If they did not, they were excluded.

Data collection

Data from selected studies were collected independently by each reviewer, using the Review Manager software (RevMan Version 5.1, Copenhagen: The Nordic Cochrane Centre, The Cochrane Collaboration, 2011) (Table 15.3). The following information was extracted: diagnostic method applied, reference test used, cut-off values, setting (*in vivo* or *in vitro* studies and if the specimens were stored frozen or not), tooth type (primary or permanent teeth),

Table 15.3 Studies included in the systematic review of the performance of LF and LFpen.

Study	Title	Year	n	D1 Sn	D1 Sp	D3 Sn	D3 Sp	Method	Primary/permanent	Tooth surface	In vitro/in vivo	Reference standard	Cut-off value
Jablonski-Momeni et al.[51]	Impact of measuring multiple or single occlusal lesions on estimates of diagnostic accuracy using fluorescence methods	2012	82	0.83	0.65	0.82	0.59	LFpen	Permanent	Occlusal	In vitro, not frozen	Histological	Sound (≤5); enamel (6–13); dentinal (≥17)
Matos et al.[52]	Influence of cross-infection control methods on performance of pen-type laser fluorescence in detecting occlusal caries lesions in primary teeth	2012	62	0.69	0.67	0.78	0.90	LFpen	Primary	Occlusal	In vitro frozen	histological	Sound (≤8); enamel (≥9); dentinal (≥31)
Novaes et al.[53]	Performance of fluorescence-based and conventional methods of occlusal caries detection in primary molars – an in vitro study	2012	113	0.703	0.837	0.526	0.904	LF	Primary	Occlusal	In vitro, frozen	Histological	Sound (≤8); enamel (>8); dentinal (≥24)
Novaes et al.[53]	Performance of fluorescence-based and conventional methods of occlusal caries detection in primary molars – an in vitro study	2012	113	0.781	0.714	0.684	0.840	LFpen	Primary	Occlusal	In vitro, frozen	Histological	Sound (≤9); enamel (>9); dentinal (≥31)
Rechmann et al.[54]	Performance of laser fluorescence devices and visual examination for the detection of occlusal caries in permanent molars	2012	1034	0.87	0.66			LF	Permanent	Occlusal	In vivo	Visual	Enamel (>15)
Seremidi et al.[55]	Comparative in vitro validation of VistaProof and DIAGNOdent pen for occlusal caries detection in permanent teeth	2012	107	0.432	0.814	0.550	0.862	LFpen	Permanent	Occlusal	In vitro, not frozen	Histological	Sound (≤8); enamel (9–24); dentinal (≥44)
Aktan et al.[56]	A novel LED-based device for occlusal caries detection	2011	129	0.65	0.97	0.33	0.60	LFpen	Permanent	Occlusal	In vitro, not frozen	Histological	Sound (0–13); enamel (14–20); dentinal (21–99)
Bittar et al.[57]	Influence of moisture and plaque on the performance of a laser fluorescence device in detecting caries lesions in primary teeth	2011	55	0.946	0.556	0.917	0.744	LFpen	Primary	Occlusal	In vitro, frozen	Histological	Sound (<9); enamel (>9); dentinal (>31)

(Continued)

Table 15.3 (Continued)

Study	Title	Year	n	D1 Sn	D1 Sp	D3 Sn	D3 Sp	Method	Primary/permanent	Tooth surface	In vitro/in vivo	Reference standard	Cut-off value
Bittar et al.[57]	Influence of moisture and plaque on the performance of a laser fluorescence device in detecting caries lesions in primary teeth	2011	58	0.611	0.682	0.846	0.978	LFpen	Primary	Proximal	*In vitro*, frozen	Histological	Sound (<8); enamel (>8); dentinal (>30)
de Paula et al.[58]	*In situ* and *in vitro* comparison of laser fluorescence with visual inspection in detecting occlusal caries lesions	2011	64	0.72	1.00	0.42	0.65	LF	Permanent	Occlusal	In vitro, not frozen	Histological	Sound (0–10); enamel (11–20); dentinal (21–99)
Diniz et al.[59]	Influence of different professional prophylactic methods on fluorescence measurements for detection of occlusal caries	2011	55	0.42	0.92	1.0	0.81	LF	Permanent	Occlusal	*In vitro*, frozen	Histological	Sound (0–15); enamel (16–25); dentinal (≥25)
Diniz et al.[59]	Influence of different professional prophylactic methods on fluorescence measurements for detection of occlusal caries	2011	55	0.71	0.58	0.92	0.77	LFpen	Permanent	Occlusal	*In vitro*, frozen	Histological	Sound (0–10), enamel (11–34), dentinal (≥34)
Jablonski-Momeni et al.[60]	Performance of laser fluorescence at tooth surface and histological section	2011	181	0.82	0.48	0.54	0.89	LF	Permanent	Occlusal	*In vitro*, not frozen	Histological	Sound (0–7); enamel (8–14); dentinal (>24)
Kavvadia et al.[61]	Combined validity of DIAGNOdent(trademark) and visual examination for *in vitro* detection of occlusal caries in primary molars	2011	111	0.87	0.38	0.39	0.87	LF	Primary	Occlusal	*In vitro*, not frozen	Histological	Sound (≤3); enamel (>3); dentinal (>40)
Matos et al.[62]	Clinical performance of two fluorescence-based methods in detecting occlusal caries lesions in primary teeth	2011	D1- 383 D3- 407	0.687	0.813	0.952	0.883	LFpen	Primary	Occlusal	*In vivo*	Visual and biopsy	Sound (0–4); enamel (>4); dentinal (>34)
Neuhaus et al.[63]	Performance of laser fluorescence devices, visual and radiographic examination for the detection of occlusal caries in primary molars	2011	37	0.74	0.81	0.68	0.84	LF	Primary	Occlusal	*In vitro*, frozen	Histological	Sound (<10); enamel (>10); dentinal (>17)

Study	Title	Year	N					Device	Dentition	Surface	Setting	Reference standard	Thresholds
Neuhaus et al.[63]	Performance of laser fluorescence devices, visual and radiographic examination for the detection of occlusal caries in primary molars	2011	37	0.70	0.90	0.76	0.80	LFpen	Primary	Occlusal	In vitro, frozen	Histological	Sound (<14); enamel (>14); dentinal (>31)
Rando-Meirelles, de Sousa[64]	Using laser fluorescence (DIAGNOdent) in surveys for the detection of noncavitated occlusal dentine caries	2011	789	0.64	0.74			LF	Permanent	Occlusal	In vivo	Radiographic	Sound (00–20); enamel (21–30); dentinal (31–99)
Rodrigues et al.[65]	Light-emitting diode and laser fluorescence-based devices in detecting occlusal caries	2011	97	0.70	0.76	0.63	0.88	LF	Permanent	Occlusal	In vitro, frozen	Histological	Sound (0–7); enamel (8–14); dentinal (>24)
Rodrigues et al.[65]	Light-emitting diode and laser fluorescence-based devices in detecting occlusal caries	2011	97	0.62	0.76	0.63	0.87	LFpen	Permanent	Occlusal	In vitro, frozen	Histological	Sound (0–7); enamel (8–14); dentinal (>24)
Chu et al.[66]	Clinical diagnosis of fissure caries with conventional and laser-induced fluorescence techniques	2010	144	0.70			0.84	LF	Permanent	Occlusal	In vivo	Biopsy	Dentinal (>40)
Huth et al.[67]	In vivo performance of a laser fluorescence device for the approximal detection of caries in permanent molars.	2010	117	0.68	0.7	0.6	0.84	LFpen	Permanent	Proximal	In vivo	Visual and radiographic	Sound (<7); enamel (>7); dentinal (>16)
Novaes et al.[68]	Influence of the discomfort reported by children on the performance of approximal caries detection methods	2010	592	0.295	0.816	0.516	0.952	LFpen	Primary	Proximal	In vivo	Visual after tooth separation	Sound (0–5); enamel (>5); dentinal (>16)
Umemori et al.[69]	The possibility of digital imaging in the diagnosis of occlusal caries	2010	100	0.89	0.84			LF	Permanent	Occlusal	In vivo	Biopsy	Sound (>16.9); enamel (>45.2); dentinal (>57.9)
Abalos et al.[70]	Performance of laser fluorescence for detection of occlusal dentinal caries lesions in permanent molars: an in vivo study with total validation of the sample	2009	102			0.89	0.75	LF	Permanent	Occlusal	In vivo	Biopsy	Dentinal (>20)
Apostolopoulou et al.[71]	Histological validation of a laser fluorescence device for occlusal caries detection in primary molars	2009	111	0.9	0.36	0.36	0.91	LF	Primary	Occlusal	In vitro, not frozen	Histological	Enamel (<16); dentinal (>59)

(Continued)

Table 15.3 (*Continued*)

Study	Title	Year	n	D1 Sn	D1 Sp	D3 Sn	D3 Sp	Method	Primary/permanent	Tooth surface	In vitro/in vivo	Reference standard	Cut-off value
Braga et al.[72]	*In vitro* performance of methods of approximal caries detection in primary molars	2009	131	0.87	0.25	0.77	0.71	LFpen	Primary	Proximal	*In vitro*, frozen	Visual and histological	Sound (0–4); enamel (4.1–38); dentinal (>38)
Diniz et al.[73]	*In vivo* evaluation of laser fluorescence performance using different cut-off limits for occlusal caries detection	2009	130			0.7	0.87	LF	Permanent	Occlusal	*In vivo*	Visual, radiographic, and biopsy	Sound (0–14); enamel (15–21); dentinal (>22)
Goel et al.[74]	Comparison of validity of DIAGNOdent with conventional methods for detection of occlusal caries in primary molars using the histological gold standard: an *in vivo* study	2009	83	0.81	1.00	0.77	0.74	LF	Primary	Occlusal	*In vivo*	Histological	Sound (0–6); enamel (7–20); dentinal (≥35)
Khalife et al.[75]	*In vivo* evaluation of DIAGNOdent for the quantification of occlusal dental caries	2009	60			0.91	0.38	LF	Permanent	Occlusal	*In vivo*	biopsy	Dentinal (>30)
Novaes et al.[76]	Performance of a pen-type laser fluorescence device and conventional methods in detecting approximal caries lesions in primary teeth: *in vivo* study	2009	621	0.16	0.96	0.65	1.00	LFpen	Primary	Proximal	*In vivo*	Temporary separation (visual)	Sound (0–5); enamel (5–16); dentinal (>16)
Rodrigues et al.[77]	*In vitro* comparison of laser fluorescence performance with visual examination for detection of occlusal caries in permanent and primary molars	2009	148	0.53	0.92	0.16	0.89	LF	Permanent	Occlusal	*In vitro*, not frozen	Histological	Sound (0–7); enamel (7.1–14); dentinal (>24)
Rodrigues et al.[77]	*In vitro* comparison of laser fluorescence performance with visual examination for detection of occlusal caries in permanent and primary molars	2009	179	0.24	0.92	0.20	0.94	LF	Primary	Occlusal	*In vitro*, not frozen	Histological	Sound (0–7); enamel (7.1–14); dentinal (>24)
Sridhar et al.[78]	A comparative evaluation of DIAGNOdent with visual and radiography for detection of occlusal caries: an *in vitro* study	2009	50	1	0.33	0.87	0.833	LF	Permanent	Occlusal	*In vitro*, not frozen	Histological	Sound (<6); enamel (6–14)
Barberia et al.[79]	A clinical study of caries diagnosis with a laser fluorescence system. (78)	2008	243	0.89	0.89			LF	Primary	Occlusal	*In vivo*	Visual	Sound (0–4); enamel (5–25); dentinal (>26)

Study	Title	Year	N					Device	Dentition	Surface	Setting	Validation	Thresholds
Barberia et al.[79]	A clinical study of caries diagnosis with a laser fluorescence system	2008	77	0.40	0.82			LF	Permanent	Occlusal	In vivo	Visual	Sound (0–4); enamel (5–25); dentinal (>26)
Costa et al.[80]	Use of Diagnodent for diagnosis of non-cavitated occlusal dentin caries	2008	151			0.93	0.75	LF	Permanent	Occlusal	In vivo	Biopsy	Sound (0–20); enamel (21–29); dentinal (>30)
Huth et al.[81]	Clinical performance of a new laser fluorescence device for detection of occlusal caries lesions in permanent molars	2008	120	0.88	0.85	0.67	0.79	LFpen	Permanent	Occlusal	In vivo	Biopsy	enamel (>12); dentinal (>25)
Kavvadia, Lagouvardos[82]	Clinical performance of a diode laser fluorescence device for the detection of occlusal caries in primary teeth	2008	405	0.43	0.88	0.78	0.63	LF	Primary	Occlusal	In vivo	biopsy	Sound (0–9); enamel (10–42); dentinal (30–99)
Rocha-Cabral et al.[83]	Autoclaving and battery capacity influence on laser fluorescence measurements	2008	120	0.88	0.63	0.77	0.74	LF	Primary	Occlusal	In vitro, not frozen	Histological	Sound (0–4); enamel (5–12); dentinal (>12)
Rodrigues et al.[84]	Performance of fluorescence methods, radiographic examination and ICDAS II on occlusal surfaces in vitro	2008	119			0.51	0.89	LF	Permanent	Occlusal	In vitro, frozen	Histological	Dentinal (>24)
Rodrigues et al.[84]	Performance of fluorescence methods, radiographic examination and ICDAS II on occlusal surfaces in vitro	2008	119			0.78	0.56	LFpen	Permanent	Occlusal	In vitro, frozen	Histological	Dentinal (>17)
Rodrigues et al.[85]	Performance of fluorescence methods, radiographic examination and ICDAS II on occlusal surfaces in vitro	2008	119			0.86	0.63	FC	1.1 Permanent	1.2 Occlusal	1.3 In vitro, frozen	1.4 Histological	Dentinal (>1.319)
Rodrigues et al.[85]	In vitro evaluation of the influence of air abrasion on detection of occlusal caries lesions in primary teeth	2008	65	0.28	0.50			LF	Primary	Occlusal	In vitro, not frozen	Histological	Sound (0–13); enamel (14–20); dentinal (30–99)
Valera et al.[86]	Comparison of visual inspection, radiographic examination, laser fluorescence and their combinations on treatment decisions for occlusal surfaces	2008	72	0.33		0.33	1.00	LF	Permanent	Occlusal	In vitro, not frozen	Histological	Sound (0–5); enamel (6–10); dentinal (>21)

(Continued)

Table 15.3 (Continued)

Study	Title	Year	n	D1 Sn	D1 Sp	D3 Sn	D3 Sp	Method	Primary/permanent	Tooth surface	In vitro/in vivo	Reference standard	Cut-off value
Krause et al.[87]	Comparison of two laser fluorescence devices for the detection of occlusal caries in vivo	2007	94			0.92	0.53	LF	Permanent	Occlusal	In vivo	Biopsy	Dentinal (>36)
Krause et al.[87]	Comparison of two laser fluorescence devices for the detection of occlusal caries in vivo	2007	94			0.88	0.53	LFpen	Permanent	Occlusal	In vivo	Biopsy	Dentinal (>23)
Manton et al.[88]	The effect of pit and fissure sealants on the detection of occlusal caries	2007	198	0.49	0.83			LF	Permanent	Occlusal	In vitro, not frozen	Histological	Enamel (>14)
Akarsu, Koprulu[89]	In vivo comparison of the efficacy of DIAGNOdent by visual inspection and radiographic diagnostic techniques in the diagnosis of occlusal caries	2006	165	0.88	0.71	0.89	0.87	LF	Permanent	Occlusal	In vivo	Biopsy	Sound(0–5.5); enamel(5.5–11.5); dentinal(>11.5)
Deery et al.[90]	Effect of placing a clear sealant on the validity and reproducibility of occlusal caries detection by a laser fluorescence device: an in vitro study	2006	37	0.93	0.07	0.89	0.73	LF	Permanent	Occlusal	In vitro	Histological	Sound(0–4.9); enamel(5–25); dentinal(>25.01)
Lussi, Hellwig[38]	Performance of a new laser fluorescence device for the detection of occlusal caries in vitro	2006	119	0.96	0.69	0.81	0.79	LF	Permanent	Occlusal	In vitro, frozen	Histological	Sound (0–7); enamel (7.1–14); dentinal (>24)
Lussi, Hellwig[38]	Performance of a new laser fluorescence device for the detection of occlusal caries in vitro	2006	119	0.88	0.77	0.79	0.84	LFpen	Permanent	Occlusal	In vitro, frozen	Histological	Sound(0–6); enamel(6.1–13); dentinal(>17)
Lussi et al.[91]	Detection of approximal caries with a new laser fluorescence device	2006	150	0.87	0.93	0.92	0.81	LFpen	Permanent	Proximal	In vitro, frozen	Histological	Sound(0–9); Enamel(9.1–13); Dentinal(>22)
Mendes et al.[92]	Use of high-powered magnification to detect occlusal caries in primary teeth	2006	110	0.61	0.93	0.73	0.88	LF	Primary	Occlusal	In vitro, not frozen	Histological	Sound(0–7); enamel(8–14); dentinal(>14)
Olmez et al.[93]	Clinical evaluation of Diagnodent in detection of occlusal caries in children	2006	92	0.93	1	0.86	0.80	LF	Permanent	Occlusal	In vivo	Biopsy	Sound(0–14); enamel(15–20); dentinal(21–99)

Study	Title	Year	N					Method	Dentition	Surface	Condition	Validation	Threshold
Reis et al.[94]	Performance of methods of occlusal caries detection in permanent teeth under clinical and laboratory conditions	2006	110	0.71	0.57	0.78	0.63	LF	Permanent	Occlusal	*In vitro*, not frozen	Histological	Sound (0–13); enamel (14–19); dentinal (>20)
Reis et al.[94]	Performance of methods of occlusal caries detection in permanent teeth under clinical and laboratory conditions	2006	110	0.8	0.43	0.75	0.52	LF	Permanent	Occlusal	*In vivo*	Histological	Sound (0–13); enamel (14–19); dentinal (>20)
Bengtson et al.[95]	Influence of examiner's clinical experience in detecting occlusal caries lesions in primary teeth	2005	87	0.29	0.98	0.33	1.00	LF	Primary	Occlusal	*In vitro*, not frozen	Histological	Sound (0–4); enamel (5–12); dentinal (>12)
Burin et al.[96]	Occlusal caries detection: a comparison of a laser fluorescence system and conventional methods	2005	105			0.72	0.67	LF	Permanent	Occlusal	*In vitro*, not frozen	Histological	Sound (<11); enamel (12–16); dentinal (>16)
Lussi et al.[97]	Influence of professional cleaning and drying of occlusal surfaces on laser fluorescence *in vivo*	2005	117			0.98	0.93	LF	Permanent	Occlusal	*In vivo*	Biopsy	Sound (0–15); enamel (16–17); dentinal (>18)
Mendes et al.[98]	Performance of DIAGNOdent for detection and quantification of smooth-surface caries in primary teeth	2005	77	0.51	0.96	0.82	0.94	LF	Primary	Smooth	*In vitro*, not frozen	Histological	Sound (<3); enamel (>3); dentinal (>8)
Virajsilp et al.[99]	Comparison of proximal caries detection in primary teeth between laser fluorescence and bitewing radiography	2005	107	0.75	0.94	0.85	0.89	LF	Primary	Proximal	*In vitro*, not frozen	histological	Sound (<2); Enamel (2); Dentinal (>4)
Reis et al.[100]	Occlusal caries detection: a comparison of DIAGNOdent and two conventional diagnostic methods	2004	45			0.46	0.9	LF	Permanent	Occlusal	*In vitro*, not frozen	Histological	Sound (0–4); enamel (5–20); dentinal (>20)
Anttonen et al.[101]	Clinical study of the use of the laser fluorescence device DIAGNOdent for detection of occlusal caries in children.	2003	613	0.92		0.92	0.82	LF	Permanent	Occlusal	*In vivo*	Visual and biopsy	Dentinal (>30)
Baseren, Gokalp,[102]	Validity of a laser fluorescence system (DIAGNOdent) for detection of occlusal caries in third molars: an *in vitro* study	2003	31	1	0.74	1	0.92	LF	Permanent	Occlusal	*In vitro*, not frozen	Histological	Enamel (14–19); dentinal (>20)

(*Continued*)

Table 15.3 *(Continued)*

Study	Title	Year	n	D1 Sn	D1 Sp	D3 Sn	D3 Sp	Method	Primary/permanent	Tooth surface	In vitro/in vivo	Reference standard	Cut-off value
Chong et al.[103]	Visual-tactile examination compared with conventional radiography, digital radiography, and Diagnodent in the diagnosis of occlusal occult caries in extracted premolars	2003	320	0.89	0.56	0.82	0.36	LF	Permanent	Occlusal	*In vitro*, not frozen	Visual and radiographic	Sound (<5); enamel (5–25); dentinal (>26)
Cortes et al.[104]	An *in vitro* comparison of a combined FOTI/Visual examination of occlusal caries with other caries diagnostic methods and the effect of stain on their diagnostic performance	2003	152	0.73	0.85	0.84	0.67	LF	Permanent	Occlusal	*In vitro*, not frozen	Histological	Sound (<17); enamel (>17); dentinal (>23)
Francescut, Lussi[105]	Correlation between fissure discoloration, Diagnodent measurements, and caries depth: an in vitro study	2003	95	0.75	0.68	0.82	0.85	LF	Primary	Occlusal	*In vitro*, not frozen	Histological	Enamel (≥5); dentinal (≥13)
Francescut, Lussi[105]	Correlation between fissure discoloration, Diagnodent measurements, and caries depth: an in vitro study.	2003	95	0.77	0.49	0.73	0.65	LF	Permanent	Occlusal	*In vitro*, not frozen	Histological	Enamel (≥6); dentinal (≥10)
Heinrich-Weltzien et al.[106]	Comparison of different DIAGNOdent cut-off limits for in vivo detection of occlusal caries	2003	248			0.95	0.58	LF	Permanent	Occlusal	*In vivo*	Biopsy	Dentinal (>18)
Rocha et al.[107]	In vivo effectiveness of laser fluorescence compared to visual inspection and radiography for the detection of occlusal caries in primary teeth	2003	50	0.6	0.90	0.73	0.95	LF	Primary	Occlusal	*In vivo*	Histological	Sound (0–5); enamel (6–14); dentinal (21–99)
Bamzahim et al.[108]	Occlusal caries detection and quantification by DIAGNOdent and Electronic Caries Monitor: *in vitro* comparison	2002	87			0.8	1.00	LF	Permanent	Occlusal	*In vitro*, not frozen	Histological	Dentinal (>18)
Ouellet et al.[109]	Detection of occlusal caries lesions	2002	100			0.73	0.55	LF	Permanent	Occlusal	*In vitro*, not frozen	Clinical exam and photograph with caries-detecting dye	Dentinal (>16)

Reference	Title	Year	N	Sn	Sp	Sn	Sp	Method	Dentition	Surface	Condition	Validation	Threshold
Attrill, Ashley[110]	Occlusal caries detection in primary teeth: a comparison of DIAGNOdent with conventional methods	2001	58	0.77			0.82	LF	Primary	Occlusal	In vitro, not frozen	Histological	Sound (0–9); enamel (10–17); dentinal (18–99)
Lussi et al.[111]	Clinical performance of a laser fluorescence device for detection of occlusal caries lesions	2001	332	0.92			0.86	LF	Permanent	Occlusal	In vivo	Biopsy	Enamel (>14); dentinal (>20)
Pereira et al.[112]	Caries detection methods: can they aid decision making for invasive sealant treatment?	2001	230	0.2			0.98	LF	Permanent	Occlusal	In vitro, not frozen	Histological	Dentinal (10–11)
Sheehy et al.[33]	Comparison between visual examination and a laser fluorescence system for in vivo diagnosis of occlusal caries	2001	170	0.94	0.70	0.87	0.90	LF	Permanent	Occlusal	In vivo	Visual	Sound (0–14); enamel (15–20); dentinal (>20)
Shi et al.[113]	Comparison of QLF and DIAGNOdent for quantification of smooth surface caries	2001	71	0.75			0.96	LF	Permanent	Smooth	In vitro, not frozen	Histological	Dentinal (>9)
Shi et al.[114]	Occlusal caries detection with KaVo DIAGNOdent and radiography: an in vitro comparison	2000	70	0.82	0.46	0.95	1	LF	Permanent	Occlusal	In vitro, not frozen	Histological	Enamel (6.8–7.1); dentinal (21.5–22.1)
Lussi et al.[115]	Performance and reproducibility of a laser fluorescence system for detection of occlusal caries in vitro	1999	105	0.84	0.83	0.72	0.79	LF	Permanent	Occlusal	In vitro, not frozen	Histological	Sound (0–4); enamel (4.01–10); dentinal (>10.01)

D1, enamel threshold; D3, dentin threshold; Sn, sensitivity; Sp, specificity.

surface evaluated, sample size, and outcome data (sensitivity and specificity). In cases where more than one condition was tested, values related to performance were collected for all conditions.

Data analysis of laser fluorescence performance

Using the systematic search described above, almost 350 studies were initially identified. However, many studies were not directly related to the LF method or were reviews or conceptual publications, and as such were excluded (Fig. 15.9). Therefore, only 174 studies were considered for inclusion. Approximately half of these were not concerned specifically with LF performance in caries detection or could not be accessed (Fig. 15.9). In total, 88 studies were finally retained for data collection in the systematic review (Fig. 15.9). Of these, 57 studies had been conducted with permanent teeth and 28 with primary teeth (Table 15.3). Two studies assessed caries lesion activity using LF[48,49] and another two studies used LF for the measurement of artificially-induced caries.[30,50]

A wide variability was observed among the methods used in the identified studies. For example, cut-off points, selected scales, reference methods, study design, and surface under evaluation were possible sources of variation among these studies (Table 15.3).

Most studies (74%) were performed with LF, which is the older device.[53] The first studies using the LFpen were published in 2006,

while the studies using LF were published from 1999 (a year after the device had been developed). It is worth emphasizing that although the LF and LFpen work according to the same principle, they gave different results in the studies in which they were both tested using the same protocol.[53,59,63,77,116] In addition, some variables, for example method of sterilization, seem to influence the readings and performances of both of these devices.[52,83] Finally, different optimal cut-off points have been found for each of the devices.[53] Therefore, it should be kept in mind that the devices are similar, but not identical, the LFpen being an evolution of the LF.

From the literature, it can be noted that different cut-off points have been used and tested in several studies. The cut-off point is the reading or value chosen to determine the threshold between sound and diseased tissues. Historically, manufacturers proposed the use of the cut-off points that had been tested in one of the first clinical studies using the LF[111] (Table 15.4). Many studies have since proposed their own cut-off point scales. The cut-off points used have been shown to exert some influence on LF performance and, additionally, the choice of optimal cut-off points in each study can overestimate the validity of the results compared to when the manufacturer's scale is used.[117]

Based on these findings, although cut-off points can potentially cause divergences among studies,[73,102,106,107–117] it is evident

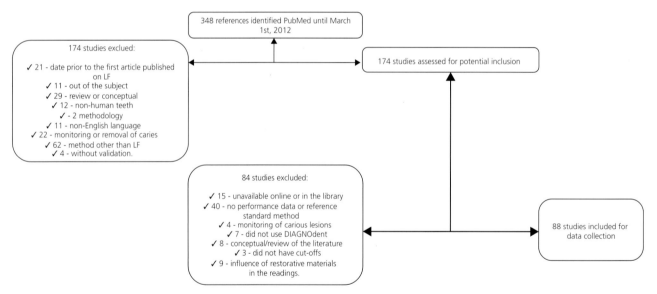

Figure 15.9 Flowchart of systematic review regarding performance of LF methods.

Table 15.4 LF cut-off points suggested by manufacturers.

Threshold	LF readings	
	Occlusal/smooth surfaces	**Approximal surfaces**
Sound or initial enamel caries	0–12	0–7
Advanced enamel caries	13–24	8–15
Dentine caries	>24	>16

LF Laser fluorescence.

that cut-off adjustment can contribute to the better use of the LF/LFpen. To choose the best cut-off point, it is important to keep in mind what the method is being used for.[117,118] If the LF/LFpen is to be used in combination with a clinical examination, to look for undetected diseased sites, the sensitivity of the method should be increased (generally by using lower cut-off points). However, if an area of low caries prevalence is being investigated, more specific methods are preferable to avoid false positives, especially at the dentin threshold, where a false-positive result could result in unnecessary operative treatment. In these cases, the use of a higher cut-off point is more sensible.

As mentioned above, LF has been encouraged as an adjunct to a thorough clinical visual examination,[39] exactly as radiographs are. Previous studies have shown similarities between the results of adjunctive methods.[76,107] Though more costly than radiographs, the device does not present the hazards of ionizing radiation[76] and is easier to use in trial conditions. The LF method could be used as an alternative to radiographic examination or as a method to identify those individuals who would benefit from radiographic examination because of the number of suspected caries lesions present.

Other important aspects found in our review were that only 33% of studies were conducted in primary teeth. Slight variations could be observed in LF performance between permanent and primary teeth. Some studies have included both primary and permanent teeth within the same design, and in these, generally, similar performances were noted for both. Therefore, these studies suggest similar cut-off points can be used for both types of teeth.[77,101,105,117,119]

In general, the performances of LF or LFpen *in vivo* were similar to those found *in vitro*. Storage solutions have been noted to influence LF performance in *in vitro* studies.[102,114,120,121] Although the majority of reviewed studies have been undertaken in laboratory settings, similarities between *in vivo* and *in vitro* results in the included studies permit extrapolation of LF/LFpen results *in vitro* to the clinical situation. This approximation between *in vitro* and *in vivo* findings could however be a result of the use of optimal cut-off points for the sample studied instead of using a standard cut-off point, which may have highlighted differences.

At this point, based on our first impressions of the results of the reviewed studies, it is important to emphasize that the conclusions drawn in the following sections are a general overview based on all data collected: some slight differences could be detected between some subgroups (e.g. primary vs. permanent teeth, *in vitro* vs. *in vivo* studies).

Overall, the LF/LFpen performance was superior at the dentin threshold compared to the enamel threshold. The method is strongly related to the measurement of fluorescence from porphyrins[29] and dentin/cavitated lesions tend to be more infected than enamel and non-cavitated dentin lesions, which is to be expected.[122] For these reasons, more advanced lesions tend to be more reliably detected by LF methods.[123] Advanced enamel lesions are also more readily detected than early ones.[123,124]

The addition of adjuncts such as LF or radiography to a clinical visual examination has been questioned, with some suggesting that a visual examination alone is adequate in low caries prevalence groups.[125] Adjuncts would be used in these populations to check that lesions have not been missed or to help where there is clinical doubt as to the presence or status of a lesion. Despite some very low specificities, in general, the LF/LFpen specificities tended to be higher than their sensitivities, corroborating previous findings restricted to the LF device.[39] A more specific method may lead to fewer false-positive results, as mentioned previously. Therefore, in order to avoid unnecessary treatment, a method whose specificity is higher than its sensitivity is useful.

There is one significant exception to the ratio of sensitivity to specificity generally being in favor of non-intervention. The devices tend to have a higher false-positive rate for the detection of occlusal dentinal caries. This is a significant drawback and could lead to over treatment.[104,126] This observation is especially important when dentin caries lesions are examined, since a false positive in these cases would result in unnecessary operative treatment. One possible reason for these false positives is the presence of occlusal staining (Fig. 15.10). It is therefore critically important that the LF/LFpen are used as adjuncts to a meticulous clinical examination and not relied upon on their own.

The assessment of caries activity has rarely been assessed using LF methods.[48,49,127] The LF has been used to monitor the activity of lesions on smooth surfaces[48] and around brackets,[127] but only the first of these studies assessed the performance of the method[48] and found moderate sensitivity and specificity (around 0.7) for this purpose. For occlusal surfaces, a variation in the methodology of application based on air drying before the LF examination was tested to see if this allowed an assessment of caries activity. Active cavitated caries lesions had higher readings than inactive ones. For non-cavitated caries lesions, the authors took readings after air drying for 3 seconds and 15 seconds: readings for the latter were higher than for the former and this procedure was able to distinguish active from inactive caries lesions (Fig. 15.11). When lesions were dried for longer (15 seconds), it is suggested that bacterial metabolites tend to concentrate, increasing the fluorescence readings. Also, active lesions are more porous and laser light will penetrate them more than inactive lesions.[49] However, this methodology is time consuming and other air drying times are being tested for caries activity assessment. At present it remains uncertain if the LF/LFpen may have a role in the clinical assessment of lesion activity.

Based on the general findings of the review, it appears that the LF/LFpen devices can be used as adjunctive methods to, but not in place of, a meticulous visual inspection in specific situations. One should bear in mind the caveats as to validity discussed above and further discussed in the next section, particularly with regard to the false-positive rate for occlusal surfaces. The clinician must balance the expected benefit, risk

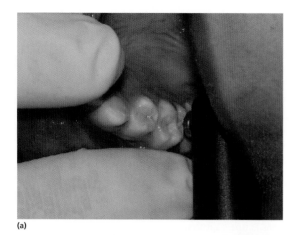

(a)

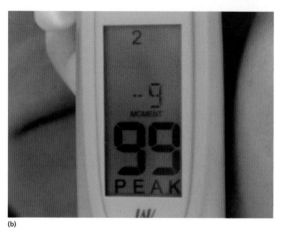

(b)

Figure 15.10 False-positive results using LFpen in a case of stained fissures: (a) LFpen examination of stained enamel caries lesion; (b) LFpen display showing a value considered as dentin caries on LFpen cut-off points scale.

of false-positives results, and additional costs related to the LF/LFpen methods, when making a decision to use these devices. In addition, LF methods can be used to monitor lesion progression over time and may have the potential to allow caries activity assessment, but further work is required to confirm this.

External factors that influence the performance of LF methods in clinical practice

Some factors related to the clinical examination have been shown to influence LF/LFpen performance. A clinician must be aware of these and take them into account when interpreting the results with the LF device used clinically.

The influence of air drying should be carefully considered. Examining moist teeth or teeth that have been air dried for a maximum of 3 seconds does not affect LF/LFpen readings.[57,116,117,128] On the other hand, longer air drying times do influence LF/LFpen readings: sensitivity is increased at the expense of specificity, which increases the number of false-positive results.[57,114,128]

The presence of plaque on surfaces can also influence the performance of LF methods.[57,108,128,129] The plaque and calculus[29] also contain bacterial porphyrins and can lead to an increase in the LF readings.[57,97,108,129] Therefore, tooth cleaning prior to LF examination should be advocated.

How surfaces are cleaned is another concern. Some prophylactic toothpastes[130,131] and some disclosing agents (unpublished data) can interfere with LF readings. It is important therefore that the influence of particles in prophylactic pastes is diminished by rinsing prior to the LF examination.[59] Alternatively, other cleaning methods can be used, for example a sodium

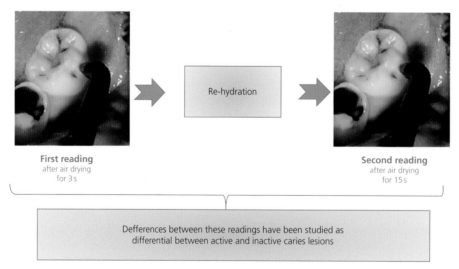

First reading
after air drying
for 3 s

Re-hydration

Second reading
after air drying
for 15 s

Defferences between these readings have been studied as differential between active and inactive caries lesions

Figure 15.11 Methodology for caries lesion activity assessment using LF.

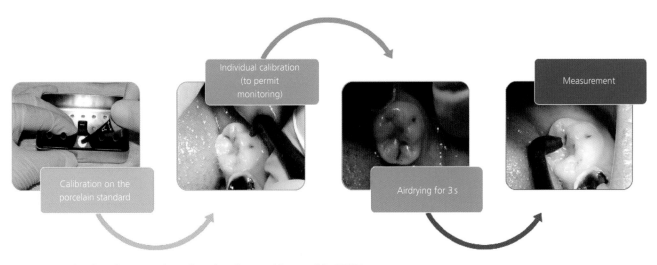

Figure 15.12 Flowchart illustrating the evidence-based protocol for use of the LF/LFpen.

bicarbonate jet, which has been shown not to significantly influence the performance of LF methods.[59] However, use of such devices will have an effect on the cost–benefit ratio.

Cross-infection control methods should also be considered with regard to interference with LF/LFpen readings. Probe tip autoclaving has been shown to be a potential influence on LF readings and LF performance.[83,132] However, for the LFpen, after successive utilization of its tips, there was a decrease in LFpen readings, independent of the autoclaving process. These findings could reflect progressive deterioration of the tip.[52]

The use of PVC barriers is another possible method to control cross-infection by LF and LFpen tips. Two studies in primary teeth showed no negative influence of a thin PVC barrier wrapped over a LF/LFpen tip.[52,132] However, another study showed that the PVC wrapping could influence the LF and LFpen performance in permanent teeth.[133] Possible explanations for these different findings include: the use of different methodologies for standard calibration of the device and histological validation; and constitution of the sample (permanent vs. primary teeth).[52] One study has shown significant differences in LF performance for primary and permanent teeth, while others have not.[134] Further studies are required to confirm the effect of PVC wrapping.

Placement of a clear fissure sealant may also interfere with the LF/LFpen readings because sealants, even clear ones, reduce LF readings and sensitivity.[90] For opaque sealants, a decrease in fluorescence readings has also been reported.[135] Recognizing this, the manufacturer recommends adjusting the cut-off point to facilitate detection of caries lesions under clear unfilled sealants.[90,135]

Finally, despite being an objective caries detection method, the use of LF devices by examiners with different levels of experience can result in different performances.[4,136] Therefore, adequate training should be undertaken by those who intend to use this method and the manufacturer's instruction should be followed closely. Figure 15.12 shows a flowchart of the important steps that must be followed when using LF/LF pen devices, in order to optimize performance.

Conclusions

Laser fluorescence methods are relatively new compared to traditional methods, such as visual inspection and radiography. However, over fewer than 20 years a considerable evidence base has accumulated. This descriptive systematic review aims to consolidate and present this evidence base in an accessible format.

Meticulous visual examination is the more complete option in caries diagnosis nowadays, but it still falls short of the ideal. LF and LFpen are at present secondary tools or adjuncts, which can be used by clinicians as appropriate to assist with diagnosis. Because of the potential for an increase in false-positive results using such devices, they should never be used alone to determine operative intervention for caries lesions.

Techniques such as the LF/LFpen offer a potential advantage as they give objective and recordable measurements. Also, the use of these devices avoids the use of ionizing radiation.

Special attention should be given to caries activity assessment. This is certainly an area of great difficulty in clinical decision-making and current evidence suggests that LF could be developed as a very useful tool in this regard, but the cost –benefit and clinical applicability of this measure needs to be verified.

The overall conclusion is that the LF and LFpen are useful caries diagnostic tools, but they need to be used by adequately trained clinicians who understand the limitations as well as the advantages of this technology.

References

1 Nyvad B. Diagnosis versus detection of caries. *Caries Res* 2004; 38(3): 192–198.

2 Baelum V, Hintze H, Wenzel A, Danielsen B, Nyvad B. Implications of caries diagnostic strategies for clinical management decisions. *Commun Dent Oral Epidemiol* 2012; 40(3): 257–66.

3 Baelum V, Heidmann J, Nyvad B. Dental caries paradigms in diagnosis and diagnostic research. *Eur J Oral Sci* 2006; 114(4): 263–277.

4 Pitts NB. Diagnostic tools and measurements--impact on appropriate care. *Commun Dent Oral Epidemiol* 1997; 25(1): 24–35.

5 Pitts NB. Modern concepts of caries measurement. *J Dent Res* 2004; 83 (Spec No C):C43-7.

6 Assaf AV, de Castro Meneghim M, Zanin L, Tengan C, Pereira AC. Effect of different diagnostic thresholds on dental caries calibration - a 12 month evaluation. *Commun Dent Oral Epidemiol* 2006; 34(3): 213–219.

7 Pitts NB, Fyffe HE. The effect of varying diagnostic thresholds upon clinical caries data for a low prevalence group. *J Dent Res* 1988; 67(3): 592–596.

8 Rimmer PA, Pitts NB. Effects of diagnostic threshold and overlapped approximal surfaces on reported caries status. *Commun Dent Oral Epidemiol* 1991; 19(4): 205–212.

9 Kidd EAM, Mejàre I, Nyvad B. Diagnóstico clínico e radiográfico. In: Fejerskov O, Kidd EAM, editors. *Cárie dentária: a doença e seu tratamento clínico. 1*. 1 ed. Sao Paulo: Editora Santos; 2005: 111–128.

10 World Health Organization. *Oral Health Surveys: Basic Methods*, 4th edn. Geneva: WHO, 1997.

11 Verdonschot EH, Angmar-Mansson B, ten Bosch JJ, et al. Developments in caries diagnosis and their relationship to treatment decisions and quality of care. *ORCA Saturday Afternoon Symposium 1997*. Caries Res 1999; 33(1): 32–40.

12 Ekstrand KR. Improving clinical visual detection--potential for caries clinical trials. *J Dent Res* 2004; 83(Spec No C): C67-71.

13 Ismail AI, Sohn W, Tellez M, Willem JM, Betz J, Lepkowski J. Risk indicators for dental caries using the International Caries Detection and Assessment System (ICDAS). *Commun Dent Oral Epidemiol* 2008; 36(1): 55–68.

14 Poulsen S, Scheutz F. Dental caries in Danish children and adolescents 1988-1997. *Commun Dent Health* 1999; 16(3): 166–170.

15 Fyffe HE, Deery C, Nugent ZJ, Nuttall NM, Pitts NB. Effect of diagnostic threshold on the validity and reliability of epidemiological caries diagnosis using the Dundee Selectable Threshold Method for caries diagnosis (DSTM). *Commun Dent Oral Epidemiol* 2000; 28(1): 42–51.

16 Ismail AI, Brodeur JM, Gagnon P, *et al.* Prevalence of non-cavitated and cavitated carious lesions in a random sample of 7-9-year-old schoolchildren in Montreal, *Quebec. Commun Dent Oral Epidemiol* 1992; 20(5): 250–255.

17 Pitts N. "ICDAS"--an international system for caries detection and assessment being developed to facilitate caries epidemiology, research and appropriate clinical management. *Commun Dent Health* 2004; 21(3): 193–198.

18 Luan W, Baelum V, Fejerskov O, Chen X. Ten-year incidence of dental caries in adult and elderly Chinese. *Caries Res* 2000; 34(3): 205–213.

19 Manji F, Fejerskov O, Nagelkerke NJ, Baelum V. A random effects model for some epidemiological features of dental caries. *Commun Dent Oral Epidemiol* 1991; 19(6): 324–328.

20 Pitts NB. Clinical diagnosis of dental caries: a European perspective. *J Dental Educ* 2001; 65(10): 972–978.

21 Angmar-Mansson BE, al-Khateeb S, Tranaeus S. Caries diagnosis. *J Dent Educ* 1998; 62(10): 771–780.

22 Nyvad B, Fejerskov O. Assessing the stage of caries lesion activity on the basis of clinical and microbiological examination. *Commun Dent Oral Epidemiol* 1997; 25(1): 69–75.

23 Basting RT, Serra MC. Occlusal caries: diagnosis and noninvasive treatments. *Quintessence Int* 1999; 30(3): 174–178.

24 Braga MM, Mendes FM, Ekstrand KR. Detection activity assessment and diagnosis of dental caries lesions. *Dent Clin North Am* 2010; 54(3): 479–493.

25 Alfano RR, Yao SS. Human teeth with and without dental caries studied by visible luminescent spectroscopy. *J Dent Res* 1981; 60(2): 120–122.

26 Foreman PC. The excitation and emission spectra of fluorescent components of human dentine. *Arch Oral Biol* 1980; 25(10): 641–647.

27 Sundstrom F, Fredriksson K, Montan S, Hafstrom-Bjorkman U, Strom J. Laser-induced fluorescence from sound and carious tooth substance: spectroscopic studies. *Swedish Dent J* 1985; 9(2): 71–80.

28 Hibst R, Gall R. Development of a diode laser-based fluorescence caries detector. *Caries Res* 1998; 32(4): 294.

29 Hibst R, Paulus R, Lussi A. Detection of occlusal caries by laser fluorescence: Basic and clinical investigations. *Med Laser Appl* 2001; 16: 205–213.

30 Mendes FM, Nicolau J, Duarte DA. Evaluation of the effectiveness of laser fluorescence in monitoring in vitro remineralization of incipient caries lesions in primary teeth. *Caries Res* 2003; 37(6): 442–444.

31 Mendes FM, Pinheiro SL, Bengtson AL. Effect of alteration in organic material of the occlusal caries on DIAGNOdent readings. *Braz Oral Res* 2004; 18(2): 141–144.

32 Buchalla W. Comparative fluorescence spectroscopy shows differences in noncavitated enamel lesions. *Caries Res* 2005; 39(2): 150–156.

33 Sheehy EC, Brailsford SR, Kidd EAM, Beighton D, Zoitopoulos L. Comparison between visual examination and a laser fluorescence system for in vivo diagnosis of occlusal caries. *Caries Res* 2001; 35(6): 421–426.

34 Braga MM, Mendes FM, Martins CR, Imparato JC. Effect of the calibration method of a laser fluorescence device for detecting occlusal caries in primary molars. *Pediatr Dent* 2006; 28(5): 451–454.

35 Reyes A, Ferreira GE, Santos J, Mendes FM, Imparato JC, Braga MM. Can the individual calibration be modified when laser fluorescence method is used for caries detection? *Int J Paediatr Dent* 2013; 23(2): 138–144.

36 Alwas-Danowska HM, Plasschaert AJM, Suliborski S, Verdonschot EH. Reliability and validity issues of laser fluorescence measurements in occlusal caries diagnosis. *J Dent* 2002; 30(4): 129–134.

37 Braun A, Krause F, Jepsen S. The influence of the calibration mode of a laser fluorescence device on caries detection. *Caries Res* 2005; 39(2): 144–149.

38 Lussi A, Hellwig E. Performance of a new laser fluorescence device for the detection of occlusal caries in vitro. *J Dent* 2006; 34(7): 467–471.

39 Bader JD, Shugars DA. A systematic review of the performance of a laser fluorescence device for detecting caries. *J Am Dent Assoc* 2004; 135(10): 1413–1426.

40 Mulrow CD. The medical review article: state of the science. *Ann Intern Med* 1987; 106(3): 485–488.

41 Cook DJ, Sackett DL, Spitzer WO. Methodologic guidelines for systematic reviews of randomized control trials in health care from the Potsdam Consultation on Meta-Analysis. *J Clin Epidemiol* 1995; 48(1): 167–171.

42 Falagas ME, Pitsouni EI, Malietzis GA, Pappas G. Comparison of PubMed, Scopus, Web of Science, and Google Scholar: strengths and weaknesses. *FASEB J* 2008; 22(2): 338–342.

43 Moher D, Pham B, Klassen TP, et al. What contributions do languages other than English make on the results of meta-analyses? *J Clin Epidemiol* 2000; 53(9): 964–972.

44 Juni P, Holenstein F, Sterne J, Bartlett C, Egger M. Direction and impact of language bias in meta-analyses of controlled trials: empirical study. *Int J Epidemiol* 2002; 31(1): 115–123.

45 Moher D, Pham B, Lawson ML, Klassen TP. The inclusion of reports of randomised trials published in languages other than English in systematic reviews. *Health Technol Assess* 2003; 7(41): 1–90.

46 Deville WL, Bezemer PD, Bouter LM. Publications on diagnostic test evaluation in family medicine journals: an optimal search strategy. *J Clin Epidemiol* 2000; 53(1): 65–69.

47 Gimenez T, Braga MM, Raggio DP, Deery C, Ricketts DN, Mendes FM. Fluorescence-based methods for detecting caries lesions: systematic review, meta-analysis and sources of heterogeneity. *PLoS One* 2013; 8(4):e60421.

48 Pinelli C, Campos Serra M, de Castro Monteiro Loffredo L. *Validity and reproducibility of a laser fluorescence system for detecting the activity of white-spot lesions on free smooth surfaces in vivo. Caries Res* 2002; 36(1): 19–24.

49 Braga MM, de Benedetto MS, Imparato JC, Mendes FM. New methodology to assess activity status of occlusal caries in primary teeth using laser fluorescence device. *J Biomed Opt* 2010; 15(4): 047005.

50 Alencar CJ, Braga MM, de Oliveira E, Nicolau J, Mendes FM. Dye-enhanced laser fluorescence detection of caries lesions around brackets. *Lasers Med Sci* 2009; 24(6): 865–870.

51 Jablonski-Momeni A, Rosen SM, Schipper HM, et al. Impact of measuring multiple or single occlusal lesions on estimates of diagnostic accuracy using fluorescence methods. *Lasers Med Sci* 2012; 27(2): 343–352.

52 Matos R, Novaes TF, Reyes A, De Benedetto MS, Mendes FM, Braga MM. Influence of cross-infection control methods on performance of pen-type laser fluorescence in detecting occlusal caries lesions in primary teeth. *Lasers Med Sci* 2013; 28(1): 185–192.

53 Novaes TF, Matos R, Gimenez T, Braga MM, De Bendetto MS, Mendes FM. Performance of fluorescence-based and conventional methods of occlusal caries detection in primary molars - an in vitro study. *Int J Paediatr Dent* 2012; 22(6): 459–466.

54 Rechmann P, Charland D, Rechmann BM, Featherstone JD. Performance of laser fluorescence devices and visual examination for the detection of occlusal caries in permanent molars. *J Biomed Opt* 2012; 17(3): 036006.

55 Seremidi K, Lagouvardos P, Kavvadia K. Comparative in vitro validation of VistaProof and DIAGNOdent pen for occlusal caries detection in permanent teeth. *Oper Dent* 2012; 37(3): 234–245.

56 Aktan AM, Cebe MA, Ciftci ME, Sirin Karaarslan E. A novel LED-based device for occlusal caries detection. *Lasers Med Sci* 2012; 27(6): 1157–1163.

57 Bittar DG, Gimenez T, Morais CC, De Benedetto MS, Braga MM, Mendes FM. Influence of moisture and plaque on the performance of a laser fluorescence device in detecting caries lesions in primary teeth. *Lasers Med Sci* 2012; 27(6): 1169–1174.

58 de Paula AB, Campos JA, Diniz MB, Hebling J, Rodrigues JA. In situ and in vitro comparison of laser fluorescence with visual inspection in detecting occlusal caries lesions. *Lasers Med Sci* 2011; 26(1): 1–5.

59 Diniz MB, Sciasci P, Rodrigues JA, Lussi A, Cordeiro RCL. Influence of different professional prophylactic methods on fluorescence measurements for detection of occlusal caries. *Caries Res* 2011; 45(3): 264–268.

60 Jablonski-Momeni A, Schipper HM, Rosen SM, et al. Performance of a fluorescence camera for detection of occlusal caries in vitro. *Odontology* 2011; 99(1): 55–61.

61 Kavvadia K, Lagouvardos P, Apostolopoulou D. Combined validity of DIAGNOdent™ and visual examination for in vitro detection of occlusal caries in primary molars. *Lasers Med Sci* 2012; 27(2): 313–319.

62 Matos R, Novaes TF, Braga MM, Siqueira WL, Duarte DA, Mendes FM. Clinical performance of two fluorescence-based methods in detecting occlusal caries lesions in primary teeth. *Caries Res* 2011; 45(3): 294–302.

63 Neuhaus KW, Rodrigues JA, Hug I, Stich H, Lussi A. Performance of laser fluorescence devices, visual and radiographic examination for the detection of occlusal caries in primary molars. *Clin Oral Invest* 2011; 15(5): 635–641.

64 Rando-Meirelles MP, de Sousa Mda L. Using laser fluorescence (DIAGNOdent) in surveys for the detection of noncavitated occlusal dentine caries. *Community Dent Health* 2011; 28(1): 17–21.

65 Rodrigues JA, Hug I, Neuhaus KW, Lussi A. Light-emitting diode and laser fluorescence-based devices in detecting occlusal caries. *J Biomed Opt* 2011; 16(10): 107003.

66 Chu CH, Lo EC, You DS. Clinical diagnosis of fissure caries with conventional and laser-induced fluorescence techniques. *Lasers Med Sci* 2010; 25(3): 355–362.

67 Huth KC, Lussi A, Gygax M, et al. In vivo performance of a laser fluorescence device for the approximal detection of caries in permanent molars. *J Dent* 2010; 38(12): 1019–1026.

68 Novaes TF, Matos R, Raggio DP, Imparato JC, Braga MM, Mendes FM. Influence of the discomfort reported by children on the performance of approximal caries detection methods. *Caries Res* 2010; 44(5): 465–471.

69 Umemori S, Tonami K, Nitta H, Mataki S, Araki K. The possibility of digital imaging in the diagnosis of occlusal caries. *Int J Dent* 2010; 2010: 860515.

70 Abalos C, Herrera M, Jimenez-Planas A, Llamas R. Performance of laser fluorescence for detection of occlusal dentinal caries lesions in permanent molars: an in vivo study with total validation of the sample. *Caries Res* 2009; 43(2): 137–141.

71 Apostolopoulou D, Lagouvardos P, Kavvadia K, Papagiannoulis L. Histological validation of a laser fluorescence device for occlusal caries detection in primary molars. *Eur Arch Paediatr Dent* 2009; 10 (Suppl 1): 11–15.

72 Braga MM, Morais CC, Nakama RC, Leamari VM, Siqueira WL, Mendes FM. In vitro performance of methods of approximal caries detection in primary molars. *Oral Surg Oral Med Oral Pathol Oral Radiol Endod* 2009; 108(4): e35–41.

73 Diniz MB, Rodrigues JA, de Paula AB, Cordeiro Rde C. In vivo evaluation of laser fluorescence performance using different cut-off limits for occlusal caries detection. *Lasers Med Sci* 2009; 24(3): 295–300.

74 Goel A, Chawla HS, Gauba K, Goyal A. Comparison of validity of DIAGNOdent with conventional methods for detection of

occlusal caries in primary molars using the histological gold standard: an in vivo study. *J Indian Soc Pedod Prev Dent* 2009; 27(4): 227–234.

75 Khalife MA, Boynton JR, Dennison JB, Yaman P, Hamilton JC. In vivo evaluation of DIAGNOdent for the quantification of occlusal dental caries. *Oper Dent* 2009; 34(2): 136–141.

76 Novaes TF, Matos R, Braga MM, Imparato JC, Raggio DP, Mendes FM. Performance of a pen-type laser fluorescence device and conventional methods in detecting approximal caries lesions in primary teeth--in vivo study. *Caries Res* 2009; 43(1): 36–42.

77 Rodrigues JA, Diniz MB, Josgrilberg EB, Cordeiro RC. In vitro comparison of laser fluorescence performance with visual examination for detection of occlusal caries in permanent and primary molars. *Lasers Med Sci* 2009; 24(4): 501–506.

78 Sridhar N, Tandon S, Rao N. A comparative evaluation of DIAGNOdent with visual and radiography for detection of occlusal caries: an in vitro study. *Indian J Dent Res* 2009; 20(3): 326–331.

79 Barberia E, Maroto M, Arenas M, Silva CC. A clinical study of caries diagnosis with a laser fluorescence system. *J Am Dent Assoc* 2008; 139(5): 572–579.

80 Costa AM, De Paula LM, Bezerra ACB. Use of diagnodent® for diagnosis of non-cavitated occlusal dentin caries. *J Appl Oral Sci* 2008; 16(1): 18–23.

81 Huth KC, Neuhaus KW, Gygax M, et al. Clinical performance of a new laser fluorescence device for detection of occlusal caries lesions in permanent molars. *J Dent* 2008; 36(12): 1033–1040.

82 Kavvadia K, Lagouvardos P. Clinical performance of a diode laser fluorescence device for the detection of occlusal caries in primary teeth. *Int J Paediatr Dent* 2008; 18(3): 197–204.

83 Rocha-Cabral RM, Mendes FM, Miura F, Ribeiro Ada C, Braga MM, Zezell DM. Autoclaving and battery capacity influence on laser fluorescence measurements. *Acta Odontol Scand* 2008; 66(2): 122–127.

84 Rodrigues JA, Hug I, Diniz MB, Lussi A. Performance of fluorescence methods, radiographic examination and ICDAS II on occlusal surfaces in vitro. *Caries Res* 2008; 42(4): 297–304.

85 Rodrigues JA, Hug I, Diniz MB, Lussi A. Performance of fluorescence methods, radiographic examination and ICDAS II on occlusal surfaces in vitro. *Caries Res* 2008; 42(4): 297–304.

86 Valera FB, Pessan JP, Valera RC, Mondelli J, Percinoto C. Comparison of visual inspection, radiographic examination, laser fluorescence and their combinations on treatment decisions for occlusal surfaces. *Am J Dent* 2008; 21(1): 25–9.

87 Krause F, Jepsen S, Braun A. Comparison of two laser fluorescence devices for the detection of occlusal caries in vivo. *Eur J Oral Sci* 2007; 115(4): 252–256.

88 Manton DJ, Messer LB. The effect of pit and fissure sealants on the detection of occlusal caries in vitro. *Eur Arch Paediatr Dent* 2007; 8(1): 43–48.

89 Akarsu S, Koprulu H. In vivo comparison of the efficacy of DIAGNOdent by visual inspection and radiographic diagnostic techniques in the diagnosis of occlusal caries. *J Clin Dent* 2006; 17(3): 53–58.

90 Deery C, Iloya J, Nugent ZJ, Srinivasan V. Effect of placing a clear sealant on the validity and reproducibility of occlusal caries detection by a laser fluorescence device: an in vitro study. *Caries Res* 2006; 40(3): 186–193.

91 Lussi A, Hack A, Hug I, Heckenberger H, Megert B, Stich H. Detection of approximal caries with a new laser fluorescence device. *Caries Res* 2006; 40(2): 97–103.

92 Mendes FM, Ganzerla E, Nunes AF, Puig AV, Imparato JC. Use of high-powered magnification to detect occlusal caries in primary teeth. *Am J Dent* 2006; 19(1): 19–22.

93 Olmez A, Tuna D, Oznurhan F. Clinical evaluation of diagnodent in detection of occlusal caries in children. *J Clin Pediatr Dent* 2006; 30(4): 287–291.

94 Reis A, Mendes FM, Angnes V, Angnes G, Grande RH, Loguercio AD. Performance of methods of occlusal caries detection in permanent teeth under clinical and laboratory conditions. *J Dent* 2006; 34(2): 89–96.

95 Bengtson AL, Gomes AC, Mendes FM, Cichello LR, Bengtson NG, Pinheiro SL. Influence of examiner's clinical experience in detecting occlusal caries lesions in primary teeth. *Pediatr Dent* 2005; 27(3): 238–243.

96 Burin C, Loguercio AD, Grande RH, Reis A. Occlusal caries detection: a comparison of a laser fluorescence system and conventional methods. *Pediatr Dent* 2005; 27(4): 307–12.

97 Lussi A, Longbottom C, Gygax M, Braig F. Influence of professional cleaning and drying of occlusal surfaces on laser fluorescence in vivo. *Caries Res* 2005; 39(4): 284–286.

98 Mendes FM, Siqueira WL, Mazzitelli JF, Pinheiro SL, Bengtson AL. Performance of DIAGNOdent for detection and quantification of smooth-surface caries in primary teeth. *J Dent* 2005; 33(1): 79–84.

99 Virajsilp V, Thearmontree A, Aryatawong S, Paiboonwarachat D. Comparison of proximal caries detection in primary teeth between laser fluorescence and bitewing radiography. *Pediatr Dent* 2005; 27(6): 493–499.

100 Reis A, Zach VL, Jr, de Lima AC, de Lima Navarro MF, Grande RH. Occlusal caries detection: a comparison of DIAGNOdent and two conventional diagnostic methods. *J Clin Dent* 2004; 15(3): 76–82.

101 Anttonen V, Seppa L, Hausen H. Clinical study of the use of the laser fluorescence device DIAGNOdent for detection of occlusal caries in children. *Caries Res* 2003; 37(1): 17–23.

102 Baseren NM, Gokalp S. Validity of a laser fluorescence system (DIAGNOdent) for detection of occlusal caries in third molars: an in vitro study. *J Oral Rehabil* 2003; 30(12): 1190–1194.

103 Chong MJ, Seow WK, Purdie DM, Cheng E, Wan V. Visual-tactile examination compared with conventional radiography, digital radiography, and Diagnodent in the diagnosis of occlusal occult caries in extracted premolars. *Pediatr Dent* 2003; 25(4): 341–349.

104 Cortes DF, Ellwood RP, Ekstrand KR. An in vitro comparison of a combined FOTI/visual examination of occlusal caries with other caries diagnostic methods and the effect of stain on their diagnostic performance. *Caries Res* 2003; 37(1): 8–16.

105 Francescut P, Lussi A. Correlation between fissure discoloration, Diagnodent measurements, and caries depth: an in vitro study. *Pediatr Dent* 2003; 25(6): 559–564.

106 Heinrich-Weltzien R, Kühnisch J, Oehme T, Ziehe A, Stösser L, García-Godoy F. Comparison of Different DIAGNOdent Cut-off Limits for In Vivo Detection of Occlusal Caries. *Oper Dent* 2003; 28(6): 672–680.

107 Rocha RO, Ardenghi TM, Oliveira LB, Rodrigues CR, Ciamponi AL. In vivo effectiveness of laser fluorescence compared to visual inspection and radiography for the detection of occlusal caries in primary teeth. *Caries Res* 2003; 37(6): 437–441.

108 Bamzahim M, Shi XQ, Angmar-Mansson B. Occlusal caries detection and quantification by DIAGNOdent and Electronic Caries Monitor: in vitro comparison. *Acta Odontol Scand* 2002; 60(6): 360–364.

109 Ouellet A, Hondrum SO, Pietz DM. Detection of occlusal carious lesions. *Gen Dent* 2002; 50(4): 346–350.

110 Attrill DC, Ashley PF. Occlusal caries detection in primary teeth: a comparison of DIAGNOdent with conventional methods. *Br Dent J* 2001; 190(8): 440–443.

111 Lussi A, Megert B, Longbottom C, Reich E, Francescut P. Clinical performance of a laser fluorescence device for detection of occlusal caries lesions. *Eur J Oral Sci* 2001; 109(1): 14–19.

112 Pereira AC, Verdonschot EH, Huysmans MC. Caries detection methods: can they aid decision making for invasive sealant treatment? *Caries Res* 2001; 35(2): 83–9.

113 Shi XQ, Tranaeus S, Angmar-Mansson B. Comparison of QLF and DIAGNOdent for quantification of smooth surface caries. *Caries Res* 2001; 35(1): 21–26.

114 Shi XQ, Welander U, Angmar-Mansson B. Occlusal caries detection with KaVo DIAGNOdent and radiography: an in vitro comparison. *Caries Res* 2000; 34(2): 151–158.

115 Lussi A, Imwinkelried S, Pitts N, Longbottom C, Reich E. Performance and reproducibility of a laser fluorescence system for detection of occlusal caries in vitro. *Caries Res* 1999; 33(4): 261–266.

116 Rodrigues JA, Hug I, Lussi A. The influence of zero value subtraction on the performance of a new laser fluorescence device for approximal caries detection. *Lasers Med Sci* 2009; 24(3): 301–306.

117 Braga MM, Mendes FM, Imparato JCP, Rodrigues CRMD. Effect of cut-off points on performance of laser fluorescence for detecting occlusal caries. *J Clin Pediatr Dent* 2007; 32(1): 33–36.

118 Astvaldsottir A, Holbrook WP, Tranaeus S. Consistency of DIAGNOdent instruments for clinical assessment of fissure caries. *Acta Odontol Scand* 2004; 62(4): 193–198.

119 Anttonen V, Seppa L, Hausen H. A follow-up study of the use of DIAGNOdent for monitoring fissure caries in children. *Commun Dent Oral Epidemiol* 2004; 32(4): 312–318.

120 Francescut P, Zimmerli B, Lussi A. Influence of different storage methods on laser fluorescence values: a two-year study. *Caries Res* 2006; 40(3): 181–185.

121 Kuhnisch J, Ziehe A, Brandstadt A, Heinrich-Weltzien R. An in vitro study of the reliability of DIAGNOdent measurements. *J Oral Rehabil* 2004; 31(9): 895–899.

122 Ricketts DN, Ekstrand KR, Kidd EA, Larsen T. Relating visual and radiographic ranked scoring systems for occlusal caries detection to histological and microbiological evidence. *Oper Dent* 2002; 27(3): 231–237.

123 Braga MM, Nicolau J, Rodrigues CRM, Imparato JCP, Mendes FM. Laser fluorescence device does not perform well in detection of early caries in primary teeth: an in vitro study. *Oral Health Prev Dent* 2008; 6(2): 165–169.

124 Mendes FM, Ganzerla E, Nunes AF, Puig AVC, Imparato JCP. Use of high-powered magnification to detect occlusal caries in primary teeth. *Am J Dent* 2006; 19(1): 19–22.

125 Mendes FM, Novaes TF, Matos R, et al. Radiographic and laser fluorescence methods have no benefits for detecting caries in primary teeth. *Caries Res* 2012; 46(6): 536–543.

126 El-Housseiny AA, Jamjoum H. Evaluation of visual, explorer, and a laser device for detection of early occlusal caries. *J Clin Pediatr Dent* 2001; 26(1):41–48.

127 Andersson A, Sköld-Larsson K, Hallgren A, Petersson LG, Twetman S. Measurement of enamel lesion regression with a laser fluorescence device (DIAGNOdent): a pilot study. *Orthodontics* 2004; 1(3): 201–205.

128 Mendes FM, Hissadomi M, Imparato JCP. Effects of drying time and the presence of plaque on the in vitro performance of laser fluorescence in occlusal caries of primary teeth. *Caries Res* 2004; 38(2): 104–108.

129 Lussi A, Hibst R, Paulus R. DIAGNOdent: an optical method for caries detection. *J Dent Res* 2004; 83(Spec No C): C80–C3.

130 Hosoya Y, Matsuzaka K, Inoue T, Marshall GW, Jr. Influence of tooth-polishing pastes and sealants on DIAGNOdent values. *Quintessence Int* 2004; 35(8): 605–611.

131 Lussi A, Reich E. The influence of toothpastes and prophylaxis pastes on fluorescence measurements for caries detection in vitro. *Eur J Oral Sci* 2005; 113(2): 141–144.

132 Cabral RM, Mendes FM, Nicolau J, Zezell DM. The influence of PVC seal wrap and probe tips autoclaving on the in vitro performance of laser fluorescence device in occlusal caries in primary teeth. *J Clin Pediatr Dent* 2006; 30(4): 306–309.

133 Rodrigues Jde A, Hug I, Lussi A. The influence of PVC wrapping on the performance of two laser fluorescence devices on occlusal surfaces in vitro. *Photomed Laser Surg* 2009; 27(3): 435–439.

134 Braga MM, Mendes FM, Imparato JC, Rodrigues CR. Effect of cut-off points on performance of laser fluorescence for detecting occlusal caries. *J Clin Pediatr Dent* 2007; 32(1): 33–36.

135 Diniz MB, Rodrigues JA, Hug I, Cordeiro RC, Lussi A. The influence of pit and fissure sealants on infrared fluorescence measurements. *Caries Res* 2008; 42(5): 328–333.

136 Fung DT, Ng GY, Leung MC, Tay DK. Therapeutic low energy laser improves the mechanical strength of repairing medial collateral ligament. *Lasers Surgery Med* 2002; 31(2): 91–96.

CHAPTER 16

Lasers in caries prevention

Lidiany Karla Azevedo Rodrigues,[1] Patrícia M. de Freitas,[2] and Marinês Nobre-dos-Santos[3]

[1]Faculty of Pharmacy, Dentistry and Nursing, Federal University of Ceará, Fortaleza, CE Brazil
[2]Special Laboratory of Lasers in Dentistry (LELO), Department of Restorative Dentistry, School of Dentistry, University of São Paulo (USP), São Paulo, SP, Brazil
[3]Department of Pediatric Dentistry, Piracicaba Dental School, State University of Campinas (UNICAMP), Piracicaba, SP, Brazil

Introduction

Since the development of the first laser by Maiman in 1960, enhancement of enamel resistance to caries using lasers has been reported. CO_2 lasers were the first to be investigated in the reduction of acid dissolution of enamel.[1–8] Other lasers have since been investigated in *in vitro/in vivo* studies, such as the Nd:YAG,[9,10] Er:YAG,[11–13] Er,Cr:YSGG,[14–16] and argon lasers.[17–20] Although this issue has been discussed for over 50 years, only a few reported *in vivo* studies have investigated the effectiveness of different lasers in decreasing the caries susceptibility of the enamel surface, restricting its clinical use. In the following sections, the mechanism of caries inhibition by CO_2, Nd:YAG, and argon lasers are summarized to help clinicians choose the appropriate lasers for caries prevention and control.

To prevent dental caries, the energy generated by the lasers must be highly absorbed by the dental substrates and efficiently converted into thermal energy, which is confined to the surface and can modify the structure and chemical composition of these substrates to promote increased acid resistance.[21] Therefore, knowledge of the mechanisms of action is relevant to determining the maximal inhibition of caries lesions with the lowest risk of pulp damage.

Carbon dioxide lasers

Several hypotheses have been proposed to explain the reduction of enamel demineralization after irradiation with CO_2 lasers. However, the actual mechanism that leads to the inhibition of the development of caries lesions has not been fully elucidated.

The first suggested explanation focused on a reduction in enamel permeability to chemical agents caused by the melting of hydroxyapatite crystals.[22] However, this hypothesis seems unlikely as in a unique experimental study that measured the permeability of irradiated enamel, permeability increased rather than decreased.[23] The authors of this study were the first to suggest that the increased enamel resistance to acid could be a result of chemical changes such as the loss of carbonate and the organic matrix.[23] In addition, the prevention of caries by laser irradiation could result from a combination of reduced permeability and solubility as a result of the melting, recrystallization, and fusion of hydroxyapatite crystals that seal the enamel surface by decreasing the interprismatic spaces.[23] However, more recent studies have shown a caries inhibitory effect in regions of no melting and fusion present on the irradiated enamel surfaces.[24] Additionally, when these areas are found, they are not homogeneous but are mostly well defined.[25,26]

Another hypothesis is based on the change in the solubility of heated apatite as less soluble compounds are formed.[25] However, the analysis of irradiated surfaces with melting zones revealed the presence of carbon tetracalcium diphosphate monoxide, also known as calcium oxide phosphate, which is less soluble than the group of phosphate minerals commonly present in enamel.[25] Reduction of carbonate content is usual in irradiated enamel and can also inhibit enamel demineralization.[24,26] In this respect, Tagliaferro et al.[24] found a lower carbonate content in the deciduous enamel after CO_2 laser irradiation even in the absence of morphological changes on the enamel surface.

Hsu et al., following research with a low energy density (0.3 J/cm²), suggested that enamel irradiation may cause a partial decomposition of the organic matrix, which leads to a blockage of the intra- and inter-prismatic spaces.[27,28] This blockage decreases the diffusion of ions and consequently reduces enamel demineralization. However, it should be emphasized that Hsu et al., used sodium hypochlorite to remove the organic matrix,[28] which may have removed ions such as magnesium and carbonate. Therefore, instead of laser irradiation, it may have been the effect of the hypochlorite that caused the inhibition of demineralization.[27,28]

Previous investigations have shown that laser irradiation combined with topical fluoride treatment can induce an even greater increase in caries resistance. There are two possible mechanisms for the laser-induced increase of fluoride uptake. In the first mechanism, the laser–fluoride treatment produces numerous spherical precipitates that morphologically resemble

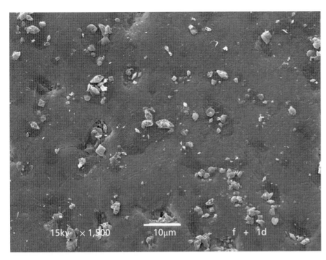

Figure 16.1 Scanning electron micrograph of the enamel surface after laser–fluoride treatment. Note the calcium fluoride-like deposits.

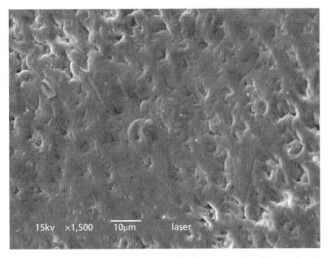

Figure 16.2 Scanning electron micrograph of the enamel surface irradiated with a CO_2 laser alone. Note the surface alterations (melting and fusion) and no evidence of calcium fluoride-like deposits.

calcium fluoride-like deposits on the dental surfaces, which serve as a reservoir to replenish fluoride.[29] Figure 16.1 shows calcium fluoride deposits on the enamel surface following the laser–fluoride treatment. However, no calcium fluoride formation is seen on the enamel surface when the CO_2 laser is used alone (Fig. 16.2).

The second mechanism emphasizes the role of lasers in enhancing fluoride uptake into the crystalline structure of the tooth in the form of firmly bound fluoride.[30]

In vivo studies using CO_2 lasers to prevent caries

The first clinical study using a CO_2 laser to prevent caries was a 4-year follow-up *in vivo* study.[31] In this study, human permanent first molars from children were used to investigate whether laser irradiation combined with the use of conventional fissure sealants promoted caries-free occlusal surfaces. The parameters used were

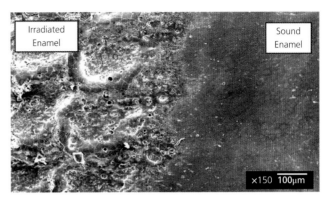

Figure 16.3 Scanning electron micrograph of the enamel surface treated with the CO_2 laser, compared with the non-irradiated enamel surface.

2 W, a pulsing emission at 7 pps, and a pulsing length of 20 ms. The authors reported that the enamel surfaces showed a milky color after irradiation and that some areas had the characteristics of carbonized material. These authors also found improved sealant retention, but there was no effect on occlusal caries prevention.[31]

Recently, a short-term clinical trial was performed with a short-pulsed 9.6-µm CO_2 laser (pulse duration 20 µs, pulse repetition rate 20 Hz, beam diameter 1100 µm, average fluence $4.1 \pm 0.3\,J/cm^2$, and 20 laser pulses per spot).[32] In this study, the bicuspid area surrounding the orthodontic brackets was irradiated. After a 4-week cariogenic challenge period, laser treatment was found to have inhibited 46% of the enamel demineralization and that this inhibition effect was higher (87%) after a 12-week period. To effectively inhibit enamel demineralization using CO_2 lasers without causing any significant damaging side effects, the temperatures should be maintained at a safe level. Temperature changes exceeding 5 °C within the pulp chamber could result in permanent damage to the dental pulp [33]. In this respect, Goodis et al. reported that a 9.6-µm wavelength laser caused no permanent/serious pulpal damage at an incident fluence of $1.5\,J/cm^2$, a repetition rate of 10 Hz, and a spot size of 1 mm in diameter, and this laser can be used safely for caries prevention treatments in humans.[34]

Rechmann et al. have also shown an 86% reduction in dental enamel smooth surface demineralization *in vivo* following short-pulsed, 9.6-µm CO_2 laser irradiation.[35] Specific microsecond short-pulsed 9.6-µm CO_2 laser irradiation markedly inhibited caries progression in pits and fissures in comparison to fluoride varnish alone over 12 months.

In conclusion, it appears that the 9.6-µm pulsed CO_2 laser can be used safely to alter the enamel surface and make it more resistant to caries, without causing dental pulp damage (Fig. 16.3).

Argon lasers

The proposed mechanism for the protective effect of argon laser irradiation against both caries initiation and progression is alteration of the characteristics of the enamel surface by creating microspaces that trap calcium, phosphate, and fluoride ions during an acid challenge.[19,36,37] The ions are incorporated into the enamel surface. In other words, in the lased enamel, the microspaces trap the released ions and act as sites for mineral repRecipitation within the enamel structure. Thus, the enamel irradiated with the argon laser has an increased affinity for calcium, phosphate, and fluoride ions.

In vivo studies using argon lasers to prevent caries

The *in vivo* effects of argon laser irradiation on human enamel demineralization were first reported by Blankenau et al. in 1999.[38] A pilot clinical study employed a model of caries production in patients who required premolar extractions as part of their comprehensive orthodontic treatment. The teeth in the experimental group were irradiated with an argon laser at approximately 12 J/cm^2 using a 250-mW and 5-mm diameter beam for 10 seconds. The control teeth on the opposite side of the mouth were not lased. After irradiation, a specially designed band was fabricated, and two sections of stainless steel wire were welded to the internal surface of the facial portion of each band to create a pocket for the accumulation of plaque and food debris. The bands were cemented in place for 5 weeks. The study found a 29.1% reduction in the average lesion depth in the lased samples compared with the controls.

In another study using the same intraoral model to develop the demineralization of human enamel *in vivo*, teeth were irradiated with a 325-mW, 5-mm diameter laser beam for 60 seconds (with an energy density of approximately 100 J/cm^2). In this study, after a 5-week intraoral exposure period, the use of the argon laser alone was found to reduce the lesion depth by 91.4% and the lesion area by 94.6% compared to the non-pumiced, non-etched control. Pumicing and etching the enamel before laser irradiation reduced the lesion depth by 89.1% and the lesion area by 92.2% compared to the control group.[39]

Due to their ability to increase the affinity of enamel for fluoride ions, argon lasers have been recommended in combination with fluoridated vehicles. The previously described intraoral model was applied in a pilot study that tested this combination.[20] The enamel surface was irradiated (12 J/cm^2, 250 mW, 10 seconds) and submitted to topical fluoride application (neutral sodium fluoride, 4 minutes). When fluoride was followed by argon laser irradiation, an even greater degree of resistance against caries development in enamel was achieved.

In a 6-month follow-up *in vivo* study, enamel was treated with fluoride gel (applied for 5 minutes followed by 1 minute of rinsing with distilled water) after irradiation with an argon laser at 10.74 J/cm^2 (beam diameter 11 mm, irradiation time 30 seconds, and output power 340 mW in continuous mode).[40] This enamel retained 14.12% of the fluoride after the fluoridation process, whereas the control enamel retained only 3.27% of the fluoride.

An *in vitro* study showed that nearly identical microhardness values for enamel surfaces were found with either argon laser irradiation alone or combined with fluoride treatment.[41] This result may indicate that argon laser exposure increases enamel

microhardness, while fluoride uptake by lased enamel, which is harder than non-lased enamel, enhances caries resistance. Thus, this result suggests that the synergistic effect of argon laser irradiation and fluoride treatment may favorably influence the critical pH at which the minerals of enamel undergo dissolution, which may improve resistance to subsequent caries development.[20]

In conclusion, the use of argon lasers with and without fluoride may be a simple technique to reduce the caries susceptibility of enamel.

Nd:YAG lasers

As studies have reported surface melting and temperatures of up to 600 °C when enamel is irradiated with Nd:YAG lasers, similar mechanisms to those for CO_2 lasers have been suggested for Nd:YAG lasers in caries prevention. However, unlike the CO_2 laser, which is the most efficiently absorbed laser by dental enamel, the Nd:YAG laser is not effectively absorbed by human enamel (the absorption coefficient is lower than $4 \times 10^{1-2}$/cm).[21] Thus, its efficient use in this substrate depends on the application of a photosensitizer.

In vivo studies using Nd:YAG lasers to prevent caries

A clinical trial was performed to investigate the effect of Nd:YAG laser irradiation on the occlusal surface. Irradiation was performed by scanning the surfaces with an Nd:YAG laser of 0.6 W, 60 mJ per pulse, repetition rate 10 Hz, spot size diameter 300 µm, and fluence 84.9 J/cm^2. The procedure of dye (triturated coal diluted in equal parts of deionized water and 99% ethanol) application followed by laser irradiation was repeated three times to assure enamel melting.[42] The teeth were then brushed with pumice paste, and a fluoride gel (1.23% F$^-$) was applied to both the lased sample and the control sample for 4 minutes. Figure 16.4 shows Nd:YAG irradiation and fluoride application on occlusal surface of a 2nd primary molar and 1st permanent molar in a high caries risk children. The application of acidulated phosphate fluoride combined with Nd:YAG laser irradiation increased enamel resistance to demineralization: caries incidence was reduced by more than 39% compared to the non-treatment control.

However, because the scientific literature provides little evidence for the clinical use of Nd:YAG lasers to prevent caries and because it is necessary to use a photosensitizer to make the enamel absorb this laser, the Nd:YAG laser has restricted usage.

Conclusion

In conclusion, based on the results of *in vitro*, *in situ*, and clinical studies, the CO_2 laser seems to be the most useful laser to prevent caries. However, from a practical standpoint, before lasers find widespread utilization among practicing dentists, a variety of well-substantiated studies and treatment modalities utilizing lasers must be developed.

Clinical case 16.1

The treatment of a patient at high caries risk with Nd:YAG irradiation and fluoride is shown in Figure 16.4 (clinical case conducted by Dr. Patrícia M. Freitas and Dr. Ricardo S. Navarro at the Special Laboratory of Lasers in Dentistry - FOUSP).

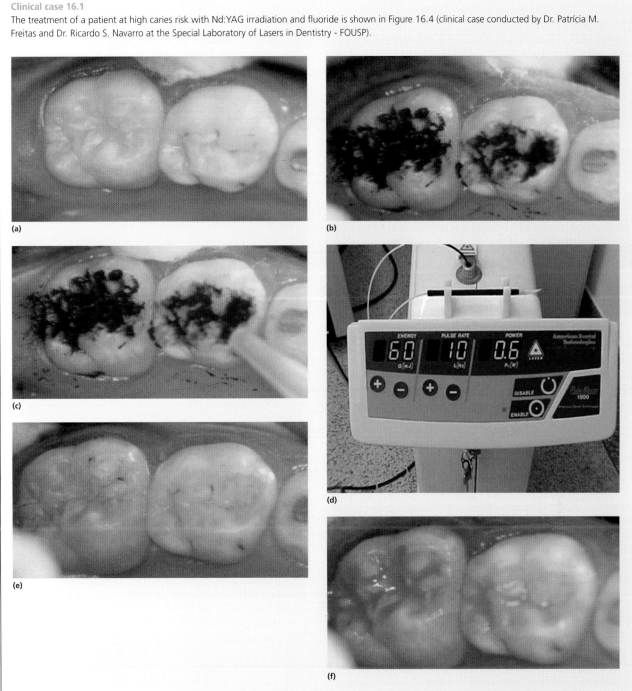

Figure 16.4 (a) Initial image of upper posterior teeth in a patient with high caries risk. (b) Mineral powder coal application to the area to be irradiated with the Nd:YAG laser. (c) Laser irradiation on the pit and fissures areas. (d) Nd:YAG laser used, showing the parameters that were selected. (e) Occlusal image of upper posterior teeth following laser irradiation. Almost all the mineral powder coal was removed due to its interaction with the laser light. (f) Topical fluoride application after the laser treatment.

References

1 Stern RH, Sognnaes RF. Laser inhibition of dental caries suggested by first tests *in vivo*. J Am Dent Assoc 1972; 85: 1087–1090.

2 Stern RH, Vahl J, Sognnaes RF. Lased enamel: ultrastructural observations of pulsed carbon dioxide laser effects. J Dent Res 1972; 51: 455–460.

3 Beeking PO, Herrmann C, Zuhrt R. Examination of laser-treated tooth surfaces after exposure to acid. Dtsch Stomatol 1990; 40: 490–492.

4 Fox JL, Yu D, Otsuka M, et al. Combined effects of laser irradiation and chemical inhibitors on the dissolution of dental enamel. Caries Res 1992; 26: 333–339.

5 Hsu J, Fox JL, Wang Z, et al. Combined effects of laser irradiation/solution fluoride ion on enamel demineralization. J Clin Laser Med Surg 1998; 16: 93–105.

6 Hossain M, Nakamura Y, Kimura Y, et al. Acquired acid resistance of dental hard tissues by CO_2 laser irradiation. J Clin Laser Med Surg 1999; 17: 223–226.

7 Featherstone JD, Barrett-Vespone NA, Fried D, et al. CO_2 laser inhibitor of artificial caries-like lesion progression in dental enamel. J Dent Res 1998; 77: 1397–1403.

8 Kantorowitz Z, Featherstone JD, Fried D. Caries prevention by CO_2 laser treatment: dependency on the number of pulses used. J Am Dent Assoc 1998; 129: 585–591.

9 Huang GF, Lan WH, Guo MK, et al. Synergistic effect of Nd:YAG laser combined with fluoride varnish on inhibition of caries formation in dental pits and fissures in vitro. J Formos Med Assoc 2001; 100: 181–185.

10 Hossain M, Nakamura Y, Kimura Y, et al. Effect of pulsed Nd:YAG laser irradiation on acid demineralization of enamel and dentin. J Clin Laser Med Surg 2001; 19: 105–108.

11 Hossain M, Nakamura Y, Kimura Y, et al. Caries-preventive effect of Er:YAG laser irradiation with or without water mist. J Clin Laser Med Surg 2000; 18: 61–65.

12 Delbem AC, Cury JA, Nakassima CK, et al. Effect of Er:YAG laser on CaF_2 formation and its anticariogenic action on human enamel: an *in vitro* study. J Clin Laser Med Surg 2003; 21: 197–201.

13 Bevilácqua FM, Zezell DM, Magnani R, et al. Fluoride uptake and acid resistance of enamel irradiated with Er:YAG laser. Lasers Med Sci 2008; 23: 141–147.

14 Hossain M, Kimura Y, Nakamura Y, et al. A study on acquired acid resistance of enamel and dentin irradiated by Er,Cr:YSGG laser. J Clin Laser Med Surg 2001; 19: 159–163.

15 Moslemi M, Fekrazad R, Tadayon N, et al. Effects of ER,Cr:YSGG laser irradiation and fluoride treatment on acid resistance of the enamel. Pediatr Dent 2009; 31: 409–413.

16 Freitas PM, Rapozo-Hilo M, Eduardo Cde P, et al. In vitro evaluation of erbium, chromium:yttrium-scandiumgallium-garnet laser-treated enamel demineralization. Lasers Med Sci 2010; 25: 165–170.

17 Westerman GH, Hicks MJ, Flaitz CM, et al. Argon laser irradiation in root surface caries: in vitro study examines laser's effects. J Am Dent Assoc 1994; 125: 401–407.

18 Flaitz CM, Hicks MJ, Westerman GH, et al. Argon laser irradiation and acidulated phosphate fluoride treatment in caries-like lesion formation in enamel: an *in vitro* study. Pediatr Dent 2005; 17: 31–35.

19 Hicks MJ, Flaitz CM, Westerman GH, et al. Enamel caries initiation and progression following low fluence (energy) argon laser and fluoride treatment. J Clin Pediatr Dent 1995; 20: 9–13.

20 Hicks J, Winn D 2nd, Flaitz C, et al. In vivo caries formation in enamel following argon laser irradiation and combined fluoride and argon laser treatment: a clinical pilot study. Quintessence Int 2004; 35: 15–20.

21 Featherstone JDB. Caries detection and prevention with laser energy. Dent Clin North Am 2000; 44: 955–969.

22 Stern RH, Vahl J, Sognnaes RF. Lased enamel: Ultrastructural observations of pulsed carbon dioxide laser effects. J Dent Res 1972; 51: 455–460.

23 Borggreven JM, van Dijk JW, Driessens FC. Effect of laser irradiation on the permeability of bovine dental enamel. Arch Oral Biol 1980; 25: 831–832.

24 Tagliaferro EP, Rodrigues LK, Soares LE, et al. Physical and compositional changes on demineralized primary enamel induced by CO_2 Laser. Photomed Laser Surg 2009; 27: 585–590.

25 Nelson DG, Wefel JS, Jongebloed WL, et al. Morphology, histology and crystallography of human dental enamel treated with pulsed low-energy infrared laser radiation. Caries Res 1987; 21: 411–426.

26 Steiner-Oliveira C, Rodrigues LK, Soares LE, et al. Chemical, morphological and thermal effects of 10.6-microm CO_2 laser on the inhibition of enamel demineralization. Dent Mater J 2006; 25: 455–462.

27 Hsu CY, Jordan TH, Dederich DN, et al. Effects of low-energy CO_2 laser irradiation and the organic matrix on inhibition of enamel demineralization. J Dent Res 2000; 79: 1725–1730.

28 Hsu CYS, Jordan TH, Dederich DN, et al. Laser-matrix-fluoride effects on enamel demineralization. J Dent Res 2001; 80: 1797–1801.

29 Chin-Ying SH, Xiaoli G, Jisheng P et al. Effects of CO_2 laser on fluoride uptake in enamel. J Dent 2004; 32: 161–167.

30 Meurman JH, Hemmerlé J, Voegel JC, et al. Transformation of hydroxyapatite to fluorapatite by irradiation with high-energy CO_2 laser. Caries Res 1997; 31: 397–400.

31 Brugnera A Jr A, Rosso N, Duarte D, et al. The use of carbon dioxide laser in pit and fissure caries prevention: clinical evaluation. J Clin Laser Med Surg 1997; 15: 79–82.

32 Rechmann P, Fried D, Le CQ, et al. Caries inhibition in vital teeth using 9.6-μm CO_2-laser irradiation. J Biomed Opt 2011; 16: 071405.

33 Zach L, Cohen G. Pulp response to externally applied heat. Oral Surg Oral Med Oral Pathol 1965; 19: 515–530.

34 Goodis HE, Fried D, Gansky S, et al. Pulpal safety of 9.6 microm TEA CO_2 laser used for caries prevention. Lasers Surg Med 2004; 35: 104–110.

35 Rechmann P, Charland DA, Rechmann BM, Le CQ, Featherstone JD. In-vivo occlusal caries prevention by pulsed CO_2-laser and fluoride varnish treatment--a clinical pilot study. Lasers Surg Med 2013; 45: 302–310.

36 Kelsey WP III, Blankenau RJ Jr, Powell GL. Application of argon laser to dentistry. Lasers Surg Med 1991; 11: 495–49.8.

37 Flaitz CM, Hicks MJ, Westerman GH, et al. Argon laser irradiation and acidulated phosphate fluoride treatment in caries-like lesion formation in enamel: an in vitro study. Pediatr Dent 1995; 17: 31–35.

38 Blankenau RJ, Powell G, Ellis RW, et al. *In vivo* caries-like lesion prevention with argon laser: pilot study. J Clin Laser Med Surg 1999; 17: 241–243.

39 Anderson AM, Kao E, Gladwin M, et al. The effects of argon laser irradiation on enamel decalcification: An in vivo study. Am J Orthod Dentofacial Orthop 2002; 122: 251–259.

40 Nammour S, Rocca JP, Pireaux JJ, et al. Increase of enamel fluoride retention by low fluence argon laser beam: a 6-month follow-up study in vivo. Lasers Surg Med 2005; 36: 220–224.

41 Westerman GH, Latta MA, Eliis RW, et al. An in vitro study of enamel surface hardness following argon laser irradiation and APF treatment. J Dent Res 2003; 82 (Special issue A): 1552.

42 Zezell DM, Boari HG, Ana PA, et al. Nd:YAG laser in caries prevention: a clinical trial. Lasers Surg Med 2009; 41: 31–35.

SECTION 3

Endodontics

CHAPTER 17

Bacterial reduction in root canals using antimicrobial photodynamic therapy

Aguinaldo S. Garcez and Silvia C. Núñez

São Leopoldo Mandic Dental Research Center, Campinas, SP, Brazil

Elimination of the pathogenic microflora from the root canal system is one of the main goals of endodontic treatment. Microbial infection plays an important role in the development of necrosis in the dental pulp and the formation of periapical lesions.[1]. It is well established in the literature that the eradication of microorganisms from root canals is problematic, and current endodontic techniques are unable to consistently disinfect the root canal systems.[2]

Contemporary treatment procedures to eliminate infection include root canal debridement and mechanical shaping, irrigation with a disinfectant solution such as sodium hypochlorite or chlorhexidine, the application of an inter-appointment dressing containing an antimicrobial agent, and finally sealing of the root canal.[3,4] The use of antibiotics and antiseptics is an alternative approach, but the long-term use of chemical antimicrobial agents can be rendered ineffective by resistance developing in the target organisms.[5-7]

Combined conventional endodontic treatment/antimicrobial photodynamic therapy

The combination of endodontic treatment and antimicrobial photodynamic therapy (aPDT) is a new strategy that involves a non-toxic photosensitizer (PS) and a harmless visible light source.[8] The excited PS reacts with molecular oxygen to produce highly reactive oxygen species, which induce injury to and death of microorganisms.[9,10]

Studies from different groups[11-16] have shown that the combination of conventional endodontic therapy followed by aPDT (endodontic/aPDT) is effective in reducing bacterial load in *ex vivo* root canals (in planktonic as well as in biofilm) and also in patients, although the success rate varies between studies and their comparison is difficult, due to the use of different PS, light parameters, and especially light delivery techniques.

Garcez et al.[16] have treated 20 patients with symptoms of necrotic pulp and periapical periodontitis, with endodontic/

aPDT. A conjugate between polyethylenimine (PEI) and chlorin e6 was used as the PS, and a diode laser coupled to a 300-μm optical fiber, emitting at 660 nm, was the light source. Microbial samples were collected from the pulp chamber after conventional treatment and after aPDT. The reduction in microbial load obtained after two sessions of endodontic/aPDT was 3.19 log of the initial load; the authors suggested that endodontic/aPDT might be an appropriate approach for the treatment of endodontic infections.

Pinheiro et al.[17] showed the same positive results for endodontic/aPDT in deciduous teeth with necrotic pulp. The antimicrobial activity of endodontic/aPDT was greater than 98%.

However, many papers have shown negative or non-significant results for endodontic/aPDT.[18-20] There are many factors that could affect the efficiency of endodontic/aPDT, such as PS concentration, diffusion of the PS through the root canal system, and light distribution during irradiation.

Photosensitizers

To perform aPDT the PS has to be able to efficiently absorb light and then convert this light into one of the several reactive oxygen species: singlet oxygen, superoxide anion, and hydroxyl radical. It also has to have some degree of affinity for microorganism membranes and be able to penetrate the microbial biofilm.[21]

Some factors limiting the elimination of bacteria by conventional treatment are the inability of chemical disinfectant to kill bacteria within the dentinal tubules and the anatomical complexities of the root canal, especially when microorganisms are organized in biofilms. Therefore, when performing aPDT it is important to assure that both the light and the PS can reach all the bacteria in the innermost parts of the root canal system.[22]

One important issue is that even if aPDT is performed, the conventional chemical irrigants still play an important role in endodontics since, besides eliminating microorganisms, these

---

Lasers in Dentistry: Guide for Clinical Practice, First Edition. Edited by Patrícia M. de Freitas and Alyne Simões.

chemical agents have tissue dissolution properties and remove debris and the smear layer. Nevertheless, no single solution is able to fulfil these actions completely; therefore, they must always be used in combination.

Some bacteria produce their own PS and can be killed by illumination alone. The PS produced is usually a porphyrin and this can be efficiently excited with red and blue light. Unfortunately, most of the organisms responsible for endodontic infection do not produce PS and therefore an external PS has to be used. In order to choose the optimal PS for any clinical condition, the characteristics of a PS should be evaluated.

Since all bacteria can be stained, the idea of using dyes for lethal photosensitization is pretty straightforward. Some dyes and other molecules have been used for aPDT in endodontics, such as methylene blue, toluidine blue, and chlorins, with good results.

External factors can affect the photoreaction; for example, the interactions between phenothiazine dyes and blood or saliva from the oral cavity may render these dyes less efficient despite correct illumination and PS concentration.[23]

Therefore, before filling the root canal with the PS, the root canal should be cleaned with a sterile water solution and/ or dried.

PS concentration is another factor to be considered during aPDT. While higher concentration provides a high number of PS molecules for the photoreaction, it also induces a phenomenon known as *optical shield*. Optical shield occurs when the concentration of the medium is high enough to block light penetration of the entire volume of the PS and the photoreaction is restricted to the surface of the PS volume (Fig. 17.1).

The use of a PS concentration between 50 and 100 µM seems to achieve a good balance between light absorption and light distribution through the PS volume, resulting in more efficient aPDT.

Regarding the preirradiation time, the literature is controversial, with some studies using times of greater than 30 minutes, which would not be clinically feasible. Times between 1 and 2 minutes are more appropriate to clinical practice and result in a good microbial reduction.[16]

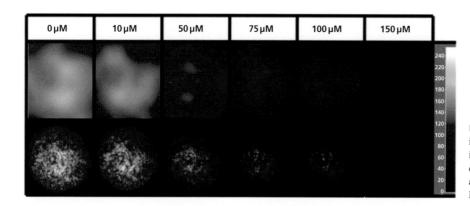

Figure 17.1 Light transmission through increasing concentrations of methylene blue in a 96-well plate (300 µL per well). At higher concentration (150 µM), light is absorbed at the surface and does not penetrate the PS volume.

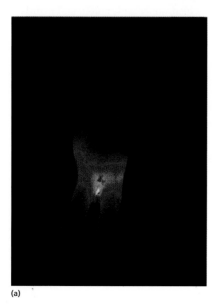

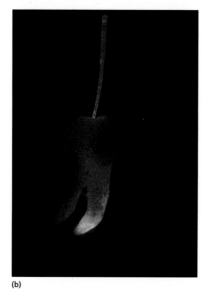

(a) (b)

Figure 17.2 Light distribution during irradiation performed inside an extracted human molar (a) with the laser tip at the pulp chamber, (b) with the optical fiber inside the root canal. Note that with the use of an optical fiber the amount of light, especially in the apex region, is higher than when no fiber is used.

Light source

The result of PDT is directly dependent on the presence of light, PS, and oxygen. Therefore, a good light distribution across the root canal improves the efficiency of the therapy. There is no consensus in the literature on the use of an optical fiber: some authors recommend its use,[15,16] but others do not.[24] Figure 17.2 shows the light distribution in an extracted human molar with and without the use of an optical fiber.

Garcez et al.[25] found that the irradiation with an optical fiber increased the uniformity of light distribution along the root canal, giving better irradiation near to the root apex and greater bacterial reduction during endodontic aPDT. The authors evaluated 50 extracted teeth contaminated with a 3-day biofilm of *Enterococcus faecalis* and submitted to endodontic aPDT with methylene blue. Bacterial reduction in the group where the laser tip was used was less than 1 log (97%), compared with a 4 log reduction (99.99%) in the group where an optical fiber was used.

Clinical case 17.1 Periapical lesion

A 62-year-old female patient presented with a periapical lesion on tooth 34. After conventional endodontic treatment with the Mtwo rotatory file system and irrigation with 2.5% sodium hypochlorite, the tooth was cleaned with EDTA and washed with sterile water solution. The root canal was filled with 1 M (3%) hydrogen peroxide for 1 minute and with 60 µM methylene blue

for another 1 minute. The root canal system was irradiated with a 40-mW diode laser emitting at 660 nm coupled with a 300-µm optical fiber (Twin laser MMOptics, São Carlos, Brazil). Helicoidal movements were performed during the 4 minute irradiation (total energy 9.6 J) to assure the entire root canal wall was irradiated. Figure 17.3 shows the sequence of the therapy.

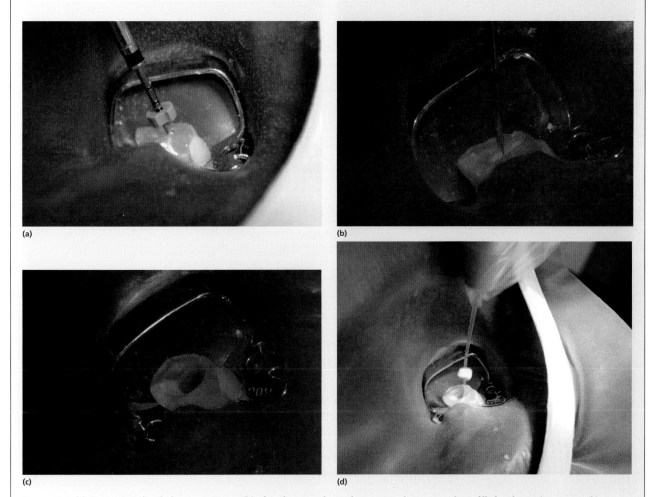

(a) (b) (c) (d)

Figure 17.3 (a) Conventional endodontic treatment, (b) after chemomechanical treatment, the root canal was filled with 1 M (3% or 10 vol.) hydrogen peroxide for 1 minute, (c) root canal filled with 60 µM methylene blue. Note the PS concentration (color) used for endodontic aPDT, (d) irradiation with a 660-nm diode laser coupled with an optical fiber.

Clinical case 17.2 Periapical periodontitis and apical bone lesion

A 55-year-old female patient presented with symptoms of periapical periodontitis and an apical bone lesion on the upper lateral incisor was detected by radiography. The clinical protocol was to conduct an endodontic surgery.

The tooth was conventionally treated with a full mucoperiosteal flap, osteotomy with a high-speed bur, manual curettage of the periapical lesion and the external surface of the root, and root-end resection of 2–3 mm with no bevel, and retrograde cavities were prepared using ultrasonic retro-tips to a depth of 3 mm.

After the conventional surgical procedure the bone cavities were filled with an aqueous solution of 60 μM methylene blue for 3 minutes, and were then irradiated with a diode laser (660 nm, 40 mW for 3 minutes;

7.2 J). The cavity was then dried and the tip of the laser was changed to allow access to the retrograde cavity. The irradiation inside the retrograde cavity was performed with an optical fiber (MMOptics, São Carlos, Brazil) with spiral movements, and the cavity was irrigated with 10 mL of sterile saline solution to remove the PS.

Subsequent to aPDT, a retrograde filling with mineral trioxide aggregate was done, and the flap repositioned and sutured. Microbiological samples were taken during the surgery. The results showed a microbiological reduction of 3 log after the conventional procedure and a further reduction of 5 log after aPDT.

Figure 17.4 shows the sequence of the treatment and the radiographic images before and after treatment.

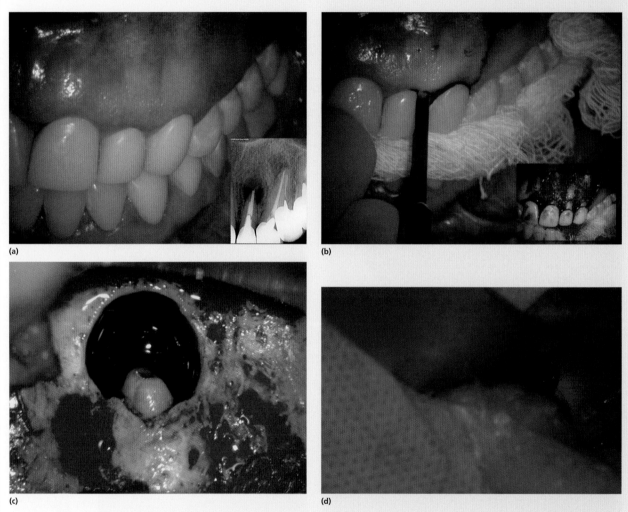

(a)

(b)

(c)

(d)

Figure 17.4 (a) Clinical and radiographic image of the lesion, (b) a full mucoperiosteal flap, allowing access to the lesion, (c) after the conventional procedure, the cavity was filled with a sterile aqueous solution of methylene blue for 3 minutes, (d) irradiation with the laser tip covering all cavity surfaces, (e) the retrograde cavity was also filled with the PS solution for 1 minute, (f) to irradiate the cavity, the laser was coupled to an optical fiber, (g) radiographic images immediately after the surgery (left) and 6 months later (right). Note the healing of the lesion compared to the initial radiographic exam (courtesy of Debora Parra Sellera).

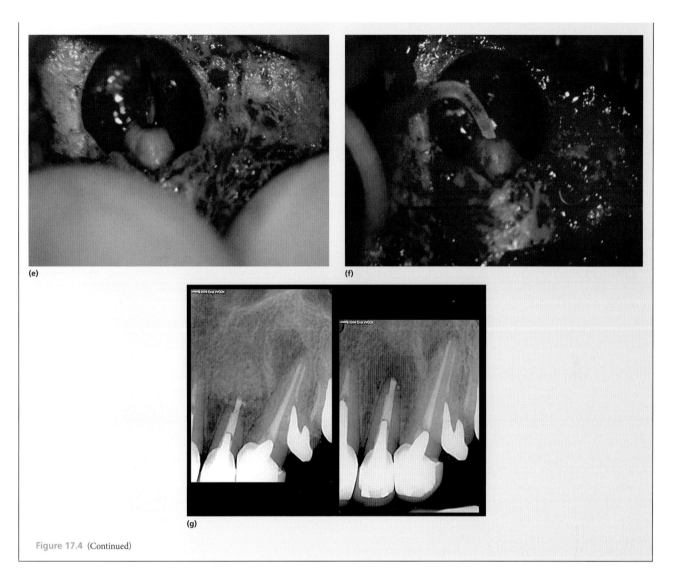

(e) (f)

(g)

Figure 17.4 (Continued)

References

1 Siqueira JF, Jr. Endodontic infections: concepts, paradigms, and perspectives. Oral Surg Oral Med Oral Pathol Oral Radiol Endod 2002; 94(3): 281–293.

2 Bonsor SJ, Nichol R, Reid TM, Pearson GJ. Microbiological evaluation of photo-activated disinfection in endodontics (an in vivo study). Br Dent J 2006; 200(6): 337–341, discussion 29.

3 Bahcall JK, Barss JT. Understanding and evaluating the endodontic file. Gen Dent 2000; 48(6): 690–692.

4 Sedgley C. Root canal irrigation--a historical perspective. J Hist Dent 2004; 52(2): 61–65.

5 Reynaud Af Geijersstam AH, Ellington MJ, Warner M, Woodford N, Haapasalo M. Antimicrobial susceptibility and molecular analysis of *Enterococcus faecalis* originating from endodontic infections in Finland and Lithuania. Oral Microbiol Immunol 2006; 21(3): 164–168.

6 Pinheiro ET, Gomes BP, Drucker DB, Zaia AA, Ferraz CC, Souza-Filho FJ. Antimicrobial susceptibility of *Enterococcus faecalis* isolated from canals of root filled teeth with periapical lesions. Int Endod J 2004; 37(11): 756–763.

7 Figdor D. Microbial aetiology of endodontic treatment failure and pathogenic properties of selected species. Aust Endod J 2004; 30(1): 11–14.

8 Hamblin MR, Hasan T. Photodynamic therapy: a new antimicrobial approach to infectious disease? Photochem Photobiol Sci 2004; 3(5): 436–450.

9 Demidova TN, Hamblin MR. Photodynamic therapy targeted to pathogens. Int J Immunopathol Pharmacol 2004; 17(3): 245–254.

10 Wainwright M. Photodynamic antimicrobial chemotherapy (PACT). J Antimicrob Chemother 1998; 42(1): 13–28.

11 Fimple JL, Fontana CR, Foschi F, et al. Photodynamic treatment of endodontic polymicrobial infection in vitro. J Endod 2008; 34(6): 728–734.

12 Garcez AS, Ribeiro MS, Tegos GP, Nunez SC, Jorge AO, Hamblin MR. Antimicrobial photodynamic therapy combined with conventional endodontic treatment to eliminate root canal biofilm infection. Lasers Surg Med 2007; 39(1): 59–66.

13 Kishen A, Upadya M, Tegos GP, Hamblin MR. Efflux pump inhibitor potentiates antimicrobial photodynamic inactivation of *Enterococcus faecalis* biofilm. Photochem Photobiol 2010; 86(6): 1343–1349.

14 Foschi F, Fontana CR, Ruggiero K, et al. Photodynamic inactivation of *Enterococcus faecalis* in dental root canals in vitro. Lasers Surg Med 2007; 39(10): 782–787.

15 Garcez AS, Nunez SC, Hamblim MR, Suzuki H, Ribeiro MS. Photodynamic therapy associated with conventional endodontic treatment in patients with antibiotic-resistant microflora: a preliminary report. J Endod 2010; 36(9): 1463–1466.

16 Garcez AS, Nunez SC, Hamblin MR, Ribeiro MS. Antimicrobial effects of photodynamic therapy on patients with necrotic pulps and periapical lesion. J Endod 2008; 34(2): 138–142.

17 Pinheiro SL, Schenka AA, Neto AA, de Souza CP, Rodriguez HM, Ribeiro MC. Photodynamic therapy in endodontic treatment of deciduous teeth. Lasers Med Sci 2009; 24(4): 521–526.

18 Meire MA, Coenye T, Nelis HJ, De Moor RJ. Evaluation of Nd:YAG and Er:YAG irradiation, antibacterial photodynamic therapy and sodium hypochlorite treatment on Enterococcus faecalis biofilms. Int Endod J 2012; 45(5): 482–491.

19 Ng R, Singh F, Papamanou DA, et al. Endodontic photodynamic therapy *ex vivo*. J Endod 2011; 37(2): 217–222.

20 Seal GJ, Ng YL, Spratt D, Bhatti M, Gulabivala K. An *in vitro* comparison of the bactericidal efficacy of lethal photosensitization or sodium hyphochlorite irrigation on *Streptococcus intermedius* biofilms in root canals. Int Endod J 2002; 35(3): 268–274.

21 Dai T, Huang YY, Hamblin MR. Photodynamic therapy for localized infections--state of the art. Photodiagn Photodyn Ther 2009; 6(3–4): 170–188.

22 Shrestha A, Friedman S, Kishen A. Photodynamically crosslinked and chitosan-incorporated dentin collagen. J Dent Res 2011; 90(11): 1346–1351.

23 Nunez SC, Garcez AS, Gomes L, Baptista MS, Ribeiro MS. Methylene blue aggregation in the presence of human saliva. Proc SPIE. 2008; 9: 684608-1–7.

24 Williams JA, Pearson GJ, Colles MJ. Antibacterial action of photoactivated disinfection (PAD) used on endodontic bacteria in planktonic suspension and in artificial and human root canals. J Dent 2006; 34(6): 363–371.

25 Garcez AS, Fregnani ER, Rodriguez HM, et al. The use of optical fiber in endodontic photodynamic therapy. Is it really relevant? Lasers Med Sci 2013; 28(1): 79–85.

CHAPTER 18

High power lasers in apical surgery

Sheila C. Gouw-Soares,[1] José Luiz Lage-Marques,[2] and Cláudia Strefezza[3]

[1] School of Dentistry, University of Cruzeiro do Sul (UNICSUL), São Paulo, SP, Brazil
[2] Discipline of Endodontics, Department of Restorative Dentistry, School of Dentistry, University of São Paulo (USP), São Paulo, SP, Brazil
[3] Faculdades Metropolitanas Unidas (FMU), São Paulo, SP, Brazil

Introduction

The main role of endodontic treatment is to clean and shape the root canal, and then to apply an apical seal, to prevent reinfection and to cure apical periodontitis caused by infection of the root canal system.[1,2]

Although root canal therapy has been shown to be a predictable procedure with a high degree of success,[3,4] recent publications have reported failure rates of 14–16% for initial root canal treatment.[3,5] Lack of healing is attributed to persistent intraradicular infection in previously uninstrumented canals, in dentinal tubules, and in the complex irregularities of the root canal system[6–9]; to foreign body reaction caused by extruded endodontic materials; and to unresolved cystic lesion.[2,10–15]

Epidemiological studies[1,3] reveal, however, that 33–60% of root-filled teeth show apical periodontitis (AP), suggesting the persistence of the primary infection or emergence of infection after treatment. The least invasive approach in these cases is orthograde retreatment, unless other factors or benefit–risk analysis suggests management with apical surgery.[16]

Apical surgery is often the last resort to maintain an endodontically treated tooth with a persistent periapical lesion. After the introduction of microsurgical principles and new materials for apical obturation in the early 1990s, healing rates following surgical procedures with root-end filling have improved, but remain around 80%. To further improve the results, three different strategies may be considered: improvement of technical equipment/instruments, changes in surgical technique, and appropriate case selection. The choice of treatment, however, is often based on individual experience and skill rather than on evidence-based prognostic factors. The latter would narrow the indications for a certain treatment by weighing various predictors and thereby increasing the likelihood of a favorable outcome.[17]

Apicoectomy normally comprises the removal of pathological tissue, periapical curettage followed by root-end resection, and retrograde filling. In specific cases where microorganisms colonize only the apical ramifications of the root canal system, or where microorganisms are present in extraradicular infection, or even where pathosis is sustained by a periapical foreign body, the surgical procedure effectively removes the infected site and enhances the chances of healing. However, in the majority of teeth, microorganisms colonize the entire root canal system and the root-end filling might not effectively prevent persistence or recurrence of apical periodontitis after the surgical procedure.[4,5]

In a study conducted in Toronto, of 261 treated teeth in the pooled sample, 96 were lost to follow-up and 31 were extracted. Of the remaining 134 teeth (85% recall, excluding 66 teeth that could not be recalled) examined for outcome, 74% were healed at follow-up 4–10 years after the surgical procedure. The outcome was better in patients aged over 45 years who had an inadequate root-filling length.[5]

Surgical endodontics success rates have improved over the years with the development of retrograde filling materials and the use of ultrasonic preparation. Rates of 60–70% have increased to more than 90% of cases (91.5% of healed cases at a follow-up of 5–7 years).[7,8]

Apicoectomy with retrograde filling is a well-established surgical procedure to treat teeth affected by persistent periapical lesions. The apical root-end is generally removed with burs and the adjacent periapical tissue is curetted. Alternatively, treatment has also been performed with ultrasound or laser technology.

Lasers for apicoectomy

In 1971, Weichman et al.[9] first demonstrated the possibility of using laser photonic energy in endodontics. Numerous other studies have since used different wavelengths and power settings in root canal disinfection: the CO_2 laser, Nd:YAG laser (1064 nm), high power diode laser (810 nm), Er:YAG laser (2940 nm), and Nd:YAP laser (1340 nm), all of them showing marked bactericidal effect.[10–13] High power lasers, used appropriately and at an optimum setting for the target tissue, reduce dentin permeability,[14] allow cavity preparation without vibration,[15] and assist in disinfection during canal instrumentation.[18]

Lasers in Dentistry: Guide for Clinical Practice, First Edition. Edited by Patrícia M. de Freitas and Alyne Simões.
© 2015 John Wiley & Sons, Inc. Published 2015 by John Wiley & Sons, Inc.

Clinical case 18.1

A male patient presented with the main complaint of a fistula on the mucosa of the apical region of tooth 11 (Fig. 18.1a). Due to periapical infection observed clinically by the presence of fistula and radiographically by an extensive radiolucent area in the apical region of teeth 11–22 (Fig. 18.1b), it was decided to perform the surgery with laser technology: Er:YAG laser (2940 nm, pulse mode), Nd:YAG laser (1064 nm, pulse mode), and GaAlAs laser (790 nm, continuous wave).[24]

The Er:YAG laser was used to perform osteotomy and root resection without vibration or discomfort, and with less contamination of the surgical site and no smear layer on the dentin surface (Fig. 18.1c,d). Nd:YAG laser irradiation through a fiber sealed the dentinal tubules on the dentin cut surface and reduced the bacterial count in the cavity bone (Fig. 18.1e,f). In addition, the GaAlAs laser improved healing and the postoperative course.

At 1-month clinical follow-up, a radiolucent area in the apical region was still present (Fig. 18.1 g). The radiographic image 6 months after surgery showed a decrease in the periapical radiolucent area, indicating bone repair (Fig. 18.1 h).

At 3-year follow-up examination, a radiographically significant decrease in the radiolucent periapical area was observed (Fig. 18.1i). Five years after apical surgery, radiographic imaging showed a complete bone repair (Fig. 18.1j). The presence of scar tissue did not infer impairment of bone tissue repair. No clinical signs or symptoms were reported by the patient during follow-up.

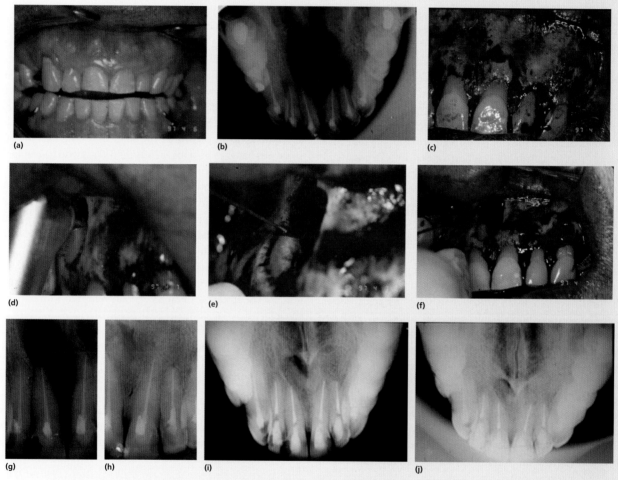

Figure 18.1 (a) Initial clinical image. Note the presence of the fistula on the mucosa of the apical region of tooth 11. (b) Initial radiograph showed a large periapical lesion. (c) After the incision (handpiece 2062, 50/10 fiber of the KAVO KEY II) and removal of the flap, the erbium laser defined the area of the cortical bone defect to be removed. (d) The Er:YAG laser (handpiece 2060, 350 mJ/4 Hz, KAVO KEY)was used to perform the apicoectomy. (e) Nd:YAG laser irradiation (1.5 W, 100 mJ, 15 Hz; 124 J/cm^2) on the cut dentin surface after apicoectomy promoted sealing of the dentinal tubules. (f) Disinfection of the periapical region with Nd:YAG laser irradiation (1.5 W, 100 mJ, 15 Hz; 124J/cm^2). (g) Radiographic imaging 1 month after apicoectomy of tooth 11, (h) 6 months after apicoectomy shows a decrease in the periapical radiolucent area, indicating bone repair, and (i) 3 years after apicoectomy shows a significant decrease in the periapical radiolucent area. (j) Radiographic imaging 5 years after apicoectomy showed bone healing, albeit with the presence of scar tissue.

One of the concerns with high power laser application inside the root canal system is the conversion of light energy into caloric energy during the interaction with dentinal structures, which could increase the temperature of the external root surface and adjacent structures. The most important possible consequence of the thermal variations is damage to the cement layer, predisposing to reabsorption of roots and periodontal ligament fibers, ankylosis, alveolar bone necrosis, and pain. The severity of these effects is determined by the quantity of heat generated and the time that it persists in the region. According to Eriksson and Albrektsson [19] an increase in temperature of more than 10 C on the external root canal surface for 1 minute causes necrosis of periodontal ligament and external root resorption.[20]

Studies evaluating the characteristics of different types of laser showed that the Er:YAG laser is suitable for root resection and apicoectomies as its wavelength is highly absorbed by the hydroxyapatite and water present in dental components. It has also been reported that with this type of laser, preparation of the retrograde cavity is significantly quicker and cleaner than with ultrasound, and there is no significant difference in the quality of seal of the retrograde cavities prepared.[13,21–26] Furthermore, clinical studies with the Er:YAG laser in periapical surgery demonstrated improvement in healing and increased postoperative patient compliance.[24,25]

To increase the success rate of endodontic surgical procedures, the combined use of three lasers in apicoectomy has been reported: Er:YAG laser (2940 nm, pulse mode), Nd:YAG laser (1064 nm, pulse mode), and GaAlAs laser (790 nm, continuous wave). The combined use of the three lasers allowed an incision to be made in the alveolar mucosa and the cortical bone to be cut, root resection and decontamination of the dentin cut surface, and the removal of the pathological tissue, which promoted a favorable prognosis following the surgical procedure[24] (see Clinical cases 18.1 and 18.2).

As the Er:YAG laser wavelength is highly absorbed by hydroxyapatite and water, may reduce microorganism load, and does not cause thermal damage, it is the laser of choice for periapical surgery.[13,21–26]

In a recent study, 65 apicoectomies on necrotic teeth with apical lesions were performed between 2000 and 2010 with the Er:YAG laser (2940 nm) and Er,Cr:YSGG laser (2780 nm). There were only nine failures, occurring at different times, and the remaining patients (86.15%) had no complications and their treatment followed a positive course. This study demonstrated that laser-assisted surgery can be added to the range of therapeutic approaches for endodontic treatment, and that apicoectomy with the erbium laser results in a high success rate with considerable benefit in terms of clinical outcome.[21]

An *in vitro* study of fibroblast adhesion to dentin surfaces treated with Er:YAG or Nd:YAG laser irradiation analyzed the morphology and roughness of dentin surfaces.[26] Laser irradiation was used for apicoectomy and retrograde cavity preparation,

---

Clinical case 18.2

A 38-year-old male patient presented with the main complaint of pain in tooth 22. The radiographic image showed a large radiolucent area in the periapical region. The Er:YAG laser was used to make an incision in the mucosa, and to remove cortical bone and resect the root resection. Radiographic imaging immediately after apical surgery on tooth 22 with the Er:YAG laser, Nd:YAG laser, and the low power diode laser, showed a large periapical lesion (Fig. 18.2a).

Radiographic 6- and 12-month follow-up showed significant bone healing (Fig. 18.2b) with a decrease in the periapical radiolucent area (Fig. 18.1c). The patient reported no signs and symptoms during clinical follow up and complete apical bone repair was observed 2 years after the surgical procedure. There had been no recurrence of the infection at 14-year follow-up (Fig.18.2d).

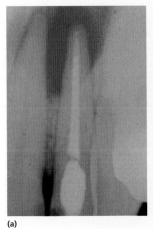 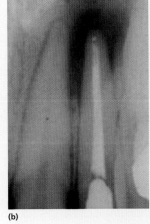 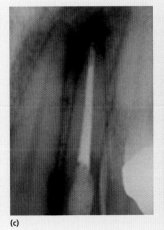 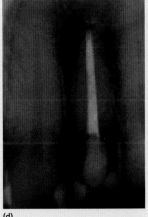

(a) (b) (c) (d)

Figure 18.2 (a) Presence of a large periapical lesion. Radiographic imaging immediately after the root resection of tooth 22. (b) Six month follow-up. (c) One year follow-up, bone healing. No symptoms reported by the patient. (d) Apical bone tissue had completely regenerated 14 years after apicoectomy and there had been no recurrence of the apical lesion.

with effective removal of the smear layer and evidence of collagen fiber on the root surface, which influenced clinical healing by enhancing periodontal ligament cell attachment. Cellular responses are greatly influenced by surface properties, including roughness and morphology. The quality of the dentin cut surface may affect the orientation of periodontal ligament cells and tissue repair as surrounding cells proliferate and migrate to the wound site. Laser irradiation causes morphological changes on the dental surface: hard tissue interactions produce surfaces with different textures and morphologies. Laser irradiation produces surfaces biocompatible with periodontal cell viability. Cutting dentin surfaces with Er:YAG lasers, combined with Nd:YAG laser irradiation or not, may have different effects on the initial cell attachment, compared with cutting with burs.[23] Morphological analysis and roughness measurement showed rougher surfaces following Er:YAG laser irradiation compared with no irradiation or irradiation with the Nd:YAG laser. The Er:YAG laser induced the greatest number of attached cells among all groups after 12 and 24 hours, with a favorable effect on the attachment of fibroblasts to dentin surfaces.[26]

References

1 Sundqvist G, Figdor D, Persson S, Sjogren U. Microbiologic analysis of teeth with failed endodontic treatment and the outcome of conservative re-treatment. *Oral Surg Oral Med Oral Pathol Oral Radiol Endod* 1998; 85: 86–93.

2 Torabinejad M, Corr R, Handysides R, Shabahang S. Outcomes of nonsurgical retreatment and endodontic surgery: A systematic review. *J Endod* 2009; 35(7): 930–937.

3 Eriksen HM, Kirkevang LL, Petersson K. Endodontic epidemiology and treatment outcome: general considerations. *Endod Topics* 2002: 1–9.

4 Friedman S. Treatment outcome: the potential for healing and retained function. In: Ingle JI, ed. *Endodontics*, 6th edn. Hamilton, Ontario: BC Decker, 2008.

5 Barone C, Dao TT, Basrani BB, Wang N, Friedman S. Treatment outcome in endodontics: The Toronto Study – Phases 3, 4 and 5: Apical surgery. *J Endod* 2010; 36: 28–36.

6 Lieblich SE. Endodontic surgery. *Dent Clin North Am* 2012; 56(1): 121–132.

7 Arx VT, Kurl B. Root-end cavity preparation after apicectomy using a new type of sonic and diamond surfaced retrotip: a 1 year follow-up study. *J Oral Maxillofac Surg* 1999; 57: 656–661.

8 Zuolo ML, Ferreira MO, Gutmann JL. Prognosis in periapical surgery: a clinical prospective study. *Int Endod* 2000; 33(2): 91–98.

9 Weichman JA, Johnson FM, Nitta LK. Laser use in endodontics. *Oral Surg Oral Med Oral Pathol Oral Radiol Endod* 1972; 34: 828–830.

10 Miserendino LJ. The laser apicectomy: endodontic application of the CO2 laser for pariapical surgery. *Oral Surg Oral Med Oral Pathol Oral Radiol Endod* 1988, 66: 615–619.

11 Franzen R, Gutknecht N, Falken S, Heussen N, Meister J. Bactericidal effect of a Nd:YAG laser on *Enterococcus faecalis* at pulse durations

12 Moritz A, Schoop U, Goharkhay K, et al. The bactericidal effect of Nd:YAG, Ho:YAG and Er:YAG laser irradiation in the root canal: an in vitro comparison. *J Clin Laser Med Surg* 1999; 17: 161–164.

13 Oliveira RG, Gouw-Soares S, Baldochi SL, Eduardo CP. Scanning electron microscopy (SEM) and optical microscopy: effects of Er:YAG and Nd:YAG lasers on apical seals after apicoectomy and retrofill. *Photomed Laser Surg* 2004; 22: 533–536.

14 Aranha AC, Domingues FB, Franco VO, Gutknecht N, Eduardo Cde P. Effects of Er:YAG and Nd:YAG lasers on dentin permeability in root surfaces: a preliminary *in vitro* study. *Photomed Laser Surg* 2005; 23: 504–508.

15 Gordon W, Atabakhsh VA, Meza F, et al. The antimicrobial efficacy of the erbium, chromium:yttrium-scandium-gallium-garnet laser with radial emitting tips on root canal dentin walls infected with Enterococcus faecalis. *J Am Dent Assoc* 2007; 138: 992–1002.

16 Friedman S. Considerations and concepts of case selection in the management of post-treatment endodontic disease (treatment failure). *Endod Topics* 2002: 54–78.

17 Arx VT, Penarrocha M, Jensen S. Prognostic factors in apical surgery with root-end filling: A meta-analysis. *J Endod* 2010; 36 (6): 957–973.

18 Gutknecht N, Apel C, Schafer C, Lampert F. Microleakage of composite fillings in Er, Cr: YSGG laser-prepared Class II cavities. *Lasers Surg Med* 2001; 28: 371–374.

19 Eriksson A, Albrektsson T, Grane B, Mcqueen D. Thermal injury to bone: a vital-microscopic description of heat effects. *Int J Oral Surg* 1982; 11: 115–121.

20 Strefezza C, Zezell DM, Bachmann L, Cecchini SC, Pinotti M, Eduardo CP. Thermal effects during in vitro intracanal application of Nd:YAG laser. *J Dent Res* 2000; 79(5): 1074.

21 Angiero F, Benedicenti S, Signore A, Parker S, Crippa R. Apicoectomies with the erbium laser: A complementary technique for retrograde endodontic treatment. *Photomed Laser Surg* 2011; 29(12): 845–849.

22 Gouw-Soares S, Lage-Marques JL, Eduardo CP. Apicoectomy by Er:YAG laser: permeability and morphological study of dentine cut surface. In: *International Laser Congress*, 1996, Greece. Proceedings. Greece: Monduzzi, 1996: 365–370.

23 Gouw-Soares SC, Stabholz A, Lage-Marques JL, Zezell DM, Groth EB, Eduardo CP. Comparative study of dentine permeability after apicectomy and surface treatment with 9.6μm TEA CO2 and Er:YAG laser irradiation. *J Clin Laser Med Surg* 2004; 22(2): 129–139.

24 Gouw-Soares SC, Tanji EY, Haypek P, Cardoso W, Eduardo CP. The use of Er:YAG, Nd:YAG and Ga-Al-As lasers in periapical surgery. Three years clinical case. *J Clin Laser Med Surg* 2001; 19(4): 193–198.

25 Gouw-Soares SC, Pelino JEP, Haypek P, Bachman L, Eduardo CP. Temperature rise in cavities prepared by Er:YAG laser. *J Oral Laser Appl* 2001; 1: 119–123.

26 Bolortuya G, Ebihara A, Ichinose S, et al. Effects of dentin surface modifications treated with Er:YAG and Nd:YAG laser irradiation on fibroblast cell adhesion. *Photomed Laser Surg* 2012; 30(2): 63–70.

CHAPTER 19

High power lasers in endodontics

José Luiz Lage–Marques,[1] Sheila C. Gouw Soares,[2] and Cláudia Strefezza[3]

[1]Discipline of Endodontics, Department of Restorative Dentistry, School of Dentistry, University of São Paulo (USP), São Paulo, SP, Brazil
[2]School of Dentistry, University of Cruzeiro do Sul (UNICSUL), São Paulo, SP, Brazil
[3]Faculdades Metropolitanas Unidas (FMU), São Paulo, SP, Brazil

Despite the availability of new instrumentation technology and advances in microscopy techniques, the search for more integrated treatments in the field of endodontics has prompted scientific research and the clinical use of both high and low power lasers, leading to considerably improved rates of success.

Dentin permeability

The use of the Nd:YAG laser in endodontics has become a favored approach following the development of finer gauge optical fibers that can access root canals (100, 200, and 300 μm). The wavelength of this laser (1064 nm) is poorly absorbed by hard and soft non-pigmented dental tissues. Irradiation of the root canal using this laser reduces microorganisms and promotes sealing of the irradiated root canal wall by melting the dentin, particularly in the apical region.

The wavelengths of the Er:YAG (2940 nm) and Er,Cr:YSGG (2790 nm) lasers match the resonant frequency of water molecule vibrations and are therefore highly absorbed by water-rich tissues.[1] The high absorbance by water of wavelengths that lie in the infrared range (Er:YAG 2940 nm, and Er,Cr:YSGG 2780 nm) induces microexplosions, which are responsible for the ablation phenomenon. Consequently, irradiation of dentin by these lasers strips the hydroxyapatite structure and smear layer from the cavity walls, thus clearing the dentinal tubules and increasing dentin permeability to intracanal medications or chemical solutions: depth of penetration into the apical third was increased by 29% following Er:YAG irradiation compared to irrigation without laser irradiation.[2]

Microorganism elimination from the endodontic system

Failure of endodontic treatment is often attributable to the persistence of viable microorganisms in the root canal system or dentinal tubules. Given the limitations of the antimicrobial procedures performed during treatment, laser irradiation has been proposed as an adjunctive therapy to achieve greater reduction in microorganisms in the root canal system.

Studies have shown promising results regarding the photothermic action of high power laser irradiation for eliminating microbial flora within root canals (see Clinical cases 19.1–19.3).[3,4] Despite the proven bactericidal effect of Nd:YAG, Er:YAG, and Er,Cr:YSGG lasers and their use in endodontic therapy, diode lasers have shown comparatively better performance, offering efficacy coupled with a lower cost–benefit ratio.[3,5] However, the effectiveness of bacterial elimination by irradiation is reduced as dentin thickness increases, and higher power laser are then required.

The percentage bacterial reduction reported after diode laser irradiation of 500-μm thick human dentin samples infected by *Streptococcus mutans* was 97.7% at a 7-W power setting. This rate fell to 50.9% for dentin thicknesses of 1 mm and 2 mm. In a study *in vitro*, the percentage bacterial reduction obtained using a 3-W laser was comparable to that achieved by irrigation with hydrogen peroxide (H_2O_2)/sodium hypochlorite (NaOCl).[6] Higher bacterial death rates were attained by irradiation using a laser at a setting of 4.5 W, or by irrigation with H_2O_2/NaOCl solution in combination with root canal irradiation using a setting of 3 W.[7] Furthermore, combined use of a diode laser (830 nm) with calcium hydroxide and camphorated paramonochlorophenol (CPMC) lead to 100% elimination of *Enterococcus faecalis* from inoculated root canals. The use of laser alone, in the absence of medication, lead to 96.5% and 57.6% reductions at 3-W and 2.5-W power settings, respectively. Reductions achieved by intracanal irradiation using the diode laser are clinically evidenced by resolution of periapical diseases of different degrees of complexity.

Treatment of the pulp chamber floor

The furcation region has a high prevalence of accessory canals in primary molars, implying a high risk of communication of inflammatory or infectious processes of the pulp with the interradicular bone region and periodontal tissues.[8]

Lasers in Dentistry: Guide for Clinical Practice, First Edition. Edited by Patrícia M. de Freitas and Alyne Simões.
© 2015 John Wiley & Sons, Inc. Published 2015 by John Wiley & Sons, Inc.

Irradiation of the furcation region in primary teeth using the Er:YAG laser was unable to reduce 0.5% methylene blue penetration since the wavelength of this laser strips the smear layer and exposes the openings of the dentinal tubules. However, irradiation of the pulp chamber floor and subsequent application of cyanoacrylate *in vitro* promoted a significant reduction in dentin permeability. This represents a highly effective approach for maintaining the effects of disinfection in this region.[9]

Clinical case 19.1 Endodontic treatment of a non-vital upper right lateral incisor using a high power diode laser

A 38-year-old male patient was referred to our clinic for evaluation and treatment of his upper right lateral incisor. The patient had experienced moderate sensitivity to percussion stimuli for the last 6 months; however, for the past 4 days, the pain had become severe, continuous, and pulsing, and had spread over the entire anterior maxilla. Tenderness upon palpation and soft periradicular swelling were observed in the region around the tooth.[10]

Clinical examination revealed a large restoration cavity on the distal aspect of the tooth. Examination of the buccal mucosa revealed a fistula, but periodontal probing was normal (Fig. 19.1a,b).

Two radiographs taken from different angles confirmed that the disease was actually centered around the upper right lateral incisor. Radiographic examination revealed a long root, with a large, irregular radiolucency around the tooth apex (Fig. 19.1c,d).

Based on the patient's symptoms, a diagnosis was made of pulpal necrosis with an acute periradicular abscess involving the upper right lateral incisor, and single-visit root canal therapy were planned.

The root was very long and moderately curved, and the root canal system was partially filled by a previous endodontic intervention.

The adhesive composite resin was removed to facilitate both the placing of the rubber dam and irrigation. The root canal opening was worn progressively using a #3 ultrasonic tip on the pulp chamber walls (Fig. 19.1e,f).

The root canal was negotiated with a #08 K-File, followed by abundant irrigation with 2.5% NaOCl,[11,12] and the working length was established with an apex locator. The root canal length was approximately 25 mm.

Initial negotiation was difficult, even with the #08 K-File, and required more than 10 minutes to complete. Abundant exudate was aspirated (Fig. 19.1 g)

After using the #8 K-File, the EndoWave MGP #15 was used at 700 rpm with a torque of approximately 4 N/cm, followed by abundant irrigation with 2.5% NaOCl.

Rotary instrumentation was then performed using an EndoWave NiTi (Morita Co.) file system up to the working length using PTC gel with NaOCl. The canal was irrigated with 2 mL of 1% NaOCl between the application of each instrument, using a disposable 10-mL syringe and a 30-gauge needle (BD Microlance; Becton Dickinson). After instrumentation, the canal was irrigated with 6 mL of 15% ethylenediaminetetraacetic acid (EDTA) for 3 minutes, followed by a final rinse with 2 mL of 2.5% NaOCl.

Next, the root canal was irradiated with a high power diode laser (Thera Lase)[13–15] set to operate in continuous mode at 2 W, with a 400-μm fiber diameter spot applied to the root canal surface in four applications of 5 seconds each, with a 20-second interval between applications. Abundant irrigation of the canal was performed with 2.5% NaOCl during the intervals, and the irrigant was maintained in the canal during the subsequent applications. The Thera Lase Surgery (DMC Importação e Exportação de Equipamentos LTDA, Brazil) is an infrared laser (808 nm ± 10 nm) used at high power (4.5 W ± 20%) in surgery and at low power (100 mW), in laser therapy (dentistry, physical therapy, and general medicine).

Finally, the canal was dried with sterile paper points and filled (Fig. 19.1 h,i). Follow-up radiograph at 90 days is shown in Figure 19.1 j. Follow-up radiograph at 180 days is shown in Figure 19.1 k.

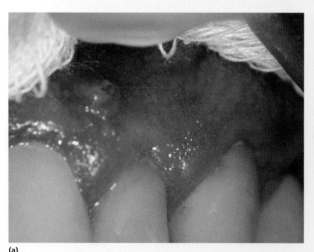
(a)

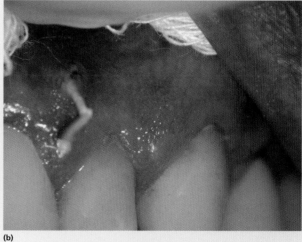
(b)

Figure 19.1 (a) Presence of a large restoration cavity on the distal aspect of the tooth. (b) Presence of a fistula at the buccal mucosa. (c) Radiograph image showing a large, irregular radiolucency around the tooth apex of the upper right lateral incisor. (d) Root canal opening was worn progressively using a #3 ultrasonic tip on the pulp chamber walls. (e) Abundant exudate aspirated throughout root canal negotiation. (f) Root canal was dried with sterile paper points and filled. (g) Follow-up radiograph at 90 days.

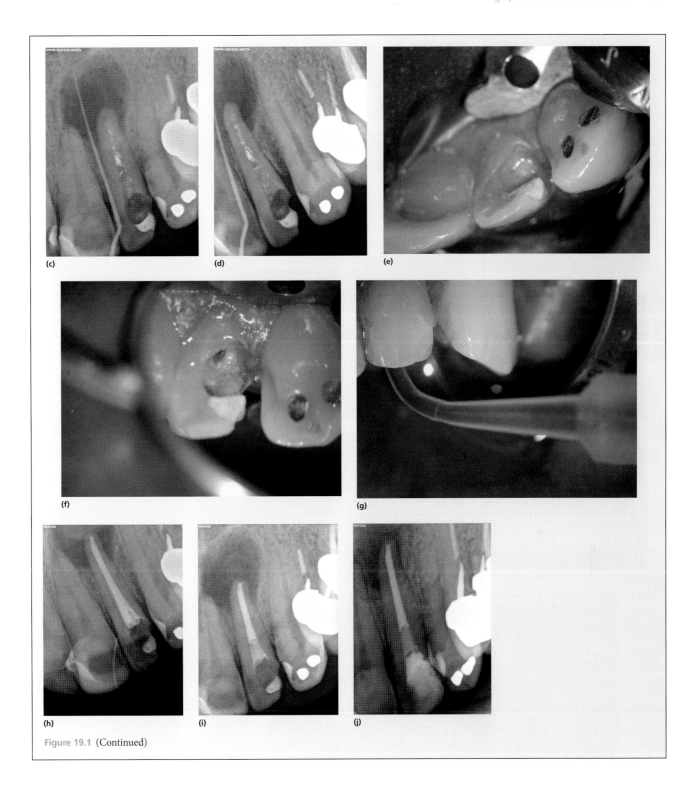

Figure 19.1 (Continued)

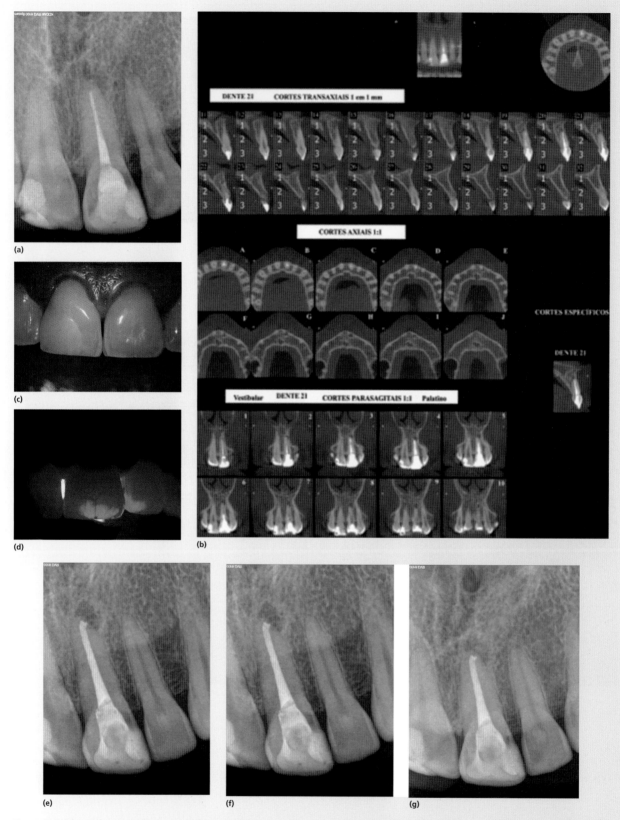

Figure 19.2 (a) Initial periapical radiograph. (b) Computed tomographic images depicting details of the apical inflammation[16,17] (Distel et al. 2002. Reproduced with permission of Elsevier). (c) Clinical image depicting details of the esthetics of the incisors. (d) Transillumination image depicting details of the crown microfractures. (e) Postoperative radiograph. After cleaning and shaping, the root canal was irradiated with a high power diode laser set to operate in continuous mode at 2 W with a 400-μm optical fiber applied to the root canal surface in four applications of 5 seconds each, with a 20-second interval between applications[18,19] (Garbuz et al. 2008. Reproduced with permission of Elsevier). (e) Abundant irrigation of the canal was performed with 2.5% NaOCl during the intervals, and the irrigant was maintained in the canal during the subsequent applications. Finally, the canal was dried with sterile paper points and filled. (f) Radiograph at 90-day follow-up (g) Radiograph at 180-day follow-up.

Clinical case 19.3 Endodontic treatment of a non-vital low molar using a high power diode laser

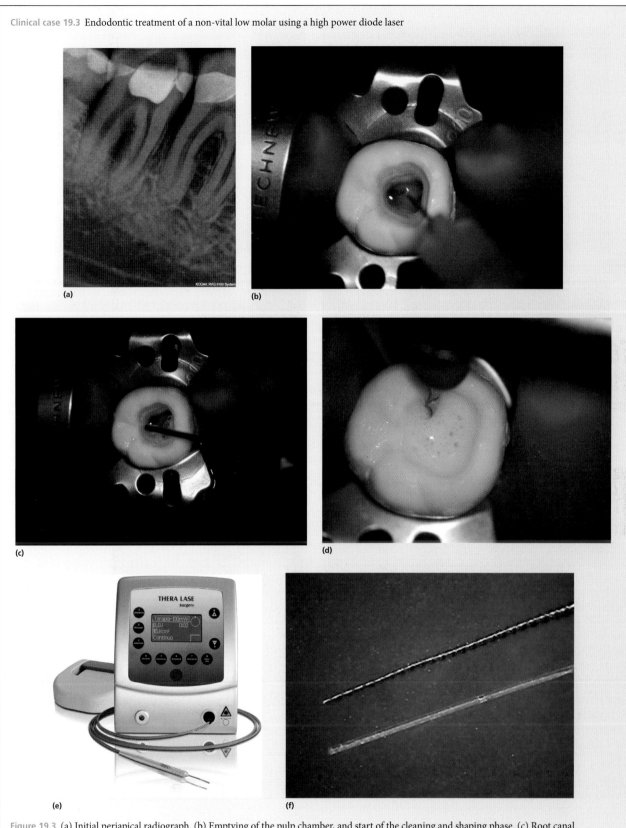

Figure 19.3 (a) Initial periapical radiograph. (b) Emptying of the pulp chamber, and start of the cleaning and shaping phase. (c) Root canal preparation with 1% NaOCl and PTC gel. (d) Instruments and chemical substances. (e) DMC Thera Lase Surgery. (f) 400-μm optical fiber and #30K-file.

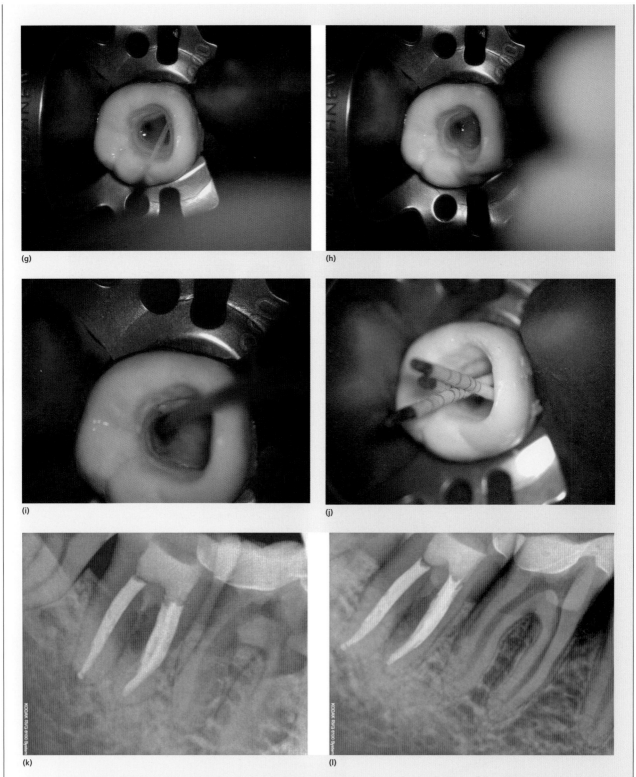

Figure 19.3 (Continued) (g,h) Continuous mode at 2 W applied to the root canal surface in four applications of 5 seconds each, with a 20-second interval between applications. (i) Draining the irrigant solution by aspiration. (j) Paper cones and drying of the canal. (k,l) Final radiographs showing complete absence of signs of infection.

References

1 Eriksson AR, Albrektsson T. Temperature threshold levels for heat-induced bone tissue injury: a vital-microscopic study in the rabbit. *J Prosthet Dent* 1983; 50(1): 101–107.

2 Raldi DP, Lage-Marques JL. *In vitro* evaluation of the effects of the interaction between irrigating solutions, intracanal medication and Er:YAG laser in dentin permeability of the endodontic system. *Pesq Odontol Bras* 2003; 17(3): 278–285.

3 Schoop U, Kluger W, Moritz A, Nedjelik N, Georgopoulos A, Sperr W. Bactericidal effect of different laser systems in the deep layers of dentin. *Lasers Surg Med* 2004; 35(2): 111–116.

4 Gouw-Soares S, Gutknecht N, Conrads G, Lampert F, Matson E, Eduardo CP. The bactericidal effect of Ho:YAG laser irradiation within contaminated root dentinal samples. *J Clin Laser Med Surg* 2000; 18(2): 81–87.

5 de Souza EB, Cai S, Simionato MR, Lage-Marques JL. High-power diode laser in the disinfection in depth of the root canal dentin. *Oral Surg Oral Med Oral Pathol Oral Radiol Endod* 2008; 106(1): 68–72.

6 Lee BS, Lin YW, Chia JS, et al. Bactericidal effects of diode laser on *Streptococcus mutans* after irradiation through different thickness of dentin. *Lasers Surg Med* 2006; 38(1): 62–69.

7 Kreisler M, Kohnen W, Beck M, et al. Efficacy of NaOCl/H2O2 irrigation and GaAlAs laser in decontamination of root canals in vitro. *Lasers Surg Med* 2003; 32(3):189–196.

8 Wrbas KT, Kielbassa AM, Hellwig E. Microscopic studies of accessory canals in primary molar furcations. *ASDC J Dent Child* 1997; 64(2): 118–122.

9 Lopes-Silva AMS, Lage-Marques JL. Evaluation of the permeability of the furcation area of deciduous molars conditioned with Er:YAG laser and cyanoacrylate. *Pesqui Odonto Bras* 2003; 17(3): 212–216.

10 Kouchi Y, Ninomiya J, Yasuda H, Fukui K, Moriyama T, Okamoto H. Location of *Streptococcus mutans* in the dentinal tubules of open infected root canals. *J Dent Res* 1980; 59(12): 2038–2046.

11 Berutti E, Marini R, Angeretti A. Penetration ability of different irrigants into dentinal tubules. *J Endod* 1997; 23(12): 725–727.

12 Moritz A, Doertbudak O, Gutknecht N, Goharkhay K, Schoop U, Sperr W. Nd:YAG laser irradiation of infected root canals in combination with microbiologic examinations. *J Am Dent Assoc* 1997; 128: 1525–1530.

13 Vaarkamp J, ten Bosch JJ, Verdonschot EH. Propagation of light through human dental enamel and dentine. *Caries Res* 1995; 29 (1): 8–13.

14 Odor TM, Watson TF, Pitt Ford TR, Mc Donald F. Pattern of transmission of laser light in teeth. *Int Endod J* 1996; 29 (4): 228–234.

15 Schoop U, Kluger W, Dervisbegovic S, et al. Innovative wavelengths in endodontic treatment. *Lasers Surg Med* 2006; 38: 624–630.

16 Distel JW, Hatton JF, Gillespie MJ. Biofilm formation in medicated root canals. *J Endod* 2002; 28: 689–693.

17 Spratt DA, Pratten J, Wilson M, Gulabivala K. An *in vitro* evaluation of the antimicrobial efficacy of irrigants on biofilms of root canal isolates. *Int Endod J* 2001; 34: 300–307.

18 Gurbuz T, Ozdemir Y, Kara N, Zehir C, Kurudirek M. Evaluation of root canal dentin after Nd:YAG laser irradiation and treatment with five different irrigation solutions: a preliminary study. *J Endod* 2008; 34(3): 318–321.

19 Beer F, Buchmair A, Wernisch J, Georgopoulos A, Moritz A. Comparison of two diode lasers on bactericidity in root canals-an in vitro study. *Lasers Med Sci* 2012; 27: 361–364.

SECTION 4

Periodontology

CHAPTER 20

Surgical and non-surgical treatment of periodontal diseases

Leticia Helena Theodoro and Valdir Gouveia Garcia

Research and Study on Laser in Dentistry Group (GEPLO), Department of Surgery and Integrated Clinic, Division of Periodontics, University Estadual Paulista (UNESP), Araçatuba, SP, Brazil

Introduction

The clinical application of high power lasers has expanded over the past two decades, yet the efficacies of many of these applications are still uncertain. High power lasers have been used in periodontics mainly for the surgical treatment of soft tissues and in non-surgical periodontal treatments such as therapy for sulcular or periodontal pocket debridement, reduction of subgingival bacteria, and scaling and root planing (SRP).[1]

CO_2 (10 600 nm), Nd:YAG and Nd:YAP (1064 nm and 1340 nm), and semiconductor diode (800–980 nm) lasers were the first to be recommended for treating soft tissues in the field of periodontics[2]; Nd:YAG and semiconductor diode lasers have also been used to reduce microbes in periodontal pockets. By contrast, Er:YAG lasers (2940 nm) and, more recently, Er,Cr:YSGG lasers (2780 nm) have been indicated for soft tissue surgery, treatment of mineralized tissues, and radicular scraping.

Surgical treatment of periodontal diseases

High power lasers have been widely utilized for conservative surgery and the management of periodontal soft tissues; these lasers provide the advantage of ablating soft tissue with effective hemostasis and a reduction of the bacterial burden.[2] Several clinical procedures can be performed using these lasers, including enlarging the clinical crown, gingivectomy, frenectomy, recontouring of the gingival tissue, removal of melanin pigmentation, proximal wedges, and excisional biopsies. CO_2 (10 600 nm), Nd:YAG (1064 nm), Er:YAG (2940 nm), and semiconductor diode (800–980 nm) lasers have been the most widely used for these procedures.

The wavelength of the CO_2 laser (10 600 nm) is rapidly absorbed by water, the energy is converted into heat, and there is little spreading and penetration of this heat into the tissues; consequently, only a narrow area of superficial necrosis occurs in the tissues that are incised using this laser.[3] The CO_2 laser thus may be useful for performing gingivectomies, bridectomies, melanin pigment removal, and excisional biopsies.

The Nd:YAG laser (1064 nm) exhibits the greatest power to penetrate tissues. It has a wavelength that is highly absorbed by pigmented tissues, and thus it is useful for the removal of tissues that have a potential for abnormal hemorrhage and for hemostasis of small capillaries and blood vessels.[3] However, when used in soft tissues, the irradiation parameters must be cautiously selected to avoid damaging the adjacent bone.

The diode laser (810–820 nm) is also absorbed by pigment in the soft tissues, making it an excellent hemostatic tool; it can also be used to remove soft tissue, reducing the amount of deep thermal damage.[3]

The Er:YAG laser (2940 nm) is highly absorbed by water, which makes it appropriate for surgery on soft tissue and mineralized tissue, which are rich in water. Because gingival tissue is rich in water, the energy is effectively absorbed without promoting undesirable thermal damage to the adjacent hard tissues (teeth and bone). This characteristic makes the procedure easy to execute and capable of conservatively and precisely removing lesions, especially in areas that involve periodontal esthetics. However, the Er:YAG lasers are not capable of promoting satisfactory hemostasis of the surgical area, as is typical of the CO_2, diode, and Nd:YAG lasers.

Resective, periodontal soft tissue surgeries (such as gingivectomies) may be performed using high power lasers, with the advantage of greater hemostasis and the achievement of a more conservative clinical procedure.[4,5] Periodontal laser surgery is also indicated for cases of enlarged clinical crowns or to remove excess gingival tissue caused by trauma, bacterial plaque, medications, or passive eruption (Fig. 20.1 and 20.2). Lasers facilitate these procedures (mainly in young patients), reducing the need for flaps and sutures.

Other clinical procedures that may utilize these lasers include frenectomies or bridectomies. These clinical techniques may be performed in the most conservative manner without requiring sutures and may achieve greater hemostasis in the treated tissues.

The lasers can also be employed for excisional biopsies. This technique requires an incision at the base of the lesion and the use of tweezers or a suture thread to grasp and remove the lesion

Lasers in Dentistry: Guide for Clinical Practice, First Edition. Edited by Patrícia M. de Freitas and Alyne Simões.
© 2015 John Wiley & Sons, Inc. Published 2015 by John Wiley & Sons, Inc.

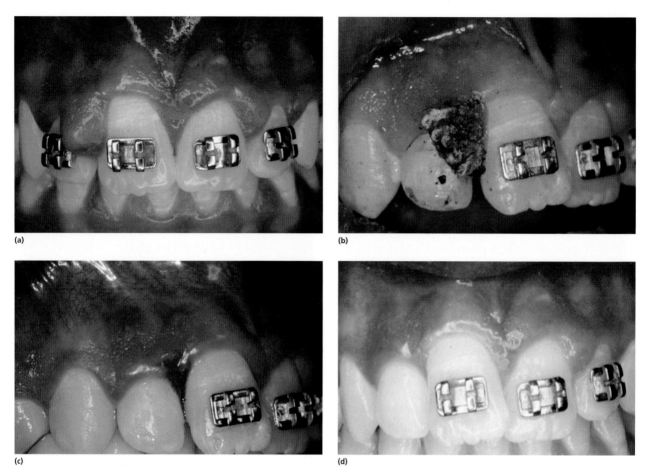

Figure 20.1 (a) Alteration of the contour of the marginal gingiva caused by orthodontic movement; (b) surgical gingivectomy performed with a CO_2 laser; (c) seven days and (d) 30 days after the operation.

without damaging it, so that the anatomopathological exam can be performed (Fig. 20.3).

The use of high power lasers during periodontal surgery has proven advantageous in the improvement of tissue repair, because these devices facilitate a more conservative technique without discomfort during or after the surgery and without postoperative sensitivity, pain, or bleeding.

Although high power lasers can incise and excise soft tissues (gingiva and alveolar mucosa), their use is limited to flap surgeries.[6] However, Er:YAG and Er,Cr:YSGG lasers can also be used during gingival curettage or SRP.

Non-surgical treatment of periodontal diseases

Several lasers have been studied for the treatment of root surfaces, including CO_2 and Nd:YAG,[7] diode,[8,9] Er:YAG,[8,9] and most recently, Er,Cr:YSGG lasers.[10–12] High power lasers have been developed using technology and fiber optics to access

periodontal pockets, with the great advantage of a strong bactericidal action. The effect of laser irradiation on tissues depends on the wavelength of the lasers and on its absorbance by the tissues. In biological tissues, the absorption is mainly due to the presence of molecules that are free of water, proteins, pigments, and other macromolecules.[8] Other irradiation parameters may also interfere with the biological response of the tissues: power, laser emission mode, fiber-optic angle, and exposure time.[13]

The CO_2 laser is not indicated for scraping the root surface because it is incapable of removing tartar from the tooth surface and causes carbonization and melting of the irradiated surfaces.[2] The diode and Nd:YAG lasers are not effective in removing mineralized bacterial deposits; therefore, the use of these lasers in periodontal therapy is based on the removal of the sulcular epithelium and the reduction of periodontal pathogenic bacteria in the periodontal pockets.

The authors of a systematic review of the clinical studies employing the Nd:YAG laser for non-surgical therapy concluded that there is no scientific evidence proving that the Nd:YAG laser when used as monotherapy or in combination

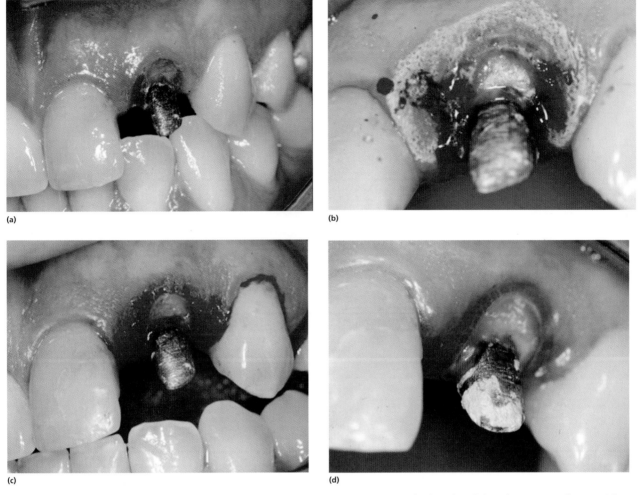

Figure 20.2 (a) Increased gingival volume covering the end of the coronal preparation; (b) surgery for the enlarged clinical crown using the Er:YAG laser (2940 nm; 400 mJ; 10 Hz); (c) immediate clinical appearance and (d) seven days after the operation.

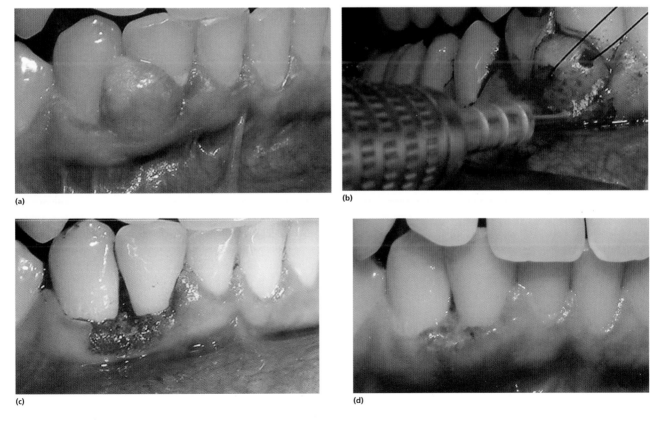

Figure 20.3 (a) Fibroid located in the interdental papilla; (b) excisional biopsy performed with the Er:YAG laser (400 mJ/10 Hz); (c) immediate clinical appearance and (d) seven days after the operation.

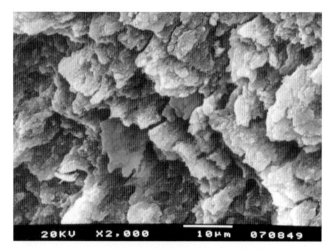

Figure 20.4 Electron photomicrography of the root surface irradiated with an Er:YAG laser set at 100 mJ and 10 Hz (original magnification 2000×).

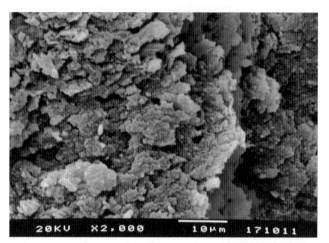

Figure 20.5 Electron photomicrography of the root surface irradiated with an Er,Cr:YSGG at a power setting of 1.5 W (original magnification 2000×).

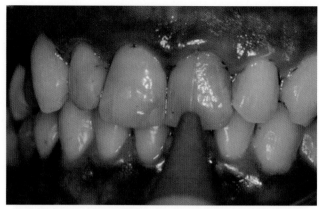

Figure 20.6 Fiber of the diode laser positioned in the periodontal pocket during decontamination of the periodontal pocket.

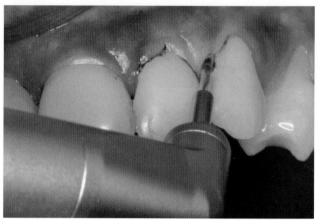

Figure 20.7 Fiber of the Er:YAG laser positioned in the periodontal pocket during root surface scaling.

with SRP procedures is superior to the conventional modalities for periodontal treatment.[14]

The use of the diode laser for adjuvant therapy with SRP has been studied by several researchers.[15–18] Some clinical studies have demonstrated a reduction of periodontal pathogenic microorganisms in pockets that are irradiated with a high power diode laser.[15,18] However, other studies have not demonstrated a greater reduction of periodontal pathogenic bacteria in irradiated pockets compared with infected pockets treated with conventional mechanical therapy.[16,19] Regarding the periodontal clinical parameters, some investigations have revealed greater reductions of probing pocket depths and the levels of clinical insertion at periodontal sites that are treated with SRP and irradiation with a diode laser[15,19]; in contrast, other studies have not demonstrated any clinical advantages of using the diode laser as adjuvant therapy with SRP.[16,17]

The ability of water molecules to absorb laser irradiation determines the radiation's penetration into the tissues and its ability to cause thermal damage to the adjacent tissues.[20] The wavelengths of the Er:YAG (2940 nm) and Er,Cr:YSGG (2780 nm) lasers are highly absorbed by the water molecules that are interspersed among the hydroxyapatite crystals, providing these lasers with the photomechanical or photothermal ability to remove mineralized tissues without heating the adjacent tissues.

In vitro experiments have revealed that this irradiation may promote the formation of an irregular and rough surface[8,9,21] that results from the explosive ablation process (Figs 20.4 and 20.5); furthermore, this roughness depends on the angle of irradiation between the tooth and the delivery of the fiber beam.[11]

The fibers of high power lasers must be positioned (in the case of the diode laser) toward the gingival surface or as parallel as possible to the root surface (Fig. 20.6). The Er:YAG laser must be positioned less than 30 degrees relative to the subgingival root surface, performing an apical-to-occlusal movement while being cooled by water (Fig. 20.7).

Use of the Er:YAG laser has been compared with SRP, and the clinical effects of the two therapies are similar,[22–28] despite promoting a greater reduction of microbes in the long term.[29] Furthermore, a limited number of studies have evaluated and

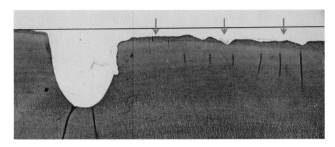

Figure 20.8 Root surface irradiated with an Er,Cr:YSGG laser at a power setting of 1.5 W (arrows) (original magnification, 5×) (De Oliveira et al. 2010 Wiley-Liss, Inc.).

investigated the clinical effects of lasers as an adjuvant therapy with SRP in the treatment of periodontitis.[28–31]

Recently, another laser has been demonstrated to act on mineralized tissues: the Er,Cr:YSGG laser with a wavelength of approximately 2780 nm. This laser's mechanism for removing mineralized tissues is called thermomechanical processing, in which the emission of light is absorbed by water within the mineralized hydroxyapatite tissues (similar to the mechanism of the Er:YAG laser) and is combined with the effect of the emitted water on the treated tissue. Other recent studies have demonstrated that 1.5 W is an appropriate power setting for the removal of root tartar without causing significant morphological alterations (Fig. 20.8).[10,32] There have been only a few controlled clinical studies of the use of the Er,Cr:YSGG laser system as adjuvant therapy with SRP, and the results reveal significant improvements in the evaluated clinical parameters.[12]

Final considerations

CO_2, Nd:YAG, diode, Er:YAG, and Er,Cr:YSGG lasers may be safely used for soft tissue surgeries for periodontitis, with the advantages of less bleeding, reduced microbial burdens, and greater postoperative comfort.

Currently, there is insufficient evidence to support the clinical application of CO_2, Nd:YAG, and semiconductor diode lasers in non-surgical periodontal therapies. In contrast, the Er:YAG laser has been proven to be the most useful device for non-surgical periodontal therapy combined with SPR for chronic periodontitis, although the majority of studies have not demonstrated clinical advantages using this laser compared with the conventional technique. Certain benefits, however, have been observed, such as a long-term reduction of the microbial burden. Furthermore, Er:YAG laser irradiation has been demonstrated to be a more comfortable therapy for patients, treating their lesions without causing thermal damage to the adjacent tissues. Furthermore, despite the existence of only a few controlled studies on the use of the Er,Cr:YSGG laser as an adjuvant therapy for the treatment of periodontal disease, this device may also become recognized as a promising auxiliary tool.

In addition to the aforementioned evaluations of the safety of therapies using the various lasers at their given wavelengths and irradiation powers, no significant adverse effects have yet been reported in the literature.

References

1 American Academy of Periodontology. Statement on the efficacy of lasers in the non-surgical treatment of inflammatory periodontal disease. *J Periodontol* 2011; 82: 513–514.

2 Ishikawa I, Aoki A, Takasaki AA, et al. Application of lasers in periodontics: true innovation or myth? *Periodontology 2000* 2009; 50: 90–126.

3 American Academy of Periodontology. Lasers in periodontics. *J Periodontol* 2002; 73: 1231–1239.

4 Pick RM, Pecaro BC, Silverman CJ. The laser gingivectomy. The use of the CO_2 laser for the removal of phenytoin hyperplasia. *J Periodontol* 1985; 56: 492–496.

5 Pick RM, Pecaro BC. Use of the CO_2 laser in soft tissue dental surgery. *Lasers Surg Med* 1987; 7: 207–213.

6 Pick RM, Colvard MD. Current status of lasers in soft tissue dental surgery. *J Periodontol* 1993; 64: 589–602.

7 Israel M, Cobb CM, Rossmann JA, et al. The effects of CO_2, Nd:YAG and Er:YAG lasers with and without surface coolant on tooth roots surfaces. An *in vitro* study. *J Clin Periodontol* 1997; 24: 595–602.

8 Theodoro LH, Haypek P, Bachmann L, et al. Effect of Er:YAG and diode laser irradiation on the root surface: morphological and thermal analysis. *J Periodontol* 2003; 74: 838–843.

9 Theodoro LH, Sampaio JE, Haypek P, et al. Effect of Er:YAG and Diode lasers on the adhesion of blood components and on the morphology of irradiated root surfaces. *J Periodontal Res* 2006; 41: 381–390.

10 Ting CC, Fukuda M, Watanabe T, et al. Effects of Er,Cr:YSGG laser irradiation on the root surface: morphologic analysis and efficiency of calculus removal. *J Periodontol* 2007; 78: 2156–2164.

11 De Oliveira GJPL, Pavone C, Sampaio JEC, et al. Influence of the angle of irradiation of the Er,Cr:YSGG laser on the morphology, attachment of blood components, roughness, and root wear: in vitro study. *Lasers Surg Med* 2010; 42: 683–691.

12 Kelbauskiene S, Baseviciene N, Goharkahay K, et al. One-year clinical results of Er,Cr:YSGG laser application in addition to scaling and root planing in patients with early to moderate periodontitis. *Lasers Med Sci* 2011; 26: 445–452.

13 Niemz MH. *Laser-Tissue Interactions: Fundamentals and Applications*. Berlin: Springer, 1996.

14 Slot DE, Kranendonk AA, Paraskevas S, et al. The effect of a pulsed Nd:YAG Laser in non-surgical periodontal therapy. *J Periodontol* 2009; 80: 1041–1056.

15 Kamma JJ, Vasdekis VG, Romanos GE. The effect of diode laser (980 nm) treatment on aggressive periodontitis: evaluation of microbial and clinical parameters. *Photomed Laser Surg* 2009; 27: 11–19.

16 De Micheli G, Andrade AK, Alves VTE, et al. Efficacy of high intensity diode laser as an adjunct to non-surgical periodontal treatment: a randomized controlled trial. *Lasers Med Sci* 2011; 26: 43–48.

17 Euzébio Alves VT, de Andrade AK, Toaliar JM, et al. Clinical and microbiological evaluation of high intensity diode laser adjutant to

non-surgical periodontal treatment: a 6-month clinical trial. *Clin Oral Investig* 2013; 17(1): 87–95.

18 Giannelli M, Bani D, Viti C, et al. Comparative evaluation of the effects of different photoablative laser irradiation protocols on the gingiva of periodontopathic patients. *Photomed Laser Surg* 2012; 30: 222–230.

19 Caruso U, Nastri L, Piccolomini R, et al. Use of diode laser 980 nm as adjunctive therapy in the treatment of chronic periodontitis. A randomized controlled clinical trial. *New Microbiol* 2008; 31: 513–518.

20 Jepsen S, Deschner J, Braun A, et al. Calculus removal and the prevention of its formation. *Periodontology 2000* 2011; 55: 167–188.

21 Oliveira GJ, Theodoro LH, Marcantonio Junior E, et al. Effect of Er,Cr:YSGG and Er:YAG laser irradiation on the adhesion of blood components on the root surface and on root morphology. *Braz Oral Res* 2012; 26: 256–262.

22 Schwarz F, Sculean A, Georg T, et al. Periodontal treatment with an Er:YAG laser compared to scaling and root planing: A controlled clinical study. *J Periodontol* 2001; 72: 361–367.

23 Schwarz F, Sculean A, Berakdar M, et al. Clinical evaluation of an Er:YAG laser combined with scaling and root planing for nonsurgical periodontal treatment: A controlled, prospective clinical study. *J Clin Periodontol* 2003; 30: 26–34.

24 Schwarz F, Sculean A, Berakdar M, et al. Periodontal treatment with an Er:YAG laser or scaling and root planing: A 2-year follow-up split-mouth study. *J Periodontol* 2003; 74: 590–596.

25 Tomasi C, Schander K, Dahlén G, et al. Short-term clinical and microbiologic effects of pocket debridement with an Er:YAG laser during periodontal maintenance. *J Periodontol* 2006; 77: 111–118.

26 Crespi R, Cappare P, Toscanelli I, et al. Effects of Er:YAG laser compared to ultrasonic scaler in periodontal treatment: A 2-year follow-up split-mouth clinical study. *J Periodontol* 2007; 78: 1195–1200.

27 Derdilopoulou FV, Nonhoff J, Neumann K et al. Microbiological findings after periodontal therapy using curettes, Er:YAG laser, sonic, and ultrasonic scalers. *J Clin Periodontol* 2007; 34: 588–598.

28 Lopes BM, Marcantonio RA, Thompson GM, et al. Short-term clinical and immunological effects of scaling and root planing with Er:YAG laser in chronic periodontitis. *J Periodontol* 2008; 79: 1158–1167.

29 Lopes BM, Theodoro LH, Melo RF, et al. Clinical and microbiologic follow-up evaluations after non-surgical periodontal treatment with erbium:YAG laser and scaling and root planing. *J Periodontol* 2010; 81: 682–691.

30 Karlsson MR, Diogo Löfgren CI, Jansson HM. The effect of laser therapy as an adjunct to non-surgical periodontal treatment in subjects with chronic periodontitis: A systematic review. *J Periodontol* 2008; 79: 2021–2028.

31 Schwarz F, Aoki A, Becker J, et al. Laser application in non-surgical periodontal therapy: a systematic review. *J Clin Periodontol* 2008; 35 (Suppl 8): 29–44.

32 Hakki SS, Berk G, Dundar N, et al. Effects of root planing procedures with hand instrument or erbium, chromium:yttrium-scandium-gallium-garnet laser irradiation on the root surfaces: a comparative scanning electron microscopy study. *Lasers Med Sci* 2010; 25: 345–53.

CHAPTER 21

Antimicrobial photodynamic therapy in the treatment of periodontal diseases

Valdir Gouveia Garcia and Letícia Helena Theodoro

Research and Study on Laser in Dentistry Group (GEPLO), Department of Surgery and Integrated Clinic, Division of Periodontics, University Estadual Paulista (UNESP), Araçatuba, SP, Brazil

Introduction

The colonization of the tooth surface and epithelial cells in the interior of the gingival sulcus or periodontal pocket by bacterial biofilms is a complex process that occurs even following adequate oral hygiene. These biofilms consist of a diverse community of bacteria that is maintained in a matrix of extracellular polymers and may lead to the onset of gingivitis and periodontitis.[1,2] Considered to be a multifactorial disease, periodontitis may be modified by different risk factors.[3] The bacterial etiology of periodontal diseases is mainly correlated with the presence of certain bacterial species, such as *Aggregatibacter actinomycetemcomitans*, *Tannerella forsythensis*, and *Porphyromonas gingivalis*.[4] Other studies demonstrate the relationships between bacterial species and different subgingival microbial complexes with clinical periodontal parameters.[5]

The mechanical control of bacterial biofilms and deposits mineralized on the root surface is the most widely used control method (gold standard) for periodontitis.[6] However, certain conditions make this procedure ineffective with regard to complete bacterial reduction, mainly in the presence of unfavorable anatomical conditions, such as root concavity; areas that are difficult to access with instruments, such as furcation areas in deep pockets[7]; and the invasion of gingival tissue by bacteria.[8]

Antimicrobial photodynamic therapy (aPDT) is a noninvasive therapy that is capable of eliminating periodontopathic bacteria; it uses a low power laser as a light source and has been used to treat periodontal and peri-implant diseases.[9]

Experimental studies on aPDT in the treatment of periodontal diseases

The results of several *in vivo* studies have demonstrated the effectiveness of aPDT in the reduction of periodontopathic bacteria.[10–13] Using histomorphometric analysis, studies have also evaluated the effects of aPDT in the control of alveolar bone loss and the extension of the inflammatory process in experimentally-induced periodontitis in animals,[12–16] whereas other studies have evaluated the immune-inflammatory response of the host.[17,18] These studies have demonstrated that aPDT is an effective therapy for controlling and treating periodontal disease, used either alone [12,14,15] or in conjunction with conventional mechanical treatment, under adverse systemic conditions or otherwise[16,17,19,20] (Figs 21.1 and 21.2).

Clinical application of aPDT in the treatment of periodontitis

In the past 5 years, several clinical studies on humans have evaluated the effect of aPDT as an adjunctive therapy in the treatment of chronic periodontitis.[21–28] Certain studies have not demonstrated any clinical advantage associated with its use.[25,28] However, upon surveying the treated sites, other studies have shown that aPDT can reduce the amount of bleeding.[23,24,27] With regard to the effect of aPDT on the reduction of periodontopathic bacteria, several authors have clinically demonstrated a greater reduction in bacteria after the use of the therapy during a period of 3 or 6 months following treatment.[24,26,28,29]

Advantages of aPDT

The great advantage of the use of aPDT as an adjunctive treatment along with conventional periodontal treatment is that it is a low cost, local therapy that has no systemic effects and does not cause bacterial resistance, particularly compared with the use of antibiotic therapy. In addition, aPDT may be very useful for patients exhibiting modifying systemic factors that are capable of altering the biological response of the periodontal tissues during the tissue repair process following conventional treatment, or even influencing the progression of the disease. Among these modifying factors, diabetes, smoking, the use of immunosuppressive medications, and acquired immunodeficiency syndrome may be cited.[30,31]

Lasers in Dentistry: Guide for Clinical Practice, First Edition. Edited by Patrícia M. de Freitas and Alyne Simões.
© 2015 John Wiley & Sons, Inc. Published 2015 by John Wiley & Sons, Inc.

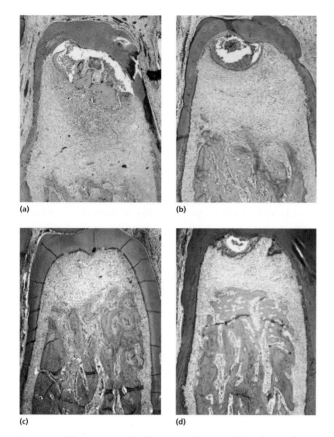

Figure 21.1 Photomicrographs illustrating the areas of bone loss in the furcation regions of the mandibular first molars in induced periodontal disease in ovariectomized rats: (a) No aPDT treatment at day 7 and (b) day 15 post scaling and root planing (SRP) (c) aPDT treatment at day 7 and (d) day 15 post treatment (SRP plus aPDT) (original magnification 100×). The sections were stained with hematoxylin and eosin (H&E).

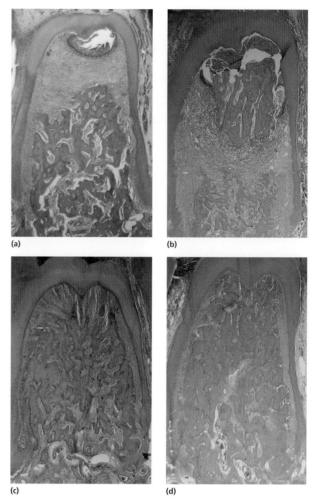

Figure 21.2 Photomicrograph illustrating the areas of bone loss in the furcation regions of the mandibular first molars in induced periodontal disease in rats: (a) SRP treatment at day 15 post treatment in a non-diabetic animal (b) SRP treatment at day 15 post treatment in a diabetic animal (c) aPDT treatment at day 7 and (d) day 30 post treatment in a diabetic animal (original magnification 100×). The sections were stained with hematoxylin and eosin (H&E).

Additionally, aPDT can be applied in the treatment of residual pockets or the treatment of patients in periodontal maintenance.[32,33] These uses are beneficial for patients because aPDT is an independent therapy that is more conservative and gentle to the periodontal tissues and root surface than are conventional treatments; thus, this treatment can decrease the dentin hypersensitivity caused by the removal of cementum through various scraping procedures on the root surfaces. In addition to chronic periodontitis, previous studies have shown that aPDT is a promising treatment for aggressive periodontitis (Fig. 21.3a–d).[34,35]

Application technique

Two important conditions should be considered with respect to aPDT: the irradiation parameters used in the studies and the photosensitizing drugs. Most published clinical studies have used a low power laser with a wavelength varying from 635 to 680 nm, and the most widely used photosensitizing drug has

been of methylene blue (10 mg/mL or 100 μg/mL). Toluidine blue has also been used at a concentration of 100 μg/mL. However, the output power of the lasers has varied, including 30, 75, 100, and 140 mW, and the energy density, when provided, has varied from 4.5 to 65 J/cm². The total irradiation of the tissues has typically been for 60 seconds per tooth or 10 seconds per site, although certain studies have employed longer irradiation times.

The clinical application of aPDT as an adjuvant for non-surgical periodontal disease therapy begins with the irrigation of the periodontal pockets with the photosensitizing drug; after 1 minute, the irradiation of these pockets is performed with a low power laser. This laser may emit radiation by means of either a small-diameter fiber that is capable of penetrating the periodontal sulcus or pocket, or a fiber with a larger diameter

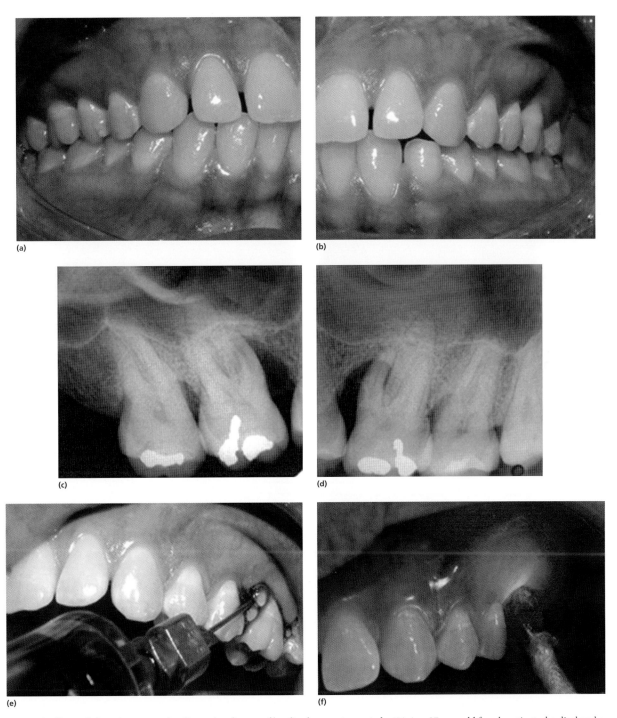

Figure 21.3 (a–d) Initial clinical images and radiographs of a case of localized aggressive periodontitis in a 27-year-old female patient who displayed a periodontal pocket with angled bone loss in the region of teeth 16 and 26. (e) Irrigation of the periodontal pocket with methylene blue solution; (f) irradiation with a low power laser for 133 seconds (660 nm, 57.14 J/cm^2).

that is positioned parallel to the periodontal pocket but which does not penetrate the interior of the pocket (Fig. 21.3e,f).

This therapy could also be used during the decontamination procedure of the periodontal tissues in surgical therapy. In this case, after forming the periodontal flap and debriding the area with manual instruments, the surgical area is irrigated with a photosensitizing agent and irradiated with a low power laser with a wavelength that is appropriate for the photosensitizer (Fig. 21.4). This technique may also be used as an adjunctive therapy in the decontamination of difficult-to-access areas, such as furcation lesion, and in regenerative periodontal surgery (Figs 21.5 and 21.6).

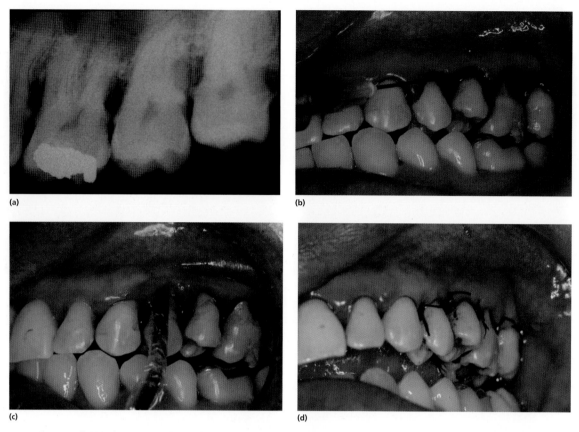

Figure 21.4 Application of aPDT during surgical periodontal therapy with the performance of a periodontal flap in areas of chronic periodontal disease. (a) Initial radiograph demonstrating bone loss in the molar region; (b) irrigation with methylene blue solution after scaling and root planing in an open field; (c) irradiation with a low power laser for 133 seconds (660 nm, 57.14 J/cm^2); (d) immediately post operation (courtesy of JM Almeida).

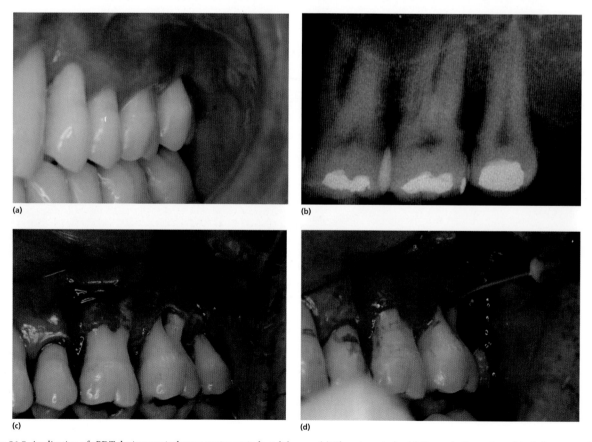

Figure 21.5 Application of aPDT during surgical regenerative periodontal therapy. (a) Chronic periodontal disease in the region of the left upper molars; (b) initial periapical radiograph demonstrating angled bone loss; (c) the periodontal flap and a view of an affected furcation area; (d) irrigation with methylene blue solution after scaling and root planing (courtesy of Almeida JM).

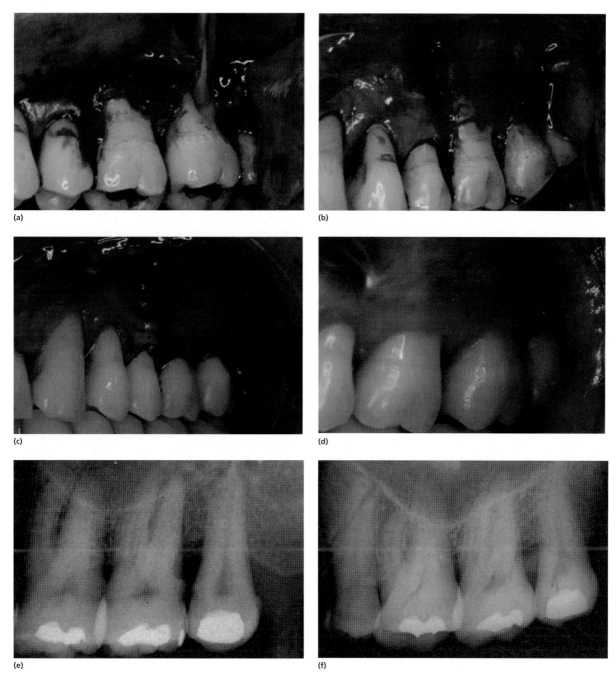

Figure 21.6 Application of aPDT during surgical regenerative periodontal therapy. (a) Irradiation of the photosensitized area with a low power laser for 133 seconds (660 nm, 57.14 J/cm²); (b) a collagen membrane in place; (c) the repositioned and sutured flap; (d) clinical image 180 days post surgery; (e) initial radiograph compared with; (f) the radiograph 180 days post surgery (courtesy of Almeida JM).

Final considerations

Meta-analyses of publications evaluating the clinical use of aPDT in humans have produced controversial results. One of these meta-analyses demonstrated that aPDT, as an adjunctive treatment to or independently of SRP, is not superior to conventional periodontal treatment.[36] Conversely, a more recent meta-analysis concluded that the use of aPDT as an adjunctive therapy

along with conventional periodontal treatment promotes beneficial effects over the short term. However, the microbiological effects are controversial, and the authors stress that there is no evidence of the effectiveness of the use of aPDT as an alternative therapy to SRP.[37] Therefore, we believe that new clinical research with microbial evaluations and longitudinal studies should be performed to standardize the parameters for radiation and the concentration of the photosensitizing agents, so that the effectiveness of aPDT as an adjunctive therapy or alternative to conventional periodontal treatment can be established. In addition, future challenges must be overcome, mainly those in establishing an appropriate protocol for periodontal treatment as well as to the development of new photosensitizers, natural or otherwise and with or without nanoparticles, that are capable of remaining in the interior of the periodontal pocket in satisfactory or stable therapeutic concentrations.

References

1 Zijnge V, Ammann T, Thurnheer T, et al. Subgingival biofilm structure. Front Oral Biol 2012; 15: 1–16.

2 Soukos NS, Goodson JM. Photodynamic therapy in the control of oral biofilms. Periodontology 2000 2011; 55: 143–166.

3 Meisel P, Kocker T. Photodynamic therapy for periodontal disease: state of the art. J Photoch Photobiol B 2005; 79: 159–170.

4 Consensus report. Periodontal diseases: Pathogenesis and microbial factors. Ann Periodontol 1996; 1: 926–932.

5 Socransky SS, Haffajee AD, Cugini MA, et al. Microbial complexes in subgingival plaque. J Clin Periodontol 1998; 25: 134–144.

6 Atieh MA Photodynamic therapy as an adjunctive treatment for chronic periodontitis: a meta-analysis. Lasers Med Sci 2010; 25: 605–613.

7 Adriaens PA, Adriaens LM. Effects of nonsurgical periodontal therapy on hard and soft tissues. Periodontology 2000 2004; 36: 121–145.

8 Thiha K, Takeuchi Y, Umeda M, et al. Identification of periodontopathic bacteria in gingival tissue of Japanese periodontitis patients. Oral Microbiol Immunol 2007; 22: 201–207.

9 Takasaki AA, Aoki A, Mizutani K, et al. Application of antimicrobial photodynamic therapy in periodontal and peri-implant diseases. Periodontology 2000 2009; 51: 109–140.

10 Kömerik N, Nakanishi H, MacRobert AJ, et al. In vivo killing of Porphyromonas gingivalis by Toluidine blue-mediated photosensitization in an animal model. Antimicrob Agents Chemother 2003; 47: 932–940.

11 Sigusch BW, Pfitzner A, Albrecht V, et al. Efficacy of photodynamic therapy on inflammatory signs and two selected periodontopathogenic species in a beagle dog model. J Periodontol 2005; 76: 1100–1105.

12 Qin YL, Luan XL, Bi LJ, et al. Comparison of toluidine blue-mediated photodynamic therapy and conventional scaling treatment for periodontitis in rats. J Periodont Res 2008; 43: 162–167.

13 Prates RA, Yamada Jr AM, Suzuki LC, et al. Histomorphometric and microbiological assessment of photodynamic therapy as an adjunctive treatment for periodontitis: a short-term evaluation of inflammatory periodontal conditions and bacterial reduction in a rat model. Photomed Laser Surg 2011; 29: 835–844.

14 Almeida JM, Theodoro LH, Bosco AF, et al. Influence of photodynamic therapy on the development of ligature-induced periodontitis in rats. J Periodontol 2007; 78: 566–575.

15 Almeida JM, Theodoro LH, Bosco AF, et al. In vivo effect of photodynamic therapy on periodontal bone loss in dental furcations. J Periodontol 2008; 79: 1081–1088.

16 Almeida JM, Theodoro LH, Bosco AF, et al. Treatment of experimental periodontal disease by photodynamic therapy in rats with diabetes. J Periodontol 2008; 79: 2156–2165.

17 Gualberto EC Jr. Histologic, histometric and immunohistochemistry evaluation of laser and photodynamic therapy effects on treatment of induced periodontal disease in rats ovariectomy treated or not with hormone replacement. [Dissertation]. Araçatuba: UNESP – São Paulo State University, 2010.

18 Carvalho AL, Napimoga MH, Campos JC Jr, et al. Photodynamic therapy reduces bone resorption and decreases inflammatory response in an experimental rat periodontal disease model. Photomed Laser Surg 2011; 29: 735–740.

19 Fernandes LA, Almeida JM, Theodoro LH, et al. Treatment of experimental periodontal disease by photodynamic therapy in immunosuppressed rats. J Clin Periodontol 2009; 36: 219–228.

20 Garcia VG, Fernandes LA, Macarini VC, et al. Treatment of experimental periodontal disease with antimicrobial photodynamic therapy in nicotine-modified rats. J Clin Periodontol 2011; 38: 1106–1114.

21 Andersen R, Loebel N, Hammond D, et al. Treatment of periodontal disease by photodisinfection compared to scaling and root planing. J Clin Dent 2007; 18: 34–38.

22 Braun A, Dehn C, Krause F, et al. Short-term clinical effects of adjunctive antimicrobial photodynamic therapy in periodontal treatment: a randomized clinical trial. J Clin Periodontol 2008; 35: 877–884.

23 Christodoulides N, Nikolidakis D, Chondros P, et al. Photodynamic therapy as an adjunct to non-surgical periodontal treatment: a randomized, controlled clinical trial. J Periodontol 2008; 79: 1638–1644.

24 Chondros P, Nikolidakis D, Christodoulides N, et al. Photodynamic therapy as adjunct to non-surgical periodontal treatment in patients on periodontal maintenance: a randomized controlled clinical trial. Lasers Med Sci 2009; 24: 681–688.

25 Polansky R, Haas M, Heschl A, et al. Clinical effectiveness of photodynamic therapy in the treatment of periodontitis. J Clin Periodontol 2009; 36: 575–580.

26 Pinheiro SL, Donegá JM, Seabra LMS, et al. Capacity of photodynamic therapy for microbial reduction in periodontal pockets. Lasers Med Sci 2010; 25: 87–91.

27 Ge L, Shu R, Li Y, et al. Adjunctive effect of photodynamic therapy to scaling and root planing in the treatment of chronic periodontitis. Photomed Laser Surg 2011; 29: 33–37.

28 Theodoro LH, Silva SP, Pires JR, et al. Clinical and microbiological effects of photodynamic therapy associated with nonsurgical periodontal treatment. A 6-month follow-up. Lasers Med Sci 2012; 27: 687–693.

29 Sigusch BW, Engelbrecht M, Völpel A, et al. Full-mouth antimicrobial photodynamic therapy in Fusobacterium nucleatum-infected periodontitis patients. J Periodontol 2010; 81: 975–981.

30 Al-Zahrani MS, Bamshmous SO, Alhassani AA, et al. Short-term effects of photodynamic therapy on periodontal status and glycemic control of patients with diabetes. J Periodontol 2009; 80: 1568–1573.

31 Noro Filho GA, Casarin RCV, Casati MZ, et al. PDT in non-surgical treatment of periodontitis in HIV patients: A split-mouth, randomized clinical trial. Lasers Surg Med 2012; 44: 296–302.

32 Lulic M, Leiggener Görög I, Salvi GE, et al. One-year outcomes of repeated adjunctive photodynamic therapy during periodontal maintenance: a proof-of-principle randomized-controlled clinical trial. J Clin Periodontol 2009; 36: 661–666.

33 Cappuyns I, Cionca N, Wick P, et al. Treatment of residual pockets with photodynamic therapy, diode laser, or deep scaling.

A randomized, split-mouth controlled clinical trial. Lasers Med Sci 2012; 27: 979–986.

34 de Oliveira RR, Schwartz-Filho HO, Novaes AB Jr, et al. Antimicrobial photodynamic therapy in the non-surgical treatment of aggressive periodontitis: a preliminary randomized controlled clinical study. J Periodontol 2007; 78: 965–973.

35 Novaes AB. Jr, Schwartz-Filho HO, de Oliveira RR, et al. Antimicrobial photodynamic therapy in the non-surgical treatment of aggressive periodontitis: microbiological profile. Lasers Med Sci 2012; 27: 389–395.

36 Azarpazhooh A, Shah PS, Tenenbaum HC, et al. The effect of photodynamic therapy for periodontitis: a systematic review and meta-analysis. J Periodontol 2010; 81: 4–14.

37 Sgolastra F, Petrucci A, Gatto R, et al. Photodynamic therapy in the treatment of chronic periodontitis: a systematic review and meta-analysis. Lasers Med Sci 2013; 28: 669–682.

CHAPTER 22

Esthetic treatment of gingival melanin hyperpigmentation with the Er:YAG laser

Daniel Simões A. Rosa[1] and Akira Aoki[2]

[1] Private Dental Practice, São Paulo, SP, Brazil

[2] Department of Periodontology, Graduate School of Medical and Dental Sciences, Tokyo Medical and Dental School, Tokyo, Japan

Introduction

Oral pigmentation is a discoloration of the oral mucosa or gingiva due to a variety of lesions and conditions, and it has been associated with endogenous and exogenous etiological factors.[1] Most pigmentation is caused by primary pigments, including melanin, melanoid, oxyhemoglobin, reduced hemoglobin, and carotene.[2] Other pigments are bilirubin and iron. Melanin, a non-hemoglobin derived brown pigment, is the most common of the endogenous pigments and is produced by melanocytes present in the basal and suprabasal cell layers of the epithelium.[2,3]

The number of melanocytes in the mucosa corresponds to that in the skin; however, in the mucosa their activity is reduced. Various stimuli can result in an increased production of melanin at the level of the mucosa, including trauma, hormones, radiation, and medications. Dummet and Barens identified many systemic and local factors as causes of changes in oral pigmentation.[4,5] High levels of oral melanin pigmentation are normally observed in individuals of African, East Asian or Hispanic ethnicity.

Melanin pigmentation

Physiological pigmentation probably is determined genetically; however, as Dummet suggested, the degree of pigmentation is partially related to mechanical, chemical, and physical stimulation. In darker skinned people, oral pigmentation increases, but there is no difference in the number of melanocytes between fair-skinned and dark-skinned individuals.[6] The variation is related to differences in the activity of melanocytes. Polycyclic amines like nicotine and benzopyrenes found in cigarette smoke are known to penetrate the oral mucosa and bind to melanin, stimulating the production of melanin by melanocytes. The term "smoker's melanin" has been used to describe this benign melanin pigmentation.[7]

The gingiva is the most frequently pigmented tissue of the oral cavity. While melanin pigmentation does not represent a medical problem, patients usually complain of "black gums" and frequently request cosmetic therapy, particularly if the pigmentation is visible during speech and smiling.[8]

Procedures for melanin depigmentation

Cosmetic therapy of gingival melanin pigmentation is common and various methods have been used with different degrees of success, including gingivectomy,[9] gingivectomy with free gingival autografting,[10] electrosurgery,[11] cryosurgery,[12] chemical agents such as 90% phenol and 95% alcohol,[13] and abrasion with diamond bur.[14] More recently, lasers have been used to ablate cells containing and producing the melanin pigment.[15]

The effectiveness of melanin hyperpigmentation removal with different types of lasers has been evaluated in several studies,[8,14,16–19] and the use of pulsed erbium-doped:yttrium–aluminum–garnet (Er:YAG) lasers has gained increasing importance and acceptance in recent years.

Since its approval for soft tissue treatment by the US Food and Drug Administration (FDA) in 1999, the Er:YAG laser has been studied and effectively applied for periodontal soft tissue management without causing major thermal side effects.[20] The Er:YAG laser emits light of a wavelength of 2940 nm and its laser energy is highly absorbed by water.[21] Theoretically, its absorption coefficient for water is 10 times that of the CO_2 laser (10 600 nm) and 15 000–20 000 times that of the Nd:YAG laser (1064 nm).[21] Due to its high absorption by water, less tissue degeneration with very thin surface interaction occurs after Er:YAG laser irradiation. The temperature rise is minimal in the presence of water irrigation, allowing hard and soft tissue removal without any carbonization.[22–25] Moreover, because of its sterilization and soft tissue ablation characteristics, the Er:YAG laser can be used as a smooth knife. Another reported advantage of Er:YAG laser irradiation is its high bactericidal effect.[26]

Lasers in Dentistry: Guide for Clinical Practice, First Edition. Edited by Patrícia M. de Freitas and Alyne Simões.
© 2015 John Wiley & Sons, Inc. Published 2015 by John Wiley & Sons, Inc.

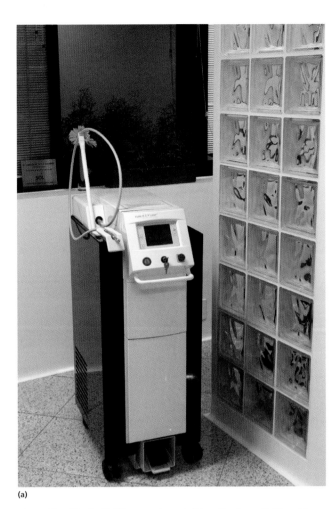

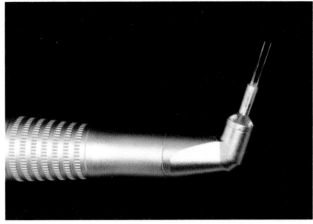

(b)

(a)

Figure 22.1 The Er:YAG laser equipment (Kavo Key Laser II; Kavo, Germany) with handpiece 2056 and chisel tip with a rectangular end of 1.65 × 0.5 mm and transmission factor of 64%.

The extensive advantages and properties of this laser, and also its capacity for excellent soft tissue ablation, make it suitable for melanin pigmentation removal.[16-19,27] It has been described as a promising device for minor periodontal soft tissue management, especially for delicate esthetic treatments, resulting in significant improvement of gingival discoloration with satisfactory wound healing and lower recurrence.

It is extremely important to obtain a complete medical history from patients and to perform a careful clinical examination before this cosmetic therapy. Moreover, patients with systemic diseases associated with healing disturbances, diabetes, autoimmune disease, pregnancy, and a history of postsurgical keloids should be particularly carefully examined.

Er:YAG laser treatment

The Er:YAG laser equipment employed is the Kavo Key Laser II (Kavo, Germany) with handpiece 2056 and contact chisel tip with a rectangular end of 1.65 × 0.5 mm; this tip has a transmission factor of 64% (Fig. 22.1). For this cosmetic therapy, patients are treated with topical and local anesthesia (2% lidocaine). Irradiation is performed with an energy output of 64 mJ per pulse (8.5 J/cm² per pulse, panel settings 100 mJ per pulse) and repetition rate of 10 Hz under water spray in an oblique contact mode. The laser beam is applied using the "brush technique" as described by Tal et al.[16] with continuous and slow movements (Fig. 22.2). As far as possible, the papillary edges and the free gingival margins are left untouched, without any irradiation, preventing any type of gingival recession. The entire surface of each upper and lower gingiva requiring treatment is generally irradiated in a single session. Patients are instructed to take paracetamol, 500 mg, after the surgery and to continue with the medication for the next 3 days in case of pain.

Wound healing and recurrence

The benefit of Er:YAG laser irradiation in soft tissue surgery is the precise cutting and easy ablation of gingival tissue, using delicate contact tips. Unlike the earlier hard lasers, the Er:YAG laser does not produce strong carbonization and marked coagulation

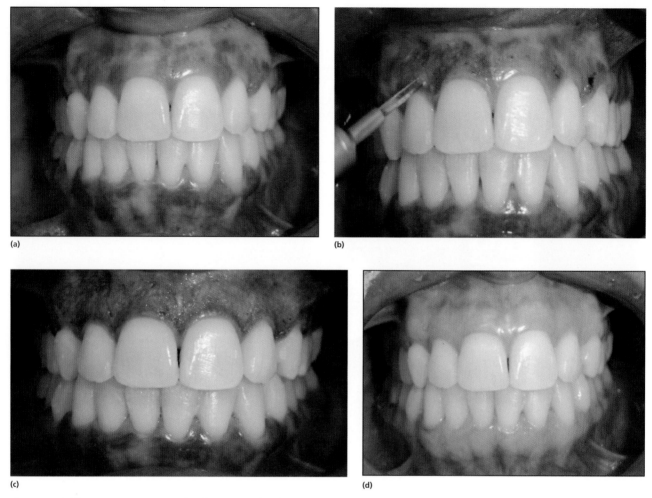

Figure 22.2 (a) Preoperative appearance of moderate gingival melanin pigmentation. (b) Irradiation of the maxillary gingiva. Note the chisel tip in oblique contact mode. The laser beam is applied using the "brush technique" as described by Tal et al.[16] (c) Immediately after irradiation of the maxillary gingiva. Note the precise and effective ablation of gingival pigmentation without any marked coagulation or carbonization on the treated surface. The papillary edges and free gingival margins were not irradiated. (d) Three months after treatment. Note the significant decrease in gingival melanin pigmentation of the maxillary and mandibular gingiva without any recurrence, or gingival recession or deformity.

on the soft tissues. The amount of soft tissue ablation can be controlled easily and tissue reshaping or recontouring can be performed.[28] Successful treatment of melanin gingival pigmentation for esthetic purposes has been reported with the Er:YAG laser.[16–19,27] It has been observed that following laser irradiation of pigmented areas, gingival tissue healing is satisfactory and there is complete regeneration of a healthy, pink, and firm tissue. These observations are common to clinical researchers who use different lasers and various techniques.[8,14,29–31]

Precise treatment with minimal thermal side effects was possible with Er:YAG laser contact irradiation because the laser wavelength is highly absorbed by water. The operation field could be visualized easily with water spray. The use of water minimized heat generation, by cooling the irradiated area and absorbing excessive laser energy. Furthermore, long intervals between pulses and an air stream also helped to keep the target cooler by avoiding heat transfer to the surrounding tissues. As a result, no side effects were observed (Fig. 22.3). The relatively speedy postoperative recovery after Er:YAG laser ablation of the gingiva probably was due to the narrow zone of thermal disruption on the laser-treated surface (Fig. 22.3).

Physiological recurrence can be seen after melanin pigmentation removal. Dummet and Bolden observed partial recurrence of pigmentation in six of eight patients at 1–4 months after gingivectomy[32] and Perlmutter and Tal described partial recurrence after 7–8 years.[33] No recurrence was found in any of the four patients treated by Atsawasuwan et al.[14] at 11–13 months after gingival depigmentation with the Nd:YAG laser. Nakamura et al. described the use of the CO_2 laser in 10 patients; repigmentation was observed 24 months after treatment.[29] Tal et al. using an Er:YAG laser, observed no recurrence at 6-month follow-up.[16]

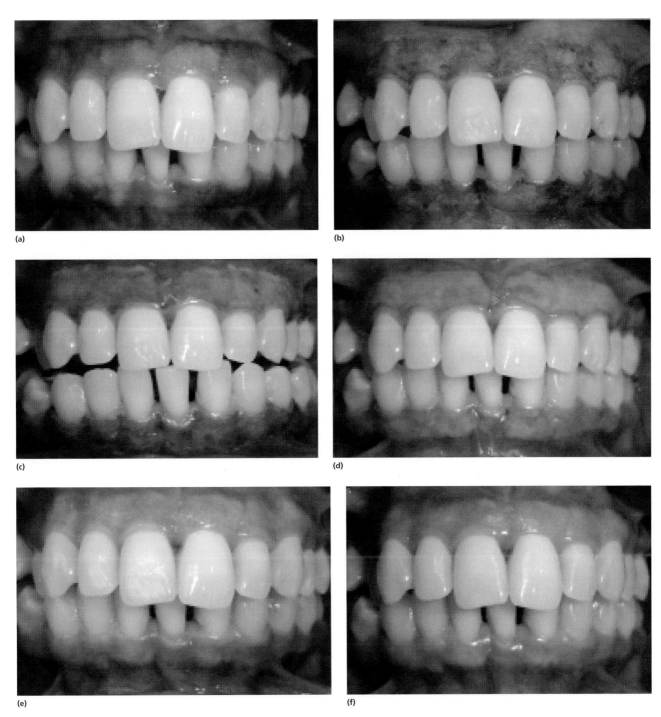

Figure 22.3 (a) Preoperative appearance of moderate gingival melanin pigmentation. (b) Immediately after irradiation of maxillary gingiva without any marked coagulation or carbonization on the treated surface. (c) Twenty-four hours after treatment of the gingiva. (d) Forty-eight hours after treatment of the gingiva. (e) Two weeks after treatment, the gingiva shows almost complete healing. (f) One month after treatment, there is significant reduction of gingival melanin pigmentation of the maxillary and mandibular gingiva without recurrence or gingival recession or deformity.

Surgical microscope monitoring during irradiation would be another advantage with the Er:YAG laser. Therefore, careful irradiation using a microscope might be helpful in preventing recurrence by detecting any remaining pigmentation during irradiation.[17,26]

As regards the irradiation method, compared with the non-contact method reported by Tal et al. in 2003,[16] the contact method with water spray used for melanin pigmentation removal[17] would be more effective and practical for Er:YAG laser treatment, especially in severe case of pigmentation, due to its precise irradiation and lower thermal effect in the clear operating field. It has been reported that the width of the thermally changed layer in dog gingival connective tissue was 5–25 μm after Er:YAG laser melanin removal in contact mode with water spray, using a conventional cylindrical contact tip.[26] Clinical results indicating safety and effective melanin pigmentation ablation have been reported with this contact method (see Fig. 22.2).[17,25,27,33] Removal of discolored gingiva together with metal fragments, namely metal tattoos caused by dental treatment procedures or restorative materials, may be another indication for this method: excellent results have been reported using an Er:YAG laser irradiation at 24–48 mJ per pulse (panel setting 40–83 mJ per pulse, 8.5–17.0 J/cm² per pulse), 10–30 Hz under water spray in contact mode, with a 600 μm diameter fiber.[28,34]

During surgery, bleeding can be controlled and since the Er:YAG laser lacks a coagulation effect, it does not delay the wound healing in any way. In addition, the low hemostatic effect of the Er:YAG laser can be advantageous for esthetic surgery of periodontal soft tissue, since it guarantees blood clot formation on the ablated gingival surface and subsequent recovery of gingival contour. At the same time, the effect of the defocused Er:YAG laser, which scatters or penetrates into the surrounding tissue during contact irradiation, like low level laser therapy (LLLT), might also promote tissue repair, as described by Quadri et al.[35] These authors concluded that additional treatment with low power lasers reduced periodontal gingival inflammation. The absorption of small quantities of energy leads to a cascade of photobiological events, which could have advantageous effects on periodontal healing. *In vitro* studies have primarily concentrated on the stimulation of fibroblast proliferation after the use of low power laser, showing that stimulated fibroblasts are better organized in parallel bundles.[36] Pourzarandian et al. also reported that low level Er:YAG laser irradiation stimulated the proliferation of cultured gingival fibroblasts.[37]

While using an Er:YAG laser, the operator must be aware of all the possible risks involved and caution must be exercised to minimize these risks, even though this laser generally shows very high safety for clinical use. Appropriate laser parameters, such as power energy, energy density, and irradiation time, should be known and studied. Even though successful experimental results have been reported, inappropriate protocols and irradiation parameters can cause major risks to the patient. Furthermore, dental practitioners should be correctly instructed with regard to the safe and effective use of the Er:YAG laser.

Conclusion

Based on its various characteristics, such as ablation, vaporization, homeostasis, and sterilizing effect, the Er:YAG laser has become one of the most promising treatments for periodontal therapy. Due to excellent tissue ablation with minimal thermal effect, the Er:YAG laser is a very useful and safe device for periodontal soft tissue management, especially for delicate esthetic treatments like gingival depigmentation of melanin or metal tattoo. The Er:YAG laser with water spray can effectively and safely remove melanin pigmentation, with fast wound healing and significant improvement of gingival discoloration; no complications or side effects have been observed following gingival pigmentation removal with this laser and patient responses have indicated satisfaction with the results.

References

1 Meyerson MA, Cohen PR, Hymes SR. Lingual hyperpigmentation associated with minocycline therapy. *Oral Surg Oral Med Oral Pathol Oral Radiol Endodont* 1995; 79: 180–184.

2 Cicek Y, Ertas U. The normal and pathological pigmentation of oral mucous membrane: a review. *J Contemp Dent Pract* 2003; 4: 76-86

3 Dummett CO. Oral tissue color changes (I). *Quintessence Int* 1979; 10: 39–45.

4 Dummet CO, Barens G. Oromucosal pigmentation: an updated literary review. *J Periodontol* 1971; 42: 726–36

5 Dummett CO, Barens G. Pigmentation of the oral tissues: a review of the literature. *J Periodontol* 1967; 38: 360–378

6 Dummett. CO. Clinical observation on pigment variations in healthy oral tissues in the Negro. *J Dent Res* 1945; 24: 7–13.

7 Brown FH, Housten GD. Smoker's melanosis. A case report. *J Periodontol* 1991; 62: 524–527.

8 Esen E, Haytac MC, Oz A, Erdogan O, Karsli E. Gingival melanin pigmentation and its treatment with the CO₂ laser. *Oral Surg Oral Med Oral Pathol Oral Radiol Endondont* 2004; 98: 522–527.

9 Bergamaschi O, Kon S, Doine AI. Melanin repigmentation after gingivectomy: a 5-year clinical and transmission electron microscopic study in humans. *Int J Periodont Restorat Dent* 1993; 13: 85–92.

10 Tamizi M, Taheri M. Treatment of severe physiologic gingival pigmentation with free gingival autograft. *Quintessence Int* 1996; 27: 555–558.

11 Gnanasekhar JD, al-Duwairi YS. Electrosurgery in dentistry. *Quintessence Int* 1998; 29: 649–654.

12 Yeh CJ. Cryosurgical treatment of melanin-pigmented gingiva. *Oral Surg Oral Med Oral Path* 1998; 86: 660–663.

13 Hasegawa A, Okagi H. Removing melagenous pigmentation using 90 percent phenol with 95 percent alcohol. *Dent Outlook* 1973; 42: 673–676.

14 Atsawasuwan P, Greethong K, Nimmanon V. Treatment of gingival hyperpigmentation for esthetic purposes by Nd:YAG laser: report of 4 cases. *J Periodontol* 2000; 71: 315–321.

15 Sharon E, Azaz B, Ulmansky M. Vaporization of melanin in oral tissues and skin a carbon dioxide laser: a canine study. *J Oral Maxillofac Surg* 2000; 58: 1387–1393.

16 Tal, H, Oegiesser D, Tal M. Gingival depigmentation by Erbium:YAG laser: clinical observations and patient response. *J Periodontol* 2003; 74: 1660–1667.

17 Kawashima Y, Aoki A, Ishii S, Watanabe H, Ishikawa I. Er:YAG laser treatment of gingival melanin pigmentation. *Int Congress Series* 2003; 1248: 245–248.

18 Ishii S, Aoki A, Kawashima Y, Watanabe H, Ishikawa I. Application of an Er:YAG laser to remove gingival melanin hyperpigmentation – Treatment procedure and clinical evaluation. *J Jpn Soc Laser Dent* 2002; 13: 89–96.

19 Azzeh MM. Treatment of gingival of gingival hyperpigmentation By erbium-doped:yttrium, aluminum, and garnet laser for esthetic purposes. *J Periodontol* 2007; 78: 177–184.

20 Watanabe H, Ishikawa I, Suzuki M, Hasegawa K. Clinical assessments of the Erbium:YAG laser for soft tissue surgery and scaling. *J Clin Laser Med Surg* 1996; 14: 67–75.

21 Hale GM, Querry MR. Optical constants of water in the 200-nm to 200um wavelength region. *Appl Opt* 1973; 12: 555–563.

22 Aoki A, Ando Y, Watanabe H, Ishikawa I. *In vitro* studies on laser scaling of subgengival calculus with as Erbium:YAG laser. *J Periodontol* 1994; 65: 1097–1106.

23 Aoki A, Miura M, Akiyama F. *In vitro* evaluation of Er:YAG laser scaling of subgingival calculus in comparison with ultrasonic scaling. *J Periodontol Res* 2000; 35: 266–277.

24 Aoki A, Sasaki KM, Watanabe H, Ishikawa I. Lasers in nonsurgical periodontal therapy. *Periodontology* 2000 2004; 36: 59–97.

25 Ishikawa I, Sasaki KM, Aoki A, Watanabe H. Effects of Er: YAG laser on periodontal therapy. *J Int Acad Periodontol* 2003; 5: 23–28.

26 Ando Y, Aoki A, Watanabe H, Ishikawa I. Bactericidal effect of Erbium YAG laser on periodontopathic bacteria. *Lasers Surg Med* 1996; 19: 190–200.

27 Rosa DSA, Aranha ACC, Eduardo CP, Aoki, A. Esthetic treatment of gingival melanin hyperpigmentation with Er:YAG laser: Short term clinical observations and patient follow-up. *J Periodontal* 2007; 78: 2018–2025.

28 Aoki A, Ishikawa I. *Application of the Er:YAG laser for esthetic management of periodontal soft tissues.* Proceedings of the 9th international Congress on Laser in Dentistry. Bologna: Monduzzi Editore, 2004: 1–6.

29 Nakamura Y, Hossain M, Hirayama K, Matsumoto K. A clinical study on the removal of gingival melanin pigmentation with the CO_2 laser. *Lasers Surg Med* 1999; 25: 140–147.

30 Yousuf Y, Hossain M, Nakamura Y, Yamada Y, Kinoshita J, Matsumoto K. Removal of gingival melanin pigmentation with the semiconductor diode laser: a case report. *J Clin Laser Med Surg* 2000; 18: 263–266.

31 Trelles MA, Vekruysse W, Segui JM, Udaeta A. Treatment of melanotic spots in the gingiva by Argon laser. *J Oral Maxillofac Surg* 1993; 51: 759–761.

32 Dummet CO, Bolden TE. Postsurgical clinical repigmentation of the gingiva. *Oral Surg Oral Med Oral Pathol* 1963; 16: 353–357.

33 Perlmutter S, Tal H. Repigmentation of the gingiva following surgical injury. *J Periodontol* 1986; 57: 48–50.

34 Ishikawa I, Aoki A, Takasaki AA. Potential applications of Erbium: YAG laser in periodontics. *J Periodontol Res* 2004; 39: 275–285.

35 Quadri T, Miranda L, Túner J, Gustafsson A. The short-term effects of low-level laser as adjunct therapy in the treatment of periodontal inflammation. *Journal of Clinical Peridontol* 2005; 32: 714–719.

36 Almeida-Lopes L, Rigau J, Zángaro RA, Guidugli-Neto J, Jaeger MM. Comparison of the low level laser therapy effects on cultured human gingival fibroblast proliferation using different irradiance and same fluency. *Lasers Surg Med* 2001; 29: 179–184.

37 Pourzarandian A, Watanabe H, Ruwanpura SM, Aoki A, Ishikawa I. Effect of low-level Er:YAG laser irradiation on cultured human gingival fibroblasts. *J Periodontol* 2005; 76: 187–193.

SECTION 5

Oral surgery

CHAPTER 23

Lasers in soft tissues surgeries

Luciane Hiramatsu Azevedo,[1] Marines Sammamed Freire Trevisan,[2,3] and Ana Maria Aparecida de Souza[2,3]

[1]Dentistry Clinic, University of São Paulo (USP), São Paulo, SP, Brazil
[2]Private Dental Practice, São Paulo, SP, Brazil
[3]Special Laboratory of Lasers in Dentistry (LELO), School of Dentistry, University of São Paulo (USP), São Paulo, SP, Brazil

Introduction

One of the first lasers to be used for soft tissue surgery in medicine was the CO_2 laser. Since 1970, this laser has also been used for oral tissue surgery and was approved for this purpose by the US Food and Drug Administration (FDA) in 1976.[1]

The CO_2 laser emits light of wavelength 10 600 nm and may operate in the pulsed or continuous mode. It is highly absorbed by the water in oral tissues, which results in precise and localized tissue removal. It is used in various soft tissue treatments: crown augmentation, treatment of ulcers (aphthas), frenectomy and gingivectomy, and re-epithelialization of gingival tissue during periodontal treatment. The characteristics of the CO_2 laser allow good hemostasis, rapid and efficient tissue removal, and good healing.[2]

The Nd:YAG laser emits light in the near-infrared range (1064 nm) and operates in the pulsed mode. It acts on tissue by coagulation and vaporization and has various applications in dentistry: endodontics, periodontics, preventive dentistry, and surgery. The Nd:YAG laser makes it possible to use a minimally invasive technique in dentistry and in procedures involving soft tissues. It is capable of penetrating deeply into the target tissue.[3]

As is the case with the Nd:YAG laser, the Argon laser has great coagulation and vaporization capacity for tissues rich in hemoglobin and melanin, and emits in the range between 457 and 502 nm in pulsed or continuous mode. However, it has superficial cutting capacity, reducing its use in oral surgery. In dentistry, its use is related to dental bleaching and resin polymerization.[4]

Two other lasers that act very well on hard tissues are the Er:YAG (2940 nm) and Er,Cr:YSGG (2780 nm) lasers. They have great affinity for water. These two wavelengths are extensively used in pediatric dentistry because of their versatility and because they can be used on both hard and soft tissues.[5] The two lasers work in the pulsed mode. The Er:YAG laser may be used in tooth preparation, endodontics, and some soft tissue surgeries.[6,7] Their use is also recommended for osteotomy in implants.[8] The Er,Cr:YSGG laser has various applications in hard tissues, such as enamel conditioning, caries removal, cavity preparations, and in endodontics. The Er,Cr:YSGG laser is considered safe for dental pulp and for caries removal or cavity preparation in dentistry, and in some cases, it is even eliminates the need for local anesthetic. It can also be used to fuse enamel, which increases enamel resistance to acid.[4]

The diode laser (high power) is a semiconductor that emits light between 805 and 980 nm. It may be used in continuous or pulsed mode, and in contact or not in contact with tissue.[9] The wavelength of the diode laser (high power) is highly absorbed by pigmented tissues (melanin) and little absorbed by hydroxyapatite and bone.[10,11] Various studies with the diode laser (high power) have demonstrated good efficiency in soft tissue surgeries, such as frenectomies, hyperplasias, and gingivectomies.[12]

Frenectomy

In dentistry, the labial frenum becomes a problem if it is inserted very close to the gingival margin. The tension on the frenum in this region may cause traction on the gingival margin and retract it, leading to exposure of the tooth root.[13] This condition may increase biofilm accumulation and make it difficult to clean in the cervical region.[14] In this case, surgical removal must be performed if there is gingival retraction, in order to prevent periodontal problems, and when the frenum causes diastemas, making it difficult to perform orthodontic, phonoaudiological, prosthetic, and esthetic treatments.[15]

It is important to evaluate the radiographic exam, in order to eliminate the possibility of the presence of supernumerary teeth, or absence of union of the maxillary processes, which are contraindications to frenectomy[16]

Frenums may be classified according to their insertion:
- Mucosal insertion: situated on the mucogingival line (causes no problems);
- Gingival insertion: situated on the inserted gingiva;
- Papillary insertion: when there is traction, this causes ischemia in the papillary region. During the procedure, the papilla must be preserved;

Lasers in Dentistry: Guide for Clinical Practice, First Edition. Edited by Patrícia M. de Freitas and Alyne Simões.
© 2015 John Wiley & Sons, Inc. Published 2015 by John Wiley & Sons, Inc.

• Interdental insertion: The attachment of the frenum passes right up to the papilla, inserting in attached gingiva. This is the cause of severe ischemia.[17]

Frenectomy or frenulectomy basically consists of the complete removal of the frenum insertion, which is very fibrous and close to the gingival margin, resulting in traction and retraction of this margin, which may lead to progressive localized recession. The insertion of a prominent frenum is associated with a narrow zone of attached gingiva. Another technique used is frenotomy or frenulotomy, with the purpose of partial removal of the frenum in order to move its insertion more into the apical direction, without interfering with the papilla, so that the final result is more esthetic.[14,18]

Labial frenum

One technique used for removal of the labial frenum is the conventional type, the precursor of all the other techniques. This is performed with a scalpel handle and blade, and the labial frenum is removed by means of an incision. This is the most commonly used technique, followed by the technique using an electric scalpel or electric cautery, which cuts tissue by means of electrically heating the blade-shaped tip of the appliance. The use of high power laser in soft tissue surgeries has demonstrated favorable results and is well accepted because of its efficiency, incisive power, ablation, and good clinical and biological responses, and it has been used for labial frenum removal[9,19] (see Clinical case 23.1)

Clinical Case 23.1

Treatment with a diode laser was proposed for a 29-year-old female patient in good general health but with an abnormal inferior labial frenum that was causing retraction of the gingival margin (Fig. 23.1a). The incision was carried out at a wavelength of 808 nm (continuous mode) and 2-W output power. Irradiation was delivered using a flexible quartz fiber 300 μm in diameter. The frenum mucosa was removed, as well as the deeper tissue comprising connective fiber and muscle fiber. Local anesthetic was given prior to surgery. No sutures were required (Fig. 23.1b) and healing with re-epithelization was complete 3 weeks after treatment (Fig. 23.1c).

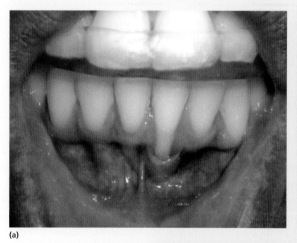

(a)

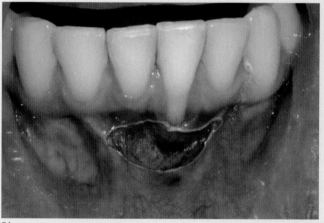

(b)

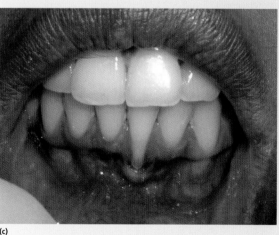

(c)

Figure 23.1 (a) Abnormal inferior labial frenum that is causing retraction of the gingival margin. (b) Clinical image immediately after the irradiation and (c) at 3 weeks follow-up.

Clinical Case 23.2

A 26-year-old white male presented with a very high lingual frenum that limited the movement of his tongue (Fig. 23.2a). Treatment options included traditional surgery with a scalpel and suturing or the use of a dental laser. After informed consent, lingual frenectomy with an Nd:YAG laser was performed. Topical and local anesthesia was administered and a horizontal releasing incision was made with the laser in pulsed wave, contact mode (100 mJ pulse energy, 2 W output power, 20 Hz), using a tip of 320-μm flexible fiber (Fig. 23.2b).

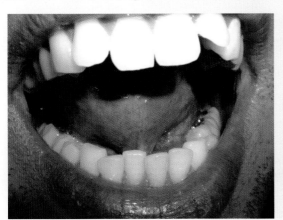
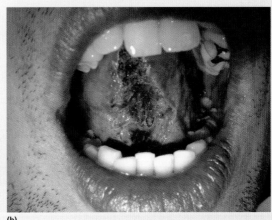

(a) (b)

Figure 23.2 (a) Abnormal inferior labial frenum that is causing retraction of the gingival frenum. (b) Clinical image immediately after irradiation.

Clinical Case 23.3

An 11-year-old female presented with a 6-month history of retention of tooth 23. months. From the clinical and radiographic examinations, the decision was made to perform an ulectomy to allow the eruption of the tooth (Fig. 23.3a). A high power 1.2-W diode laser (808 nm) was used in contact mode under local anesthesia. Irradiation was delivered using a flexible quartz fiber of 300 μm in diameter in continuous wave mode (Fig. 23.3b).

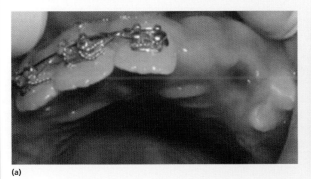
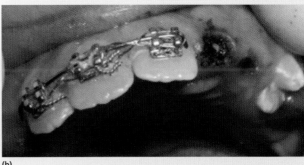

(a) (b)

Figure 23.3 (a) Patient who presented with a 6-month history of retention of tooth 23. (b) Clinical picture immediately after irradiation.

Lingual frenum

According to Basile,[20] the short lingual frenum changes the functional mechanics of other oral structures. The frenum of the tongue is made up of conjunctive tissue rich in collagen and elastic fibers, fatty cells, some muscle fibers, and blood vessels. These tissues are covered by stratified pavimentous epithelial tissue.

Ankyloglossia is a developmental anomaly characterized by a short, thick lingual frenum, which limits movements of the tongue.

In patients with a normal frenum, it has been observed that orofacial functions and the mobility of the tongue are better if the frenum insertion is short or anteriorized. It has also been observed that when it is short, the tip of the tongue is elevated and in general, this elevation raises the floor of the mouth or the mandible. In addition, short frenums are thicker than other types.

In a phonoaudiological evaluation, a partially or completely united lingual frenum will determine the treatment: surgical frenuloplasty for the partial or complete removal of the frenum from the tongue (see Clinical case 23.2).

Ulectomy/ulotomy

The periods of tooth eruption, in general, differ among populations and geographical areas, as they may be influenced by several factors, such as environmental conditions, socioeconomic level, race, gender, and local disturbances, such as gingival fibrosis and eruption cysts. Gingival fibrosis is caused by friction of foods during mastication, and occurs more frequently on the maxillary central incisor due to premature exfoliation or early loss of primary teeth. The dentist may perform an ulectomy, which consists of excision of the tissues that line the incisal or occlusal face of the tooth crown of an unerupted primary or permanent tooth. The aim of this procedure is to facilitate the eruption of the tooth. For a precise indication of the surgical technique, meticulous clinical and radiographic examination of the region is required. Once ulectomy has been indicated, it must be performed immediately, because postponement of the surgery may lead to closure of the space, due to inclination of the neighboring teeth, which will prevent later orthodontic treatment to recover the lost space (see Clinical case 23.3).

References

1 Haytac MC, Ozcelik O. Evaluation of patient perceptions after frenectomy operations: a comparison of carbon dioxide laser and scalpel techniques. *J Periodontol* 2006; 77: 1815–1819.

2 Fulton JE, Shitabata PK. CO_2 laser physics and tissue interactions in skin. *Lasers Surg Med* 1999; 24: 113–121.

3 Vesnaver A, Dovsak DA. Treatment of large vascular lesions in the orofacial region with the Nd:YAG laser. *J Craniomaxillofac Surg* 2009; 37: 191–195.

4 Dederich DN, Bushick RD. Lasers in dentistry: separating science from hype. *J Am Dent Assoc* 2004; 135: 204–212.

5 Romeo U, Libotte F, Palaia G, et al. Histological *in vitro* evaluation of the effects of Er:YAG laser on oral soft tissues. *Lasers Med Sci* 2012; 27: 749–753.

6 Sperandio FF, Meneguzzo DT, Ferreira LS, da Ana PA, Azevedo LH, de Sousa SC. Different air-water spray regulations affect the healing of Er,Cr:YSGG laser incisions. *Lasers Med Sci* 2011; 26: 257–265.

7 Borsatto MC, Torres CP, Chinelatti MA, Pécora JD, Corona SA, Palma-Dibb RG. Effect of Er:YAG laser parameters on ablation capacity and morphology of primary enamel. *Photomed Laser Surg* 2009; 27: 253–260.

8 Roper MJ, White JM, Goodis HE, Gekelman D. Two-dimensional changes and surface characteristics from an erbium laser used for root canal preparation. *Lasers Surg Med* 2010; 42: 379–383.

9 Stübinger S, Biermeier K, Bächi B, Ferguson SJ, Sader R, von Rechenberg B. Comparison of Er:YAG laser, piezoelectric, and drill osteotomy for dental implant site preparation: a biomechanical and histological analysis in sheep. *Lasers Surg Med* 2010; 42: 652–661.

10 Correa-Afonso AM, Ciconne-Nogueira JC, Pécora JD, Palma-Dibb RG.Influence of the irradiation distance and the use of cooling to increase enamel-acid resistance with Er:YAG laser. *J Dent* 2010; 38: 534–540.

11 Romanos G, Nentwig GH. Diode laser (980 nm) in oral and maxillofacial surgical procedures: clinical observations based on clinical applications. *J Clin Laser Med Surg* 1999; 17:193–197.

12 Azevedo LH, Galletta VC, Eduardo Cde P, Migliari DA. Venous lake of the lips treated using photocoagulation with high-intensity diode laser. *Photomed Laser Surg* 2010; 28: 263–265.

13 Angiero F, Benedicenti S, Romanos GE, Crippa R. Treatment of hemangioma of the head and neck with diode laser and forced dehydration with induced photocoagulation. *Photomed Laser Surg* 2008; 26: 113–118.

14 Saleh HM, Saafan AM Excision biopsy of tongue lesions by diode laser. *Photomed Laser Surg* 2007; 25: 45–49.

15 Kara C. Evaluation of patient perceptions of frenectomy: a comparison of Nd:YAG laser and conventional techniques. *Photomed Laser Surg* 2008; 26: 147–152.

16 Pereira PF, Aranega MA, Lacoski KM, Silva LJ, Garcia RI, KIna RJ. Advantages and limitations of the technique of frenulectomy to laser Er: YAG. *Revista Odonto* 2006; 14(27/28): 56–62.

17 Placek M, Skach M, Mrklas L. Problems with the lip frenulum in paradontology. I. Classification and epidemiology of tendons of the lip frenulum. *Ceskoslovenská Stomatol* 1974; 74: 385–389.

18 Olivi G, Signore A, Olivi M, Genovese MD. Lingual frenectomy: functional evaluation and new therapeutical approach. *Eur J Paediatr Dent* 2012; 13(2): 101–106.

19 Gargari M, Autili N, Petrone A, Prete V. Using the diode laser in the lower labial frenum removal. *Oral Implantol (Rome)* 2012; 5(2–3): 54–57.

20 Klockars T. Short lingual frenulum. *Duodecim* 2013; 129(9): 947–949.

CHAPTER 24

Implantodontology

Juliana Marotti[1] and Georgios E. Romanos[2]
[1]Department of Prosthodontics and Biomaterials, Center for Implantology, Medical School of the RWTH Aachen University, Aachen, Germany
[2]Stony Brook University, School of Dental Medicine, Stony Brook, NY, USA

Introduction

The use of low and high power lasers (LPLs and HPLs) has increased in implant dentistry due to a large spectrum of applications in soft and hard tissues. There are several clinical indications for laser therapy and laser surgery in modern implantology, aiming to improve the dental implant procedures and to provide more comfort to patients.[1,2]

While LPLs are used for tissue biomodulation, with no increase of temperature, HPLs work at higher powers in tissues in order to promote incision, vaporization or coagulation. The HPLs most used in implantology are the Er:YAG (2940 nm), Er,Cr:YSGG (2780 nm), Nd:YAG (1064 nm), CO_2 (9600 nm or 10 600 nm), and diode lasers (810 nm or 980 nm). To determine which laser is most suitable for each clinical procedure, the appropriate wavelength must be first chosen according to the target tissue/procedure and then the other laser parameters must be determined, like the energy density (fluence), output power, repetition rate, and how the laser is operated. In continuous mode, the laser provides a constant and stable delivery of energy. Pulsed laser systems, in contrast, provide bursts of energy. Lasers that emit in the ultraviolet region (100–380 nm) ionize tissues, a process known as photochemical desorption. Lasers that emit longer wavelengths, especially those emitting within the infrared region of the spectrum (700–10 000 nm), cause significant tissue heating (photothermal reaction). Most surgical lasers belong to this group and comprise the "thermal" lasers. The light of these lasers is rapidly converted to thermal energy, causing denaturation of proteins, decomposition of tissue, microexplosion of cell water, and charring.[2]

One of the benefits of laser surgery is the optimization of the wound healing process. Only the target tissue is ablated, avoiding damage to the adjacent tissue and reducing complications of wound healing. Laser surgery also reduces the inflammatory response, promoting release of enzymatic inhibitors of the inflammatory process. However, the most interesting property of lasers in implantology is the killing of bacteria, reducing or eliminating the problems of infection, when combined with conventional therapies. Finally, they stimulates the healing of hard and soft tissue.[3]

The main clinical applications of lasers in implantology range from bone biomodulation, management of postoperative inflammatory signs, surgical procedures, and the treatment of peri-implantitis, and are described in this chapter.

Clinical applications

Improvement of osseointegration

Treatment with dental implants is only considered a complete success when these are fully osseointegrated, with absence of pain and inflammation, lack of mobility, absence of continuous periapical radiolucency, and return of esthetics and function.[4–6] Bone formation at the implant–bone interface is a complex physiological process, regulated by systemic hormones and local factors produced by the skeletal cells. It involves sequential events such as cellular attachment, proliferation, differentiation, and deposition of bone matrix.[7]

Many studies have attempted to accelerate the osseointegration process, but most have focused on modifying the texture of the titanium implant surface or the implant design and using other methodologies for immediate loading therapeutic protocols. The use of LPLs has been suggested as a possible technique to accelerate and improve the bone tissue healing process.[8–14] Laser light irradiation has been shown to have biomodulatory effects on wound healing, fibroblast proliferation, and collagen synthesis.[10,15,16] The infrared lasers are known to have a greater depth of tissue penetration in comparison to red or blue light; thus, the osteoblasts cells can better absorb the laser energy because of the low absorption by water at infrared wavelengths.[17–19] For this reason, the infrared wavelengths are indicated for the improvement of the osseointegration process, showing increased osteoblastic proliferation, collagen deposition, and new bone formation.[20–23] Considering that osteoneogenesis is determined by the available local blood flow and by neovascularization, the vascular response to laser therapy can

Lasers in Dentistry: Guide for Clinical Practice, First Edition. Edited by Patrícia M. de Freitas and Alyne Simões.
© 2015 John Wiley & Sons, Inc. Published 2015 by John Wiley & Sons, Inc.

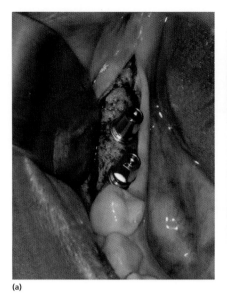 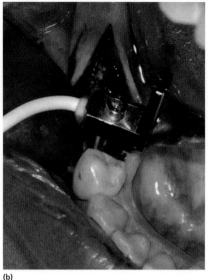 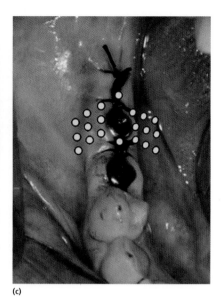

(a)   (b)   (c)

Figure 24.1 (a) Implant placement (b) transducer fitted intraorally (c) point distribution of infrared laser irradiation per implant (courtesy of Dr Joelle Marie García-Morales, Prosthodontic Department of the Dental School of the University of São Paulo, Brazil).

be considered as one of the reasons for the positive clinical results.[24–26] Nonetheless, laser light seems to increase mitochondrial respiration and adenosine triphosphate (ATP) synthesis.[27,28] In addition, better and more effective results can be achieved when the laser therapy is carried out at early stages when cellular proliferation is high.[8,25]

Laser parameters play an important role in achieving the desired results.[8] Nissan et al. compared laser irradiation at $4 \, \text{mW/cm}^2$ and $22.4 \, \text{mW/cm}^2$, and concluded that the lower power density significantly increased radio-calcium accumulation 2 weeks after surgery, whereas the higher power density had no effect.[29] Nevertheless, Silva et al. concluded that a greater volume of newly formed bone was observed with irradiation at a higher energy density of $10.2 \, \text{J/cm}^2$, when compared with only $5.1 \, \text{J/cm}^2$.[30]

Bisphosphonates are currently being widely used in the treatment of osteoporosis in postmenopausal women, as inhibitors of bone resorption, so dental implant surgeries must be performed with even more caution in order to avoid postoperative complications. As laser light, particularly low level laser therapy (LLLT), may play a positive role in bone defect healing, Garcia et al. analyzed the histological effect of LLLT in combination with bisphosphonate on bone healing in surgically created critical size defects in rat calvaria. The defects were submitted to GaAlAs laser irradiation at 660 nm, 24 J, and $0.42 \, \text{W/cm}^2$.[31] Histomorphometric assessments using image analysis software and histological analyses were performed. The authors concluded that LLLT alone or combined with bisphosphonate treatment effectively stimulated bone formation in these critical size defects in the calvaria of rats.[31]

García-Morales et al. performed a randomized clinical study to assess the effect of LLLT on implant stability by means of resonance frequency analysis.[9] Thirty implants were distributed bilaterally in the posterior mandible of eight patients. On the experimental side, the implants were submitted to LLLT (GaAlAs, 830 nm, 86 mW, $92.1 \, \text{J/cm}^2$, 0.25 J per point, 3 seconds per point, at 20 points), and on the control side, the irradiation was simulated (placebo). The first irradiation was performed in the immediate postoperative period, and it was repeated every 48 hours in the first 14 days (Fig. 24.1). The authors concluded that LLLT had no effect on the stability of implants. Two hypotheses were proposed to explain the lack of stability improvement: (1) since the control and test implants were paired in the same patient, laser irradiation could have induced a systemic effect; (2) the effect of the laser could have been masked by the high initial stability attained in bone type II. Further studies should be performed in areas with type IV bone quality and in patients with systemic diseases like diabetes and those who are heavy smokers.[9]

In osteogenesis, *in vitro* studies have previously demonstrated the beneficial effects of LPL irradiation in promoting new bone formation by inducing proliferation and differentiation of osteoblasts.[25,43–45] Based on these findings, Aleksic et al. investigated the potential photobiomodulatory effects of low power Er:YAG laser irradiation on osteoblasts, focusing on *in vitro* cell proliferation.[35] The osteoblastic cells were treated with low power Er:YAG laser irradiation at different settings (fluence: $0.7 \pm 17.2 \, \text{J/cm}^2$) and in the presence or absence of culture medium during irradiation. Higher proliferation rates were found with various combinations of irradiation parameters on days 1 and 3. Significantly higher proliferation was also observed in laser-irradiated cells at a fluence of approximately $1.0–15.1 \, \text{J/cm}^2$. Further, low power Er:YAG irradiation induced the phosphorylation of extracellular signal-regulated protein kinase

(MAPK/ERK) 5–30 minutes after irradiation. The authors concluded that low power Er:YAG laser irradiation increases osteoblast proliferation mainly by activation of MAPK/ERK, suggesting that the Er:YAG laser may be able to promote bone healing following periodontal and peri-implant therapy.

These preliminary studies suggested that HPLs could be used as LPLs, since the irradiation parameters can be controlled, in order to promote greater osteoblast proliferation and adhesion to dental implants, improving the osseointegration process. However, more clinical studies need to be performed in order to determine optimal parameters of laser irradiation.[36]

Postoperative treatment

Considering the benefits of LPL irradiation described above, the postoperative phase, when the biomodulation process of hard and soft tissues occurs, with higher cellular proliferation, appears to the optimal timing of the application of laser irradiation. The laser light accelerates wound healing, collagen synthesis, and fibroblast proliferation.[4,25] Moreover, the laser also has an important effect on analgesia, reducing the need for analgesics.[37] Both laser red and infrared wavelengths are suitable for postoperative treatment. While the red laser can be used for soft tissue, the infrared wavelength is indicated for bone and nervous system tissue.[8,21]

A study performed by Dörtbudak et al. showed that when the laser irradiation (690 nm, 100 mW, 1 minute, 6 J) was performed immediately after implant placement, viable osteocytes were found in 41.7% versus 34.4% in the non-irradiated group (P <0.027).[26] The bone resorption rate, in contrast, was not affected by laser irradiation. According to the authors, the results suggested that more vital bone tissue is present in the irradiated area than in the non-irradiated area, and that wound healing may be expected to be faster. Moreover, the LPL irradiation appears to produce highly reactive and vital peri-implant bone tissue, reducing healing time and accelerating osseointegration of dental implants.[26]

Figure 24.2 shows a clinical case, 4 days post irradiation with an LPL emitting an infrared wavelength (810 nm, spot area 0.028 cm^2, 70 mW, 20 J/cm^2, 0.56 J per point, 8 seconds per point, contact mode) with six points of laser irradiation for each implant, three on the vestibular side and three on the palatal side. The laser irradiation was performed in the immediate postoperative period, after 48 hours, and 4 and 6 days later. The red laser light shown in Figure 24.2 can only been seen with the photographic camera, since this wavelength is invisible to the human eye.

Second-stage surgery

The second-stage surgery of submerged dental implants and the removal of hyperplasic peri-implant tissue are traditionally performed with a scalpel, but they can also be performed using electrosurgery or with lasers. Using the scalpel for incision or excision, there is always some bleeding, and the patient can experience some pain and discomfort during and after the

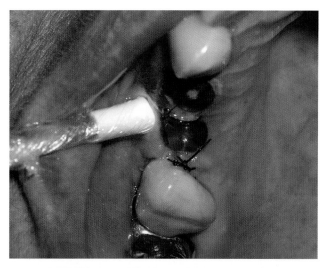

Figure 24.2 Postoperative infrared laser irradiation of dental implants.

surgical procedure. Electrosurgery may damage the implant surface, hindering the osseointegration process and leading to overheating, which may lead to implant failure.[1] On the other hand, laser surgery has some advantages: simplicity of manipulation, absence of bleeding, a reduced need for local anesthesia, obviation of need for sutures, and increased patient comfort during and after the operation. Disadvantages include the high cost of the laser procedures in comparison to the traditional methods and the risk of thermal damage to tissues when the irradiation parameters are not controlled.[1,36,38]

The erbium lasers (Er:YAG and Er,Cr:YSGG) have been the most reported systems for use in second-stage implant surgery.[39] These lasers have a negligible thermal effect and allow precise sectioning of both hard and soft tissues around the implant, without implant surface damage or effect on osseointegration.[40] The diode and Nd:YAG lasers, which are commonly used systems in oral surgery, have been rarely recommended for use in implant surgery,[41] since they can promote an undesirable increase in temperature, which may damage implants and peri-implant tissues.[36,40]

Titanium reflects incident light energy, so a temperature elevation in bone between 44 °C and 47 °C can lead to osteonecrosis.[2,42] The thermal increase generated on the implant surface appears to be influenced by the wavelength and power settings of the laser,[43] as well as by the surface characteristic of the implant.[44]

The wavelength of the Er:YAG laser is well absorbed by water and hydroxyapatite. The CO_2 laser emitting at 9.6 µm has a high absorption coefficient for water and for hydroxyapatite with phosphate, carbonate, and hydroxyl groups; furthermore, it is also highly absorbed by collagen.[2] Therefore, it is promising for use in implantology, but more studies are needed. Figure 24.3 shows a clinical case in whom the CO_2 laser was used to uncover a submerged implant. One of the advantages of this laser is the good hemostasis and low penetration depth.

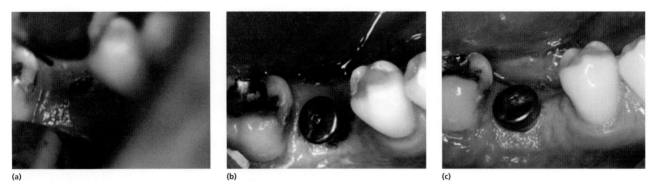

(a) (b) (c)

Figure 24.3 Second-stage surgery using a CO_2 laser for (a) implant uncovering and (b) placement of a sulcus former. (c) Excellent wound healing 2 weeks after surgery.

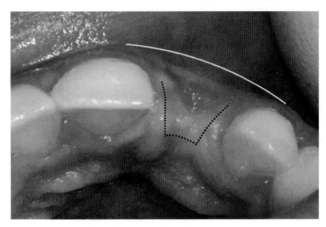

Figure 24.4 Proposed flap design. Occlusal view of the severe vestibular bone loss often responsible for unsatisfactory results following prosthetic rehabilitation and thus this case is a candidate for mucogingival surgery to restore lost volume (courtesy of Dr Josep Arnabat-Domínguez, Department of Oral Surgery and Implantology of the Dental School of the University of Barcelona, Spain).

Parker suggested irradiation parameters of 1–2 W for the diode laser, 150 mJ/15 pps for the Nd:YAG laser, 200–250 mJ/10 pps for the erbium lasers, and 1–2 W for the CO_2 laser, which seem to be appropriate for removing gingival tissue overlying the implant cover screw.[42]

Arnabat-Domínguez et al. used the Er,Cr:YSGG laser for second-stage surgery of submerged implants in the anterior area and compared this treatment with the traditional scalpel technique.[40] The laser was used with 1 W of power and 10% water/15% air spray. A trapezoidal full-thickness flap was raised to uncover the implant, allowing the apical repositioning and transpositioning of keratinized gingiva to the buccal side (Fig. 24.4). The authors presented three clinical cases (Figs 24.6, 24.7, and 24.8) and reported a reduced healing time with the laser, possibly through the avoidance of sutures when compared to the control group (Fig. 24.5). The authors reported that for

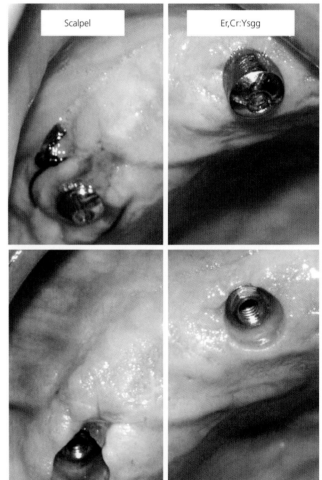

Scalpel Er,Cr:Ysgg

Figure 24.5 Comparison of postoperative healing after second-stage implant surgery with that after use of the cold scalpel, based on the conventional technique versus the Er,Cr:YSGG laser. Upper panel: 1 week after surgery; lower panel: 2 weeks after surgery (courtesy of Dr Josep Arnabat-Domínguez, Department of Oral Surgery and Implantology of the Dental School of the University of Barcelona, Spain).

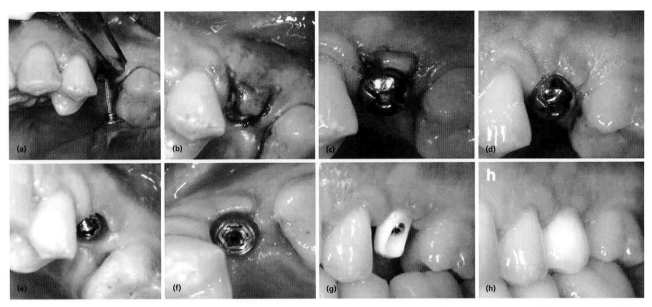

Figure 24.6 General surgical technique. (a,b) Design and raising of the trapezoidal flap, exposing the cover screw of the implant (c) substitution with the healing abutment: the flap rests on the latter to allow healing by secondary intention (d) 1 week after surgery; (e,f) appearance of the newly formed papilla on removal of the healing abutment: vestibular and occlusal views (g) rehabilitation using an esthetic zirconium post (h) final result (courtesy of Dr Josep Arnabat-Domínguez, Department of Oral Surgery and Implantology of the Dental School of the University of Barcelona, Spain).

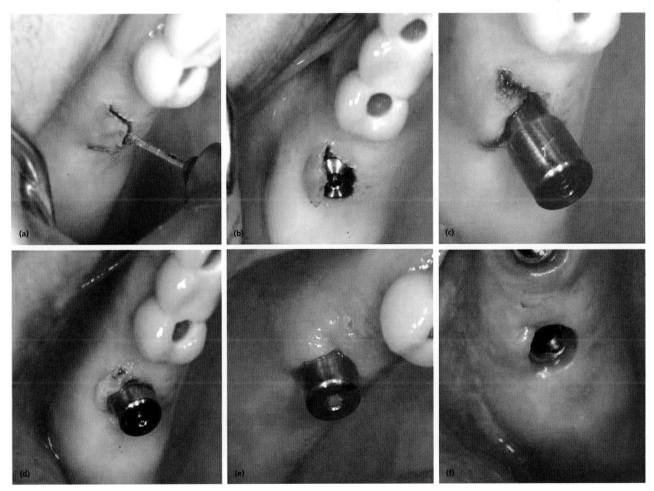

Figure 24.7 Rehabilitation of a right superior molar. (a) Trapezoidal incision with the Er,Cr:YSGG laser (b) flap and the cover screw, (c) insertion of the healing abutment (d) use of a rolling flap to gain volume in the affected area. Note that after preparation and before placement of the flap folded onto itself, the external surface was vaporized with the laser to secure de-epithelialization; (e,f) healing 1 week after surgery (courtesy of Dr Josep Arnabat-Domínguez, Department of Oral Surgery and Implantology of the Dental School of the University of Barcelona, Spain).

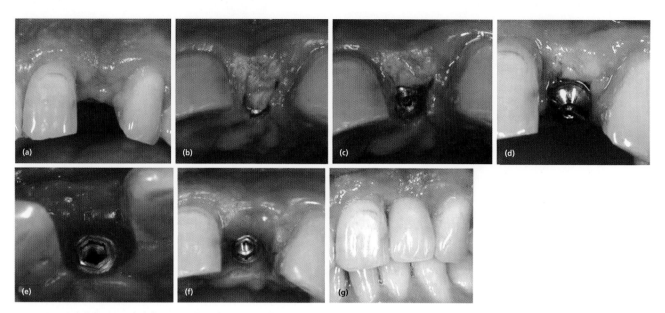

Figure 24.8 Rehabilitation of a left superior lateral incisor. (a) Preoperative appearance, showing important vestibular bone loss secondary to a chronic infection; (b,c) use of a rolling flap to gain volume in the affected area. Note that after preparation and before placement of the flap folded onto itself, the external surface was vaporized with the Er,Cr:YSGG laser to secure de-epithelialization (d) healing 1 week after surgery; (e,f) occlusal and vestibular view of the peri-implant soft tissue contour achieved (g) final result (courtesy of Dr Josep Arnabat-Domínguez, Department of Oral Surgery and Implantology of the Dental School of the University of Barcelona, Spain).

the clinical cases where the laser was used, postoperative pain was minimized, the time to prosthetic rehabilitation was shortened, and the esthetic results were far superior than with the conventional scalpel technique. In addition, no complications were recorded.[40]

Based on laser–tissue interaction characteristics, all laser wavelengths are suitable for the second-stage recovery of implants, provided care is taken to avoid prolonged contact with the implant surface to prevent an undesired increase in temperature in peri-implant tissues.

Implant bed preparation

For most patients, drills and handpieces are the cause of most discomfort in dentistry. Therefore, laser osteotomy could be an attractive alternative.[2]

The preparation of the implant bed demands a technique in which the local temperature does not exceed 47 °C.[38,45] The super-pulsed CO_2 laser was compared to the Er:YAG laser and the conventional drill with regard to thermal effects on human bone, and it was found that lasers caused less increase in temperature than conventional drilling for osteotomies on larger bone segments compared to small bone slices. Moreover, the laser showed acceptable efficacy, with drilling times comparable to those with a conventional drill.[46] Kimura et al. analyzed morphological changes in bovine mandibular bone after Er,Cr:YSGG laser irradiation. In the fixed position and contact mode group, thermal damage was apparent, but it was minimal (<10 μm) in the non-fixed position and non-contact mode group.[47]

Kim et al. investigated the accuracy and effectiveness of implant bed preparation in pig rib bone using an Er,Cr:YSGG laser.[48] The laser was employed at 5.75 W, 30 Hz, and 70 μs, with a 50% water/60% air spray. The groups were divided according to the laser tip: group 1: parallel shaped sapphire tip; group 2: parallel shaped zirconia tip; and group 3: tapered sapphire tip. The Er,Cr:YSGG laser tip was applied for 15 seconds in non-contact mode (1 mm away from the bone). After irradiation, the bone was sectioned for specimens. Histological measurements were determined by computerized morphometry. Results showed that the prepared length for group 3 was longer than that for group 2. In all groups, the prepared bone width was larger than the width of the laser tip. Different cutting effects were observed according to the laser tip, emphasizing the importance of proper tip selection in the clinical setting. Moreover, bone removal was observed adjacent to the areas that received direct laser application. The authors speculated that this was due to a hydrokinetic effect on the surrounding bone. Lasers, by their nature, focus their energy directly forward in a straight beam, but the sprayed water interacting with the laser does not necessarily follow the same direction. As a result, excited water molecules with new vectors may impact the adjacent bone, especially if the bone is weak. To compensate, laser implant bed preparation should be less compared with drill bed preparation in clinical applications. Special care needs to be taken in patients with weak bones. In clinical applications, the laser should not be applied continuously to the same area, and the irradiation time should be reduced to when the laser tip reaches the final depth for implant placement.[48]

It was reported that bone healing following Er:YAG laser irradiation in an inferior border defect of the rat mandible appeared to be equivalent or even faster than that following bur drilling.

These data seem to indicate that an Er:YAG laser may also be a promising tool for bone ablation during implant bed preparation. Indeed, preliminary results from experimental studies in rats have indicated that titanium screws were able to osseointegrate in an Er:YAG laser-prepared bone defect.[49,50] Implant channels of 0.7 mm in diameter were prepared on both sides of the calvarium using either an Er:YAG laser or a conventional metal bur, followed by the insertion of 1-mm diameter self-threading titanium screws. After healing periods of 3 and 12 weeks, the titanium screws in both groups were successfully osseointegrated and surrounded by vital woven or lamellar bone-like tissue structures, respectively.[50] Even though these data suggest that osseointegration of titanium screws may not be compromised following implant bed preparation using an Er:YAG laser, it must be emphasized that the results for small diameter osteotomy holes prepared in the calvarium or tibia of rats may not be transferable to the oral cavity. Indeed, most common titanium implants used for the replacement of missing teeth have a diameter of at least 3.3 mm and a length of 8 mm. Therefore, the amount of bone ablation needed for the insertion of commonly used dental titanium implants is far higher than that for experimentally modified titanium screws. Accordingly, it might be hypothesized that the risk for potential thermal damage to the adjacent alveolar bone might increase with the amount of ablated bone volume.[51]

Schwarz et al. evaluated the influence of implant bed preparation using an Er:YAG laser on the osseointegration of titanium implants.[63] A total of 24 implant channels were prepared in the lower jaws of four beagle dogs using either an Er:YAG laser device or conventional drill (CD) according to a split-mouth design (six implant channels per animal). Three screw-type titanium implants from different manufacturers were randomly inserted in both groups to evaluate submerged healing at 2 and 12 weeks. Width of the peri-implant gap (WPG) and bone–implant contact (BIC) were assessed histomorphometrically. There were no identifiable signs of any thermal side effects in either group. Er:YAG osteotomy frequently resulted in wide peri-implant gaps, particularly in the apical area of the implant-supporting bone. The mean scores (±SD) were: WPG (2 weeks) – Er:YAG 0.89 ± 0.48 mm and CD 0.27 ± 0.09 mm (P <0.001); BIC (2 weeks) – Er:YAG $34.5 \pm 7.76\%$ and CD $48.5 \pm 11.08\%$ ($P < 0.001$); BIC (12 weeks) –Er:YAG $64.1 \pm 8.97\%$ and CD $68.94 \pm 11.23\%$ (P >0.05). The authors concluded that the Er:YAG laser may represent a promising tool for implant bed preparation.[51]

Most of the studies in the literature were performed *in vitro* or in animals. Thus, more clinical studies are necessary in order to determine which lasers and parameters are most suitable for implant bed preparation, allowing enhanced safety and efficacy.

Sinus lift procedures

Insufficient bone volume is a common problem in the rehabilitation of the edentulous posterior maxilla with implant-supported prostheses. The bone available for implant placement is usually limited due to the presence of the maxillary sinus associated with loss of alveolar bone height. Bone volume can be increased by means of augmentation, and the sinus cavity is commonly augmented with autogenous bone and/or biomaterials.[52] Carbide burs or piezosurgery tips are usually used for bony window osteotomy in direct sinus grafting procedures.[53,54]

Recently, lasers have also been used for sinus grafting procedures, as reported in a study performed with an Er,Cr:YSGG laser.[54] The advantages of using the erbium laser include straight clean cuts and precise hard tissue cuts by virtue of the laser's energy interaction with water at the tissue interface.[54] Also, it increases hemostasis, minimizes damage to the surrounding tissue, reduces the probability of infection, and reduces pain postoperatively.[3] However, Er,Cr:YSGG laser light and the water spray do not penetrate to the deep regions of the thick lateral wall of the sinus, so the osteotomy efficiency is compromised.

The Er,Cr:YSGG laser was used by Sohn et al. for osteotomy in 12 sinus lift procedures (Fig. 24.9).[54] For soft tissue incision, the laser was set with a light water spray and the parameters of $4 J/cm^2$, 700 μs, and 30 Hz, using the MT4 tip. For osteotomy, the parameters were $6 J/cm^2$, 140 μs, and 20 Hz, using the MG6 tip. When the bone of the lateral wall was less than 2 mm thick, the bony window was made with the Er,Cr:YSGG laser only. The time for complete osteotomy was 2–7 minutes (average, 3 minutes 24 seconds). When the bone thickness was 3 or 4 mm, piezoelectric surgery was added in the final stage, followed by laser irradiation. For window osteotomy, the time was 4–9 minutes (average 6 minutes 30 seconds). Membrane perforation was reported in four of 12 sinuses during window osteotomy (perforation rate 33.3%). No implants failed during the follow-up period.

When using laser irradiation there should be no contact with tissues, unlike when using the drill or in piezoelectric surgery, but the risk of membrane perforation may be increased if the laser comes into direct contact with the membrane during window osteotomy. Partial osteotomy and bony window detachment are recommended in laser-assisted sinus bone grafting, to reduce the rate of membrane perforation. Furthermore, during erbium laser irradiation, the bone tissue should be positioned 0.5–1 mm away from the laser tip to yield maximum cutting power.[54]

Peri-implantitis treatment

Bacterial contamination of dental implants leads to inflammatory reactions, resulting in loss of osseointegration. Peri-implant disease is a general term used to describe host tissue inflammatory reactions. Two major types of peri-implant diseases are described: peri-implant mucositis and peri-implantitis.[55,56]

Peri-implant mucositis is defined as a reversible inflammation of the soft tissue surrounding the dental implant without loss of the supporting bone. Clinical signs are bleeding and/or suppuration and probing depths of more than 3 mm.

Peri-implantitis is defined as a progressive, inflammatory process affecting the tissues surrounding an osseointegrated implant,

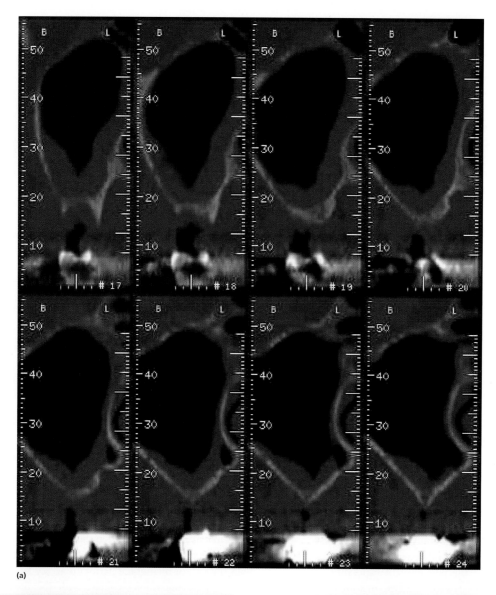

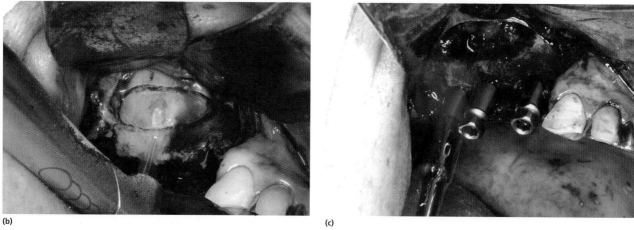

Figure 24.9 (a) Computerized tomograph showing thin lateral wall and low bone height of right maxillary sinus (b) window osteotomy with the Er,Cr:YSGG laser (c) implant placement and simultaneous sinus grafting (d) a bony window was repositioned over the bone graft as a barrier membrane to prevent ingrowth of soft tissue into the sinus cavity (e) allograft and implants placed; – (f) postoperative panoramic radiograph; – (g,h) placement of the final restorations 7 months after surgery and periapical X-ray control (courtesy of Dr Dong-Seok Sohn, Department of Dentistry and Oral and Maxillofacial Surgery of the Catholic University of Medical Center of Daegu, Republic of Korea).

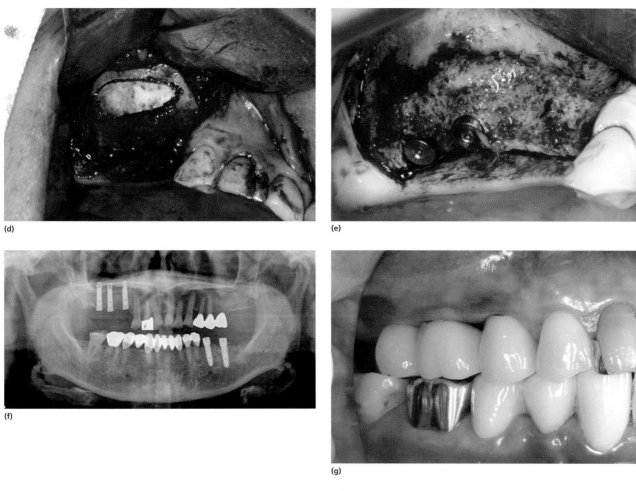

(d)

(e)

(f)

(g)

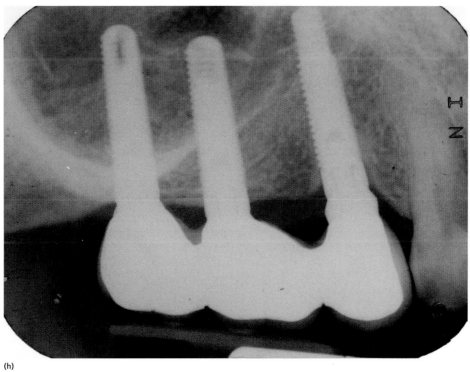

(h)

Figure 24.9 (Continued)

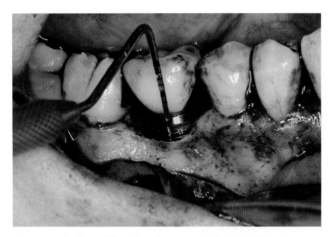

Figure 24.10 Advanced bone loss due to peri-implantitis, with a circumferential crater defect.

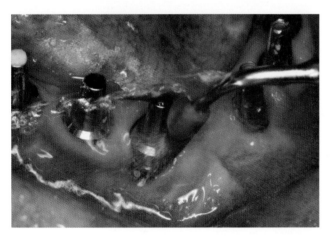

Figure 24.11 Cleaning of the abutments using a special ultrasonic device with a plastic tip.

resulting in loss of the supporting bone. Clinical signs are deep probing depths (>5 mm) and bleeding and/or suppuration on probing. Loss of supporting bone resulting from peri-implantitis usually forms a circumferential crater defect (Fig. 24.10).[57]

As microbial colonization plays a major etiological role,[58] it was assumed that the removal of bacterial plaque biofilms from the implant surface is a prerequisite for the therapy of peri-implant infections.[59] In recent years, several maintenance regimens and treatment strategies (i.e. mechanical, chemical) have been proposed for the treatment of peri-implant infections.[60,61] Correct diagnosis is critical for appropriate management of peri-implant disease.[62]

Mechanical debridement (Fig. 24.11) is usually performed using specific instruments made of materials that are softer than titanium (i.e. plastic curettes, polishing with rubber cups) to avoid the roughening the metallic surface that may favor bacterial colonization.[63,64]

Because mechanical methods alone have proven to be insufficient for the elimination of bacteria on roughened implant surfaces, the adjunctive use of chemical agents (i.e. irrigation with local disinfectants, local or systemic antibiotic therapy) has been recommended to enhance healing after treatment.[56,65]

A variety of antimicrobial treatment regimens in combination with non-surgical or surgical debridement, with and without regenerative therapy, have been proposed for peri-implantitis treatment. Use of systemic or local antibiotics in conjunction with non-surgical mechanical debridement has been shown to be effective in the resolution of the peri-implant infection in the majority of patients and implants with moderate peri-implantitis.[65] Nevertheless, in these studies some implants in some patients had persistent peri-implantitis and required surgical intervention. One of the difficulties in treating peri-implantitis is obtaining access for adequate implant surface decontamination.[57] Decontamination procedures include the use of sterile saline, chlorhexidine, citric acid, hydrogen peroxide, mechanical debridement, and, more recently, lasers.[57,61]

The use of different laser systems has been proposed for both cleaning and decontamination of implant surfaces for peri-implantitis treatment (Fig. 24.12).[41,66–68] The results from a recent *in vitro* studies have demonstrated that, in an energy-dependent manner, only the CO_2 laser, diode lasers, and Er:YAG laser may be suitable for the instrumentation of implant surfaces because their specific wavelength is poorly absorbed by titanium and the implant body temperature does not increase significantly during irradiation.[41,67,68] In contrast, the Nd:YAG laser resulted in extensive melting and damage to the porous titanium surface and coating.[41,67]

So far, bactericidal effects on common dental implant surfaces *in vitro* have only been reported for the CO_2 and Er:YAG lasers, indicating that both systems may be useful in removing bacterial contaminants from textured titanium surfaces.[69] Since neither CO_2 nor diode lasers were effective in removing calculus from root surfaces or titanium implants, both types of lasers were only used as an adjunct to mechanical treatment procedures.[70] In contrast, the ability of the Er:YAG laser to effectively ablate dental calculus without producing thermal side effects to adjacent tissue has been demonstrated in some *in situ* studies.[70,71] Controlled clinical trials have also indicated that non-surgical periodontal treatment with an Er:YAG laser may lead to significant clinical improvements as evidenced by probing depth reduction and improved clinical attachment.[72–74] These improvements were comparable to those obtained following treatment with hand instruments.[73,74] The clinical results were maintained for a period of up to 2 years.[72] Preliminary results have also shown that non-surgical instrumentation of titanium implants with an Er:YAG laser, used with a special application tip, resulted in the effective removal of subgingival calculus without leading to any thermal damage. The attachment of human osteoblast-like cells to differently coated titanium discs after irradiation at an energy density of $12.7 J/cm^2$ was not reduced when compared to untreated control specimens, indicating that the biocompatibility of the titanium surface was not affected.[66,75]

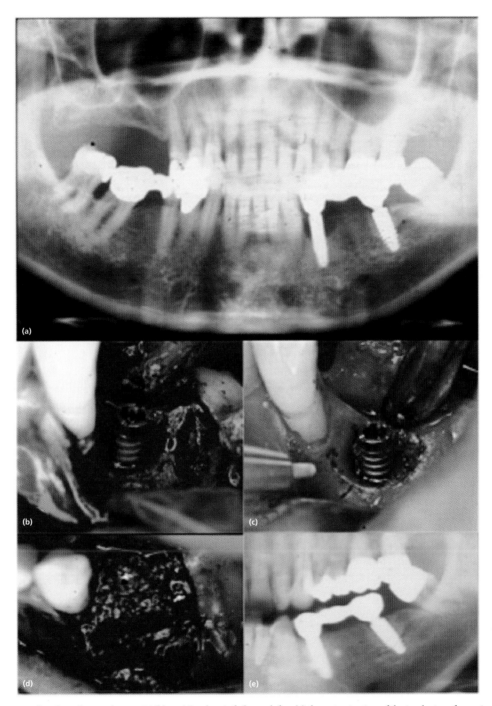

Figure 24.12 (a) Peri-implant bone loss at element 34 (b) peri-implant infrabony defect (c) decontamination of the implant surface using a CO_2 laser (d) augmentation with mineral bovine bone (e) radiological fill 4 years after treatment.

In a study by Schwarz et al. it was concluded that at 6 months following treatment, both Er:YAG and chlorhexidine treatment lead to significant improvements of the investigated clinical parameters, and the Er:YAG laser resulted in a statistically significant higher reduction of bleeding on probing.[66]

Despite the advantages of the bactericidal effect, hemostatic properties, and selective calculus ablation of HPLs, they can promote an undesirable increase in temperature and damage the implant surface.[76,77] The high cost of HPL equipment is another disadvantage. An alternative approach to decontamination of the implant surface is the combination of conventional treatment with antimicrobial photodynamic therapy (aPDT).[36,76,77]

In a study in dogs, Hayek et al. compared the effects of aPDT, using paste-based azulene and irradiation with a 50 mW diode laser, with a conventional technique, which included mucoperiosteal flap surgery and irrigation with chlorhexidine, on microbial reduction following ligature-induced peri-implantitis.[78] Periodontal pathogens, such as *Prevotella* ssp., *Fusobacterium* ssp., and β-hemolytic *Streptococcus*, were effectively reduced by aPDT to a level equivalent to that achieved with conventional treatment. Application of the photosensitizer in a paste instead of a liquid solution allowed it to be easily removed after treatment without compromising esthetics. Similar results were described by Shibli et al., who reported that aPDT (toluidine blue O + 50 mW diode laser) reduced the bacterial count of *Prevotella intermedia*, *P. nigrescens*, *Fusobacterium* spp. and β-hemolytic *Streptococcus* in ligature-induced peri-implantitis in dogs and, in some cases, complete elimination of those bacteria was achieved.[79]

In a clinical case series study, Haas et al. investigated the clinical effects of the combination of aPDT (toludine blue O + diode laser) with guided bone regeneration using autogenous bone grafts on 24 dental implants diagnosed with peri-implantitis in 17 patients.[80] Twenty-one of the 24 implants showed improvements in the bone defect after a mean observation period of 9.5 months.

Dörtbudak et al. analyzed the effectiveness of aPDT in contaminated implant surfaces by evaluating the remaining levels of *Aggregaticater actinomycetemcomitans*, *Porphyromonas gingivalis*, and *P. intermedia*.[81] Microbiological samples were taken from the same implants of 15 patients diagnosed with peri-implantitis before and after application of toluidine blue O and then after the laser irradiation. A significant decrease of all species of bacteria was observed following aPDT compared with baseline levels. However, the use of toluidine blue O alone without laser light also resulted in a decrease of all bacterial species, and complete bacterial reduction was not achieved with either the application of toluidine blue O alone or of aPDT alone. Furthermore, in a case report, effective bone regeneration within bone defects around implants affected by peri-implantitis was demonstrated following surgical therapy using aPDT (tolonium chlorine + 100 mW diode laser) to decontaminate the implant surface and the use of recombinant human bone morphogenetic protein-2.[82]

Figure 24.13 shows a clinical case of a patient in an advanced stage of peri-implantitis. The patient, a 58-year-old man referred to the Clinic for Maxillofacial Surgery and Implant Center of the Katharinenhospital, Stuttgart, Germany, had peri-implantitis at the elements 13, 11, 21, and 23. On clinical examination, signs of bleeding and suppuration were present, with probing depths of greater than 10 mm. The treatment proposed was aPDT combined with conventional peri-implantitis treatment. After surgical incision, the implants were exposed, and mechanical debridement was performed with carbon curettes. All implant surfaces were irrigated with 0.01% (m/V) methylene blue dye for 5 minutes, and then irradiated with a 660-nm LPL (120 J/cm^2, 100 mW, 3.36 J per point, 34 seconds per point, eight points per implant, laser spot area 0.028 cm^2, continuous mode, in contact). Despite the bone defect, the patient did not show signs of bleeding and suppuration at 6-month follow-up.

The results of the above studies indicate that aPDT can effectively reduce the prevalence of pathogens on implant surfaces without causing any side effects on the implant and bone surfaces.[77] Nevertheless, combined treatment with aPDT and conventional treatments may achieve better results for peri-implantitis.

Implant surface modification

After the discovery of osseointegration by Brånemark, there was an exponential increase in the demand for implants with surfaces that could accelerate the osseointegration process. Today there are probably thousands of dental implants on the market, and each manufacturer will try to convince the dentist of the superiority of their implant in terms of faster and better osseointegration. Each year new types of implant surfaces are presented to the market. Besides these being of commercial value to the implant companies, new and/or improved dental implant surfaces are still required due to the challenging cases still presenting in daily practice. Different loading protocols, anatomically compromised alveolar ridges, or patients with impaired wound healing (e.g. diabetic, osteoporotic, or irradiated patients) are some of the daily challenges that clinicians face in their practice. As a consequence, there is a need for new titanium surfaces that give a predictable improvement in the osseointegration process.[83,84]

The surface can be roughened with chemical modification, hydroxyapatite plasma spray, acid etching, acid etching associated with sandblasting, and laser ablation. These methods are responsible for an improved bone–implant contact and the possibility of early implant loading.[84]

Laser irradiation increases the temperature of the titanium surface to its melting point, followed by fast cooling, which results in unique microstructures with increased hardness and corrosion resistance, associated with a high degree of purity, standard roughness, and a thick titanium oxide layer.[84–86] The titanium oxide layer formed is composed of different titanium oxides, including TiO_2, which when exposed to body fluids is deprotonized. Negative Ti–O groups are also formed, attracting Ca^{2+} ions from the body fluids, which bond to the surface. The layer of Ca^{2+} ions attracts negatively charged phosphate ions, which also bond to the surface, and a metastable phase of calcium phosphate is formed.[87] This biochemical process forms a more stable hydroxyapatite coating layer that is strongly bonded to the titanium implant surface.[84]

Faster bone formation within cavities by means of titanium laser ablation can be explained by the fact that osteoblast precursors migrate into the pores of the rough surface, reaching confluence earlier within the enclosed spaces, ceasing proliferation, and then differentiating.[84,88,89]

Considering that titanium surface texture and chemical modification can successfully improve the host response and consequently the bone–implant contact surrounding dental implants,

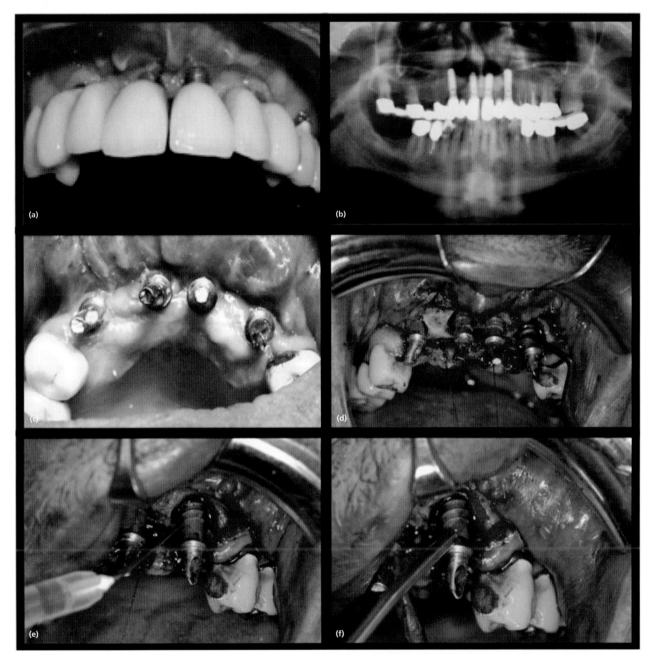

Figure 24.13 (a) Clinical and (b) radiographic view of a patient with peri-implantitis at elements 13, 11, 21, and 23 (c) exposition of the implants due to bone loss. (d) After mechanical debridement of the implant surfaces, (e) methylene blue dye was applied for 5 minutes, and then (f) LPL irradiation was performed for aPDT.

Faeda et al. investigated the effects of titanium surface modification by laser ablation (Nd:YAG) followed by the thin chemical deposition of hydroxyapatite.[84] The tibiae of 48 rabbits received one implant with a machined (MS), laser-modified (LMS), or biomimetic hydroxyapatite-coated (HA) surface. Bone–implant contact (BIC) and bone area (BBT) were evaluated after 4, 8, and 12 weeks in cortical and cancellous regions. The results showed that the average BIC in the cortical region was higher ($P < 0.001$) for the LMS and HA implants at all time points, with no differences between LMS and HA implants. For the cancellous area, the LMS and HA implants showed a higher ($P < 0.01$) BIC than MS implants at the initial time point. The LMS and HA implants showed similar values in the cortical region, but there was a tendency to higher values for HA implants in the cancellous region at all time points. Differences in the BBT were found only between HA and MS implants in the cortical region after 4 weeks ($P < 0.05$), and in the cancellous area after 12 weeks ($P < 0.05$). The authors concluded that HA biomimetic coating

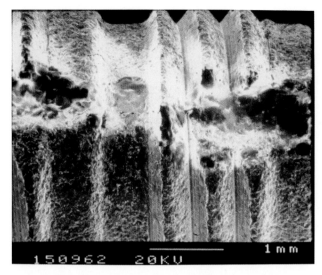

Figure 24.14 Implant irradiation using a Nd:YAG (2W pulsed) laser achieves significant melting of the implant surface.

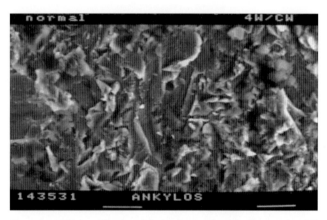

Figure 24.15 No modification of the implant surface after the use of a 4-W, continuous wave CO_2 laser (right) in comparison with the non-irradiated surface (left).

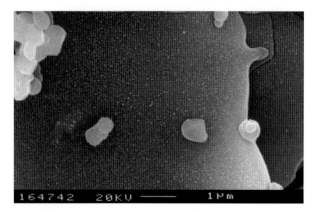

Figure 24.16 No changes to the implant surface after irradiation with a continuous wave diode laser (980 nm, 10 W).

preceded by laser treatment induced contact osteogenesis and allowed the formation of a more stable bone–implant interface, even at the earlier time points.[84]

Romanos et al. evaluated osteoblast attachment to titanium discs irradiated with either a CO_2 (10 600 nm, output power varying from 4 to 6 W, frequency 20 Hz) or an Er,Cr:YSGG (2780 nm, output power 1.25 W, 42% air/41% water spray, frequency 20 Hz) laser and compared them with non-irradiated discs.[90] The results showed that osteoblasts grew on all discs; however, the cellular density was higher in the laser-irradiated specimens. No difference was found between the discs irradiated with the different lasers.

For optimization of the surface of a zirconia dental implant, Delgado-Ruíz et al. analyzed a femtosecond laser.[108] As far as roughening of the zirconia surface is concerned, electrical techniques are precluded and acid or alkaline etching techniques do not give rise to high surface roughness levels, because the original material is manufactured using high isostatic pressure to make it resistant to chemical, physical, or wear changes. Femtosecond laser microtexturing increases surface roughness and reduces the presence of residual elements, and these surface characteristics are permanent. It is also a technique that has much potential for automation and therefore reproducibility. The authors aimed to generate high quality microstructures (grooves and pores) on the surface of cylindrical zirconia dental implants by means of ultrafast laser ablation. The modified implant surfaces were analyzed to evaluate their potential to improve implant performance. The laser system delivered 120-fs linearly polarized pulses with a wavelength of 795 nm and a repetition rate of 1 kHz. The transverse mode was TEM00 and the laser beam width was 9 mm ($1/e^2$ criterion). Pulse energy could reach a maximum of 1.1 mJ and this was reduced with neutral filters and a half wave plate and polarizer system, to generate the most suitable fluence on the surface of the material for producing ablation with minimal damage to the surrounding area. The authors concluded that femtosecond laser microstructuring of zirconia implants increases surface roughness and removes contaminants incorporated in earlier stages of manufacturing, which could improve the biocompatibility of the implant. Additionally, analysis of the processed surfaces by X-ray diffraction and Raman spectrometry showed that the material surrounding the microstructures does not exhibit phase transformation due to a possible strong thermal load.[91]

Figures 24.14, 24.15, and 24.16 show the changes promoted by the Nd:YAG, CO_2 and 980 nm diode lasers in dental implant surface, respectively.

Final considerations

Different laser devices and different irradiation parameters may give different results for osseointegration. No standardized laser parameters have been reported for improvement of osseointegration. It is usually difficult to compare the different studies, especially because in most, laser irradiation parameters are not reported. No standard protocol for laser irradiation has yet been defined for implant dentistry.[13] It has been observed that there is a very large variation in the choice of energy density and wavelengths for LPL irradiation of bone tissue.[9,13]

The LLLT has been demonstrated to be a non-invasive method for the stimulation of osteogenesis and for the reduction of the time for bone consolidation through bioenergetic, bioelectrical, biochemical, and biostimulatory effects on cells.[92]

Some advantages of laser use in second-stage surgery of dental implants are increased hemostasis, facilitating easier visual access to the cover screw, production of a protective coagulum as an aid to healing, and patient comfort during and after treatment.[42]

Clinicians must be aware that despite the many advantages of lasers in implantology, such as straight, clean, precise cuts in both soft and hard tissues, increased hemostasis, minimal damage to the surrounding tissues, reduced infection, and reduced postoperative pain, a learning period is required to ensure best treatment is given.

Acknowledgments

The authors are grateful to Dr Josep Arnabat-Domínguez, Department of Oral Surgery and Implantology of the Dental School of the University of Barcelona, Spain; Dr Dong-Seok Sohn, Department of Dentistry and Oral and Maxillofacial Surgery of the Catholic University of Medical Center of Daegu, Republic of Korea; and Dr Joelle Marie García-Morales, Prosthodontic Department of the Dental School of the University of São Paulo, Brazil, for having kindly provided some images for illustration and enrichment of this chapter.

References

1 Romanos GE, Gutknecht N, Dieter S, et al. Laser wavelengths and oral implantology. *Lasers Med Sci* 2009; 24: 961–970.

2 Deppe H, Horch HH. Laser applications in oral surgery and implant dentistry. *Lasers Med Sci* 2007; 22: 217–221.

3 Martin E. Lasers in dental implantology. *Dent Clin North Am* 2004; 48: 999–1015, viii.

4 Branemark PI, Hansson BO, Adell R, et al. Osseointegrated implants in the treatment of the edentulous jaw. Experience from a 10-year period. *Scand J Plast Reconstr Surg Suppl* 1977; 16: 1–132.

5 Albrektsson T, Sennerby L, Wennerberg A. State of the art of oral implants. *Periodontology 2000* 2008; 47: 15–26.

6 Buser D, Weber HP, Lang NP. Tissue integration of non-submerged implants. 1-year results of a prospective study with 100 ITI hollow-cylinder and hollow-screw implants. *Clin Oral Implants Res* 1990; 1: 33–40.

7 Khadra M, Lyngstadaas SP, Haanaes HR, et al. Effect of laser therapy on attachment, proliferation and differentiation of human osteoblast-like cells cultured on titanium implant material. *Biomaterials* 2005; 26: 3503–3509.

8 Kazem Shakouri S, Soleimanpour J, Salekzamani Y, et al. Effect of low-level laser therapy on the fracture healing process. *Lasers Med Sci* 2010; 25: 73–77.

9 Garcia-Morales JM, Tortamano-Neto P, Todescan FF, et al. Stability of dental implants after irradiation with an 830-nm low-level laser: a double-blind randomized clinical study. *Lasers Med Sci* 2012; 27: 703–711.

10 Eduardo FP, Mehnert DU, Monezi TA, et al. Cultured epithelial cells response to phototherapy with low intensity laser. *Lasers Surg Med* 2007; 39: 365–372.

11 Guzzardella GA, Torricelli P, Nicoli-Aldini N, et al. Osseointegration of endosseous ceramic implants after postoperative low-power laser stimulation: an in vivo comparative study. *Clin Oral Implants Res* 2003; 14: 226–232.

12 Pinheiro AL, Martinez Gerbi ME, Carneiro Ponzi EA, et al. Infrared laser light further improves bone healing when associated with bone morphogenetic proteins and guided bone regeneration: an in vivo study in a rodent model. *Photomed Laser Surg* 2008; 26: 167–174.

13 Khadra M, Ronold HJ, Lyngstadaas SP, et al. Low-level laser therapy stimulates bone-implant interaction: an experimental study in rabbits. *Clin Oral Implants Res* 2004; 15: 325–332.

14 Lopes CB, Pinheiro ALB, Sathaiah S, et al. Infrared laser photobiomodulation (lambda 830 nm) on bone tissue around dental implants: A Raman spectroscopy and scanning electronic microscopy study in rabbits. *Photomed Laser Surg* 2007; 25: 96–101.

15 Conlan MJ, Rapley JW, Cobb CM. Biostimulation of wound healing by low-energy laser irradiation. A review. *J Clin Periodontol* 1996; 23: 492–496.

16 Pourzarandian A, Watanabe H, Ruwanpura SM, et al. Effect of low-level Er:YAG laser irradiation on cultured human gingival fibroblasts. *J Periodontol* 2005; 76: 187–193.

17 Bouvet-Gerbettaz S, Merigo E, Rocca JP, et al. Effects of low-level laser therapy on proliferation and differentiation of murine bone marrow cells into osteoblasts and osteoclasts. *Lasers Surg Med* 2009; 41: 291–297.

18 Blaya DS, Guimaraes MB, Pozza DH, et al. Histologic study of the effect of laser therapy on bone repair. *J Contemp Dent Pract* 2008; 9: 41–48.

19 Pretel H, Lizarelli RF, Ramalho LT. Effect of low-level laser therapy on bone repair: histological study in rats. *Lasers Surg Med* 2007; 39: 788–796.

20 da Silva RV, Camilli JA. Repair of bone defects treated with autogenous bone graft and low-power laser. *J Craniofac Surg* 2006; 17: 297–301.

21 Fujihara NA, Hiraki KR, Marques MM. Irradiation at 780 nm increases proliferation rate of osteoblasts independently of dexamethasone presence. *Lasers Surg Med* 2006; 38: 332–336.

22 Kim YD, Kim SS, Hwang DS, et al. Effect of low-level laser treatment after installation of dental titanium implant-immunohistochemical study of RANKL, RANK, OPG: an experimental study in rats. *Lasers Surg Med* 2007; 39: 441–450.

23 Pyo SJ, Song WW, Kim IR, et al. Low-level laser therapy induces the expressions of BMP-2, osteocalcin, and TGF-beta1 in hypoxic-cultured human osteoblasts. *Lasers Med Sci* 2013; 28: 543–550.

24 Campanha BP, Gallina C, Geremia T, et al. Low-level laser therapy for implants without initial stability. *Photomed Laser Surg* 2010; 28: 365–369.

25 Pinheiro AL, Gerbi ME. Photoengineering of bone repair processes. *Photomed Laser Surg* 2006; 24: 169–178.

26 Dörtbudak O, Haas R, Mailath-Pokorny G. Effect of low-power laser irradiation on bony implant sites. *Clin Oral Implants Res* 2002; 13: 288–292.

27 Morimoto Y, Arai T, Kikuchi M, et al. Effect of low-intensity argon laser irradiation on mitochondrial respiration. *Lasers Surg Med* 1994; 15: 191–199.

28 Karu T. Photobiology of low-power laser effects. *Health Phys* 1989; 56: 691–704.

29 Nissan J, Assif D, Gross MD, et al. Effect of low intensity laser irradiation on surgically created bony defects in rats. *J Oral Rehabil* 2006; 33: 619–924.

30 Silva RV, Camilli JA, Bertran CA, et al. The use of hydroxyapatite and autogenous cancellous bone grafts to repair bone defects in rats. *Int J Oral Maxillofac Surg* 2005; 34: 178–184.

31 Garcia VG, da Conceicao JM, Fernandes LA, et al. Effects of LLLT in combination with bisphosphonate on bone healing in critical size defects: a histological and histometric study in rat calvaria. *Lasers Med Sci* 2013; 28: 407–414.

32 Shimizu N, Mayahara K, Kiyosaki T, et al. Low-intensity laser irradiation stimulates bone nodule formation via insulin-like growth factor-I expression in rat calvarial cells. *Lasers Surg Med* 2007; 39: 551–559.

33 Stein A, Benayahu D, Maltz L, et al. Low-level laser irradiation promotes proliferation and differentiation of human osteoblasts *in vitro*. *Photomed Laser Surg* 2005; 23: 161–166.

34 Aleksic V, Aoki A, Iwasaki K, et al. Low-level Er:YAG laser irradiation enhances osteoblast proliferation through activation of MAPK/ERK. *Lasers Med Sci* 2010; 25: 559–569.

35 Aleksic V, Aoki A, Iwasaki K, et al. Low-level Er:YAG laser irradiation enhances osteoblast proliferation through activation of MAPK/ERK. *Lasers Med Sci* 2010; 25: 559–569.

36 Marotti J, Tortamano-Neto P, Campos TT, et al. Recent patents of lasers in implant dentistry. *Recent Patents Biomed Eng* 2011; 4: 103–105.

37 Doshi-Mehta G, Bhad-Patil WA. Efficacy of low-intensity laser therapy in reducing treatment time and orthodontic pain: a clinical investigation. *Am J Orthod Dentofacial Orthop* 2012; 141: 289–297.

38 Geminiani A, Caton JG, Romanos GE. Temperature increase during CO(2) and Er:YAG irradiation on implant surfaces. *Implant Dent* 2011; 20: 379–382.

39 Arnabat-Dominguez J, Espana-Tost AJ, Berini-Aytes L, et al. Erbium:YAG laser application in the second phase of implant surgery: a pilot study in 20 patients. *Int J Oral Maxillofac Implants* 2003; 18: 104–112.

40 Arnabat-Dominguez J, Bragado-Novel M, Espana-Tost AJ, et al. Advantages and esthetic results of erbium, chromium:yttrium-scandium-gallium-garnet laser application in second-stage implant surgery in patients with insufficient gingival attachment: a report of three cases. *Lasers Med Sci* 2010; 25: 459–464.

41 Romanos GE, Everts H, Nentwig GH. Effects of diode and Nd:YAG laser irradiation on titanium discs: a scanning electron microscope examination. *J Periodontol* 2000; 71: 810–815.

42 Parker S. Surgical laser use in implantology and endodontics. *Br Dent J* 2007; 202: 377–386.

43 Kreisler M, Al Haj H, d'Hoedt B. Temperature changes at the implant-bone interface during simulated surface decontamination with an Er:YAG laser. *Int J Prosthodont* 2002; 15: 582–587.

44 Wooten CA, Sullivan SM, Surpure S. Heat generation by super-pulsed CO2 lasers on plasma-sprayed titanium implants: an in vitro study. *Oral Surg Oral Med Oral Pathol Oral Radiol Endod* 1999; 88: 544–548.

45 Geminiani A, Caton JG, Romanos GE. Temperature change during non-contact diode laser irradiation of implant surfaces. *Lasers Med Sci* 2012; 27: 339–342.

46 Eyrich G. *Hard-tissue drilling and cutting with a 9.6 μm CO$_2$ laser.* Med Habililationsschrift 2004, Zurich.

47 Kimura Y, Yu DG, Fujita A, et al. Effects of erbium,chromium:YSGG laser irradiation on canine mandibular bone. *J Periodontol* 2001; 72: 1178–1182.

48 Kim SK, Heo SJ, Koak JY, et al. Effects of the Er,Cr:YSGG laser on bone bed preparation with various laser tips. *J Kor Acad Prosthodont* 2008; 43: 255–259.

49 Kesler G, Romanos G, Koren R. Use of Er:YAG laser to improve osseointegration of titanium alloy implants--a comparison of bone healing. *Int J Oral Maxillofac Implants* 2006; 21: 375–379.

50 el-Montaser M, Devlin H, Dickinson MR, et al. Osseointegration of titanium metal implants in erbium-YAG laser-prepared bone. *Implant Dent* 1999; 8: 79–85.

51 Schwarz F, Olivier W, Herten M et al. Influence of implant bed preparation using an Er:YAG laser on the osseointegration of titanium implants: a histomorphometrical study in dogs. *J Oral Rehabil* 2007; 34: 273–281.

52 Esposito M, Grusovin MG, Rees J, et al. Effectiveness of sinus lift procedures for dental implant rehabilitation: a Cochrane systematic review. *Eur J Oral Implantol* 2010; 3: 7–26.

53 Sohn DS, Ahn MR, Lee WH, et al. Piezoelectric osteotomy for intraoral harvesting of bone blocks. *Int J Periodont Restor Dent* 2007; 27: 127–131.

54 Sohn DS, Lee JS, An KM, et al. Erbium, chromium:yttrium-scandium-gallium-garnet laser-assisted sinus graft procedure. *Lasers Med Sci* 2009; 24: 673–677.

55 Norowski PA, Jr, Bumgardner JD. Biomaterial and antibiotic strategies for peri-implantitis: a review. *J Biomed Mater Res B Appl Biomater* 2009; 88: 530–543.

56 Schwarz F, Bieling K, Bonsmann M, et al. Nonsurgical treatment of moderate and advanced periimplantitis lesions: a controlled clinical study. *Clin Oral Investig* 2006; 10: 279–288.

57 Heitz-Mayfield LJ. Diagnosis and management of peri-implant diseases. *Aust Dent J* 2008; 53 (Suppl 1): S43–48.

58 Quirynen M, De Soete M, van Steenberghe D. Infectious risks for oral implants: a review of the literature. *Clin Oral Implants Res* 2002; 13: 1–19.

59 Schwarz F, Papanicolau P, Rothamel D, et al. Influence of plaque biofilm removal on reestablishment of the biocompatibility of contaminated titanium surfaces. *J Biomed Mater Res A* 2006; 77: 437–444.

60 Mombelli A, Lang NP. Microbial aspects of implant dentistry. *Periodontology 2000* 1994; 4: 74–80.

61 Schou S, Berglundh T, Lang NP. Surgical treatment of peri-implantitis. *Int J Oral Maxillofac Implants* 2004; 19 (Suppl): 140–149.

62 Heitz-Mayfield LJ. Peri-implant diseases: diagnosis and risk indicators. *J Clin Periodontol* 2008; 35: 292–304.

63 Ruhling A, Kocher T, Kreusch J, et al. Treatment of subgingival implant surfaces with Teflon-coated sonic and ultrasonic scaler tips and various implant curettes. An *in vitro* study. *Clin Oral Implants Res* 1994; 5: 19–29.

64 Matarasso S, Quaremba G, Coraggio F, et al. Maintenance of implants: an *in vitro* study of titanium implant surface modifications subsequent to the application of different prophylaxis procedures. *Clin Oral Implants Res* 1996; 7: 64–72.

65 Heitz-Mayfield LJ, Lang NP. Antimicrobial treatment of peri-implant diseases. *Int J Oral Maxillofac Implants* 2004; 19 (Suppl): 128–139.

66 Schwarz F, Sculean A, Rothamel D, et al. Clinical evaluation of an Er:YAG laser for nonsurgical treatment of peri-implantitis: a pilot study. *Clin Oral Implants Res* 2005; 16: 44–52.

67 Kreisler M, Al Haj H, Gotz H, et al. Effect of simulated CO2 and GaAlAs laser surface decontamination on temperature changes in Ti-plasma sprayed dental implants. *Lasers Surg Med* 2002; 30: 233–239.

68 Kreisler M, Gotz H, Duschner H. Effect of Nd:YAG, Ho:YAG, Er:YAG, CO2, and GaAIAs laser irradiation on surface properties of endosseous dental implants. *Int J Oral Maxillofac Implants* 2002; 17: 202–211.

69 Kreisler M, Kohnen W, Marinello C, et al. Bactericidal effect of the Er:YAG laser on dental implant surfaces: an in vitro study. *J Periodontol* 2002; 73: 1292–1298.

70 Schwarz F, Sculean A, Berakdar M, et al. *In vivo* and *in vitro* effects of an Er:YAG laser, a GaAlAs diode laser, and scaling and root planing on periodontally diseased root surfaces: a comparative histologic study. *Lasers Surg Med* 2003; 32: 359–366.

71 Eberhard J, Ehlers H, Falk W, et al. Efficacy of subgingival calculus removal with Er:YAG laser compared to mechanical debridement: an in situ study. *J Clin Periodontol* 2003; 30: 511–518.

72 Schwarz F, Sculean A, Berakdar M, et al. Periodontal treatment with an Er:YAG laser or scaling and root planing. A 2-year follow-up split-mouth study. *J Periodontol* 2003; 74: 590–596.

73 Schwarz F, Sculean A, Berakdar M, et al. Clinical evaluation of an Er:YAG laser combined with scaling and root planing for non-surgical periodontal treatment. A controlled, prospective clinical study. *J Clin Periodontol* 2003; 30:26-34.

74 Schwarz F, Sculean A, Georg T, et al. Periodontal treatment with an Er: YAG laser compared to scaling and root planing. A controlled clinical study. *J Periodontol* 2001; 72: 361–367.

75 Schwarz F, Rothamel D, Sculean A, et al. Effects of an Er:YAG laser and the Vector ultrasonic system on the biocompatibility of titanium implants in cultures of human osteoblast-like cells. *Clin Oral Implants Res* 2003; 14: 784–792.

76 Marotti J, Pigozzo MN, Nakamae EDM, et al. Terapia fotodinâmica no tratamento da periimplantite. *Implant News* 2008; 5: 401–405.

77 Takasaki AA, Aoki A, Mizutani K, et al. Application of antimicrobial photodynamic therapy in periodontal and peri-implant diseases. *Periodontology 2000* 2009; 51: 109–140.

78 Hayek RR, Araujo NS, Gioso MA, et al. Comparative study between the effects of photodynamic therapy and conventional therapy on microbial reduction in ligature-induced peri-implantitis in dogs. *J Periodontol* 2005; 76: 1275–1281.

79 Shibli JA, Martins MC, Ribeiro FS, et al. Lethal photosensitization and guided bone regeneration in treatment of peri-implantitis: an experimental study in dogs. *Clin Oral Implants Res* 2006; 17: 273–281.

80 Shibli JA, Martins MC, Nociti FH, Jr, et al. Treatment of ligature-induced peri-implantitis by lethal photosensitization and guided bone regeneration: a preliminary histologic study in dogs. *J Periodontol* 2003; 74: 338–345.

81 Haas R, Baron M, Dortbudak O, et al. Lethal photosensitization, autogenous bone, and e-PTFE membrane for the treatment of peri-implantitis: preliminary results. *Int J Oral Maxillofac Implants* 2000; 15: 374–382.

82 Dörtbudak O, Haas R, Bernhart T, et al. Lethal photosensitization for decontamination of implant surfaces in the treatment of peri-implantitis. *Clin Oral Implants Res* 2001; 12: 104–108.

83 Schuckert KH, Jopp S, Muller U. De novo grown bone on exposed implant surfaces using photodynamic therapy and recombinant human bone morphogenetic protein-2: case report. *Implant Dent* 2006; 15: 361–365.

84 Junker R, Dimakis A, Thoneick M, et al. Effects of implant surface coatings and composition on bone integration: a systematic review. *Clin Oral Implant Res* 2009; 20 (Suppl 4): 185–206.

85 Faeda RS, Spin-Neto R, Marcantonio E, et al. Laser ablation in titanium implants followed by biomimetic hydroxyapatite coating: Histomorphometric study in rabbits. *Microsc Res Tech* 2012; 75: 940–948.

86 Faeda RS, Tavares HS, Sartori R, et al. Evaluation of titanium implants with surface modification by laser beam. Biomechanical study in rabbit tibias. *Braz Oral Res* 2009; 23: 137–143.

87 Cho SA, Jung SK. A removal torque of the laser-treated titanium implants in rabbit tibia. *Biomaterials* 2003; 24: 4859–4863.

88 Forsgren J, Svahn F, Jarmar T, et al. Formation and adhesion of biomimetic hydroxyapatite deposited on titanium substrates. *Acta Biomater* 2007; 3: 980–984.

89 Mangano C, Raspanti M, Traini T, et al. Stereo imaging and cytocompatibility of a model dental implant surface formed by direct laser fabrication. *J Biomed Mater Res A* 2009; 88: 823–831.

90 Shibli JA, Mangano C, D'Avila S, et al. Influence of direct laser fabrication implant topography on type IV bone: a histomorphometric study in humans. *J Biomed Mater Res A* 2010; 93: 607–614.

91 Romanos G, Crespi R, Barone A, et al. Osteoblast attachment on titanium disks after laser irradiation. *Int J Oral Maxillofac Implants* 2006; 21: 232–236.

92 Delgado-Ruiz RA, Calvo-Guirado JL, Moreno P, et al. Femtosecond laser microstructuring of zirconia dental implants. *J Biomed Mater Res B Appl Biomater* 2011; 96: 91–100.

93 Ribeiro DA, Matsumoto MA. Low-level laser therapy improves bone repair in rats treated with anti-inflammatory drugs. *J Oral Rehabil* 2008; 35: 925–933.

CHAPTER 25

Bone biomodulation

Antonio Luiz Barbosa Pinheiro,[1,2] Aparecida Maria Cordeiro Marques,[1,2] Luiz Guilherme Pinheiro Soares,[1,2] and Artur Felipe Santos Barbosa[1–3]

[1] Center of Biophotonics, School of Dentistry, Federal University of Bahia (UFBA), Salvador, BA, Brazil
[2] National Institute of Optics and Photonics, São Carlos, SP, Brazil
[3] Laboratory of Immunomodulation and New Therapeutic Approaches (LINAT), Recife, PE, Brazil

Introduction

Bone loss is a major problem in many medical and dental specialties and may occur due to several physiological and pathological conditions. Physiological bone loss occurs mainly due to aging. Bone tissue has an enormous capacity to regenerate, and most of the time it is able to restore its usual architecture and mechanical properties. However, there are limits to this capacity, and complete recovery may not occur if there is a deficient blood supply, mechanical instability, or competition with highly proliferating tissues. The loss of bone fragments or the removal of necrotic or pathological bone, or even some surgical procedures may lead to bone defects. These defects may be too large for spontaneous and physiological repair.[1]

Several methods can be used to ameliorate bone repair, and these include the use of grafts and more recently low level laser therapy (LLLT). LLLT has been reported as an important tool to positively stimulate bone both *in vivo* and *in vitro*. These results indicate that the photophysical and photochemical properties of some wavelengths are the primary factors responsible for the tissue responses. The use of correct and appropriate parameters has been shown to be effective in the promotion of a positive biomodulatory effect on the repairing bone.[1]

The results of our studies and those of others indicate that bone irradiated mostly with infrared wavelengths shows increased osteoblastic proliferation, collagen deposition, and bone neoformation when compared to non-irradiated bone. The results of our studies indicate that a good outcome with LLLT is observed when the treatment is carried out at early stages when there is high cellular proliferation. Vascular responses to LLLT have also been suggested as a possible mechanism for the positive clinical results observed following LLLT. It still remains uncertain if bone stimulation by laser light is a general effect or if it is the isolated stimulation of osteoblasts that is responsible for the effect.[1]

Bone is an adaptable tissue with a structure that develops according to both the type of mechanical forces exerted on it and its metabolic needs. Bone metabolism responds to hormonal regulation and biomechanics; these two regulatory mechanisms act antagonistically.[2]

Nowadays, a major problem in dentistry is the repair of bone defects caused by trauma, surgical procedures, or pathologies. A wide range of biomaterials has been used to improve the repair of these defects. Both autogenous and xenogenous grafts provide good structure and stimulation of bone neoformation, beyond that achieved through their association with membranes in the guided bone regeneration (GBR) technique.[3,4]

Biomaterials used in the repair of bone loss can be classified as those obtained from human bone tissue (autologous and allogeneic) and those of animal origin (xenograft). Among the synthetically produced (alloplastic) biomaterials, the most widely used are the hydroxyapatites, followed by tricalcium phosphate, bioglass, and polymers.[5–7]

The use of bone morphogenetic proteins (BMPs) is not new in dentistry. These proteins are extensively used in the reconstruction of alveolar bone, the filling of gaps left by bone loss, and the repair of several types of bone defects, as well as GBR.[8] Despite the successful use of biomaterials and BMPs in the bone repair process, other treatments, including the use of laser energy in combination with biomaterials, have been evaluated with the aim of achieving a more effective result.[8,9]

Bone tissue

Bone, which forms the rigid, resistant structure of the skeleton, is a specialized and complex connective tissue, of which a third is an organic matrix composed of type I collagen (28%) and non-collagenous proteins, including osteonectin, osteocalcin, BMPs, bone proteoglycans, and bone sialoprotein.

Despite appearing inert, bone grows; it is continuously remodeled and remains active throughout the lifespan of the individual. This continued vitality is demonstrated by the repair

Lasers in Dentistry: Guide for Clinical Practice, First Edition. Edited by Patrícia M. de Freitas and Alyne Simões.
© 2015 John Wiley & Sons, Inc. Published 2015 by John Wiley & Sons, Inc.

of bone when it is injured, as in a fracture. Bone tissue homeostasis is controlled by mechanical and humoral factors, both local and general.[6,7]

Bone remodeling is mediated primarily by two cell types: the osteoblasts and osteoclasts. Biological and mechanical restoration, unlike in most other organs and tissues, is possible.[10] Bone response to trauma consists of an ordered and well-differentiated sequence of events that results in the repair of the damaged tissue, resulting in a structure quite similar to the initial one.[11,12]

Under physiological conditions, bone tissue has considerable regenerative potential. However, certain situations limit this potential, such as some systemic disorders that interfere with bone metabolism: in these, repair occurs by formation of fibrous tissue, which hinders or even prevents bone tissue regeneration, a phenomenon known as fibrosis.[13]

Several factors may modify the process of osteogenesis and cause, for example, delay in the consolidation of fractures and/or a pseudoarthrosis.[14] In this context, animal models of diabetes mellitus have demonstrated the effect of this condition on the morphology of skeletal tissue by delaying bone repair and alveolar bone remodeling.[15]

Bone repair

Bone repair, regardless of the cause of the injury, consists of a series of events similar to those that occur during the healing of soft tissue wounds: inflammation, fibroplasia, and remodeling. However, in contrast to soft tissue healing, osteoblasts and osteoclasts participate in the reconstruction and remodeling of the injured bone tissue. Initially, the injured site is filled with an embryonic bone tissue, which is highly cellular and is quickly formed, but is relatively less mineralized with randomly oriented fibers and of low resistance. Over time, this bone is replaced by mature lamellar bone, capable of bearing loads, such as an implant, without being compromised.[4–8]

The bone repair process is classically divided into three consecutive phases: inflammatory, repair, and remodeling.

The inflammatory phase is initially characterized by the formation of a blood clot, which involves the bone surfaces in the injured area and extends through the periosteum near the medullary cavities, together with more or less intense edema. This initiates the acute inflammatory process, which involves a significant mobilization of neutrophils.

Inflammation is followed by the repair phase with the appearance of a large number of fibroblasts that produce and secrete collagen in order to form the fibrous callus. A new capillary network is also formed, as well as a process of endochondral or intramembranous ossification. This phase will result in the formation of immature bone.

In the remodeling phase, the callus undergoes a process of resorption and bone formation until it takes on the morphology it had before the lesion.[8]

Bone grafts

Bone grafts may be classified based on both morphological and immunological aspects. According to morphological criteria, they are classified as cancellous, cortical, or cortico-spongeous. The latter is characterized by faster revascularization than cortical bone grafts, with thin trabeculae separated by large marrow spaces filled with hematopoietic cells, which facilitates cell migration, but does not provide significant mechanical support.[11]

Bone grafts may be used to improve the repair of bone defects. These grafts may be autologous, allogenic, heterogenous or alloplastic (biomaterials).[16] Biomaterials are natural or synthetic substances. They are biocompatible and may be used to replace various tissues temporarily or permanently, stimulating chemical and biological reactions that are favorable to the tissues' function.[17]

Biomaterials may act on bone repair by osteoconduction, osteoinduction or osteostimulation. Osteoconduction enables angiogenesis and growth of bone cells from osteoprogenitor cells of the recipient bed, through the surface of the graft, giving rise to osteoblasts; these are responsible for bone formation at the wounded site. Osteostimulation promotes bone growth by transferring osteoblasts together with the graft or by stimulation of osteoblasts in the receiver site. Autogenous bone grafts, both intra- and extra-oral, are examples of biomaterials with this property. Osteoinduction promotes the differentiation of mesenchymal stem cells into perivascular osteoprogenitor cells, under the stimulation of one or more substances released by the bone graft matrix, such as the BMPs.[17]

Bone morphogenetic proteins

The growth and maintenance of bone tissue is a complex process that is influenced by systemic hormones and growth factors. Bone tissue contains several growth factors, including BMPs, which are produced by osteoblasts in a cascade of events initiated by the proliferation of undifferentiated mesenchymal cells and ending with bone formation.[18]

BMPs are members of the transforming growth factor (TGF) superfamily and can stimulate bone formation in various clinical situations, such as tibial fractures, maxillofacial reconstruction, and postsurgical defects. This activity stimulated interest in their clinical applicability and, consequently, industrial production, originally in small quantities from bone extracts. The advent of molecular techniques made possible the production of large quantities of BMPs.[18]

There are over 30 types of BMPs, and the most studied are BMP-1 to BMP-7. However, not all members of this family of proteins are involved in osteoinduction. BMP-2, -4, -6, and -7 are considered potent inducers of odontoblastic differentiation.[19,20] These proteins have been identified as responsible for the development of the acellular cementum, regeneration of the periodontal ligament, and alveolar bone formation in the embryo. *In vitro*, these proteins have been shown to improve cell migration and proliferation of the periodontal ligament, suggesting that they may be clinically used in the repair of periodontal bone defects.[15]

Guided bone regeneration

Membranes or biological barriers have become a hallmark of the guided or directed tissue repair technique. These structures serve to prevent the ingrowth of connective tissue or junctional epithelium into the bone defect. There are basically two types of membranes: resorbable and non-resorbable.[11,12]

The main obstacle to bone regeneration is the faster formation of connective tissue compared to osteogenesis. In the last decade, several animal studies have documented the ability of certain tissues to use membranes to select the cells that repopulate the wound site. This principle has been exploited in the regeneration of periodontal tissues lost due to periodontal disease in the technique called guided periodontal regeneration, the effectiveness of which has been evaluated in both animal and human studies.[19]

A procedure called guided bone regeneration (GBR) has been developed from studies using membranes for the regeneration of bone tissue.[8] Bone defects of the "side-by-side" type created in rats with a 5-mm diameter on the mandible angle were covered with an expanded polytetrafluoroethylene (e-PTFE) membrane extending from the buccal to lingual sides, and complete bone refill was observed after 6 weeks, whereas no bone formation was observed in the controls.

Light therapies in bone repair

Several therapeutic techniques are used in clinical practice to accelerate and/or improve bone repair, including the use of coherent or non-coherent light sources. Among these light sources, we highlight the laser light used for LLLT. This therapeutic approach has been shown to be very effective in the biomodulation of both soft tissue wound healing and the bone repair process. However, many researchers believe that further studies are needed in this area, because photobiostimulation in humans is still controversial.[3,8]

Over the past 10 years, light sources have been used in a number of procedures for the repair of soft tissue wounds in both animals and humans. These treatments are now used also to promote the efficient repair of mineralized tissues, as suggested by a study that concluded that LLLT accelerates the bone repair by directly affecting new bone formation.[21]

Pinheiro and Gerbi,[1] in a comprehensive retrospective study of photobioengineering in bone repair, concluded that the effect of LLLT on bone regeneration depends not only on the total irradiation dose, but also the irradiation time and irradiation

mode. The threshold energy density and intensity are biologically independent of each other. This independence accounts for the success and the failure of LLLT at low energy density levels.

In a study evaluating the effect of LLLT (830 nm, 40 mW, continuous wave) in the repair of standardized rat femur bone defects grafted with inorganic bovine bone, a dose of $4 J/cm^2$ was applied at four points around the wound (a total of $16 J/cm^2$ per session and $112 J/cm^2$ by the end of treatment).[3] The authors observed more advanced repair in irradiated subjects and concluded that LLLT resulted in a positive biomodulatory effect.

In another study, the histological effect of LLLT (830 nm, 50 mW, continuous wave) on the repair process in autogenous bone grafts was assessed.[22] Bone defects were created in the femurs of Wistar rats and the bone fragments removed were used as autologous graft. The animals were divided into four groups according to the radiation protocol during surgery: G1 (control group), G2 (irradiation of the surgical cavity), G3 (irradiation of the bone graft), and G4 (irradiation of the surgical bed and bone graft). The radiation dose applied to the surgical cavity and bone graft was $10 J/cm^2$. All animals, except the control group, were irradiated every 48 hours for 15 days, at four different sites, with observation on days 15, 21, and 30. The results demonstrated that in those groups for which the laser was applied to the surgical cavity during surgery, the bone remodeling activity was qualitatively and quantitatively superior to that in the other groups. The results showed that LLLT has a positive effect on the bone repair process.

A histological study evaluated the effectiveness of LLLT (830 nm, 40 mW) on the bone repair of surgical defects in femurs of rats grafted with lyophilized bovine bone (organic matrix), with or without lyophilized demineralized bovine membrane.[23] The groups were treated with laser radiation at 48-hour intervals from the completion of surgery. The irradiation dose was $16 J/cm^2$ per session, divided between four points ($4 J/cm^2$ per point). The results showed that a greater concentration of collagen fibers was evident in the irradiated surgical wounds at 15 days post surgery, as well as increased bone neoformation with denser and more organized trabeculae at 30 days post surgery, compared to non-irradiated controls. The authors concluded that LLLT had a positive effect on the bone repair process in surgical defects.

Another study evaluated bone cell activity after LLLT (660 nm, $10 J/cm^2$) close to the site of femur injury in rats.[24] The animals were divided into two groups: an irradiated experimental group and a non-irradiated control group. The experimental group was irradiated on days 2, 4, 6, and 8 post surgery. The results were evaluated by bone histomorphometry. Cellular activity was higher in the irradiated group compared to controls and the authors concluded that LLLT increased the activity of bone cells, both in terms of formation and resorption around the site of repair, without changing the bone structure.

The effect of LLLT (830 nm, 40 mW, continuous wave, $16 J/cm^2$ per session) was assessed on the repair of bone defects in Wistar rats.[4] The rats were divided into five groups: control;

Gen-ox®; Gen-ox® + laser; Gen-ox® + Gen-derm®; Gen-ox® + Gen-derm® + laser. The defects were grafted with lyophilized bovine bone (Gen-ox®) with or without GBR (Gen-derm®). The animals were treated with 16 J/cm² divided between four points around the defect (4 × 4 J/cm²), with the first application performed immediately after surgery and then repeated at 48-hour intervals. By day 30, the histological results showed an increase in the deposition of collagen fibers and the presence of more organized trabecular bone in the specimens treated with LLLT.

Another study compared the effects of LLLT (780 nm, 30 mW, 112.5 J/cm²) and ultrasound (1.5 MHz, 30 mW/cm²) on the repair of bone defects in rats.[21] Assessment was carried out by histomorphometry. Animals treated with LLLT showed increased numbers of osteoblasts as well as volume of osteoid tissue, while animals treated with ultrasound showed increased numbers of osteoclasts.

Another histological study evaluated the repair of defects created in femurs of rats treated or not treated with BMPs and bovine bone grafts.[8] The animals were divided into four groups: control; laser; BMPs + GBR; GBR + laser + BMPs. The groups treated with LLLT (830 nm, 40 mW, continuous wave) received seven irradiations, starting immediately after GBR and BMP treatment and then every 48 hours (16 J/cm² per session divided between four equidistant points on the periphery of the defect). The authors found an increase in the collagen deposition on both days 15 and 21 and a better organization of trabecular bone in day 30 in LLLT-treated animals. It was concluded that laser irradiation in combination with BMPs, bovine bone grafts, and GBR had a positive effect on bone repair.

In another study, the efficacy of LLLT (790 nm, 50 mW, continuous wave, 10 J/cm²) was histologically investigated by light microscopy.[25] Twenty-four animals were divided into four groups: group 1 control; group 2 LLLT of the bone graft; group 3 BMPs and bone graft); and group 4 LLLT of the bed and the bone graft and BMPs. When appropriate, the bed was filled with lyophilized bovine bone and BMPs were used with or without GBR. The animals in the irradiated groups received 10 J/cm² per session divided between four points around the defect (4 × 2.5 J/cm²), with the first irradiation given immediately after surgery, and then repeated every other day on seven occasions. The animals were humanely killed after 40 days. In all treatment groups, new bone formation was quantitatively and qualitatively better than in the untreated animals. The less advanced repair in controls after 40 days was characterized by the presence of medullary tissue, small amounts of bone trabeculi, and some cortical repair. It was concluded that LLLT had a positive biomodulatory effect on the repair of bone defects, and that this effect was more evident when LLLT was performed on the surgical bed intraoperatively, prior to the placement of the autologous bone graft.

Another recent report evaluated the effect of LLLT (830 nm, 40 mW, continuous wave) on the repair of surgical wounds in the femur of rats.[9] In this study, animals were divided into four groups: control; LLLT; hydroxyapatite + GBR; GBR + hydroxyapatite + LLLT. The treated animals received the first dose of laser irradiation immediately after surgery and then on every day for 2 weeks at four points, totaling 16 J/cm². Rats were sacrificed at 15, 21, and 30 days. It was concluded that LLLT combined with hydroxyapatite and GBR had a positive effect, mainly in the early stages of repair.

Our group carried out a histological analysis on bone defects grafted with mineral trioxide aggregate (MTA) treated with or without laser irradiation, BMP, and GBR.[26] Benefits of the use of MTA, laser, BMPs, and GBR on bone repair are well known, but there is no report on their use in combination. Ninety rats were divided into ten groups, and each of these subdivided into three subgroups. Defects in groups 1 and 2 were filled with blood clot, in groups 3 and 4 with MTA, in groups 5 and 6 with MTA and covered with a membrane (GBR), in groups 7 and 8 with MTA and BMPs, and in groups 9 and 10 the MTA + BMP graft was covered with a membrane (GBR); groups 2, 4, 6, 8, and 10 were additionally irradiated with laser. Laser light (850 nm, 150 mW, 4 J/cm²) was applied over the defect at 48-hour intervals over 15 days. Specimens were processed, cut and stained with H&E and Sirius red, and subjected to histological analysis. The results showed different tissue responses in all groups over the course of the study. Major changes were seen in the irradiated animals, including marked deposition of new mature bone. It was concluded that combining near infrared LLLT with MTA improved the effects on bone defects.[26]

In another histological analysis, grafted bone defects (MTA) were treated with or without LED irradiation, BMPs, and membrane (GBR).[27] Their benefits individually or combined on bone repair were reported. Ninety rats were divided into ten groups and these groups were treated exactly as in the above study,26 with the exception that groups 2, 4, 6, 8, and 10 were additionally irradiated with LED rather than laser light. LED irradiation was applied over the defect at 48-hour interval over 15 days. Specimens were processed, cut, and stained with H&E and Sirius red and underwent histological analysis. The use of LED light alone dramatically reduced inflammation. However, its use with MTA combined with BMP and/or GBR increased the inflammatory reaction. Regarding bone reabsorption, the poorest result was seen when the LED light was combined with the MTA + BMP graft. In the groups 1 (clot) and 5 (MTA + GBR), no bone reabsorption was detectable. Increased collagen deposition was observed when the LED irradiation was combined with the use of MTA and BMP and/or GBR. Increased new bone formation was observed when the LED light was used alone or combined with the use of MTA + GBR, MTA + BMP, and MTA + BMP + GBR. These results indicate that the use of LED light alone or in combination with MTA, MTA + BMP, MTA + GBR, and MTA + BMP + GBR caused less inflammation, and an increase of both collagen deposition and bone deposition, as observed on both histological and morphometric analysis.

Our team has used Raman analysis to assess bone repair in these different models. Benefits of the isolated or combined use of MTA, BMPs, GBR, and laser on bone repair have been reported. Peaks of hydroxyapatite and CH groups on defects grafted with MTA, treated with or without laser, BMPs, and GBR, were studied. Laser irradiation (850 nm) was applied every other day for 2 weeks. Raman readings were taken at the surface of the defect. Statistical analysis showed significant differences between all groups ($P=0.001$) and between Group 2 and all other groups ($P <0.001$), with the exception of group 10 ($P=0.09$). At day 21, differences were seen between all groups ($P=0.031$) and between groups 8 and 10 when compared with groups 6 ($P=0.03$), 5 ($P <0.001$), 4 ($P <0.001$), and 9 ($P=0.04$). At the end of the experimental period, no significant differences were seen between the groups. With regards to CH groups, significant differences were seen by the 15th day ($P=0.002$) between group 2 and all other groups ($P <0.0001$), but not with the control. Advanced maturation of irradiated bone is due to increased secretion of calcium hydroxyapatite (CHA), which is indicative of greater bone calcification and resistance. It was concluded that the combination of MTA with LLLT and/or with GBR resulted in a better bone repair. The use of MTA combined with infrared LLLT resulted in a more advanced and better quality bone repair.[28]

Fractures have different etiologies and treatment may or may not be associated with bone loss. Laser light has been shown to improve bone repair. We aimed to assess, through Raman spectroscopy, the level of CHA ($\sim$958 cm^{-1}) in complete tibial fracture animals treated with infrared irradiation combined with or without LPT, BMPs, and GBR. Animals with complete tibial fractures were divided into five treatment groups. LLLT (790 nm, 4 J/cm^2 per point, 40 mW, continuous wave, 16 J/cm^2 per session) was started immediately after surgery and repeated at 48-hour intervals for 2 weeks. Animals were killed after 30 days. Raman spectroscopy was performed at the surface of the fracture. Our results showed significant differences between the groups internal rigid fixation (IRF) + bone loss (BL) and IRF-no bone loss (IRF_NBL) ($P=0.05$); between all experimental groups and untreated bone; bone/IRF + BL; IRF + BL + Bio + GBR; IRF + BL + LLLT; IRF + BL + Bio + GBR + LLLT; IRF_NBL ($P <0.001$, all); IRF_NBL/IRF + BL + LLLT ($P=0.03$); IRF_NBL/IRF + BL + Bio + GBR + LLLT ($P=0.02$); IRF + BL/IRF + BL + LLLT ($P=0.04$); IRF + BL/IRF + BL + Bio + GBR + LLLT ($P=0.002$); IRF + BL + Bio + GBR/IRF + BL + Bio + GBR + LLLT ($P=0.05$). It was concluded that the use of near infrared LLLT combined with BMPs and GBR was effective in improving the repair of fractured bones due to increased levels of CHA.[29]

Raman spectroscopy and fluorescence at the fracture surface were used to measure the levels of CHA, lipids, and proteins in complete fractures in animals treated with IRF with or without LLLT, BMPs, and GBR. The fluorescence data for the group IRF + LLLT + BMP were similar to those for the group IRF_NBL. Significant differences were seen between the groups IRF + LLLT + BMP and IRF + LLLT; IRF + LLLT + BMP; and IRF + BMP; and between the groups IRF + LPT + BMP and IRF. There were decreased levels of CH groups of lipids and proteins in animals treated with LPT + BMP + GBR. Pearson correlation showed that fluorescence readings for both CHA and CH groups of lipids and proteins correlated negatively with the Raman data. The use of both methods indicates that the use of the biomaterials combined with infrared LLLT resulted in a more advanced and higher quality of bone repair in fractures treated with miniplates and that the DIAGNOdent® may be used to perform optical biopsy of bone.[30]

The step-by-step procedures for the use of laser light and the effect on bone tissue are illustrated in Figure 25.1. Figure 25.1a shows the initial receptor bed of a mandible before the fixation of two different types of grafts (autologous and xenograft). After decortication with burs, the surface was irradiated with the laser light (Fig. 25.1b). After the irradiation, the blocks of grafts were fixed with screws (Fig. 25.1c,d). The grafts were then irradiated every other day for 15 days with infrared laser light (780 nm, 70 mW, continuous wave, 21.5 J/cm^2). Nine weeks after the initial procedure, the grafted site was re-exposed, the fixation was removed, and a 3.5 × 7-mm dental implant was inserted in each of the previously inserted grafts (Fig. 25.1e,f). LLLT (780 nm, 70 mW, 0.5 cm^2 spot, 4 J/cm^2 per spot [four], 16 J/cm^2 per session, 48-hour intervals between 12 sessions, continuous wave, contact mode) was used as previously described for a further 2 weeks. Histological analysis of both implants sites was carried out and showed that newly-formed mature bone involving the threads of the implants was present (Fig. 25.1 g,h).

The procedures in humans follow the same sequence. Figure 25.2a shows the inserted dental implants, and Figure 25.2b the points irradiated immediately after surgery. Usually it is recommended that at least three points along the length of the implant are irradiated, and where possible four points around the implant head on the occlusal surface. For bone, infrared laser light is recommended due to its higher penetration. After suturing, a visible laser light may be used to improve soft tissue healing. Again, the implants were irradiated with infrared light every other day for 15 days (Fig. 25.2c).

Tooth movement is closely related to the process of bone remodeling. The application of a force to the tooth results in bone absorption on the pressure side and neoformation on the traction side of the alveolar bone. Hyalinization, that is the sterile necrosis at the pressure zone of the periodontal ligament, is observed during the initial stages of the orthodontic movement and when extensive, may cause an important delay in tooth movement. Changes in alveolar bone during orthodontic movement in rats have also being studied as orthodontic movement is affected by LLLT. In a series of studies involving the use of LLLT during tooth movement in rodents, an increase in cellular metabolism, blood flow, and lymphatic drainage was observed.

We have studied young-adult Wistar rats receiving orthodontic devices calibrated to release a force of 40 g/F to move the first upper molar mesially. In the experimental group of animals, LLLT (790 nm, 4.5 J/cm per point, mesial and distal, on the palatal side; 11 J/cm^2 per point on the buccal side) was

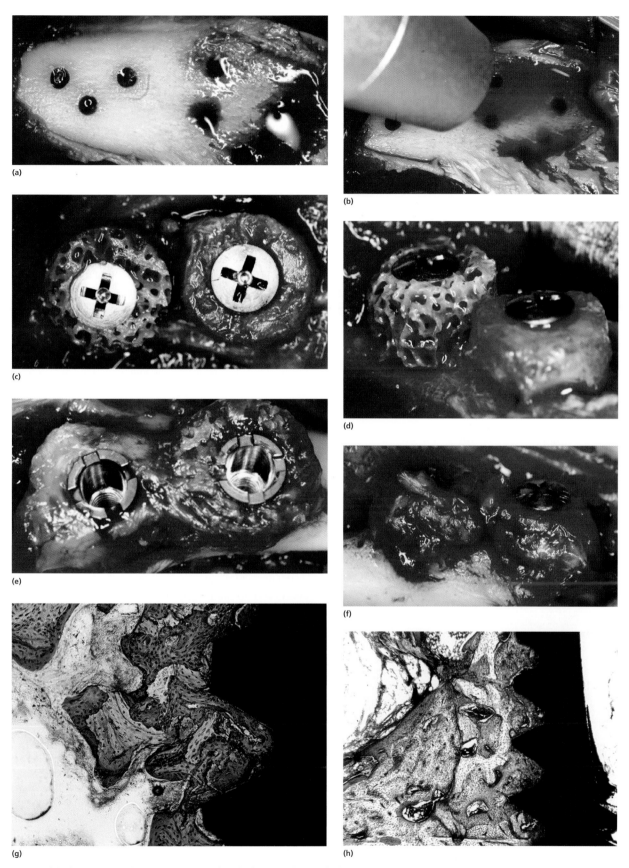

Figure 25.1 (a) The decorticated receptor site. (b) Before the fixation of the graft, the receptor bed is irradiated with infrared light (visible light is shown for the purpose of illustration). (c,d) The grafted site immediately after surgery. Following fixation, the blocks are irradiated with infrared light for 15 days. (e,f) The grafts at 9 weeks; already incorporated and ready to receive the implants. (g,h) Histology of the newly formed bone around the threads of the implants at 30 days after insertion. Note that the bone is mature and in close association with the implants.

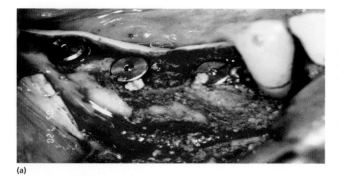

(a)

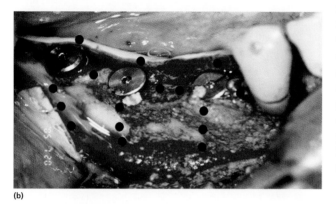

(b)

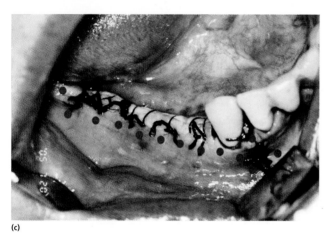

(c)

Figure 25.2 (a) Clinical image of the implants inserted in the jaw. (b) Before suturing, the implanted area is irradiated with infrared laser light at points along the length of the implant and at the occlusal surface. (c) The soft tissues are also irradiated with visible red light to improve wound healing. After surgery, irradiation with infrared light is carried out for 15 days.

repeated every 48 hours, totaling nine applications. The active movement was clinically evaluated after 7, 13, and 19 days. The results showed no statistically significant difference ($P = 0.079$ T0–T7, $P = 0.597$ T7–T13, and $P = 0.550$ T13–T19) between the laser and control groups in the amount of tooth movement at the different times evaluated. We also found that LLLT-irradiated specimens showed significantly higher numbers of osteoclasts when compared with controls at both 7 ($P = 0.015$) and 19 ($P = 0.007$) days, as well as significant

increases in the number of osteoblasts ($P = 0.015$) between days 7 and 13. The amount of collagen matrix was significantly reduced between days 7 and 13 at both pressure and tension sites in the controls ($P = 0.015$), but not in the LLLT-treated animals. The latter showed significantly greater deposition of collagen matrix at the pressure site on both days 13 ($P = 0.007$) and 19 ($P = 0.001$). At the tension site, a significant increase in the amount of collagen matrix was observed in non-irradiated specimens ($P = 0.048$) between days 7 and 19. In addition, it was demonstrated that LLLT positively affected an important aspect of dental movement – hyalinization was significantly reduced after 19 days. In irradiated animals, hyalinization was increased at day 7 with significant reduction at day 13. Despite these studies indicating that LLLT using the stated parameters did not significantly increase the amount of tooth displacement during induced orthodontic movement in rodents, it did cause significant histological changes in the alveolar bone during induced tooth movement, including alterations in the number of both osteoclasts and osteoblasts; collagen deposition in both pressure and tension areas; and histological alterations in the hyalinization at early stages and late reduction when compared to non-irradiated animals.[31–33]

Concluding remarks

Bone repair is an important homeostatic process that depends on specialized cell activation and bone immobility. A variety of factors such as age, nutrition, and medical co-morbidities may mediate the repair process.

Although bone tissue shows good regeneration, with restoration of its structure and mechanical properties, this capacity for repair may be impaired by poor blood supply, mechanical instability, and the presence of other tissues with higher proliferative activity. Large bone losses result in large defects, which are too big for routine bone repair. Several techniques have been extensively studied to accelerate the bone repair process and improve the recovery of large bone defects, including photobioengennering.[1]

The physiological effects of low level lasers occur at the cellular level, and may stimulate or inhibit biochemical and physiological mechanisms by altering intercellular communication. The possibility of selectively influencing bone formation by controlling both the quality and quantity of new bone has become a reality due to the technological development of biomaterials and methods and the evolution of knowledge of the cellular and molecular biology of bone formation. However, the development of the ideal graft material to replace autogenous bone graft still remains one of the great challenges of modern dentistry.[25,33]

Initially, *in vitro* studies of the interaction between osteoblasts and biomaterials were essentially concerned with the effect of the cellular response to various types of materials, with little attention being given to the influence of the physicochemical characterization of the surfaces. The extrinsic properties of biomaterials have a critical role in the establishment of the interface between the cell and biomaterials and the manufacturing conditions that affect their surface properties.[33,34]

The biological response to materials indicates whether or not they are biocompatible. The absence of a foreign body reaction, proliferation of osteoblastic cells, and ability to function as a substrate for bone regeneration are important characteristics for biomaterials intended for use in osteogenic modulation.[34–36]

There are several studies that demonstrate the effectiveness of the use of BMPs in the bone repair process both *in vivo*[4,5,8] and *in vitro*, as well as the benefit of using biological membranes.[4,9] In contrast, studies of the combined use of LLLT and biomaterials in bone repair that use similar parameters are limited.[3,4]

Recent studies have investigated methods to achieve quicker bone repair. Several investigations have shown that BMPs serve as an osteoinductive agent in bone repair due to their osteogenic effect; the principal function of BMPs is the induction of bone formation. These proteins are effective in large bone defects, and this effect is synergistic with that of an organic matrix.[3,4,9]

According to some authors,[2] the presence of the grafted material interferes with the normal course of the repair and may exacerbate the inflammatory response to a moderate level, delaying repair. Other authors have also observed this delay and a mononuclear inflammatory reaction in the presence of grafted material.[7] However, other authors consider the initial delay in the repair process to be a natural physiological reaction due to the presence of bone graft particles and the slower deposition of new bone around the material, which is directly proportional to its reabsorption.[22,23]

Laser irradiation possesses a wavelength-dependent capacity to alter cellular behavior in the absence of significant heating. The dispersion of the laser light in tissues is very complex as it is influenced by many tissue components. The results of our studies and those of others indicate that bone irradiated mostly with infrared wavelengths shows increased osteoblastic proliferation, collagen deposition, and bone neoformation when compared to non-irradiated bone. It is known that the stimulant effect of the laser light on bone occurs during the initial phase of proliferation of both fibroblasts and osteoblasts, as well as the initial differentiation of mesenchymal cells. Fibroblastic proliferation and increased fibroblast activity have been detected in irradiated subjects and cells cultures and these are responsible for the higher concentration of collagen fibers seen within irradiated bone.[1]

LLLT is an interesting therapeutic approach. However, the protocols proposed so far have not allowed a full determination of the optimal parameters. The wide range of possible laser parameter combinations make the establishment of an effective protocol very complex.[1,3,4,9,37]

Laser light has a positive effect on bone formation. This effect is more evident around defects also treated with hydroxyapatite grafts[1,37]: the thickness of the newly formed cortical bone is similar to that of the untreated bone.

The literature has demonstrated that the combined use of LLLT and BMPs, though these act differently, has a positive effect on bone repair. They accelerate bone repair without adverse effects.[1,3,4,9,37] The laser effects appear to be due to increased levels of growth factors, such as fibroblast growth factor, which are found in repairing bone tissue and act on differentiated cells to increase the rate of proliferation and stimulate the maturation and secretion of bone matrix. It is also accepted that LLLT may accelerate the repair process by promoting the synthesis of bone matrix due to increased vascularization and early onset of the inflammatory response.

Our experience supports the idea that LLLT can induce undifferentiated mesenchymal cells to differentiate into osteoblasts that then differentiate more rapidly into osteocytes. However, LLLT seems to be less effective or ineffective on undamaged tissues as its positive biomodulatory effect demands some level of tissue deficiency. It is known that the osteogenic potential of mesenchymal cells depends on several genetic factors and also on systemic and local inducer factors. LLLT improves bone matrix production due to both its vascularization and anti-inflammatory effect. These aspects would result in an increase in both the release of mediators and microvascularization, which would subsequently accelerate bone repair.[1,3,4,6,8,9,22,23,25–33,37–45]

Improved bone maturation in irradiated subjects is due to increased deposition of CHA. During the early stages of repair, the osteoblastic activity is chiefly proliferative, with later deposition of immature bone still poor in CHA. LLLT appears to improve the ability of mature osteoblasts to secrete CHA. However, the effect of LPT is poorly detected before 30 days after treatment because, during the early stages of bone repair, the cellular component is more prominent and more prone to be affected by the light. With the progression of the repair process, the bone matrix becomes the main component of the repair tissue. This also explains why LLLT is effective when carried out during the cellular phase when the number of osteoblasts is increasing. Later, the higher number of cells results in a larger deposition of bone matrix, which later incorporates CHA.[1,3,4,6,8,9,22,23,25–33,37–45]

Deposition of CHA characterizes bone maturation and is indicative of more resistant bone. The observed differences in the rate of deposition of CHA between irradiated and control subjects is probably due to the choice of a laser wavelength that penetrates bone and increases changes at the cellular level, such as improved ATP synthesis, early osteoblastic differentiation, and the release of growth factors.[1,3,4,6,8,9,22,23,25–33,37–45]

The use of phototherapies has been reported to improve bone repair under different conditions.[1,3,4,6,8,9,22,23,25–33,37–45] The effects of light irradiation on bone are still controversial, as there have been different or conflicting results. It is possible that the effect of different light sources on bone regeneration depends not only on the total dose of irradiation, but also on the irradiation time and the irradiation mode.[1,3,4,6,8,9,22,23,25–33,37–45]

Many studies have indicated that irradiated bone, mostly irradiated with infrared wavelengths, shows increased osteoblastic proliferation, collagen deposition, and bone neoformation when compared to non-irradiated bone.[1,3,4,6,8,9,22,23,25–33,37–45] Our group has shown, using different models, that the combined use of bone grafts, BMPs, and GBR improves the repair of bone.[1,3,4,6,8,9,22,23,25–33,37–45]

Despite all the different protocols, models, and parameters that have been tested, we have demonstrated that near infrared LLLT causes important tissue responses during healing and these are responsible for a quicker repair process as well as improved quality of the newly formed bone.[1,3,4,6,8,9,22,23,25–33,37–45] However, other studies have reported mixed results, with some observing an acceleration of fracture repair after LLLT,[46–50] and others delayed fracture repair.[51,52]

Many studies have reported a positive effect of LLLT on bone repair,[53–55] while others have reported negative results.[52]

Teng et al.[54] reported improvement in the composition and biomechanical properties of bone following irradiation for 35 days with two types of laser, compared to controls. An earlier study[52] may have reported false-negative findings as a result of the systemic effects of LLLT.[56,57] In addition, it has to be considered that the surgery on or fracture of both hind limbs of the animals in David et al.'s study[52] excessively limited the mobility of the animals and this may have affected the bone repair process.[58]

Bashardoust Tajali et al.[59] found a statistically significant impact of laser irradiation on the biomechanical properties of healed bone, particularly when more than 14 sessions of irradiation were given. Furthermore, they commented that their fail-safe calculation indicated that a large number of contradictory studies would be required to refute this finding. This would suggest that sufficient animal research is available to support the experimental use of laser irradiation for bone repair in humans. [1,3,4,6,8,9,22,23,25–33,37–45]

Findings of improved bone repair in animal models with adjunctive LLLT are consistent with other previously reported LLLT effects. The cellular reactions such as ATP synthesis promotion, electron transport chain stimulation, and cellular pH reduction,[60,61] as well as biochemical and cell membrane changes may increase the activities of macrophages, fibroblasts, lymphocytes, and other cells involved in the repair process.[62,63]

Increased collagen and DNA synthesis, faster removal of necrotic tissue,[64] increased of Ca^{2+} deposition,[28–30,41–43,46–48] increased periosteum cell function,[65] increased osteoblast and osteocyte function,[46,65] improved neovascularization,[47,48] stimulation of endochondral ossification, earlier differentiation of mesenchymal cells, increased preosteogenic cells,[49] stimulation of callus formation,[47,48] stimulation of bone formation when combined with autologous bone grafts[22,25] and allografts and GBR,[3,4,6,8,9,23,26–28,40,44,45] improved integration of dental implants,[38,41,43] induced changes in bone, decreased hyalinization during orthodontic movement,[32,33] and accelerated repair of fractures[38,41,43,65] are some of the reported positive effects of LLLT on the bone repair process and may explain the stimulation of bone repair by LLLT.[1,3,4,6,8,9,22,23,25–33,37–45]

LLLT is a modern tool that in the future can be expected to be commonly found among a dentist's equipment, widening treatment options. However, the mechanism of the effect of LLLT is complex and difficult to understand. Our experimental results revealed a significant increase in the amount of collagen fibers and the deposition of bone with a compact and conspicuous lamellar arrangement associated with increased vascularity when bone is irradiated.

The use of biomaterials is well established in bone repair, but new therapies, particularly those involving LLLT, and other materials are constantly being tested with the aim of achieving better results.

LLLT may achieve excellent results in the postoperative period, such as the reduction of inflammation and pain, and the acceleration of the healing time of surgical wounds. The positive effects of biomodulation or biostimulation of the healing process in soft and hard tissues have been shown in several reported studies. Therefore, it is believed that in the case of bone mechanical imbrication of dental implants, laser light may accelerate the process of implant integration into the bone due to a positive biomodulation of the bone repair process in the peri-implant tissue.

The number of studies on the use of lasers in dentistry is growing and it is extremely important that dentists access the specific literature showing the great benefits of the technique in the bone repair process. LLLT improves most dental surgical procedures by reducing postsurgical symptoms (pain, swelling, and inflammation) and accelerating new bone formation (by 30–35%). However, as in any other area of expertise, when using LLLT an adequate knowledge of the properties of laser irradiation is essential, as well as the irradiation parameters such as wavelength, power density, energy density, frequency of irradiation, emission modes, and application form, among others.

It is established that LLLT stimulates and accelerates bone repair, although more studies are being conducted to elucidate the mechanism of action of laser light in the bone repair process. At present, it remains uncertain whether the stimulation of bone formation by LLLT is the result of a general effect on mesenchymal cells or a direct stimulation of osteoblasts, or both.

References

1 Pinheiro ALB, Gerbi MEMM. Photobioengineering of the bone repair process. *Photomed Laser Surg* 2006; 24: 169–178.

2 Misch CE. Implantes dentários contemporâneos [Contemporary dental implants]. In: *Reações do Osso as Cargas Mecânicas [Bone Reactions to Mechanical Loads]*. Sao Paulo: Editora Santos, 2001: 317–328.

3 Pinheiro ALB, Limeira Jr, FA, Gerbi MEMM, et al. Effect of 830 nm laser light on the repair of bone defects grafted with inorganic bovine bone and decalcified cortical osseous membrane. *J Clin Laser Med Surg* 2003; 21: 383–388.

4 Gerbi MEMM, Pinheiro ALB, Marzola C, et al. Assessment of bone repair associated with the use of organic bovine bone and membrane irradiated at 830 nm. *Photomed Laser Surg* 2005; 23: 382–388.

5 Carpio L, Loza, J, Samuel L, et al. Guided bone regeneration around endosseous implants with anorganic bovine bone mineral: A randomized controlled trial comparing bioabsorbable versus non-resorbable barriers. *J Periodontol* 2000; 71: 1743–1749.

6 Limeira Jr FA. *Estudo do Reparo ósseo após irradiação com laser 830 nm associada a implante de hidroxiapatita e membrana de osso [tese] [A study on the bone repair following irradiation with 830 nm laser light associated to grafting with hydroxyapatite and osseous membrane – Thesis].* Salvador: Universidade Federal da Bahia, 2004.

7 Pinto LP, Brito JHM, Oliveira MG. Avaliação histológica do processo de reparo ósseo na presença da proteína morfogenética óssea (Gen-Pro) associada com membrana biológica (Gen-Derm) [Histological assessment of bone repair on the presence of bone morphogenetic protein (Gen-Pro) associated to biological membrane (Gen-Derm)]. *Rev Bras Cir Protese Implant* 2003; 10: 25–32.

8 Pinheiro ALB, Gerbi MEMM, Ponzi EAC, et al. Infrared laser light further improves bone healing when associated with bone morphogenetic proteins and guided bone regeneration: An *in vivo* study in a rodent model. *Photomed Laser Surg* 2008; 26: 167–174.

9 Pinheiro ALB, Gerbi MEMM, Limeira Jr FA, et al. Bone repair following bone grafting hydroxyapatite guided bone regeneration and infra-red laser photobiomodulation: a histological study in a rodent mode. *Lasers Med Sci* 2009; 24: 234–240.

10 Einhorn TA. The cell and molecular biology of fracture healing. *Clin Orthop* 1998; 355: 7–21.

11 Day SM, Ostrum RF, Chao EYS, et al. Bone injury, regeneration, and repair. In: Buckwalter JA, Einhorn TA, Simon SR, eds. *Orthopaedic Basic Science.* Chicago: AAO, 2000: 371–399.

12 Mendonça RG, Freitas AC, Ramalho LP, et al. Avaliação Histológica do Processo de Reparo Ósseo após Implantação de BMPs [Histological assessment of bone repair following the implantation of BMPs]. *Pesq Bras Odontoped Clin Integr* 2007; 7: 291–296.

13 Seal BL, Otero TC, Panith A. Polymeric biomaterials for tissue and organ regeneration. *Mater Sci Eng* 2001; 34: 147–230.

14 Giordano V. *Influência do tenoxicam no processo de consolidação de fratura. Estudo experimental em tíbia de ratos [tese] [Influence of tenoxican on the consolidation of fractures. Experimental study on the tibia of rats – (Thesis)].* Rio de Janeiro: Universidade Federal do Rio de Janeiro, 1999.

15 Funk JR, Hale JE, Carmines D, et al. Biomechanical evaluation of early fracture healing in normal and diabetic rats. *J Orthop Res* 2000; 18: 126–132.

16 Bernard GW. Healing and repair of osseous defects. *Dent Clin North Am* 1991; 35: 469–477.

17 Carvalho PSP, Bassi APF, Violin LA. Revisão e proposta de nomenclatura para os biomateriais [Review and proposal of nomenclature for biomaterials]. *Implant News* 2004; 1: 255–259.

18 Wozney JM. Biology and clinical applications of BMP-2. In: Lyinch SE, Genco RJ, Marx RE, eds. *Tissue engineering applications in maxillofacial surgery and periodontics.* Illinois: Quintessence Books, 1999: 103–123.

19 Partridge K, Yang X, Clarke NMP, et al. Adenoviral BMP-2 gene transfer in mesenchymal stem cells: *in vitro* and *in vivo* bone formation on biodegradable polymer scaffolds. *Biochem Biophys Res Commun* 2002; 292: 144–152.

20 Yoon ST, Boden SD. Osteoinductive molecules in orthopaedics: basic science and preclinical studies. *Clin Orthop Relat Res* 2002; 395: 33–43.

21 Galvão LAP, Jorgetti V, da Silva OL. Comparative study of how low-level laser therapy and low-intensity pulsed ultrasound affect bone repair in rats. In: Casalechi VL, Casalechi HL, Sonnewend D, Nicolau RA, eds. XI Encontro Latino Americano de Iniciação Científica e VII Encontro Latino Americano de Pós-Graduação – Universidade do Vale do Paraíba, 2006: 1841–1844.

22 Weber JBB, Pinheiro ALB, De Oliveira MG, et al. Laser therapy improves healing of bone defects submitted to autologous bone graft. *Photomed Laser Surg* 2006; 24: 38–44.

23 Gerbi M, Limeira FA Jr, Pinheiro ALB, et al. Assessment of bone repair associated to the use of organic bone graft and membrane with 830 nm. *SPIE Lasers Dent* 2003; 4950: 137–143.

24 Nicolau RA, Jorgetti V, Rigau J, et al. Effect of low-power GaAlAs laser (660 nm) on bone structure and cell activity: an experimental animal study. *Lasers Med Sci* 2003; 18: 49–94.

25 Torres CS, Santos JN, Pinheiro ALB, et al. Does the use of laser photobiomodulation, bone morphogenetic proteins, and guided bone regeneration improve the outcome of autologous bone grafts? An *in vivo* study in a rodent model. *Photomed Laser Surg* 2008; 26: 371–377.

26 Pinheiro ALB, Soares LGP, Aciole GTS, et al. Light microscopic description of the effects of laser phototherapy on bone defects grafted with mineral trioxide aggregate, bone morphogenetic proteins, and guided bone regeneration in a rodent model. *J Biomed Mat Res Part A* 2011; 98: 212–221.

27 Pinheiro ALB, Soares LGP, Barbosa AFS, et al. Does LED phototherapy influence the repair of bone defects grafted with MTA, bone morphogenetic proteins, and guided bone regeneration? A description of the repair process on rodents. *Lasers Med Sci* 2012; 27(5): 1013–1024.

28 Pinheiro ALB, Aciole GTS, Cangussú MCT, et al. Effects of laser phototherapy on bone defects grafted with mineral trioxide aggregate, bone morphogenetic proteins, and guided bone regeneration: A Raman spectroscopic study. *J Biomed Mat Res Part A* 2010; 95: 1041–1047.

29 Lopes CB, Pacheco MTT, Silveira L, et al. The effect of the association of near infrared laser therapy, bone morphogenetic proteins, and guided bone regeneration on tibial fractures treated with internal rigid fixation: A Raman spectroscopic study. *J Biomed Mat Res Part A* 2010; 94: 1257–1263.

30 Pinheiro ALB, Lopes CB, Pacheco MTT, et al. Raman spectroscopy validation of DIAGNOdent-assisted fluorescence readings on tibial fractures treated with laser phototherapy, BMPs, guided bone regeneration, and miniplates. *Photomed Laser Surg* 2010; 28 (Suppl 2): S89–97.

31 Gama SKC, Habib FAL, de Carvalho JSM, et al. Tooth movement after infrared laser phototherapy: Clinical study in rodents. *Photomed Laser Surg* 2010; 28 (Suppl 2): S79–83.

32 Habib FAL, Gama SKC, Ramalho LMP, et al. Laser-induced alveolar bone changes during orthodontic movement: A histological study on rodents. *Photomed Laser Surg* 2010; 28: 823–830.

33 Habib FAL, Gama SKC, Ramalho LMP, et al. Effect of laser phototherapy on the hyalinization following orthodontic tooth movement in rats. *Photomed Laser Surg* 2012; 30: 179–185.

34 Carbonari M, Ludtke J, Santos PCV, et al. Caracterização físico-química e biológica de enxerto ósseo bovino, Bonefill, em bioensaios. *Implant News* 2010; 7: 103–110.

35 Anselme K, Bigerelle M, Noel B, et al. Qualitative and quantitative study of human osteoblast adhesion on materials with various surface roughnesses. *J Biomed Mater Res* 2000; 49: 155–166.

36 Luk KD, Chen Y, Cheung KM, et al. Adeno-associated virus-mediated bone morphogenetic protein-4 gene therapy for in vivo bone formation. *Biochem Biophys Res Commun* 2006; 308: 636–645.

37 Pinheiro ALB, Brugnera A Jr, Zanin FAA. *Aplicação do Laser na Odontologia [Laser Applications in Dentistry]*. Sao Paulo: Santos Ltd, 2010: 351–379.

38 Pinheiro ALB, Oliveira MAM, Martins PPM. Biomodulação da cicatrização óssea pós-implantar com o uso da laserterapia não-cirúrgica: estudo por microscopia eletrônica de varredura [Biomodulation of peri-implant bone repair associated to the use of non-surgical laser therapy: MEV study]. *Rev FOUFBA* 2001; 22: 12–19.

39 Silva Junior AN, Pinheiro ALB, Oliveira MG, et al. Computerized morphometric assessment of the effect of low-level laser therapy on bone repair: an experimental animal study. *J Clin Laser Med Surg* 2002; 20: 83–88.

40 Pinheiro ALB, Limeira Junior FA, Gerbi MEMM, et al. Effect of low level laser therapy on the repair of bone defects grafted with inorganic bovine bone. *Braz Dent J* 2003; 14: 177–181.

41 Lopes CB, Pinheiro ALB, Sathaiah S, et al. Infrared laser light reduces loading time of dental implants: a Raman spectroscopy study. *Photomed Laser Surg* 2005; 23: 27–31.

42 Lopes CB, Pacheco MTT, Silveira L Jr, et al. The effect of the association of NIR laser therapy BMPs, and guided bone regeneration on tibial fractures treated with wire osteosynthesis: Raman spectroscopy study. *J Photochem Photobiol B Biol* 2007; 89: 125–130.

43 Lopes CB, Pinheiro ALB, Sathaiah S, et al. Infrared laser photobiomodulation (830 nm) on bone tissue around dental implants: a Raman spectroscopy and scanning electron microscopy study in rabbits. *Photomed Laser Surg* 2007; 25: 96–101.

44 Gerbi MEMM, Marques AMC, Ramalho LMP, et al. Infrared Laser light further improves bone healing when associated with bone morphogenic proteins: an in vivo study in a rodent model. *Photomed Laser Surg* 2008; 26: 55–60.

45 Gerbi MEMM, Pinheiro ALB, Ramalho LMP. Effect of IR laser photobiomodulation on the repair of bone defects grafted with organic bovine bone. *Lasers Med Sci* 2008; 23: 313–317.

46 Yamada K. Biological effects of low power laser irradiation on clonal osteoblastic cells (MC3T3-E1). *J Jpn Orthop Assoc* 1991; 65: 101–114.

47 Tang XM, Chai BP. Effect of CO_2 laser irradiation on experimental fracture healing: A transmission electron microscopic study. *Lasers Surg Med* 1986; 6(3): 346–352.

48 Motomura K. Effects of various laser irradiation on callus formation after osteotomy. *Nippon Reza Igakkai Shi [J Jpn Soc Laser Med]* 1984; 4(1): 195–196.

49 Nagasawa A, Kato K, Takaoka K. Experimental evaluation on bone repairing activation effect of lasers based on bone morphologic protein. *Nippon Reza Igakkai Shi [J Jpn Soc Laser Med]* 1988; 9(3): 165–168.

50 Pourreau-Schneider N, Soudry M, Remusat M, et al. Modifications of growth dynamics and ultrastructure after helium-neon laser treatment of human gingival fibroblasts. *Quintessence Int* 1989; 20: 887–893.

51 Gordjestani M, Dermaut L, Thierens H. Infrared laser and bone metabolism: A pilot study. *Int J Oral Maxillofac Surg* 1994; 23: 54–56.

52 David R, Nissan M, Cohen I, et al. Effect of low power He-Ne laser on fracture healing in rats. *Lasers Surg Med* 1996; 19: 458–464.

53 Tajali SB, Ebrahimi E, Kazemi S, et al. Effects of He-Ne laser irradiation on osteosynthesis. *Osteosynth Trauma Care* 2003; 11: S17–20.

54 Teng J, Liu YP, Zhang Y, et al. Effect of He-Ne laser versus low level CO_2 laser irradiation on accelerating fracture healing. *Chin J Clin Rehabil* 2006; 10: 179–181.

55 Luger EJ, Rochkind S, Wollman Y, et al. Effect of low power laser irradiation on the mechanical properties of bone fracture healing in rats. *Lasers Surg Med* 1998; 22: 97–102.

56 Mester E, Mester AF, Mester A. Biomedical effects of laser application. *Lasers Surg Med* 1985; 5: 31–39.

57 Schultz RJ, Krishnamurthy S, Thelmo W, et al. Effects of varying intensities of laser energy on articular cartilage: A preliminary study. *Lasers Surg Med* 1985; 5: 577–588.

58 Buckwalter JA, Einhorn TA, Bolander ME, et al. Healing of the musculoskeletal tissues. In: Rockwood CA, Green DP, et al., eds. *Fracture in Adults*, 4th edn. New York: Lippincott-Raven, 1996: 261–304.

59 Bashardoust Tajali S, MacDermid JC, Houghton P, et al. Effects of low power laser irradiation on bone healing in animals: a meta-analysis. *J Orthop Surg Res* 2010; 5: 1.

60 Cameron MH, Perez D, Otano Lata S. Electromagnetic radiation. In: Cameron MH, ed. *Physical Agents in Rehabilitation, From Research to Practice*. Philadelphia: WB Saunders, 1999: 303–344.

61 Karu TI. Molecular mechanisms of the therapeutic effects low intensity laser radiation. *Lasers Life Sci* 1989; 2: 53–74.

62 Young S, Bolton P, Dyson M, et al. Macrophage responsiveness to light therapy. *Lasers Surg Med* 1989; 9: 497–505.

63 Passarella S, Casamassima E, Quagliariello E, et al. Quantitative analysis of lymphocyte-Salmonella interaction and effects of lymphocyte irradiation by He-Ne laser. *Biochem Biophys Res Commun* 1985; 130: 546–552.

64 Gordjestani M, Dermaut L, Thierens H. Infrared laser and bone metabolism: A pilot study. *Int J Oral Maxillofac* 1994; 23: 54–56.

65 Trelles MA, Mayayo E. Bone fracture consolidate faster with low power laser. *Lasers Surg Med* 1987; 7: 36–45.

CHAPTER 26

Use of low level laser therapy in lymphatic drainage for edema

Luciana Almeida-Lopes and Attilio Lopes
Research and Education Center for Photo Therapy in Health Sciences, São Carlos, SP, Brazil

Introduction

Low level laser therapy (LLLT) was developed in Hungary in the 1960s by Mester,[1] who sought better tissue repair in the treatment of patients with wounds, and this was the first clinical indication for LLLT. Currently, LLLT is widely used in the treatment of the initial phases of the tissue repair process, and as an extension of this, in the treatment of the tissue inflammation process.

The first papers concerning this theme were published in the late 1980s and early 1990s.[2-5] LLLT was believed to be of use in the treatment of inflammation scenarios by activating lymphatic flow in the irradiated region[3,6] and stimulating local immunity.[7] It then began to be used for the treatment of inflammation, both acute (exudative inflammation) and chronic (proliferating inflammation). The mechanism of action of laser irradiation in the inflammatory process and its clinical deployment are described in Chapter 5. Here, the repair process that contains the inflammation, and consequently, the edema, is briefly described.

Tissue injury (infectious, chemical, physical, ischemic or mechanical) may trigger a local inflammation. Its purpose is to eliminate the aggressive agent and dead cells, and to allow extracellular matrix destruction in the area of injury. Mechanisms to heal local aggression-induced injuries begin very early in this inflammation process, and result in the repair and replacement of dead or injured cells with healthy cells. However, the repair process is not a simple, linear process, activated by growth factors and cytokines that trigger cell proliferation. It is characterized by the integration of dynamic interactive processes involving soluble mediators, figurative elements of the blood, extracellular matrix production, and parenchymatous cells. When triggered, these processes occur simultaneously and are an inherent part of the inflammation process that results from tissue injury.

Tissue repair occurs in three phases: inflammation, granulation tissue formation with extracellular matrix deposit, and tissue remodeling[8]; these phases also are superimposed in time.

The inflammatory phase is characterized by five cardinal signs of inflammation: edema, pain, erythema, heat, and loss of function. LLLT does not act as a traditional anti-inflammatory treatment, but rather as a modulator of different inflammatory mediators and enzymes. It does not inhibit inflammation, but rather accelerates the next phase of the inflammation process – repair (or healing), thus also accelerating the resolution of inflammation.

Research into the complex mechanism of action of LLLT on tissues and biological events has provided evidence that laser irradiation acts at the cellular level: increased supply of adenosine triphosphate (ATP)[9]; increased cell membrane permeability, allowing Ca^{2+} influx[10]; regulation of inflammatory cytokines and growth factors[11]; stimulation of cell differentiation and proliferation[12,13]; induction of collagen synthesis and remodeling[14]; increased tensile resistance[15]; angiogenesis,[16] among others. Additionally, LLLT modulates the activity of various cell types involved in the tissue repair process, including macrophages,[17] fibroblasts,[18,19] keratinocytes,[20] mastocytes,[21] and endothelial cells.[22,23]

These actions are the result of a dual mechanism involving cellular photosensitization and photoresponse, and may manifest clinically in various ways, such as with a primary or immediate effect with increased cell metabolism, increased endorphin synthesis, and reduced release of nociceptive transmitters, such as bradykinin and serotonin. The cell membrane will also be stabilized. Clinically, a stimulating and analgesic action of LLLT is observed. Next, a secondary or indirect effect increases blood flow and lymphatic drainage and the mediating action of laser irradiation on the inflammation is observed. Finally, later effects include an analgesic action (by inhibiting or reducing the production of phlogogen substances) and general therapeutic effects such as activation of the immune system.

In summary, it can be said that LLLT has important anti-inflammatory effects in the initial healing processes: reduction of chemical mediators, cytokines, edema, and migration of inflammatory cells, and increased growth factors, which directly contribute to the tissue rehabilitation process, as well as indirectly through the resolution of the inflammation inherent

Lasers in Dentistry: Guide for Clinical Practice, First Edition. Edited by Patrícia M. de Freitas and Alyne Simões.
© 2015 John Wiley & Sons, Inc. Published 2015 by John Wiley & Sons, Inc.

in the process. It should also be remembered that inflammation is not a disease, but rather is a defense mechanism that promotes the repair of daily damage to tissues; it is the process through which vascularized tissues react to aggression.[24]

Laser irradiation has a broad set of simultaneous actions and has also been used in the activation of lymphatic drainage.[25]

Edema

The word edema in the context of hemodynamic disorders refers to the accumulation of abnormal amounts of fluid in the intercellular spaces or in anatomic body cavities.[26] Two main types of edema are of particular interest within the scope of this chapter: (1) *inflammatory edema*, consequent to an increase in vascular permeability, and (b) *non-inflammatory edema*, resulting from increased capillary pressure, also called *hemodynamic edema*.

Edema may occur as a generalized or localized disorder. The term *anasarca* is used when the disorder is serious and generalized, and results in a marked volumetric increase of subcutaneous tissues. The fluid in non-inflammatory edema is a *transudate*, which contains no significant level of protein and other colloids. In inflammatory edema, however, the *inflammatory exudate* has a high protein content.

Exudate is formed so that mediators maintain inflammation and attract leukocytes to the region. Some of its components also act against the aggressor, eliminating it or weakening it, so that it can be phagocytosed by the cells in the inflammatory infiltrate.[24] Thus, it has crucial importance in determining the quality and agility of tissue repair in the edematous region.

Edema can be viewed as the result of an increase in the pressures that tend to move fluid from a vascular compartment to the interstitial environment. The normal interchange of fluids is regulated by the hydrostatic and osmotic pressures in and out of the vascular compartment. The opposing effects of intravascular hydrostatic pressure and plasma colloid oncotic pressure are the main factors to be considered in the pathology of edema.

Volumetric or morphological changes with edema are more evident from objective clinical examination than microscopic examination. Even though it is considered that any body organ or tissue may be affected by the edema, the three most susceptible tissues are the subcutaneous tissues (particularly those in the lower malleolar extremities), lungs, and brain.

Edema may lead to trivial clinical problems or be lethal. For instance, *Ludwig's angina*, which is relatively commonly seen in the clinical practice of the professionals concerned with the dental and head and neck areas, is an edema initiated by infection of the sublingual region due to inappropriately given local anesthesia; infection spreads through the neck into the mediastinum and culminates in a mediastinitis, with bacterial endocarditis then exposing the patient to the risk of death.[27]

For dental surgeons, oral and maxillofacial surgeons, and head and neck surgeons, it is subcutaneous tissue edema from viral infections or post surgery that is of interest.

Head and neck lymphatic system

The circulation comprises a closed system through which blood flows, and another more complex system, the lymphatic system, through which lymph flows. Both are intimately connected through a collecting duct, the *chyle system,* which comprises the finest roots of the initial portion of the lymphatic system and the end of in the venous system.[28]

The tissue liquid is partly returned through the blood capillaries, with the other part returned through the lymphatic routes, which constitute a blind lateral route of the venous system. Lymphatic vessels transport *lymph*, which is a viscous and colorless liquid, constituted of droplets of fat and lower levels of proteins and carbohydrates compared with blood plasma.

The lymphatic vessels originate, mostly, in the organs and tissues. The lymphatic capillaries are blind-ended tubes with a very thin endothelium, though slightly thicker than that of blood capillaries; their dilatations are irregular. The function of the lymphatic capillaries is to collect excess of fluid from the tissues. They unite to form thicker vessels with valves, and eventually form the main stem, the *thoracic duct*. The lymphatic routes are interrupted by lymph nodes, which act as a type of purifying filter for the lymph, and these are where lymphocytes are produced. While the blood capillaries supply fluid, oxygen, and nutrients to the tissues that they irrigate, the only purpose of the lymphatic system is to collect the fluid from the blood capillaries and transport it to the thoracic duct, after being filtered when passing through the lymph nodes. The human body is completely covered by the tangled network of lymphatic vessels (Fig. 26.1); their number and length are four times greater than those of blood vessels.[29]

Verlag[30] considers the lymph nodes as secondary lymphoid organs which, intercalated with the large lymphatic vessels, constitute the lymphovascular organs. Their main functions are (1) lymphopoiesis (lymphocyte production) and (2) capture and filtration (they are reticular organs of lymph capture and filtration).

They are also the site of proliferation of conglomerates of T and B lymphocytes. They are formed by the external cortex and internal medulla. The cortex contains the lymphoid follicles with their germinating centers and the medulla is comprised of rows of lymphatic cells (medullar cords). In addition to lymph node cells, they contain macrophages, more numerous in the medulla. B lymphocytes (related to humoral immunity) can be found mainly in the cortical follicles, while T lymphocytes (related to cellular immunity) can be found in the paracortical and medullar areas.[31]

Head and neck lymph node networks
While no part of the body is devoid of lymphatic vessels, their distribution throughout the body is not even. There are regions, such as the groin, armpits, mesentery, and viscerocranium, with larger numbers of lymph nodes. Only lymph nodes located

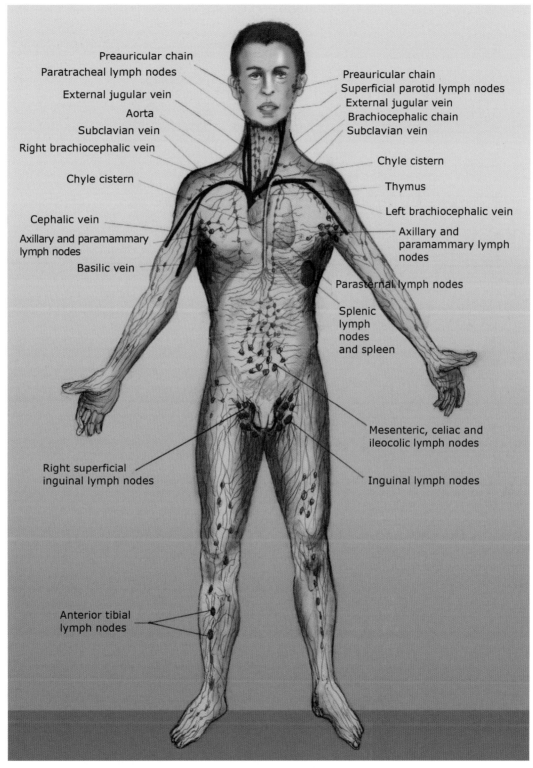

Figure 26.1 Lymphatic system comprised of lymph, vessels, and lymphatic organs (tonsils, thymus, lymph nodes, and spleen).

superficially or in cavities accessible to palpation may be detected by the examiner's tactile sensitivity. Digital palpation can detect changes in some surface lymph nodes. Tactile sensation depends on: (1) the thickness of the skin's adipose panicle, (b) the patient's age and general health, and (3) the anatomy of the particular patient. Figure 26.2 shows the palpable neck and head lymph nodes that are of interest in dental treatments, and these are described further later in this chapter.

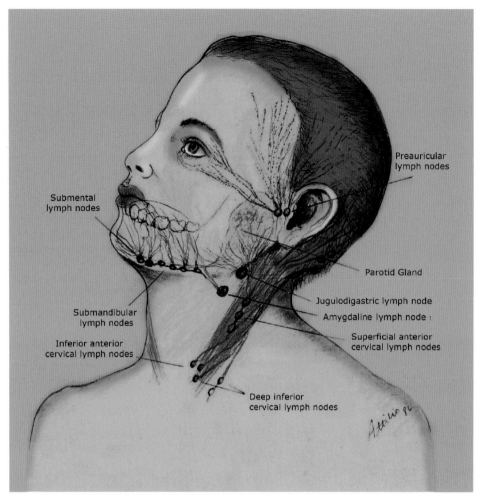

Figure 26.2 Some palpable lymph node chains used in LLLT for lymphatic drainage.

Normal lymph nodes have the approximate size of a pea, are not painful on palpation, and are smooth, mobile, and of a soft consistency. Their size and morphology may be modified by the patient's immune responses. As they are involved in a secondary line of defense, they continuously respond to stimulation, even when there is no clinical manifestation of disease. Modifications in the histology of a lymph node in response to aggressors and infections may be almost imperceptible. However, bacterial and viral infections may induce a significant increase in the size of lymph nodes, which can be detected by palpation. The presence of greater or smaller lymph node formations defines and gives names to the respective chains of lymph nodes, and these have well-defined structures surrounded by a capsule comprised of connective tissue and some elastic fibrils.[32]

Changes in lymph nodes with inflammation

With infection, there is usually a volume increase in lymph nodes, which may be intensely painful when compressed, mobile, and of slightly increased temperature. The proliferation of the lymph node cells caused by the presence of bacteria or foreign substances/organisms determines the increase in size of

the lymph nodes. Infarcted lymph node, called "inguinal bubo," are easily palpable.

However, the volume increase sensed by palpation does not always indicate an established inflammation. Sometimes lymph nodes remain inflamed even after an acute infection has been overcome. Such lymph nodes are known as *residual lymph nodes*, and there is no need, in such cases, for intervention with LLLT.

Main palpable head and neck lymph node networks

The presence of greater or smaller lymph node formations defines and define the name of the chains, even though there is wide variation of distribution, form, and number of lymph nodes from individual to individual. The International Anatomical Terminology (FCAT), published in 2001, classified regional neck and head lymph nodes; this classification has been illustrated in the drawings of Lopes.[28]

The most important regional head and neck lymph nodes for the laser lymphatic drainage technique[29,33] will be described, that is those directly involved in the drainage of the oral cavity or indirectly draining the face itself, as well as

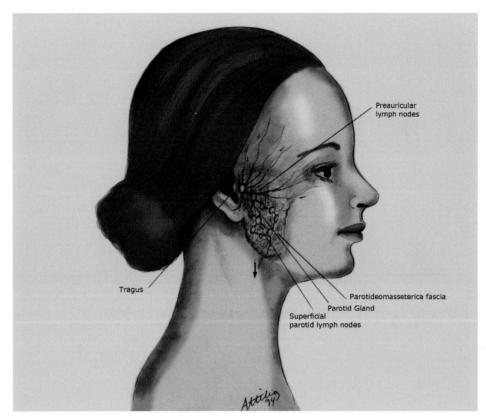

Figure 26.3 Surface parotid lymph nodes and the areas they drain, as well as the direction of this drainage.

being palpable and possible targets for the clinical application of the laser.

Surface parotid lymph nodes

The lateral anterior regions and the region above the tragus correspond topographically with the deep and surface parotid lymph nodes and with the preauricular lymph nodes. Part of these lymph nodes is located over the parotid gland (surface parotid lymph nodes) and can be sensed through palpation. The other part is comprised of the parotid intragland lymph nodes and is not perceptible through palpation (Fig. 26.3). This chain is important because it protects the parotid, the largest of the salivary glands, which explains the high concentration of lymph nodes in this region. Its drainage area is limited to the cutaneous surface, corresponding to the temporomandibular joint (TMJ) and to the insertion of the masseter into the zygomatic arch. Its compromise may result in the repercussion of an infection or trauma in the TMJ, in impacted or embedded mandibular third molars, or also in a disease or compromise of the parotid, including a sialoadenopathy of that gland.

These lymph nodes receive part of the lymph of the parotid gland, the conjunctivae, lateral region of the eyelids, nose root, tympanum membrane, outer hearing duct, and anterior surface of the ear. Lymph is drained down through the lateral surface cervical chains of the lymph nodes. Figure 26.4 shows irradiation with LLLT of these lymph nodes.

Facial lymph nodes

These are, from top to bottom: mandibular, buccinator, nasolabial or subcortical, and zygomatic lymph nodes, also known as the genian (Fig. 26.5). They have a subcutaneous location and are little observed because not all individuals who possess all these lymph nodes.

Overall, the mandibular lymph node, due to it being directly involved with various dental infections, is the most frequently infarcted and can be treated with infrared irradiation that can penetrate the tissues of the region. It is generally formed from a single lymph node, and is located in the lower lip lowering muscle, a little in front of the facial vein.

Figure 26.6 shows the irradiation of the facial lymph nodes.

Lingual lymph nodes

These are highly complex and difficult to assess clinically. However, their regional lymph nodes run from the submental lymph nodes to the neck. The tongue is the site of a broad union of the lymphatic routes from both sides, and also the lateral sublingual lymph nodes (which follow the path of the lingual vessels, under the outer surface of the genioglossus muscle) and the median or intralingual lymph nodes (throughout the central lymphatic vessels, between the two genioglossus muscles Fig. 26.7).

Figure 26.8 shows the irradiation of these lymph nodes.

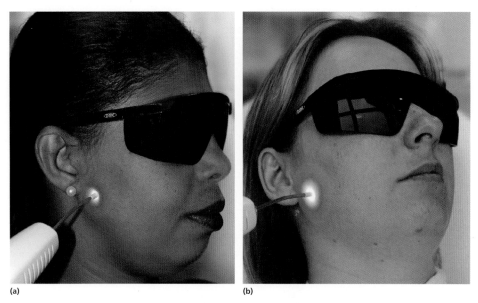

(a)   (b)

Figure 26.4 (a,b) Application of the lymphatic drainage technique with LLLT on the surface parotid lymph nodes.

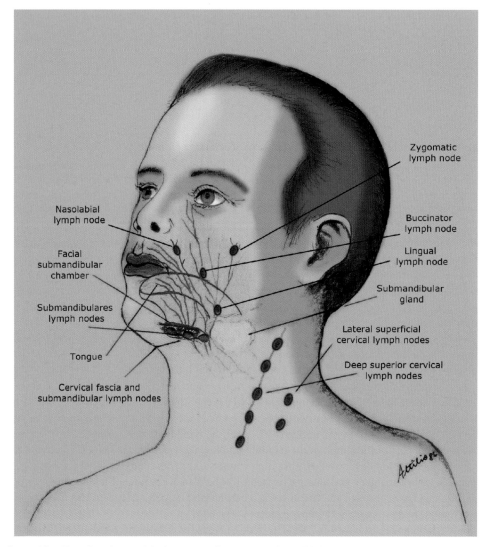

Figure 26.5 Little observed facial lymph nodes: nasolabial, zygomatic, buccinator, and mandibular. The submandibular and surface cervical lymph nodes are also shown.

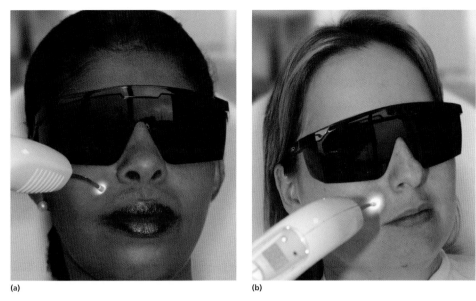

Figure 26.6 (a,b) Application of the lymphatic drainage technique with LLLT on the facial lymph nodes.

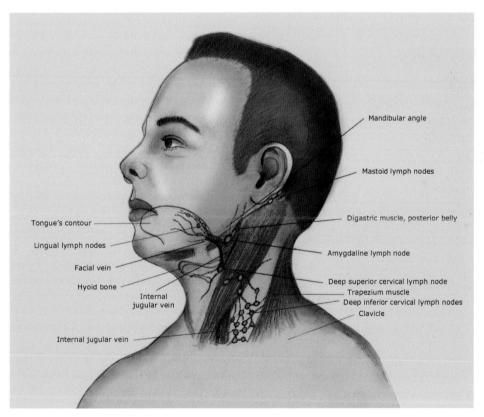

Figure 26.7 Lingual and deep lower cervical lymph nodes.

Submental lymph nodes

These are small in number (between two and four) and in dimensions, and are located in the median sagittal plan, within the *submental trigon*, their location coinciding with the milo-hyoideous muscle exactly below the chin (Fig. 26.9). All the lymph originating from the lower lip drains into these lymph nodes; that from the whole mental region, part of the sublingual region, and the anterior part of the mandible body. They are infarcted when there are neoplasic changes or infections in the sublingual region, tongue's ventral surface, and mandibular incisors, in addition to sialo-adenopathies of the glands of that region. Their infarction also precedes acute

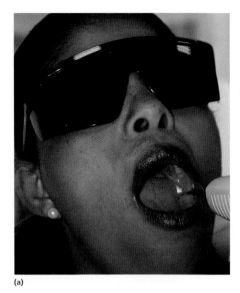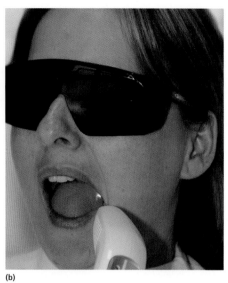

(a)   (b)

Figure 26.8 (a,b) Application of the lymphatic drainage technique with LLLT on the lingual lymph nodes.

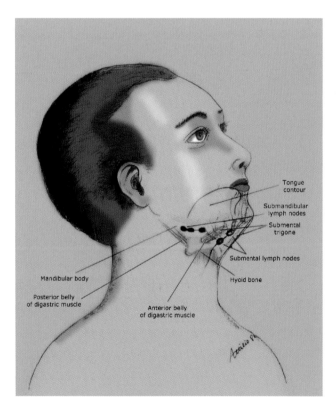

Figure 26.9 Submental and submandibular lymph nodes.

inflammatory changes of the sublingual region, including Ludwig's angina.

Irradiation of these lymph nodes is shown in Figure 26.10.

Submandibular lymph nodes

These are found in pairs within the medial face of the mandible body, on either side of the lower third of the face, following the direction of the submandibular salivary glands. These lymph drainage routes are much more important than those originating from the nasal pits; they join at a point just ahead and below the pharyngeal orifice of the *auditory tube*. From this point, there are two routes. The most important has two or four small drains that cross below the mucosa of the *pharynx recess*, pierce the superior constrictor muscle of the pharynx, and end at the retropharynx lymph nodes. They drain the face from the lower part of the medial commissure of the eyelids, lip mucosa, parotid and submandibular salivary glands, tongue, and part of the neck (Figs 26.2, 26.5, 26.9, and 26.11). Their enlargement denotes infection or neoplasia of the sublingual region, ventral surface of the tongue, and vestibular face of the lower lip. They are usually most affected when the tongue, sublingual region, and molars (both maxillary and mandibular) are infected.

Figure 26.12 shows the irradiation of these lymph nodes.

Surface cervical lymph nodes

These must be considered an accessory and inconstant drainage route of parotid lymphatic circulation. The chains of lymph nodes constituting this route form the chain of the outer jugular vein, and comprise one or two lymph nodes located along the route of that vein, of which the upper seems to be confused with the group of the subaponeurotic lower parotid lymph nodes, which ends in the jugular chain or in the transverse cervical chain (Fig. 26.13). They drain the scalp and sometimes the mouth and pharynx.

Figure 26.14 shows the irradiation of these lymph nodes.

Lateral cervical lymph nodes (surface lymph nodes)

These may be considered as belonging to the upper and lower lateral cervical chains of lymph nodes and include the infra-auricular and infragland lymph nodes.

Infra-auricular lymph nodes are found in the region of the sternocleidomastoid muscle, a little below the ear lobe. There may be two or three. They drain the lymph of the whole parotid

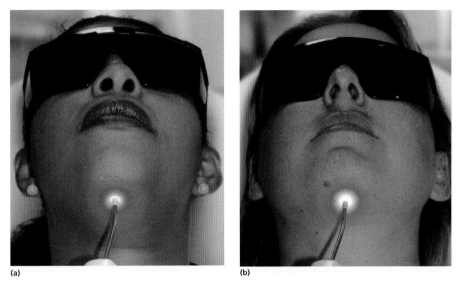

Figure 26.10 (a,b) Application of the lymphatic drainage technique with LLLT on the submental lymph nodes.

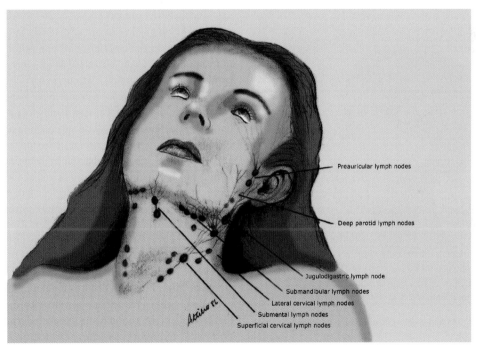

Figure 26.11 Surface and preauricular, submental, submandibular, and cervical lymph nodes.

gland, through the intragland and preauricular chains of lymph nodes. Their drainage area includes the pretragus region, the whole region of the gland above, and the inner structures of the carotid trigon and mastoid process (Fig. 26.13).

Surface cervical lymph nodes (Fig. 26.15), both anterior and lateral, may be enlarged with scalp infections and sometimes with mouth or pharynx infections. The large volume of the trapezium muscle prevents the assessment of lymph nodes located in the posterior part of the neck, but the chains of lymph nodes located in the anterior part of the neck, both in the supra-hyoid and in the infra-hyoudeous region, until the clavicle, may be assessed by digital palpation, both with the finger pulp and with the bi-digital method.

Figure 26.16 shows the irradiation of these lymph nodes.

Use of LLLT in head and neck lymph node lymphatic drainage

On the one hand, LLLT has been shown to be capable of reducing the inflammation in a wide variety of clinical situations,[34] whether reducing the development of the edema and migration

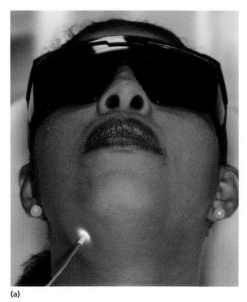 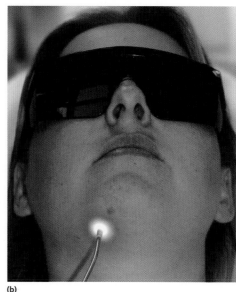

(a) (b)

Figure 26.12 (a,b) Application of the lymphatic drainage technique with LLLT on the submandibular lymph nodes.

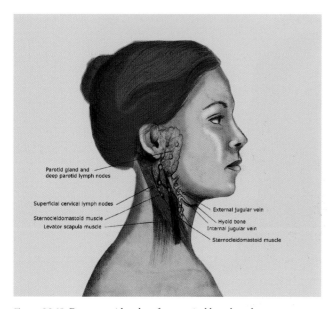

Figure 26.13 Deep parotid and surface cervical lymph nodes.

of inflammatory cells,[35] or modulating the formation of inflammation-mediating substances.[36] Authors have demonstrated that LLLT modifies some fundamental processes of aneurysm of the aorta, progressively increasing the cell proliferation of the smooth muscle and of the protein matrix, as well as the secretion of the matrix metalloproteinase.[37] In this study, it was observed that LLLT inhibits the generic expression of pro-inflammatory cytokines and interleukin-1β from irradiated cells.

On the other hand, it has been suggested that LLLT promotes the early activation of the inflammatory phase of the tissue repair process, causing an exacerbation of signs and symptoms thereof.[38]

An important observation is that the inflammatory edema results initially from the action of histamine, followed by the effect of kinins, and is potentiated by the action of prostaglandins (after approximately 5–6 hours). Throughout the first 24 hours, the prostaglandins are largely responsible for the extent of edema.[24] As with pain, the action of anti-inflammatory drugs is dependent on the reduction of the local production of prostaglandins. Prostaglandins are also important in the repair process. The efficacy of LLLT lies in the fact that it modulates the local production of such prostaglandins, and does not inhibit their production.

In clinical situations where LLLT is used as early as possible (e.g. immediately post surgery), the inflammation scenario will exist, but the patient will experience less discomfort and pain, and faster and more esthetic resolution of the inflammatory event during the repair.

Interesting clinical situations occur when patients present with low immunity as a result of systemic diseases or organic stress (e.g. a hospital admission), or with injuries infected by highly virulent microorganisms. Repeated irradiation of the site of the infected injury is contraindicated because of the risk of exacerbating the injury due to the activation of the microorganisms, or even of the inflammatory process itself. However, LLLT can be routinely used with herpes simplex and zoster infections. Classically, these infections can be divided into three well-defined clinical phases:

1 Subclinical: pruritus phase, when the injury is not clinically visible. Some patients report neuralgia or discomfort when the area is touched;

2 Vesicular: hatched vesicles are visible;

3 Post-vesicular: this is the phase when the vesicles are no longer present and the injury is no longer infectious. Once the vesicles have ulcerated, crusts begin to develop. In this phase, it is important to reduce pain and promote esthetics.

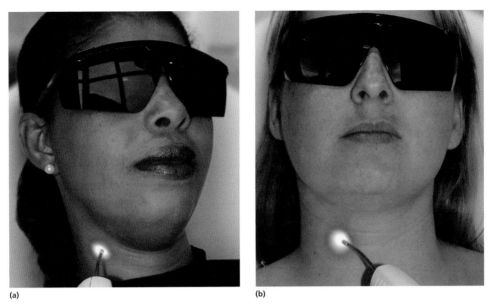

(a)   (b)

Figure 26.14 (a,b) Application of the lymphatic drainage technique with LLLT on the surface cervical lymph nodes.

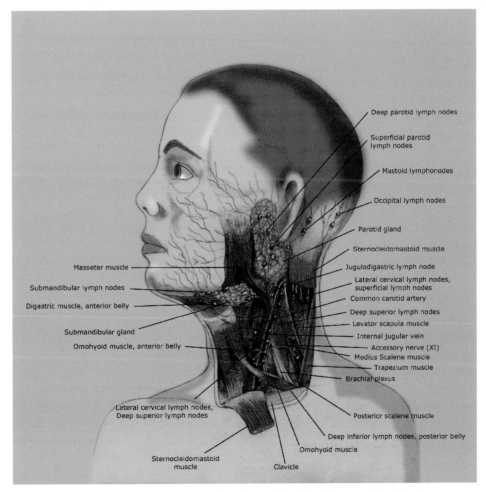

Figure 26.15 Panoramic view of the main head and neck surface lymph nodes, including the surface cervical lymph nodes.

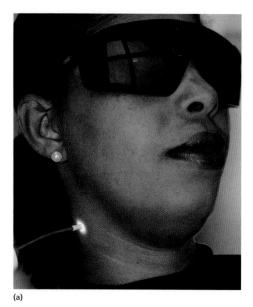 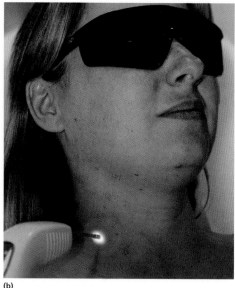

(a)   (b)

Figure 26.16 (a,b) Application of the lymphatic drainage technique with LLLT on the surface cervical lymph nodes.

In the latest decades, LLLT has been widely used to treat herpetic injuries, both in medical practice and dental practice.[39–42] Studies have been carried to clarify the mechanisms of action of LLLT on herpes simplex virus (HSV)-1 and HSV-2.[43,44] However, the indication for LLLT in the treatment of herpes treatment is limited to the first and third phase of the injury to, respectively, prevent or minimize the appearance of vesicles and to treat the crusts on the ulcerated vesicles. The second phase is critical, as this is when the patient experiences most pain, is highly contagious and esthetically compromised. However, LLLT directly on the vesicles in this phase is contraindicated. In this phase, professionals working in specialized centers usually use the surgical laser, but this technique is not available outside these specialist centers. It should be noted that low level laser irradiation can be used in photodynamic therapy in the vesicle phase.

There is also concern regarding the application of the laser directly on very contaminated injuries as LLLT can activate microorganisms.[45–48] Therefore, indirect treatment of the injury has been proposed: the lymph node chains responsible for draining the region affected are irradiated rather than the contaminated injury itself, to accelerate the resolution of the local inflammatory process and consequently improve healing.

According to this reasoning, difficult to access injuries, for example pericoronitis, could also be treated by irradiation of sites remote from the injury, as could injuries presenting with a very active infection (as can be the case with fistulas, gingivitis, and periodontitis) or those in an immunodepressed host, whose treatment would normally be contraindicated without a previous trial of antibiotic therapy. This technique is indicated in patients with acute edema resulting from mechanical, trismus, and surgical traumas. Another very practical indication would be patients with mucositis or other diseases which often

prevent them from opening their mouth because of intense pain or mechanical limitation due to the presence of crusts. Patients who asleep or sedated when the health professional arrives to perform the intraoral irradiation also fit into this indication. Thus, the use of LLLT to drain the main lymph node chains may be chosen to treat such oral injuries.

Irradiation parameters for the lymphatic drainage technique with LLLT

The technique described in this chapter aims to activate the lymphatic drainage of a region where inflammation is established.[25,29,33,49,50] This activation is achieved with LLLT by placing the tip of the laser equipment directly on the lymph nodes responsible for the drainage of the region affected. Digital palpation of the lymph node chains will detect any altered surface lymph nodes (Fig. 26.17) where irradiation should be applied. These lymph node chains can also be identified by standing behind the patient and asking the patient to gently move their head from side to side.

A laser that emits in the proximal infrared (preferably between 808 and 830 nm) region is indicated. The tip of the equipment must be placed on the lymph nodes responsible for draining the affected region, as perpendicular to them as possible. An energy dose of approximately 2 J, giving a fluency of approximately 70 J/cm², is given at each application point. The number of sessions will depend on the duration of the inflammation, but we generally use two to six sessions, with an interval of 2 days between sessions The placement of the laser must always avoid the irradiation of critical regions such as the thyroid gland. Therefore, when positioning the laser to irradiate the submental lymph nodes, for instance,

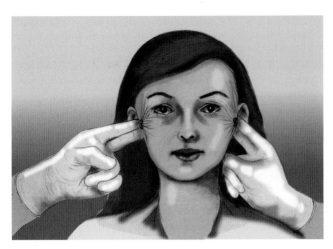

Figure 26.17 Detection of altered lymph nodes: Digital palpation.

care must be taken to direct the laser beam upwards, towards the sublingual region, and never downwards towards the thyroid gland.

Discussion

The biggest advantage of the technique described in this chapter, which avoids the direct handling and irradiation of an injury, is the reduced risk of activation of microorganisms in highly contaminated injuries (such as HSV in the vesicle phase), apical, acute or purulent injuries, pericoronitis, and alveolitis settings. This technique aims to activate the local immunity of the patient directly and indirectly by activating the drainage of the region, resulting in less edema, and as a consequence less pain and discomfort.

Concerning aseptic injuries, as exemplified by postsurgical wounds, the technique is strongly indicated to prevent postsurgical edema. It should be given immediately postoperatively.

This technique has, therefore, proven effective in the treatment of inflammation, by activating local drainage, reducing local edema, and increasing the supply of cellular specific blood elements to the region, and may be used postoperatively, in highly contaminated acute injuries, as well as in the treatment from a distance of injuries that are difficult or impossible to access.

References

1 Mester E, Spiry T, Szende B, Tota JG. Effect of lasers rays on wound healing. Am J Surg 1971; 122: 532–535.
2 Lievens P. The influence of laser-irradiation on the motricity of the lymphatic system and on the wound healing process. In: Proceedings of the International Congress on Laser in Medicine and Surgery, Bologna, Italy, 1986: 171–174.
3 Lievens P. Effects of laser treatment on the lymphatic system and wound healing. Laser. J Eur Med Laser Assoc 1988; 1(2): 12.
4 Lievens PC. The effect of a combined He:Ne and I.R. laser treatment on the regeneration of the lymphatic system during the process of wound healing. Laser News 1990; 3(3): 3–9.
5 Lievens PC. The effect of I.R. Laser irradiation on the vasomotricity of the lymphatic system. Laser Med Sci 1991; 6: 189–191.
6 Labajos M. Effects of the IR radiation of the GaAs diode laser on intestinal absorption in vitro and in vivo studies. Laser 1986; 2: 21–25.
7 Tunér J, Hode L. Laser Therapy in Dentistry and Medicine. Stockholm: Prima Books, 1996.
8 Clark RAF. Biology of dermal wound repair dermatological clinics. J Invest Dermatol 1993; 11(4): 647–661.
9 Karu T, Pyatibrat L, Kalendo G. Irradiation with He-Ne laser increases ATP level in cells cultivated in vitro. J Photochem Photobiol B 1995; 27: 219–233.
10 Lubart R, Friedmann H, Levinshal T, Lavie R, Breitbart H. Effect of light on calcium transport in bull sperm cells. J Photochem Photobiol B1992; 15: 337–341.
11 Boschi ES, Leite CE, Saciura VC, et al. Anti-inflammatory effects of low-level laser therapy (660 nm) in the early phase in carrageenan-induced pleurisy in rat. Lasers Surg Med 2008; 40: 500–508.
12 Pourreau-Schneider N, Ahmed A, et al. Helium-neon laser treatment transforms fibroblasts into myofibroblasts. Am J Pathol 1990; 137: 171–178.
13 Almeida-Lopes L, Rigau J, Zangaro RA, Guidugli-Neto J, Jaeger MMM. LLLT acts by improving the in vitro fibroblast proliferation – comparison of the low level laser therapy effects on cultured human gingival fibroblasts proliferation using different irradiance and same fluence. Lasers Surg Med 2001; 29: 179–184.
14 Araújo CE, Ribeiro MS, Favaro R, Zezell DM, Zorn TM. Ultrastructural and autoradiographical analysis show a faster skin repair in He-Ne laser-treated wounds. J Photochem Photobiol B 2007; 86: 87–96.
15 Vasilenko T, Slezák M, Kovác I, et al. The effect of equal daily dose achieved by different power densities of low-level laser therapy at 635 and 670 nm on wound tensile strength in rats: a short report. Photomed Laser Surg 2010; 28: 281–283.
16 Melo VA, Anjos DC, Albuquerque R Jr, Melo DB, Carvalho FU. Effect of low level laser on sutured wound healing in rats. Acta Cir Bras 2011; 26: 129–134.
17 Young S, Bolton P, Dyson M, Harvey W, Diamantopoulos C. Macrophage responsiveness to light therapy. Lasers Surg Med 1989; 9: 497–505.
18 Almeida-Lopes L, Rigau J, Zângaro RA, Guidugli-Neto J, Jaeger MMM. Comparison of the low level laser therapy on cultured human gingival fibroblasts proliferation using different irradiance and same fluence. Lasers Surg Med 2001; 29: 179–184.
19 Kreisler M, Christoffers AB, Willerstausen B, d'Hoedt B. Effect of low-level GaAlAs laser irradiation on the proliferation rate of human periodontal ligament fibroblasts: an in vitro study. J Clin Periodontol 2003; 30: 353–358.
20 Haas AF, Isseroff RR, Wheeland RG, Rood PA, Graves PJ. Low-energy helium-neon laser irradiation increases the motility of cultured human keratinocytes. J Invest Dermatol 1990; 94: 822–826.
21 Pereira MC, de Pinho CB, Medrado AR, Andrade Zde A, Reis SR. Influence of 670 nm low-level laser therapy on mast cells and vascular response of cutaneous injuries. J Photochem Photobiol B 2010; 98: 188–192.

22 Kipshidze N, Nikolaychik V, Keelan MH, et al. Low-power helium: neon laser irradiation enhances production of vascular endothelial growth factor and promotes growth of endothelial cells in vitro. Lasers Surg Med 2001; 28: 355–364.

23 Schindl A, Merwald H, Schindl L, Kaun C, Wojta J. Direct stimulatory effect of low-intensity 670 nm laser irradiation on human endothelial cell proliferation. Br J Dermatol 2003; 148: 334–336.

24 Consolaro A. Inflamação e Reparo. Maringá: Dental Press Editora, 2009.

25 Almeida-Lopes L, Lopes A. Técnica da Drenagem Linfática Ativada por Laserterapia. Livro de Resumos do 24° Congresso Internacional de Odontologia de São Paulo. Tomo de Estomatologia-Pacientes Especiais – Laser. Sao Paulo, 2005: 328–338.

26 Cotran RS, Kumar V, Robbins SL. Robbins Patologia Estrutural e Funcional. Inflamação e Reparação, 5th edn. Rio de Janeiro: Editora Guanabara Koogan, 1996.

27 Robbins SL, Cotran RS, Kumar V. Patologia estrutural e funcional, 6th edn. Rio de Janeiro: Guanabara Koogan, 2000.

28 Lopes A. Anatomia Cabeça e Pescoço. Sistema Linfático da Cabeça e do Pescoço. Rio de Janeiro: Editora Guanabara Koogan, 2004.

29 Almeida-Lopes A, Figueiredo ACR, Lopes A. O uso do laser terapêutico no tratamento da inflamação na clínica odontológica, através da drenagem linfática. Rev APCD 2002; 56: 27.

30 Verlag GT. Terminologia Anatômica Internacional (Sociedade Brasileira de Anatomia) (FCAT). Ed Manole, 2001.

31 Michalany J. Anatomia Patológica Geral na Prática Médico Cirúrgica. Artes Médicas Ltd, 1995.

32 Spalteholz W. Atlas de Anatomia Humana, Vol.III. Barcelona: Labor S.A, 1984.

33 Almeida-Lopes A. Present Situation of the Dental Word Regarding the Use of LLT. Anais do IV WALT Congress, Japan, 2002.

34 Pejcic A, Mirkovic D. Anti-inflammatory effect of low level laser treatment on chronic periodontitis. Med Laser Appl 2011; 26: 27–34.

35 Albertini R, Villaverde AB, Aimbire F, et al. Anti-inflammatory effects of low-level laser therapy (LLLT) with two different red wavelengths (660 nm and 684 nm) in carrageenan-induced rat paw edema. J Photochem Photobiol B Biol 2007; 89: 50–55.

36 Bjordal JM, Lopes-Martins RAB, Joensen J, Iversen VV. The anti-inflammatory mechanism of low level laser therapy and its relevance for clinical use in physiotherapy. Phys Ther Rev 2010; 15(4): 286–293.

37 Gavish L, Perez LS, Reissman P, Gertz SD. Irradiation with 780 nm diode laser attenuates inflammatory cytokines but upregulates nitric oxide in lipopolysaccharide-stimulated macrophages: Implications for the prevention of aneurysm progression. Lasers Surg Med 2008; 40: 371–378.

38 Viegas VN, Abreu ME, Viezzer C, et al. Effect of low-level laser therapy on inflammatory reactions during wound healing: Comparison with meloxicam. Photomed Laser Surg 2007; 25: 467–463.

39 Marotti J, Corrêa AC, Paula EC. The use of laser in the treatment of herpes labialis. RPG Rev Postgrad 2007; 14(4): 314–320.

40 Schindl A, Neumann R. Low-intensity laser therapy is an effective treatment for recurrent herpes simplex infection. Results from a randomized double-blind placebo-controlled study. J Invest Dermatol 1999; 113: 221–223.

41 Rallis TM, Spruance SL. Low-intensity laser therapy for recurrent herpes labialis. J Invest Dermatol 2000; 115: 131–132.

42 Muñoz Sanchez PJ, Capote Femenías JL, Díaz Tejeda A, Tunér J. The effect of 670-nm low laser therapy on herpes simplex type 1. Photomed Laser Surg 2012; 30(1): 37–40.

43 Palamara AT, Perno CF, Ciriolo MR, et al.. Evidence for antiviral activity of glutathione: in vitro inhibition of herpes simplex virus type 1 replication. Antiviral Res 1995; 27(3): 235–253.

44 Donnarumma G, De Gregorio V, Fusco A, et al. Inhibition of HSV-1 replication by laser diode-irradiation: possible mechanism of action. Int J Immunopathol Pharmacol 2010; 23(4): 1167–1176.

45 Karu T. Photobiological fundamentals of low-power laser therapy. IEEE J Quantum Electron 1987; 23(10): 1703 1717.

46 Kisuk K, Hun LD, Kun KS. Effects of low incident energy levels of infrared laser irradiation on the proliferation of Streptococcus mutans. Laser Ther 1992; 4(2): 81–85.

47 Karu T, Tiphlova O, Esenaliev R, Letokhov V. Two different mechanisms of low-intensity laser photobiological effects on Escherichia coli. J Photochem Photobiol B Biol 1994; 24(3): 155–161.

48 Nussbaum EL, Lilge L, Mazzulli T. Effects of low-level laser therapy (LLLT) of 810 nm upon in vitro growth of bacteria: Relevance of irradiance and radiant exposure. J Clin Laser Med Surg 2003; 21(5): 283–290.

49 Almeida-Lopes L, Lopes L. Using laser therapy on the lymphatic drainage technique. Photomed Laser Surg 2005; 23(1): 100 (Abstr 042).

50 Almeida-Lopes L, Lopes A, Tunér J, Calderhead RG. Infrared diode laser therapy-induced lymphatic drainage for inflammation in the head and neck. Laser Ther 2005; 14(2): 67–74.

SECTION 6

Orthodontics and orofacial pain

CHAPTER 27

Temporomandibular disorders

Caroline Maria Gomes Dantas and Carolina Lapaz Vivan
Private Dental Practice, São Paulo, SP, Brazil

Introduction

Temporomandibular dysfunction (TMD) is a group of disorders that affect the masticatory muscles, temporomandibular joint (TMD), and associated structures.[1,2] It is the most prevalent clinical entity involving the masticatory apparatus, and is the main cause of pain of non-dental origin in the facial region.[2,3] The patient can present with unilateral or bilateral symptoms, associated or not with other disorders.

TMJ has multifactorial causes, such as emotional changes, occlusal dysfunction, and parafunctional habits. Basic functions of the stomatognathic system, such as speech, chewing, and swallowing, can be impared,[4] leading to direct impacts on quality of life,[4,5] job performance, learning, and social interaction.[4–6] The patient should receive multidisciplinary treatment since the dysfunction has a known multifactorial etiology. A correct evaluation of the patient is essential to define the appropriate treatment.

Numerous non-surgical therapies can be used for the treatment of TMD, aiming to reduce the symptoms and improve the function of the masticatory system. Among them, the most common are physical therapy,[7,8] drug therapy,[9] occlusal splints,[7,9] occlusal adjustments,[10] acupuncture,[8,9] and low level laser therapy (LLLT).[8,9,11–13]

Although there is no consensus on the mechanism by which LLLT reduces pain associated with TMD, it is known that biomodulation, analgesic and anti-inflammatory response are some of the therapeutic effects observed in the irradiated tissues. It is expected, therefore, that direct irradiation of symptomatic spots contributes to pain remission.[7,12,13] Demirkol et al. and Fouda proved that LLLT is efficient at relieving the symptoms of patients with TMD.[9,14] Furthermore, LLLT has high effectiveness[12,13] and minimal contraindications, clinical management with it is easy, and usually it is not an uncomfortable intervention for the patient.[10]

LLLT as an adjuvant in the treatment of TMD is discussed in this chapter.

Temporomandibular joint anatomy

The TMJ is the joint that connects the jaw to the skull and regulates mandibular movement. It is a bicondylar joint in which the condyles function at the same time. These bones (condyle and articular fossa of the temporal bone) are surrounded by the articular capsule, with the articular fibrocartilaginous disc between them. The disc functions as a cushion, absorbing stress and allowing the condyle to move easily, mainly due to its shape. This articular complex is filled with synovial fluid, produced by the synovial membrane, which provides nutrition and lubrication to the joint structures. The disc posterior region is connected to the joint capsule by the retrodiscal tissue, which is the source of the innervation and blood supply of the whole structure.[7,15]

The muscles responsible for TMJ function are part of a complex system involving global posture balance.[16] Thus, the masticatory muscles are closely related to body posture, through muscular chains.[16] It has been proven, for example, that global postural re-education is associated with significant relief of TMD physical and psychological symptoms, related to body alignment and symmetry.[17]

The lateral pterygoid muscle is active in mandibular protrusion, opening, and laterality; the median pterygoid and masseter muscles in closing the jaw and allowing mandibular retrusion; the temporal muscle in promoting closure of the jaw and excursion movements (protrusion and laterality).[15] There are also ligaments, such as the temporomandibular, sphenomandibular and estylomandibular ligaments, which protect these structures against excessive mandible mobility.[5,15]

Temporomandibular dysfunction

Temporomandibular dysfunction, which often leads to anatomical and functional masticatory system damage, is caused by a group of diseases that do not necessarily affect only the TMJ, but

Lasers in Dentistry: Guide for Clinical Practice, First Edition. Edited by Patrícia M. de Freitas and Alyne Simões.
© 2015 John Wiley & Sons, Inc. Published 2015 by John Wiley & Sons, Inc.

also commonly the masticatory muscles and related structures. Usually there are signs and symptoms such as joint sounds, muscle pain, joint pain, and restricted mandibular excursion.[8,18] It can frequently be associated with head, ear and cervical–spinal pain.[8]

There is still no definitive consensus on TMD classification, mostly because its etiology is unclear and the clinical findings can result from different causes, including psychological causes. To standardize the clinical examination of TMD patients, Research Diagnostic Criteria for TMD (RDC/TMD) have become one of the most reliable and commonly used schemes.[19]

The implications of pain, the main symptom of TMD, go far beyond incorrect masticatory system function.[5] Chronic pain can disturb sleep, cause fatigue, alter concentration, modify mood and behavior, and hinder activities of daily living, compromising the patient's quality of life.[5]

Oliveira et al. showed that TMD pain affected work and school activities (59.09%), sleep (68.18%), and appetite/feeding (63.64%).[5] Lacerda et al. proved that orofacial pain was the main odontologic risk factor in the adult population for altered daily performance.[20]

Nowadays, the aim is to restore the musculoskeletal system with multifocal conservative treatment, based on the ideal biomechanical model of the TMJ and taking into account the multifactorial etiology of the disorder.[3,20] Due to the variety of clinical presentations and etiology, diverse therapies are commonly applied: acupuncture, massage, ultrasound, transcutaneous electric nerve stimulation (TENS), use of occlusal splints and LLLT, among others.[8,21] These adjuvant and complementary treatments could decrease the demand for invasive treatments such as drug therapy or surgery.[22]

Low level laser therapy

The use of lasers in medicine has increased, especially in conditions involving chronic pain such as in TMD. Patients tend to be receptive to LLLT and positive psychological effects are frequently reported.[23,24]

Treatment of TMD is based primarily on the pain control by non-invasive methods.[7] LLLT has been used as an anti-inflammatory, analgesic, and biomodulatory agent on the physiological, cellular, and systemic responses. Its effectiveness in reducing muscular pain and tension has been of great interest in the recent literature.[12,13,25]

It is worth pointing out that the success of the LLLT relies on the appropriate parameters of the equipment and anatomical position during the irradiation, since each wavelength has its own absorption characteristics and mechanism of action.[12,26–28]

The wavelengths used in dentistry nowadays are in the range of the visible red (630–700 nm) and near infrared (700–904 nm) parts of the spectrum, with the former being used more for tissue repair and the latter for neural repair and analgesia, according to the depth of the target tissue.[27]

Mechanism of action

Arthroscopic studies have confirmed the concept that capsular, synovial,[29] and retrodiscal tissue inflammation is the basis of pain in the joint region in TMD. In addition, in muscle pain due to increased muscle activity, the circulatory system does not support the drainage of metabolites and oxygen supply to the hypoxic areas, leading to a local accumulation of toxins and subsequent inflammatory response.[30]

If the correct parameters are used, LLLT can provide analgesic and anti-inflammatory effects by different mechanisms, such as stimulation of endogenous opiate release, decrease of the neuronal cell membrane permeability, decrease in the release of pain agents at pathological sites, and increase in ATP production and local oxygenation.[31]

The pain relief mechanism has not been fully elucidated. The most accepted theory suggests that the reduction of pain is due to a drop in the level of prostaglandin E_2 (PGE$_2$), one of the most important inflammatory mediators. Studies using varying doses of energy and power output have shown a reduction in PGE$_2$ after LLLT in ligament cell cultures and the articulation of animals, probably due to the inhibition of the enzyme that synthesizes PGE$_2$, the cyclooxygenase-2.[32,33]

Another widespread theory emphasizes the action of LLLT on neuronal cells. It is proposed that analgesia occurs as a result of a selective inhibition of nociceptive signals and regulation of the microcirculation,[34,35] which interrupts the development of pain.[36] A reduction in edema and increase in cellular metabolism have also been reported.[37] Furthermore, it has been discussed that LLLT has a systemic effect that may decrease the perception of pain by altering the sensorial input to a patient's central nervous system.[26]

When applied to cases of muscle pain in TMD, studies have described its analgesic effect: it increases the level of beta-endorphins, decreases release of histamine and bradykinin, increases lymphatic flow, decreases edema and pain substance release, increases blood supply, decreases duration of inflammation, and consequently relaxes muscles.[24,26,33,35,37]

LLLT has several uses in dentistry, and it is important to keep in mind that its effects depend on appropriate dosimetry employment and the individual systemic conditions.[38]

Clinical trials

Although recognition of the benefit of a treatment does not require a sound understanding of the mechanism, this lack of understanding with regards to LLLT makes it harder to assess clinical outcomes. In addition, the excellent therapy parameters (frequency, power output, irradiance, energy density, energy per point, irradiation time, number of sessions, among others) have not yet been determined.[22,39]

Some studies have shown great effectiveness of LLLT in TMD. However, the heterogeneity of the standardization regarding the parameters of laser calls for caution in interpretation of these results.

In 1988, Bezzur et al. observed improvement in 80% of TMD patients with painful symptoms treated with LLLT for a period of 6 days.[40] Hansson et al. demonstrated a fast reduction in TMJ intra-articular inflammation in TMD patients treated with low power laser. Bertolucci et al. and Gray et al. concluded that LLLT promotes considerable pain relief in TMD patients, compared with a group of patients undergoing a placebo treatment.[24,41,42] Simunovic et al. observed significant improvement in patients with orofacial pain related to the TMD who were treated with LLLT.[43] Kulekcioglu et al. showed that both TMD patients treated with 15 sessions of LLLT as well as the placebo group experienced a reduction in pain. However, only the irradiated group showed improvement in range of mouth opening, sideways motion, and number of trigger points.[44] Çetiner et al. reported statistically significant differences in the extent of mouth opening between patients undergoing LLLT or placebo, both immediately post irradiation and at 1-month follow-up.[45]

As in any therapy, patients may respond differently to the same stimulus. It is important when determining the ideal protocol for LLLT to consider the laser used, the target tissue, and the systemic condition of the patient. Reported unsatisfactory results may be due to the use of very low or too high doses, incorrect diagnosis or insufficient number of sessions, among other factors.[22,39]

Maia et al. conducted a systematic review and have shown that, within 14 studies that fitted the criteria, a great variety of parameters were presented. The energy density used ranged from 0.9 to 105 J/cm^2, power density from 9.8 to 500 mW, number of sessions from 1 to 20, and frequency of applications from daily for 10 days to once per week for 4 weeks.[22]

Petrucci et al. reviewed trials that considered optimal doses between 0.5 and 15 J for infrared irradiation of 780 nm, 830 nm and 1060 nm; 0.2–1.4 J for infrared irradiation of 904 nm; and 6–30 J for irradiation with the HeNe laser (632.8 nm). The optimal irradiance was reported to be between 15 and 105 mW/cm^2, 6–42 mW/cm^2, and 30–210 mW/cm^2, respectively.[11]

None of the above studies has reported adverse reactions or side effects related to exposure to the laser during or after the treatment. However, Beckerman et al. have reported adverse effects with LLLT, such as transitional tingling, mild erythema, burning sensation, pain increase, and exanthems.[28]

Evaluation of the outcome of LLLT treatment for TMD is not easy, leading to possible over- or under-interpretation of results. Some have reported a placebo effect, not knowing if the relief of pain was a real outcome of the therapy or a cyclic spontaneous remission of the symptoms.[46] However, it is worthwhile continuing to test the effectiveness of LLLT for TMD because it is a rapid, non-invasive, aseptic treatment that does not cause harm to the patient.

Suggested parameters

The LLLT parameters for TMD treatment should be determined according to the level of commitment of the articular or muscular structures, clinical signs and symptoms, time of evolution of the disease, and individual physical aspects.[47]

Table 27.1 Treatment protocol for articular symptoms.

Active medium	Diode laser (AsGaAl)
Wavelength	808 nm (infrared)
Power output	100 mW
Spot size	0.028 cm^2
Irradiance	3.5 W/cm^2
Energy per point	2.8 J
Energy density	100 J/cm^2
Time	28 s
Number of points	4
Frequency	Continuous
Mode	In contact
Number of sessions	12 (three a week)

Table 27.2 Treatment protocol for muscular symptoms.

Active medium	Diode laser (AsGaAl)
Wavelength	808 nm (infrared)
Power output	100 mW
Spot size	0.028 cm^2
Irradiance	3.5 W/cm^2
Energy per point	2.8 J
Energy density	100 J/cm^2
Time	28 s
Number of points	1 per 1.5 cm^2 of the muscle in pain
Frequency	Continuous
Mode	In contact
Number of sessions	12 (three a week)

Research groups have achieved good results with the following parameters for TMD cases: infrared diode low power laser (AsGaAl, 808 nm, spot size 0.028 cm^2), 100 J/cm^2, 2.8 J per point, 28 seconds, 100 mW, punctual, continuous mode, perpendicular to the plane of application. Table 27.1 shows a protocol for articular symptoms and Table 27.2 for muscular symptoms.

The TMJ is located anterior to the tragus and next to the external ear canal. In agreement with previous studies of LLLT for TMD, the suggested points of laser application are shown in Fig. 27.1.

The LLLT should be applied around the articular capsule with consideration for the presence of numerous nociceptors in the periauricular tissue (disc, capsular ligaments, and retrodiscal tissue), which are the structures highly related to the pain process in TMD. Similar irradiation points has been described in several papers.[43,48,49] TMJ internal derangements are often associated with pain due to the inflammatory process stretching or disrupting the TMJ collateral ligaments. The most common areas affected by muscle pain in TMD are the masseter and anterior temporal muscles. Therefore, every mandibular movement leads to pain, which can be elicited on muscle and TMJ palpation.

The precise points of applications should be determined according to the complaint and the anatomy of each patient. The LLLT can be applied to the muscle that the patient indicates is painful upon compression, or to trigger points or acupuncture

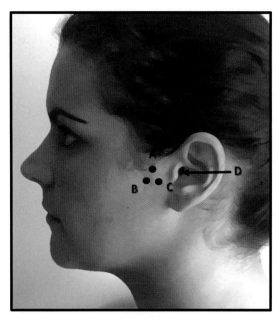

Figure 27.1 Points of laser application for the TMJ: (a) above, (b); anterior, and (c) posterior to the condyloid process; (d) an intra-auricular point towards the joint.

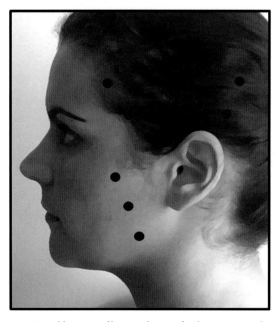

Figure 27.2 Possible points of laser application for the masseter and temporalis muscles.

Clinical case 27.1

A 48-year-old female patient reported orofacial pain upon waking and during mouth opening for 3 months. After anamnesis and physical examination, bilateral capsulitis and bilateral myositis of the masseter muscle was diagnosed, possibly caused by parafunctional habits. She received information about TMD evolution and counseling for habit and behavioral changes. While waiting for an interocclusal splint to be manufactured, she was treated with LLLT.

The patient underwent three sessions of LLLT per week for during 2 weeks with an infrared diode low power laser (AsGaAl, 808 nm, spot size 0.028 cm^2), 100 J/cm^2, 2.8 J per point, 28 seconds, 100 mW, punctual, continuous mode, perpendicular to the plane of application. The points irradiated were selected according to the areas referred to as painful during the RDC-TMD exam (Fig. 27.3).

Initially, the patient presented a passive mouth opening range of 26 mm and severe pain (3 on the 0–3 scale in the RDC-TMD questionnaire) during palpation of the TMJ and masseter muscle. After six LLLT sessions, the passive mouth opening range was 31 mm and the pain during palpation was mild (score 1) in the TMJ and moderate (score 2) in the masseter muscle.

Therapy with the interocclusal splint began and LLLT was given for a further 2 weeks. At the end of 12 sessions (1 month of treatment), the passive mouth opening range reached 36 mm, there was no pain on TMJ palpation and only mild pain (score 1) on masseter muscle palpation.

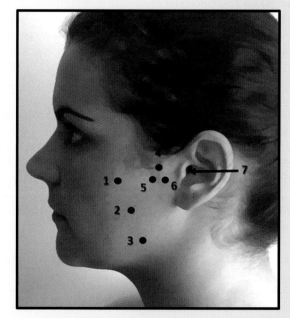

Figure 27.3 Case study: irradiated points.

points. Usually irradiation is applied between the origin, body or insertion of the masseter muscle (up to three irradiation points) and the anterior, middle, and posterior temporal muscle (up to two points each) (Fig. 27.2). Based on the scattering pattern of infrared low power lasers, the application points should be 1.5 cm^2 apart to avoid energy overlap.

The World Association for Laser Therapy recommends two to three sessions of LLLT per week, over 3–5 weeks. It is also important that the treatment is sequential, so the cumulative effect of LLLT can be achieved.[50]

Conclusion

TMD treatment is complex due its multifactorial etiology. LLLT has been accepted as a good adjuvant therapy in the control of pain and improvement of functional limitations.

Further research is necessary to define the exact role of LLLT in relieving pain and the inflammatory process in TMD cases. Future studies should be based on broad samples and their design should be longitudinal, random, and double-blinded with control groups. These are essential in order to obtain consensus regarding the best application protocol and more results with this therapy.

References

1 Di Fabio RP. Physical therapy for patients with TMD: a descriptive study of treatment, disability, and health status. *J Orofac Pain* 1998; 12(2): 124–135.

2 De Leeuw R, ed. Orofacial pain; guidelines for assessment, diagnosis, and management. 4th edn. *Chicago: Quintessence*, 2008: 129–204.

3 McNeil C. History and evolution of TMD concepts. *Oral Surg Oral Med Oral Pathol Oral Radiol Endod* 1997; 83: 51–60.

4 Murray H, Locker D, Mock D, Tenenbaum H. Pain and the quality of life in patients referred to a craniofacial pain unit. *J Orofac Pain* 1996; 10(4): 316–323.

5 Oliveira AS, Bermudez CC, Souza RA, et al. Pain impact on life of patients with temporomandibular disorder. *J Appl Oral Sci* 2003; 11(2): 138–143.

6 Okeson JP. Diagnostico diferencial e consideracões sobre o tratamento das desordens temporomandibulares: In: Okeson JP, ed. *Dor Orofacial: Guia de Avaliacao*, Diagnostico e Tratamento, 3rd edn. Sao Paulo: Quintessence Editora Ltd, 1998: 113–183.

7 Ingawalé S, Goswami T. Temporomandibular joint: disorders, treatments, and biomechanics. *Ann Biomed Eng* 2009; 37(5): 976–996.

8 McNeely ML, Armijo Olivo S, Magee DJ. A systematic review of the effectiveness of physical therapy interventions for temporomandibular disorders. *Phys Ther* 2006; 86(5): 710–725.

9 Demirkol NI, Sari F, Bulbul M, Demirkol M, Simsek I, Usumez A. Effectiveness of occlusal splints and low-level laser therapy on myofascial pain. Lasers Med Sci 2014 Feb 7 [Epub ahead of print].

10 Koh H, Robinson PG. Occlusal adjustment for treating and preventing temporomandibular joint disorders [systematic review]. *Cochrane Database Syst Rev* 2003; (1): 003812.

11 Petrucci A, Sgolastra F, Gatto R, Mattei A, Monaco A. Effectiveness of low-level laser therapy in temporomandibular disorders: a systematic review and meta-analysis. *J Orofac Pain* 2011; 25(4): 298–307.

12 Bjordal JM, Couppé C, Chow RT, Tunér J, Ljunggren AE. A systematic review of low level laser therapy with location-specific doses for pain from joint disorders. *Aust J Physiother* 2003; 49(2): 107–116.

13 Santos T de S, Piva MR, Ribeiro MH, Antunes AA, Melo AR, Silva ED. Laser therapy efficacy in temporomandibular disorders: control study. *Braz J Otorhinolaryngol* 2010; 76(3): 294–249.

14 Fouda A. Comparison between four treatment modalities for active myofascial triggers points. *Plast Aesthetic Res* 2014; 1: 21–28.

15 Fehrenbach MJ, Herring SW, Thomas P. A articulação temporomandibular: Anatomia da articulação temporomandibular. *Tradução: Edson A. Liberti. Anatomia ilustrada da cabeça e do pescoço*, 2nd edn. Sao Paulo: Manole, 2005: 135–143.

16 Myers TW. *Meridianos Miofasciais para terapeutas manuais e do movimento. Trilhos anatômicos. Tradução: Edson A. Liberti*. Sao Paulo: Manole, 2003.

17 Basso D, Correa E, da Silva AN. Efeito da reeducação postural global no alinhamento corporal e nas condições clínicas de indivíduos com disfunção temporomandibular associada a desvios posturais. *Fisioterapia e Pesquisa* 2010; 17(1): 63–68.

18 Benoit P. History and physical examination for TMD. In: Kraus SL, ed. *Clinics in Physical Therapy: Temporomandibular Disorders*, 2nd edn. New York: Churchill Livingstone, 1994: 71–98.

19 Dworkin SF, LeResche L. Research diagnostic criteria for temporomandibular disorders: review, criteria, examinations and specifications, critique. *J Craniomandib Disord* 1992; 6(4): 301–355.

20 Lacerda JT, Simionato EM, Peres KG, Peres MA, Traebert J, Marcenes W. Dental pain as the reason for visiting a dentist in a Brazilian adult population. *Rev Saúde Pública* 2004; 38(3): 453–458.

21 Fikácvoká H, Dostálová T, Vosická R, Peterová V, Navrátil L, Lesák J. Arthralgia of the temporomandibular joint and low-level laser therapy. *Photomed Laser Surg* 2006; 24(4): 522–527.

22 Maia ML1, Bonjardim LR, Quintans Jde S, Ribeiro MA, Maia LG, Conti PC. Effect of low-level laser therapy on pain levels in patients with temporomandibular disorders: a systematic review. *J Appl Oral Sci* 2012; 20(6): 594–602.

23 Carlsson GE. Epidemiology and treatment need for temporomandibular disorders. *J Orofac Pain* 1999; 13(4): 232–237.

24 Bertolucci I.E, Grey T. Clinical analysis of mid-laser vs placebo treatment of arthralgic TMJ degenerative joints. *Cranio* 1995; 13(1): 26–29.

25 Pinheiro ALB, Cavalcanti ET, Pinheiro TI, et al. Low-level laser therapy is an important tool to treat disorders of the maxillofacial region. *J Clin Laser Med Surg* 1998; 16(4): 223–226.

26 Mazzetto MO, Carrasco TG, Bidinelo EF, Pizzo RCA, Mazzetto RG. Low intensity laser application in temporomandibular disorders: a phase I double-blind study. *Cranio* 2007; 25(3): 186–192.

27 Lizarelli R. *Protocollos clínicos odontológicos: Uso do laser de baixa intensidade*, 2nd edn. Sao Carlos: Bons Negócios Editora Ltd, 2005.

28 Beckerman H, de Bie RA, Bouter LM, Cuyper HJ, Oostendorp RA. The efficacy of laser therapy for musculoskeletal and skin disorders: a criteria-based meta-analysis of randomized clinical trials. *Phys Ther* 1992; 72(7): 483–491.

29 Israel HA, Diamond B, Saed-Nejad F, Ratcliffe A. Osteoarthritis and synovitis as major pathoses of the temporomandibular joint: comparison of clinical diagnosis with arthroscopic morphology. *J Oral Maxillofac Surg* 1998; 56(9): 1023–1027.

30 Farias VHA. Análise da ação do laser de baixa potência em pacientes com dor muscular portadores de desordens temporomandibulares empregando a eletromiografia. (Dissertação de mestrado apresentada ao programa de pós-graduação em engenharia biomédica do Instituto de Pesquisa e Desenvolvimento da Universidade do Vale do Paraíba.) São José dos Campos: UNIVAP, 2005.

31 Walker J. Relief from chronic pain by low-power laser irradiation. *Neurosci Lett* 1983; 43(2-3): 339–344.

32 Shimizu N, Yamaguchi M, Goseki T, et al. Inhibition of prostaglandin E2 and interleukin 1-beta production by low-power laser irradiation in stretched human periodontal ligament cells. *J Dent Res* 1995; 74(7): 1382–1388.

33 Sandoval MC, Mattiello-Rosa SM, Soares EG, Parizotto NA. Effects of laser on the synovial fluid in the inflammatory process of the knee joint of the rabbit. *Photomed Laser Surg* 2009; 27(1): 63–69.

34 Jarvis D, MacIver MB, Tanelian DL. Electrophysiologic recording and thermodynamic modeling demonstrate that helium-neon laser

irradiation does not affect peripheral Adelta or C-fiber nociceptors. *Pain* 1990; 43(2): 235–242.

35 Makihara E, Masumi S. Blood flow changes of a superficial temporal artery before and after low-level laser irradiation applied to the temporomandibular joint area. *Nihon Hotetsu Shika Gakkai Zasshi* 2008; 52(2): 167–170.

36 Koes BW, Assendelft WJ, Van der Heijden GJ, Bouter LM. Spinal manipulation for low back pain. *An updated systematic review of randomized clinical trials. Spine* 1996; 21(24): 2860–2871.

37 Wilder-Smith P. The soft laser: therapeutic tool or popular placebo? *Oral Surg Oral Med Oral Pathol* 1988; 66(6): 654–658.

38 Kubota J, Ohshiro T. The effects of diode laser low reactive level laser therapy (LLLT) on flap survival in a rat model. *Laser Ther* 1989; 1: 127–135.

39 Melis M, Di Giosia M, Zawawi KH. Low level laser therapy for the treatment of temporomandibular disorders: A systematic review of the literature. *Cranio* 2012; 30(4): 304–312.

40 Bezuur NJ, Habets LL, Hansson TL: The effect of therapeutic laser treatment on patients with craniomandibular disorders. *J Craniomandib Disord* 1998; 2(2): 83–86.

41 Bertolucci LE, Grey T. Clinical comparative study of microcurrent electrical stimulation to mid-laser and placebo treatment in degenerative joint disease of the temporomandibular joint. *Cranio* 1995; 13(2): 116–120.

42 Gray RJ, Quayle AA, Hall CA, Schofield MA. Physiotherapy in the treatment of temporomandibular joint disorders: a comparative study of four treatment methods. *Br Dent J* 1994; 176(7): 257–261.

43 Simunovic Z. Low level laser therapy with trigger points technique: A clinical study on 243 patients. *J Clin Laser Med Surg* 1996; 14(4): 163–167.

44 Kulekcioglu S, Sivrioglu K, Ozcan O, Parlak M. Effectiveness of low-level laser therapy in temporomandibular disorder. *Scand J Rheumatol* 2003; 32(2): 114–118.

45 Çetiner S, Kahraman SA, Yücetas S. Evaluation of low-level laser therapy in the treatment of temporomandibular disorders. *Photomed Laser Surg* 2006; 24(5): 637–641.

46 Salmos-Brito JA, de Menezes RF, Teixeira CE, et al. Evaluation of low-level laser therapy in patients with acute and chronic temporomandibular disorders. *Lasers Med Sci* 2013; 28(1): 57–64.

47 Venancio R de A, Camparis C, Lizarelli Rde F. Low intensity level therapy in the treatment of temporomandibular disorders: a double-blind study. *J Oral Rehab* 2005; 32(11): 800–807.

48 Mazzetto MO, Hotta TH, Pizzo RC. Measurements of jaw movements and TMJ pain intensity in patients treated with GaAlAs laser. *Braz Dent J* 2010; 21(4): 356–360.

49 Carrasco TG, Mazzetto MO, Mazzetto RG, Mestriner W Jr. Low intensity laser therapy in temporomandibular disorder: a phase II double-blind study. *Cranio* 2008; 26(4): 274–281.

50 Conti PC. Low level laser therapy in the treatment of temporomandibular disorders (TMD): a double blind pilot study. *Cranio*.1997; 15(2):144–149.

CHAPTER 28

Low level lasers in orthodontics

Marinês Vieira S. Sousa

Department of Orthodontics, Bauru Dental School, University of São Paulo (USP), Bauru, SP, Brazil

Introduction: Principles of orthodontic movement

Tooth movement is closely related to the process of bone remodeling, which can occur quickly or slowly depending on the physical force and the biological response of the periodontal ligament (PDL).[1]

The biological results of force application to the tooth are bone resorption by osteoclasts on the pressure side and bone formation by osteoblasts on the traction side of the alveolar bone. Bone resorption and regeneration occur simultaneously around the roots[1-4] (Fig. 28.1).

The tooth movement obtained by the application of forces of different degrees of magnitude, frequency, and duration induce extensive micro and macroscopic changes in the dental and periodontal tissues, including the dental pulp, PDL, alveolar bone, and gingiva.[5]

The acute inflammatory process that defines the initial stage of orthodontic tooth movement is predominantly exudative, in which plasma and leukocytes exit the blood capillaries and enter the PDLs. One or two days later, the acute inflammation stage is replaced by a mainly proliferative chronic process involving fibroblasts, endothelial cells, osteoblasts, and osteoprogenitor cells.[6,7] During this period, leukocytes continue to migrate to the periodontal tissues and modulate the remodeling process.[7]

Changes in the remodeling of periodontal tissues are considered essential for orthodontic tooth movement. The tissue stretching produces local changes in vascularity and in the organization of the cellular and extracellular matrix, leading to the synthesis and release of various neurotransmitters, cytokines (primarily bradykinin), growth factors, colony stimulating factors (granulocytes, macrophages, and other cell types related to bone remodeling), and arachidonic acid metabolites. These cellular and molecular reactions in response to orthodontic forces are the biological basis for tooth movement.[8,9]

This process of orthodontic tooth movement causes pain and discomfort. The time required for fixed orthodontic treatment

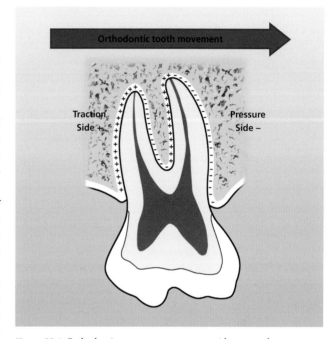

Figure 28.1 Orthodontic movement: –, pressure side – osteoclast activation; +, tension side – osteoblast activation.

is around 2–3 years and the patient will experience pain for this duration. Other disadvantages of long-term orthodontic treatment are the increased risks of gingival inflammation, dental caries, and root resorption.[10]

Although several aspects of orthodontics have significantly developed in the last decades, pain and the need for long-term treatment remain concerns for professionals and patients undergoing orthodontic treatment. Low level laser therapy (LLLT) seems to have proven its effectiveness in addressing these two main complaints.

In orthodontics, LLLT can be used for the reduction of post-adjustment pain,[11-17] bone regeneration in the midpalatal suture area after rapid maxillary expansion,[18] and acceleration of tooth movement.[14,19-22]

Effects of LLLT on the rate of orthodontic movement

The use of LLLT in orthodontics has been demonstrated to be effective in effecting biomodulation, with stimulation of tissue repair.[18,23,24] This stimulatory effect is due to the capacity of LLLT to accelerate metabolic changes[25-27] and, regarding the bone tissue, promote faster bone resorption and neoformation, which are both necessary for orthodontically-induced tooth movement.

Previous studies have tested other methods for their effectiveness in increasing the tooth movement rate without damage to the tooth and periodontium. Several investigations have shown that acceleration of tooth movement can be achieved by local injection of prostaglandins,[28] $1,25 (OH)_{2,3}$ (the active form of vitamin D)[29] or osteocalcin,[30] which is a protein exclusively produced by osteoclasts during the process of bone matrix synthesis. Although these injectable substances increased the speed of tooth movement, they also caused side effects, such as pain and discomfort.

In contrast, to date LLLT has shown beneficial effects with no negative side effects for the patient.

The exact mechanism of biostimulation promoted by LLLT is still unknown, but according to some reports it promotes the appearance of intracellular reactive oxygen species (ROS),[31-34] which increase the formation of adenosine triphosphate (ATP) at the irradiated spots,[35-38] and accelerates cell metabolism. Moreover, the Ca^{2+} ion concentration in the cytoplasm is increased[39-41] by LLLT (wavelength in the infrared band) acting on the Na^+/K^+ pump in the cell membrane.[42-44] This promotes greater protein synthesis and accelerates DNA duplication and RNA replication, accelerating cell metabolism.[45]

The type of laser device is chosen according to the target tissue and effect desired. The best wavelength for biostimulation is between 550 and 950 nm. Because infrared absorption by hemoglobin is lower than that of visible red, lasers that emit infrared light (780–820 nm) are the best at stimulating bone cells because their wavelengths penetrate the soft tissue more deeply, reaching the bone tissue.[46]

Both *in vitro*[47-50] and *in vivo* (animal)[51-56] studies have demonstrated the efficiency of LLLT as a tool to stimulate orthodontic movement, but few clinical trials have confirmed this.[10,14,19-22]

Table 28.1 shows the parameters reported in the scientific literature for LLLT in humans to accelerate the speed of orthodontic tooth movement. The points of laser application used in the studies in Table 28.1 are shown in Figure 28.2. Despite the different parameters used, all studies with the exception of that by Limpanichkul et al.,[10] reported the same conclusions, that is greater stimulation of orthodontic tooth movement with laser application. These data affirm previous studies showing that LLLT is dose dependent.

It is also noted that, when only one tooth is to be moved orthodontically, as in the case of initial retraction of canines, the energy densities ranging from 0.71 to 8 J/cm^2, corresponding to 0.2–2 J per point and 2–8 J per tooth, with three to six monthly applications, are effective in accelerating orthodontic movement. This effectiveness across this range of energy densities is related to differences in the area of the laser equipment tip (spot size).

When the movement of all teeth is to be stimulated, as in the study by Camacho and Cujar,[21] an energy density of around 80 J/cm^2, corresponding to 4.4 J per tooth or approximately 52.8 J per arch, is effective.

The assumption that the effect of LLLT is proportional to the amount of energy irradiated on the tissues is not true, because reports in the literature mention that higher doses of LLLT may have an inhibitory effect on orthodontic tooth movement[57,58]; further studies are needed to confirm this.

In addition to the dosage, another variable is the amount of skin pigmentation in different ethnic groups.[59] Individuals of African descent, for example, have more melanin pigment in the skin or mucosa and for this reason, when these tissues are irradiated, the laser parameters should be adjusted to increase the dosage by approximately 20%, to compensate for the greater amount of energy absorbed by the melanin pigment and ensure the deeper tissues receive the ideal amount of energy.

Effect of LLLT on pain after orthodontic activation

According to the scientific literature, 90–95% of orthodontic patients report pain and 8–30% of these patients interrupt their treatment for this reason.[60-62]

Due to the great discomfort caused by pain in orthodontic treatment, several treatments have been proposed to minimize it. The principal treatment is drugs such as anti-inflammatories or analgesics. However, studies have shown that, besides the side effects of these drugs, tooth movement can be inhibited by administering non-steroidal anti-inflammatory drugs (NSAIDs).[63-67] Also, currently there is a tendency to use natural therapies rather than pharmacological drugs.

In clinical practice, there is almost a consensus that LLLT has an analgesic effect.[11-13,15-17,68-70] However, there is still some controversy because the reported application protocols differ in the irradiation doses delivered for the same procedure, and an analgesic effect has not been reported with some protocols.[71,72]

LLLT reduces pain through different mechanisms from those proposed to be involved in movement: stimulation of the production of beta-endorphin, a natural mediator produced to reduce pain[73]; and inhibition of the release of arachidonic acid by damaged cells, which would generate metabolites that interact with pain receptors (prostaglandin E_2 and interleukin-1β).[68,74-76] While arachidonic acid produces a local effect, beta-endorphin has an analgesic effect throughout the body.

Table 28.1 Doses of low level laser irradiation and their effects on the rate of orthodontic movement in clinical studies ordered according to energy per point (decreasing values): literature review.

Authors	WaveLength (nm) Spot area	Energy density per point (J/cm²)	Power output (mW)	Energy per point (J)	Number of points per tooth	Total Energy per day (J)	Time per point (s)	Total energy per month (J)	Frequency of application	Acceleration of tooth movement
Limpanichkul et al.[10]	860 0.09 cm²	25	100	2.3	8 points: 4 buccally, 4 lingually	18.4	23	55.2	Days 1, 2, and 3 consecutives days after activation	No
Youssef et al.[14]	809 ?	8	100	1 (×2) 2	6 points: 3 buccally, 3 lingually	8	2 points: 10 4 points: 20	32	Days 0, 3, 7, and 14 after activation	Yes
Doshi-Mehta and Bhad-Patil[22]	800 4 mm²	5	100 0.25 ?	0.8	10 points: 5 buccally, 5 lingually	8	40 10 ?	32	Days 0, 3, 7, and 14 after activation (first mouth) and then every 15 days until complete retraction	Yes
Genc et al.[93]	808 0.28 cm²	0.71	20	0.2	10 points: 5 buccally, 5 lingually	2	10	12	Days 0, 3, 7, 14, 21, and 28 after activation	Yes
Cruz et al.[20]	780 0.04 cm²	5	20	0.2	10 points: 5 buccally, 5 lingually	2	10	8	Days 0, 3, 7, and 14 after activation	Yes
Sousa et al.[19]	780 0.04 cm²	5	20	0.2	10 Points: 5 buccally, 5 lingually	2	10	6	Days 0, 3, and 7 after activation	Yes
Camacho and Cujar[21]	830 0.028 cm²	78.57	100	2.2	2 point: 1 buccally, 1 lingually	4.4 × 12 teeth per dental arch (approximately)	22	52,8 per dental arch (approximately)	Unique day after activation	Yes

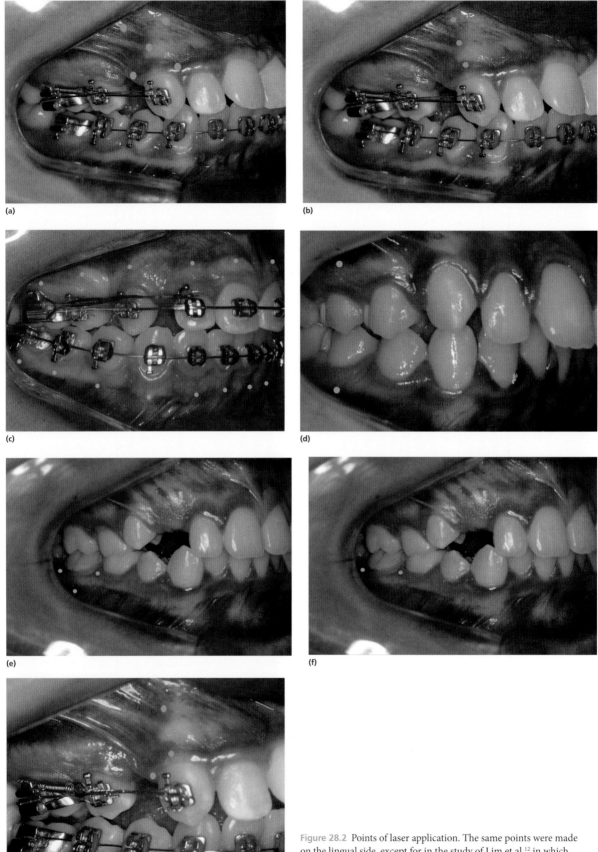

Figure 28.2 Points of laser application. The same points were made on the lingual side, except for in the study of Lim et al.[12] in which the laser was only applied at buccal points. (a) Cruz et al.,[20] Sousa et al.,[19] Angelieri et al.,[71] Tortamano et al.,[15] Genc et al.,[93] and Doshi-Mehta and Bhad-Patil[22]; (b) Youssef et al.[14]; (c) Camacho and Cujar[21] and Turhani et al.[13]; (d) Lim et al.[12]; (e) Artés-Ribas et al.[17]; (f) Bicakci et al.[16] and Esper et al.[72]; (g) Limpanichkul et al.[10]

Table 28.2 Doses of low level laser irradiation and their effects on the inhibition of pain when only one tooth is irradiated ordered according to energy per point (decreasing values): literature review.

Authors	Wavelength (nm) Spot area (cm²)	Energy density per point (J/cm²)	Power output (mW)	Energy per point (J)	Number of points	Total energy (J)	Time per point (s)	Frequency of application	Pain inhibition
Angelieri et al.[71]	780 0.04	5	20	0.2	10 points: 5 buccal, 5 lingual	2	10	Days 0, 3, and 7 after activation	No
Bicakci et al.[16]	820 0.0314	7.96	50	0.25	4 points: 2 buccal, 2 lingual	1	30	Immediately and 24 h after activation	No (immediately) Yes (24 h)
Lim et al.[12]	830 0.53	0.9	30	0.45	1 point	0.45	15	Days, 1, 2, 3, 4 and 5 after activation	No
Esper et al.[72]	660 19	4	30	0.7	4 points: 2 buccal, 2 lingual	2.8	25	Unique day after activation	No
Lim et al.[12]	830 0.53	0.9	30	0.9	1 point	0.9	30	Days, 1, 2, 3, 4 and 5 after activation	Yes NS
Lim et al.[12]	830 0.53	0.9	30	1.8	1 point	1.8	60	Days, 1, 2, 3, 4 and 5 after activation	Yes NS
Youssef et al.[14]	809 ?	10	100	1 (×2) 2	6 points: 3 buccal, 3 lingual	8	2 points:10 1 point: 20	Days 0, 3, 7, and 14 after activation	Yes
Artés-Ribas et al.[17]	830 0.4	5	100	2	6 points: 3 buccal, 3 lingual	12	20	Immediately after activation	Yes

NS, inhibition of pain but no statistically significant difference.

Table 28.3 Doses of low level laser irradiation and their effects on the inhibition of pain when all teeth in the dental arch are irradiated, ordered according to energy per point (decreasing values): literature review.

Authors	Wavelength(nm)/ Spot area (cm²)	Energy density per point (J/cm²)	Power output (mW)	Energy per point (J)	Number of points per tooth	Time per point (s)	Frequency of application	Pain inhibition
Tortamano et al.[15]	830 0.03	16	30	0.5	10 points: 5 buccal, 5 lingual	16	Unique day after activation	Yes
Turhani et al.[13]	670 0.53	4.25	75	2.25	1 point	30	Unique day after activation	Yes

Laser irradiation also suppresses the conduction of nerve impulses at peripheral nerve endings, acting on the Na⁺/K⁺ pump[25,77] or by sensitization of nociceptive transmitters such as bradykinin, histamine, serotonin, and others, in order to inhibit the transmission of the local pain impulse after low level laser irradiation.[78,79]

Few clinical studies have demonstrated the efficiency of LLLT in suppressing pain. Most of those studies that have been reported have evaluated the effects of LLLT on pain suppression in one tooth compared with the non-irradiated tooth on the opposite side (placebo), or in molars/premolars[12,72] separated with elastomers, or in canines in the initial phase of retraction[14,71] (Table 28.2). Other studies have evaluated the effects of LLLT on pain suppression in all teeth in the dental arch after placement of the first archwire (experimental group) compared with a control group[13,15] (Table 28.3).

The points of laser application for analgesia after orthodontic activation are variable and the literature presents several options (Fig. 28.2).

The ability of phototherapy to promote pain relief is dose dependent. Table 28.2 shows that, when only one tooth is irradiated, the energy recommended per point ranges from 0.9 J to 2 J and energy density from 0.9 J/cm² to 10 J/cm². When all teeth in the dental arch are irradiated (Table 28.3), the recommended energy ranges from 0.5 J to 2.25 J per point and the energy density from 4.25 J/cm² to 16 J/cm².

The positive analgesic effects obtained when the entire dental arch is irradiated with low energy doses per point, as demonstrated by Tortamano et al.,[15] probably occur due to irradiation effects throughout the dental arch innervations and PDL cells.[5]

In all the studies cited in Tables 28.2 and 28.3, the laser beam emitted a continuous wave, with the exception of the study by Fujiyama et al., who used a pulsed wave.[11] The latter authors concluded that pulsed LLLT seems to be efficient in promoting analgesia during the first four days after force application, when 20 pulses of 2-W output and five pulses per 1000 seconds were applied at a 2-mm defocus, 30 seconds after separator placement and for a period of 30 seconds.[11]

Effect of LLLT on rapid maxillary expansion

Rapid maxillary expansion (RME) is the treatment of choice to correct a constricted maxillary dental arch.[80–83] This treatment can be surgical, called surgically-assisted rapid maxillary expansion (SARME), in young adults with skeletal maturity; or orthodontic expander appliances can be used in growing patients.[84] Relapse after expansion should be avoided with the use of retainers to guarantee the success of therapy.[83,85]

The suture neoformation and the maxilla should be maintained in the new position for a period to achieve stability. The retention period required for complete ossification of the midpalatal suture is about 8–9 months, keeping the expander in place for 3 months, followed by 6 months of retention with a removable appliance or transpalatal bar[80,86,87] for young patients, and even longer for adult patients undergoing SARME.[88]

Thus, acceleration of the bone regeneration in the midpalatal suture after expansion would be beneficial in reducing the retention period. The use of laser irradiation in bone regeneration is justified by the possibility of reducing the retention period, while ensuring stability after treatment.

There are few studies on the effects of LLLT on the speed of regeneration of the midpalatal suture,[18,89–92] but there is consensus that LLLT increases the bone regeneration rate.

Table 28.4 shows the parameters reported in studies of LLLT in humans to accelerate the regeneration of the midpalatal suture, and Figure 28.3 shows the points of laser application for RME and SARME.

Table 28.4 Doses of low level laser irradiation in humans undergoing rapid maxillary expansion maxillary (RME) or surgically assisted rapid maxillary expansion (SARME):- literature review.

Authors	Wavelength (nm) Spot area (cm²)	Energy density per point (J/cm²)	Power output (mW)	Energy per point (J)	Number of points per tooth	Time per point (s)	Frequency of application
Cepera et al.[89] RME	780 0.04	10	40	0.4	10	10	Days 1, 2, 3, 4, and 5 from start of expansion screw activation Days 1, 2, and 3 immediately after end of expansion Days 11, 15, 19, 22, 27, and 29 from first day of expansion with screw activation
Abreu et al.[92] SARME	824 0.28	1.5	20	0.4	4	20	8 sessions at 48-h intervals

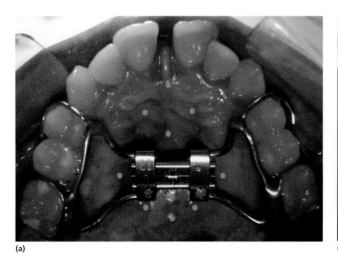
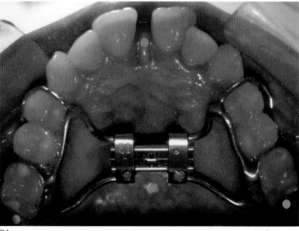

(a)   (b)

Figure 28.3 Points of laser application. (a) Cepera et al.[87] for rapid maxillary expansion (RME); (b) Abreu et al.[90] for surgically assisted rapid maxillary expansion (SARME).

Future prospects

Among the advantages of LLLT are the simplicity of its application, the facts it is painless and does not cause side effects, as well as its few contraindications.

Concerning the clinical implications, faster tooth movement and reduction of retention time after RME or SARME can significantly reduce the treatment time, being especially advantageous for adults who require longer treatment times, which increase the risk of alveolar bone loss and caries recurrence.

A decrease of sensitivity due to orthodontic movement can also be obtained by LLLT, depending on the doses employed.

Besides those facts, LLLT might also stimulate and facilitate tooth movement in difficult clinical situations, such as non-erupted teeth that will undergo orthodontic traction, in molar distalization, or in anterior teeth retraction mechanics. Laser application at stimulation levels, especially on the aforementioned teeth, probably facilitates tooth movement and consequently reduces the treatment time.[19]

There is some evidence that higher doses of LLLT have the opposite effect, that is decrease the speed of orthodontic movement. If this is confirmed, this could be clinically valuable in cases of teeth that require anchorage. Further research is still required, but laser therapy combined with orthodontics seems to have a promising future.

References

1 Consolaro A. Movimentação dentária induzida: biologia aplicada à prática clínica. In: Consolaro A, ed. *Reabsorções Dentárias nas Especialidades Clínicas*. Maringá: Dental Press Editora, 2002: 221–257.

2 Burstone CJ. The biomechanics of tooth movement. In: Kraus BS, Riedel RA, eds. *Vistas in Orthodontics*. Philadelphia: Lea & Febiger, 1962: 197–213.

3 Klein-Nulend J, Bacabac RG, Mullender MG. Mecanobiology of bone tissue. *Pathol Biol* 2005; 53(10): 576–580.

4 Smith RJ, Burstone CJ. Mechanics of tooth movement. *Am J Orthod Dentofacial Orthop* 1984; 85(4): 294–307.

5 Davidovitch Z, Finkelson MD, Steigman S, Shanfeld JL, Montgomery PC, Korostoff E. Electric currents, bone remodeling, and orthodontic tooth movement. *Am J Orthod Dentofacial Orthop* 1980; 77(1): 14–31.

6 Consolaro A. Biologia da movimentação dentária. In: Interlandi S, ed. *Ortodontia: bases para iniciação*, 4th edn. Sao Paulo: Artes Médicas, 1999: 435–439.

7 Krishnan V, Davidovitch Z. Cellular, molecular, and tissue-level reactions to orthodontic force. *Am J Orthod Dentofacial Orthop* 2006; 129(4): 469e.1–e.32.

8 Rody WJ Jr, King GJ, Gu G. Osteoclast recruitment to sites of compression in orthodontic tooth movement. *Am J Orthod Dentofacial Orthop* 2001; 120(5): 477–489.

9 Sodek J, Mckee MD. Molecular and cellular biology of alveolar bone. *Periodontology* 2000; 24: 99–126.

10 Limpanichkul W, Godfrey K, Srisuk N, Rattanayatikul C. Effects of low-level laser therapy on the rate of orthodontic tooth movement. *Orthod Craniofac Res* 2006; 9(1): 38–43.

11 Fujiyama K, Deguchi T, Murakami T, Fujii A, Kushima K, Takano-Yamamoto T. Clinical effect of CO_2 laser in reducing pain in orthodontics. *Angle Orthod* 2008; 78(2): 299–303.

12 Lim HM, Lew KKK, Tay DKL. A clinical investigation of the efficacy of low level laser therapy in reducing orthodontic postadjustment pain. *Am J Orthod Dentofacial Orthop* 1995; 108(6): 614–622.

13 Turhani D, Scheriau M, Kapral D, Benesch T, Jonke E, Bantleon HP. Pain relief by single low-level laser irradiation in orthodontic patients undergoing fixed appliance therapy. *Am J Orthod Dentofac Orthop* 2006; 130(3): 371–377.

14 Youssef M, Ashkar S, Hamade E, Gutknecht N, Lampert F, Mir M. The effect of low-level laser therapy during orthodontic movement: a preliminary study. *Lasers Med Sci* 2008; 23: 27–33.

15 Tortamano A, Lenzi DC, Haddad ACSS, Bottino MC, Dominguez GC, Vigorito JW. *Low-level laser therapy for pain caused by placement of the first orthodontic archwire: A randomized clinical trial Am J Orthod Dentofacial Orthop* 2009; 136(5): 662–667.

16 Bicakci AA, Kocoglu-Altan B, Toker H, Mutaf I, Sumer Z. Efficiency of low-level laser therapy in reducing pain induced by orthodontic forces. *Photomed Laser Surg* 2012; 30(8): 460–465.

17 Artés-Ribas M, Arnabat-Dominguez J, Puigdollers A. Analgesic effect of a low-level laser therapy (830 nm) in early orthodontic treatment. *Lasers Med Sci* 2013; 28(1): 335–341.

18 Saito S, Shimizu N. Stimulatory effects of low-power laser irradiation on bone regeneration in mid palatal suture during expansion in the rat. *Am J Orthod Dentofacial Orthop* 1997; 111(5): 525–532.

19 Sousa MVS, Scanavini MA, Sannomiya EK, Velasco LG, Angelieri F. Influence of low-level laser on the speed of orthodontic movement. *Photomed Laser Surg* 2011; 29(3): 191–196.

20 Cruz DR, Kohara EK, Ribeiro MS, Wetter NU. Effects of low-intensity laser therapy on the orthodontic movement velocity of human teeth: a preliminary study. *Lasers Surg Med* 2004; 35(2): 614–622.

21 Camacho AD, Cujar SAV. Acceleration effect of orthodontic movement by application of low-intensity laser. *J Oral Laser Applications* 2010; 10: 99–105.

22 Doshi-Mehta G, Bhad-Patil WA. Efficacy of low-intensity laser therapy in reducing treatment time and orthodontic pain: A clinical investigation. *Am J Orthod Dentofacial Orthop.* 2012; 141: 289–297.

23 Dortbudak O, Hass R, Mailath-Pokorny G. Biostimulation of bone marrow cells with a diode soft laser. *Clin Oral Impl Res* 2000; 11: 540–545.

24 Volpato LER, Oliveira RC, Espinosa MM, Bagnato VS, Machado AAM. Viability of fibroblasts cultured under nutritional stress irradiated with red laser, infrared laser, and red light-emitting diode. *J Biomed Opt* 2011; 16(7): 075004.

25 Kasai S, Kono T, Yamamoto Y, Kotani H, Sakamoto T, Mito M. Effect of low-power irradiation on impulse conduction in anesthetized rabbits. *J Clin Laser Med Surg* 1996; 14(3): 107–113.

26 Karu TI. Molecular mechanism of the therapeutic effect of low-intensity laser radiation. *Lasers Life Sci* 1988; 2(1): 53–74.

27 Karu TI, Kalendo GS, Ketokhov VS, Lobko VV. Bioestimulation of HeLa cells by low intensity visible light. II Stimulation of DNA and RNA synthesis in a wide spectral range. *Ikvantovaya Elektronika* 1983; 10: 1138–1144.

28 Yamasaki K, Shibata Y, Imai S, Tani Y, Shibasaki Y, Fukuhara T. Clinical application of prostaglandin E1 (PGE1) upon orthodontic tooth movement. *Am J Orthod Dentofacial Orthop* 1984; 85: 508–510.

29 Collins MK, Sinclair PM. The local use of vitamin D to increase the rate of orthodontic tooth movement. *Am J Orthod Dentofacial Orthop* 1988; 94(4): 278–284.

30 Kobayashi Y, Takagi H, Sakai H, Hashimoto F, Mataki S, Kobayashi K, et al. Effects of local administration of osteocalcin on experimental tooth movement. *Angle Orthod* 1998; 68(3): 259–266.

31 Callaghan GA, Riordan C, Gilmore WS, McIntyre IA, Allen JM, Hannigan BM. Reactive oxygen species inducible by low-intensity laser irradiation alter DNA synthesis in the haemopoietic cell line U937. *Lasers Surg Med* 1996; 19: 201–206.

32 Grossman N, Schneid N, Reuveni H, Halevy S, Lubart R. 780 nm low power diode laser irradiation stimulates proliferation of keratinocyte cultures: involvement of reactive oxygen species. *Lasers Surg Med* 1998; 22: 212–218.

33 Lavi R, Shainberg A, Friedmann H, et al. Low energy visible light induces reactive oxygen species generation and stimulates an increase of intracellular calcium concentration in cardiac cells. *J Biol Chem* 2003; 278: 40917–40922.

34 Zang J, Xing D, Gao X. Low-power laser irradiation activates Src tyrosine kinase through reactive oxygen species-mediated signaling pathway. *J Cell Physiol* 2008; 217: 518–528.

35 Benedicenti S, Pepe IM, Angiero F, Benedicenti A. Intracellular ATP level increases in lymphocytes irradiated with infrared laser light of wavelength 904 nm. *Photomed Laser Surg* 2008; 26(5): 451–453.

36 Karu T, Pyatibrat L, Kalendo G. Irradiation with HeNe laser increases ATP level in cells cultivated *in vitro*. *J Photochem Photobiol* 1995; 27: 219–223.

37 Karu T. Mitochondrial mechanisms of photobiomodulation in context of new data about multiple roles of ATP. *Photomed Laser Surg* 2010; 28(2): 159–160.

38 Oron U, Ilic S, De Taboada L, Streeter J. Ga-As (808 nm) laser irradiation enhances ATP production in human neuronal cells in culture. *Photomed Laser Surg* 2007; 25: 180–182.

39 Wu ZH, Zhou Y, Chen JY, Zhou LW. Mitochondrial signaling for histamine releases in laser-irradiated RBL-2H3 mast cells. *Lasers Surg Med* 2010; 42: 503–509.

40 Zungu IL, Evans DH, Abrahamse H. Mitochondrial responses of normal and injured human skin fibroblasts following low level laser irradiation—an *in vitro* study. *Photochem Photobiol* 2009; 85: 987–996.

41 Karu T. Structure of mitochondria and activity of their respiratory chain in subsequent generations of yeast cells exposed to He-Ne laser light. *Izv Akad Nauk Ser Biol* 2005; 6: 672–683.

42 Kassák P, Sikurová L, Kvasnicka P, Bryszewska M. The response of Na⁺/K⁺-ATPase of human erythrocytes to green laser light treatment. *Physiol Res* 2006; 55: 189–194.

43 Konstantinović L, Cernak I, Prokić V. Influence of low level laser irradiation on biochemical processes in brainstem and cortex of intact rabbits. *Vojnosanit Pregl* 1997; 54(6): 533–540.

44 Kujawa J, Zavodnik L, Zavodnik I, Buko V, Lapshyna A, Bryszewska M. Effect of low-intensity (3.75-25 J/cm²) near-infrared (810 nm) laser radiation on red blood cell ATPase activities and membrane structure. *J Clin Laser Med Surg* 2004; 22(2): 111–117.

45 Karu T. Primary and secondary mechanisms of action of visible to near-IR radiation on cells. *J Photochem Photobiol* 1999; 49: 1–17.

46 Gutknecht N, Franzen R. O laser: função, interação e segurança. In: Gutknecht N, Eduardo CP, eds. *A odontologia e o laser*. Berlin: Quintessence Editora Ltd, 2004: 25–60.

47 Fujita S, Yamaguchi M, Utsunomiya T, Yamamoto H, Kasai K. Low-energy laser stimulates tooth movement velocity via expression of RANK and RANKL. *Orthod Craniofac Res* 2008; 11: 143–155.

48 Dominguez A, Castro P, Morales M. An *in vitro* study of the reaction of human osteoblasts to low-level laser irradiation. *J Oral Laser Appl* 2009; 9: 21–28.

49 Aihara N, Yamaguchi M, Kasai K. Low-energy irradiation stimulates formation of osteoclast-like cells via RANK expression *in vitro*. *Lasers Surg Med* 2006; 21: 24–33.

50 Coombe AR, Ho CTG, Philips JR, et al. The effects of low level laser irradiation on osteoblastic cells. *Clin Orthod Res* 2001; 4(1): 3–14.

51 Kawasaki K, Kawasaki K, Shimizu N. Effects of low-energy laser irradiation on bone remodeling during experimental tooth movement in rats. *Lasers Surg Med* 2000; 26(3): 282–291.

52 Kim YD, Kim SS, Kim SJ, Kwon DW, Jeon ES, Son WS. Low-level laser irradiation facilitates fibronectin and collagen type I turnover during tooth movement in rats. *Lasers Med Sci* 2010; 25: 25–31.

53 Yamaguchi M, Fujita S, Yoshida N, Oikawa K, Utsunomiya T, Yamamoto H, et al. Low-energy laser irradiation stimulates the tooth movement velocity via expression of M-CSF and c-fms. *Orthodont Waves* 2007; 66: 139–148.

54 Yamaguchi M, Hayashi M, Fujita S, et al. Low-energy laser irradiation facilitates the velocity of tooth movement and the expressions of matrix metalloproteinase-9, cathepsin K, and alpha(v) beta(3) integrin in rats. *Eur J Orthod* 2010; 32: 131–139.

55 Yoshida T, Yamaguchi M, Utsunomiya T, et al. Low-energy laser irradiation accelerates the velocity of tooth movement via stimulation of the alveolar bone remodeling. *Orthodont Craniofac Res* 2009; 12: 289–298.

56 Altan BA, Sokucu O, Ozkut MM, Inan S. Metrical and histological investigation of the effects of low-level laser therapy on orthodontic tooth movement. *Lasers Med Sci* 2012; 27(1): 131–140.

57 Goulart CS, Nouer PRA, Martins LM, Garbin IU, Lizarelli RFZ. Photoradiation and orthodontic movement: experimental study with canines. *Photomed Laser Surg* 2006; 24(2): 192–196.

58 Seifi M, Shafeei HA, Daneshdoost S, Mir M. Effects of two types of low-level laser wave lengths (850 nm and 630 nm) on the orthodontic tooth movements in rabbits. *Lasers Med Sci* 2007; 22: 261–264.

59 Pinzan A, Pinzan-Vercelino CRM, Martins DR, et al. Atlas de crescimento craniofacial. editora Santos, 2006: 88.

60 Krishnan V. Orthodontic pain: from causes to management – a review. *Eur J Orthod* 2007; 29: 170–179.

61 Bergius M, Kiliaridis S, Berggren U. Pain in orthodontics. *J Orofac Orthop* 2000; 61: 125–137.

62 Polat O, Karaman A. Pain control during fixed orthodontic appliance therapy. *Angle Orthod* 2005; 75(2): 210–215.

63 Carlos F, Cobo J, Díaz-Esnal B, Arguelles J, Vijande M, Costales M. Orthodontic tooth movement after inhibition of cyclooxygenase-2. *Am J Orthod Dentofacial Orthop* 2006; 129: 402–406.

64 Gonzales C, Hotokezaka H, Matsuo KI, et al. Effects of steroidal and nonsteroidal drugs on tooth movement and root resorption in the rat molar. *Angle Orthod* 2009; 79(4): 715–726.

65 Arias OR, Marquez-Orozco MC. Aspirin, acethaminophen, and ibuprofen: their effects on orthodontic tooth movement. *Am J Orthod Dentofacial Orthop* 2006; 130(3): 364–370.

66 Bernhardt MK, Southard KA, Batterson KD, Logan HL, Baker KA, Jakobsen JR. The effect of preemptive and/or postoperative ibuprofen therapy for orthodontic pain. *Am J Orthod Dentofacial Orthop* 2001; 120(1): 20–27.

67 Chumbley AB, Tuncay OC. The effect of indomethacin (an aspirin-like drug) on the rate of orthodontic tooth movement. *Am J Orthod Dentofacial Orthop* 1986; 89(4): 312–314.

68 Shimizu N, Yamaguchi T, Goseki T, et al. Inhibition of prostaglandin E2 and interleukin 1-β production by low-power laser irradiation in stretched human periodontal ligament cells. *J Dent Res* 1995; 74(7): 1382–1388.

69 Harazaki M, Takahashi H, Ito A, Isshiki Y. Soft laser irradiation induced pain reduction in orthodontic treatment. *Bull Tokyo Dent Coll* 1998; 39(2): 95–101.

70 Saito S, Mikikawa Y, Usui M, et al. Clinical application of a pressure-sensitive occlusal sheet for tooth pain—time-dependent pain associated with a multi-bracket system and the inhibition of pain by laser irradiation. *Orthod Waves* 2002; 61: 31–9.

71 Angelieri F, Sousa MVS, Kanashiro LK, Siqueira DF, Maltagliati LA. Efeitos do laser de baixa intensidade na sensibilidade dolorosa durante a movimentação ortodôntica. *Dental Press J Orthod* 2011; 16(4): 95–102.

72 Esper MALR, Nicolau RA, Arisawa EALS. The effect of two phototherapy protocols on pain control in orthodontic procedure—a preliminary clinical study. *Lasers Med Sci* 2011; 26: 657–663.

73 Benedicenti A. *Manuale di laser del cavo orale.* Gênova: Castelo Maggioli, 1982.

74 Mizutani K, Musya Y, Wakae K, et al. A clinical study on serum prostaglandin e2 with low-level laser therapy. *Photomed Laser Surg* 2004; 22(6): 537–539.

75 Iwatsuki K, Yoshimine T, Sasaki M, Yasuda K, Akiyama C, Nakahira R. The effect of laser irradiation for nucleus pulposus: an experimental study. *Neurol Res* 2005; 27(3): 319–323.

76 Ferreira DM, Zângaro RA, Balbin Villaverde A, et al. Analgesic effect of He-Ne (632.8 nm) low-level laser therapy on acute inflammatory pain. *Photomed Laser Surg* 2005; 23(2): 177–181.

77 Tsuchiya K, Kawatani M, Takeshige C, Sato T, Matsumoto I. Diode laser irradiation selectively diminishes slow component of axonal volleys to dorsal roots from the saphenous nerve in the rat. *Neurosci Lett* 1993; 161: 65–68.

78 Ataka I. Studies of Nd:YAG low power laser irradiation on stellate ganglion. In: Ataka I, ed. *Laser in Dentistry*. Amsterdam: Elsevier, 1989: 271.

79 Jimbo K, Noda K, Suzuki K, Yoda K. Suppressive effects of low-power laser irradiation on bradykinin evoked action potentials in cultured murine dorsal root ganglion cells. *Neurosci Lett* 1998; 240: 93–96.

80 Bell RA. A review of maxillary expansion in relation to rate of expansion and patient's age. *Am J Orthod Dentofacial Orthop* 1982; 81: 32–37.

81 Atac ATA, Karasu HA, Aytac D. Surgically assisted rapid maxillary expansion compared with orthopedic rapid maxillary expansion. *Angle Orthod* 2006; 76: 353–359.

82 Babacan H, Sokucu O, Doruk C, Ay S. Rapid maxillary expansion and surgically assisted rapid maxillary expansion effects on nasal volume. *Angle Orthod* 2006; 76: 66–71.

83 Hass AJ. Palatal expansion: just the beginning of dentofacial orthopedics. *Am J Orthod Dentofacial Orthop* 1970; 57: 219–255.

84 Proffit WR, Turvey TA, Phillips C. Orthognathic surgery: a hierarchy of stability. *Int J Othognathic Surg* 1996; 11: 191–204.

85 Nicholson PT, Plint DA. A long term study of rapid maxillary expansion and bone grafting in cleft lip palate patients. *Eur J Orthod* 1989; 11: 186–192.

86 Bishara SE, Staley R. Maxillary expansion: clinical implications. *Am J Orthod Dentofacial Orthop* 1987; 91: 3–14.

87 Betts NJ, Vanarsdall RL, Barber HD, Higgins-Barber K, Fonseca RJ. Diagnosis and treatment of transverse maxillary deficiency. *Int J Adult Orthod Orthognath Surg* 1995; 10: 75–96.

88 Gurgel JA, Malmstrom MFV, Pinzan-Vercelino CRM. Ossification of the midpalatal suture after surgically assisted rapid maxillary expansion. *Eur J Orthod* 2011; 34: 39–43.

89 Cepera C, Torres FC, Scanavini MA, Paranhos LR, Capelloza Filho L, Cardoso MA, et al. Effect of a low-level laser on bone regeneration after rapid maxillary expansion. *Am J Orthod Dentofacial Orthop* 2012; 141: 444–450.

90 Silva APRB, Petri AD, Crippa GE, Stuani AS, Rosa AL, Stuani MBS. Effect of low-level laser therapy after rapid maxillary expansion on proliferation and differentiation of osteoblastic cells. Lasers Med Sci 2011.

91 Angeletti P, Pereira MD, Gomes HC, Hino CT, Ferreira LM. Effect of low-level laser therapy (GaAlAs) on bone regeneration in midpalatal anterior suture after surgically assisted rapid maxillary expansion. *Oral Surg* 2010; 109(3): e38–e46.

92 Abreu MER, Viegas VN, Pagnoncelli RM, et al. Infrared laser therapy after surgically assisted rapid palatal expansion to diminish pain and accelerate bone healing. *World J Orthod* 2010; 11: 273–277.

93 Genc G, Kocadereli I, Tasar F, Kilinc K, El S, Sarkarati B. Effect of low-level laser therapy (LLLT) on orthodontic tooth movement. *Lasers Med Sci* 2013; 28(1): 41–47.

CHAPTER 29

Traditional Chinese medicine and laser therapy

Mario Pansini,[1] Fabiano Augusto Sfier de Mello,[2] and Andrea Malluf Dabul de Mello[2]

[1] Private Dental Practice, Curitiba, PR, Brazil
[2] Herrero Faculty, Curitiba, PR, Brazil

Traditional Chinese medicine (TCM) emphasizes the relationship between humans and their environment, and takes this into account in determining the etiology, diagnosis, and treatment of disease.[1]

The diagnostic tools and therapeutic techniques that have been incorporated into the healing arts for centuries have not altered the therapeutic principles of TCM. The set of theoretical and empirical knowledge of TCM therapy aimed at curing diseases has for centuries been transmitted from generation to generation. Needles, phytotherapy, and moxas have been used for this.

Even today, given the method of teaching and the difficulty in understanding the terminology, TCM still does not fit easily within conventional medical practice, restricting its full acceptance by Western clinicians. Although acupuncture is an ancient practice, it is only in recent decades that neuroscience and recent studies have begun to demonstrate that TCM is invaluable in the treatment of much pathology. Despite its long history and tradition, acupuncture is a dynamic discipline that allows the incorporation of other techniques,[2] such as ultrasound, infrasound, electric current, infrared light, sound (tuning forks), and lasers. According to Wen,[3] TCM has enriched the therapeutic resources available in health care in general.

The use of sunlight in a natural way for the benefit of health, heliotherapy, has been used to cure some diseases since the dawn of the oldest civilizations. According to Jorge Melo, a holistic therapist and member of the International Scientific Research of the Ancestry Natural Medicines, therapies that employ the resources of nature have been gaining strength.[4] Ancient healers in India, Greece, the Roman Empire, and Mesopotamia used the sunbath. The spectrum of sunlight is composed of different colors, or different wavelengths, some of which penetrate the skin and induce chemical reactions that may result in cure. Conventional medicine uses the benefits of sunlight, as stated Shirlei Borelli and the Brazilian Society of Dermatology. Dermatologists point out the anti-inflammatory and immune-modulatory effects of the sun,[4] Science recognizes some therapeutic properties of sunlight in combating pain and inflammation, and preventing osteoporosis, among other uses.

Among the physical properties of laser monochromatic light is its ability to be directed to a point or a selected area, magnifying the therapeutic effect of light. Different lasers have different wavelengths and can be used to treat different diseases.

In dentistry, laser therapy is used as an auxiliary tool in a variety of procedures and even as a unique resource in the treatment of paresthesia,[5] glossitis, and paresthesia.[6] The laser technique is non-invasive, painless, and can be combined with other treatments.[7]

Laser therapy is applied to the diseased areas, and therefore differs from acupuncture. Tou Wu Kwang has likened laser therapy to the practice of a kind of "small acupuncture."[8] However, the application of laser light to points traditionally recognized in acupuncture gives better results compared with local application alone.[8]

In laser acupuncture, acupuncture points are stimulated by laser irradiation. There are similarities and differences in the mechanisms of action of needles and lasers on tissues. The advantages and disadvantages of one technique over another for a particular patient need to be weighed by the practitioner to give the best therapeutic results and greater patient comfort. The use of needles can invoke fear in patients, and for this reason laser irradiation is advocated by some authors for children; also laser therapy can be used in areas where needles are impractical, such as lesions of the oral mucosa and tongue.[8]

One of the therapeutic principles of acupuncture is to restore the flow of energy (Qi) in the patient, because its obstruction or stagnation in the channels or meridians results in pain. This same principle of distribution of hydrodynamic energy (Qi) can be applied to the study of therapeutic lasers in the treatment of pain, because laser-irradiated biological tissues undergo vasodilatation, favoring the restoration of blood flow; using the language of TCM, lasers unblock the channels through which Qi and Xue (energy and blood, respectively) circulate, locally and systemically.

For the repair of any damaged tissue, systemic and local blood circulation is vital. From the viewpoint of TCM, "boredom, annoyance, and frustration" that reach the organs, especially the liver, are responsible for the distribution of energy and blood. Stress leads to an altered emotional state, with loss of sleep and other physiological changes. The stagnation of Qi (energy) of Xue (blood) and stress should be eliminated. By recovering movement and sleep, and calming the mind, acupuncture can facilitate other local treatments.

According to Maciocia,[1] all Chinese medical physiology, pathology, and treatment can eventually be reduced to the theory of Yin–Yang. The concept of Yin and Yang should be seen as an extremely simple yet profound one, and is regarded as fundamental to TCM. Disruption of the balance between Yin (negative) and Yang (positive) will lead to disease. Therefore, restoring the balance between Yin and Yang will restore an unhealthy organism to its normal state of health: "When Yin predominates, Yang is unbalanced, when Yang predominates, Yin is unbalanced."[9] Thus, all aspects of the theory of TCM – organic structure, physiological functions, and pathological changes of the human body – are explained by the theory of Yin–Yang, and this theory also serves as a guide to diagnosis and clinical treatment.

Light is Yang: laser irradiation at an acupuncture point delivers Yang energy. However, the Yang energy of the laser is often used without regard to the above theory, which can sometimes result in undesirable side effects from its systemic action on the meridians, exacerbating pain, and causing dizziness and headaches due to increased blood pressure. However, this does not mean that laser therapy cannot be used to treat hypertension; studies from the USSR between 1970 and 1972 have supported the benefit of laser therapy in the treatment of hypertension and asthma.[5] However, it is important to know how to control a patient's increase in blood pressure if it occurs, such as by bleeding from the ear and even the use of laser Yin meridian points (points P7 and R6, linked to the lung and kidney, are often used to open the passages of water and nourish the Yin). In the patient with a history of high blood pressure, the balance should be restored before the laser treatment and or laser acupuncture.

The therapeutic effectiveness of laser treatment has been demonstrated in studies from all around the world. Mast cells tend to degranulate during the acute inflammation phase and release biologically active substances such as histamine, serotonin, heparin, and active enzymes, which have been suggested to mediate an increase in vascular permeability.[10] Almeida[11] cited studies of low power lasers in animal models that showed a marked increase in the degranulation of mast cells and levels of histamine, resulting in vasodilatation. The increased blood flow reported by Kami et al.[12] following irradiation with a diode laser makes it clear that the dilation of blood vessels, as a result of the increased release of histamine, accelerates the dispersion of toxic substances and therefore the resolution of inflammatory processes.

Other studies have shown the ability of laser irradiation, both visible and near infrared, to restore the activity of enzymes that have been partially degraded in damaged tissues. Such enzymes may interrupt toxic mediators of pain. For example, superoxide dismutase degrades the superoxide free radical that can accumulate in chronic pathology in skeletal muscle.[13]

Based on the above work, it can be proposed that the toxic substances mediating pain are degraded by the activation of enzymes and more easily removed from the acute inflammatory processes by the increased blood flow induced by the release of histamine, thus favoring pain control.

Laser acupuncture is used in the treatment of diseases such as hypertension, asthma, labyrinthitis, shingles, cold sores, tingling, facial paralysis, dysesthesia, trigeminal neuralgia, chronic pharyngitis, chronic sinusitis, chronic tonsillitis, rheumatic diseases, osteoarthritis, inflammatory processes, neuritis, temporomandibular joint disorders, depression, and hypersensitivity after dental treatment, including tooth whitening; this list overlaps with the disorders commonly treated by traditional acupuncture. The combined use of laser therapy and acupuncture adds the anti-inflammatory, analgesic, antispasmodic, vasodilatory, and regenerative effects inherent in laser therapy to the results obtained with traditional acupuncture.

According to Tou Wu Kwang,[14] laser therapy is not appropriate for the following diseases: peripheral ischemia, preclinical stages of preinfarction or stroke, acute inflammation with septicemia, and neoplasic diseases.

Based on the ancient principles of TCM, an important component of the methodology of needling is the technique of toning and sedation. Chen has stated: "diseases must be drained by excess and deficiency diseases should be toned."[15] In needling, many of the manipulation techniques were developed by ancient practitioners to tone and soothe; today only seven of them are still used in daily clinical practice.

Studies reporting the use of laser therapy in acupuncture have used different equipment and there does not appear to be a standard technique. Laser use in continuous mode, with fluencies, frequencies, and higher powers are suggested for sedation, whereas pulsed or interrupted mode, with fluencies, frequencies, and lower powers are suggested for toning. As suggested by some authors, the oblique positioning of the needle in the opposite direction to the meridian for sedation, and in the same direction for toning, can also be adopted for a laser pointer. However, as these suggestions for laser acupuncture are also contraindicated in the literature, it would seem sensible for the practitioner to adopt the better studied laser protocols that have been developed for laser therapy rather than laser acupuncture specifically.

Two specific conditions are discussed below to illustrate the use of laser acupuncture.

Acute herpes zoster and post-herpetic neuralgia

Laser irradiation has a beneficial effect on both acute herpes zoster and post-herpetic neuralgia (PHN). When used on acupuncture points and locally, it relieves symptoms and reduces pain (see Clinical case 29.1). There are also reasons to believe that treatment in the acute phase reduces the risk PHN. Kemmotsu et al.[16] have suggested that by restoring blood flow, laser therapy prevents the death of a large number of nerve fibers, thereby decreasing the possibility of the development of PHN.

The ability of infrared laser irradiation to promote relief of pain in the treatment of PHN has been demonstrated by Moore[17]; conventional therapy had failed to do so. Mckibbin et al. treated 39 patients suffering from PHN with a GaAs laser.[18] The average pain value for the whole group prior to the treatment, based on the VAS pain scale, was 8.5; at the end of treatment it was 3.3 and 1 year after treatment it was 2.8 (44% of the treated patients were completely free of symptoms).

According to a study by Wang et al.,[19] the application of acupuncture needles stimulates specific nerve fibers that produce

---

Clinical case 29.1 Herpes zoster and post-herpetic neuralgia

A male patient who has undergone renal transplantation was hospitalized for an acute manifestation of herpes zoster. After 3 days pain relief with conventional treatments was poor.

Two dentists who use acupuncture in their practice discussed the possibility of using laser acupuncture with the clinician responsible for this patient, as well as the laser protocol. Acupuncture points were irradiated with infrared light and the injured tissue with visible red light (Fig. 29.1a).

Acupuncture points were chosen to promote the blood circulation, remove heat, reduce pain, tone organs, and increase immunity (Fig. 29.1b).

The patient improved rapidly and after the second application of laser therapy (2 days after the first) the patient was discharged (Fig. 29.1c). After 4 days of treatment the patient could return to work. Maintenance treatment was given every 30 days, and at nearly 2 years follow-up, no other events had required intervention.

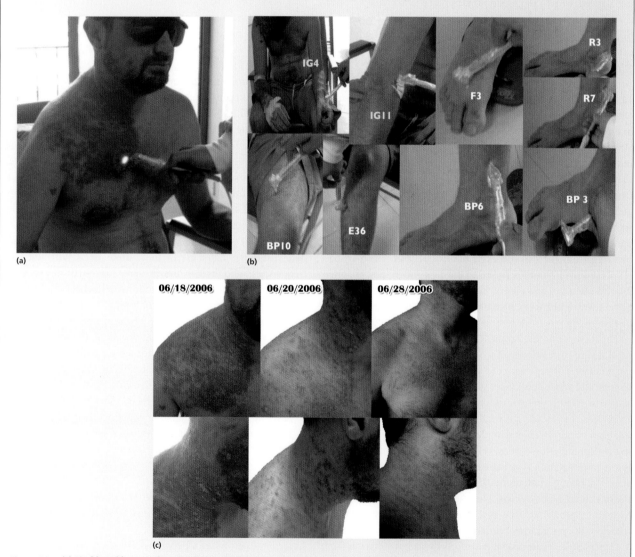

Figure 29.1 (a) Visible red laser application all over the injured area. (b) Laser (infrared) acupuncture points. (c) Treatment evolution over 10 days.

Clinical case 29.2 Paresthesia caused by a mandibular third molar tooth extraction

Tooth 48 was extracted in a 32-year-old female patient (Fig. 29.2). Laser therapy was initiated after 60 days after surgery, preceded by the use of B vitamins, with no real results.

During the initial assessment, the patient was informed about the laser treatment and also that the partial lesion recovery rate for this treatment is on average 80% and that the risk of total disruption of the alveolar nerve is small. Ten laser applications were sufficient for full recovery of the patient. The irradiation points with an infrared laser light (830 nm) are shown in Figure 29.3; a total of 24 J was delivered per application (6 J per point).

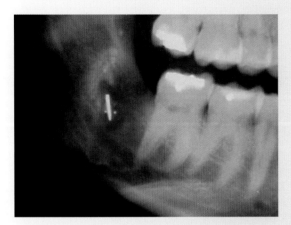

Figure 29.2 Roots of the third molar in relation to the inferior alveolar nerve.

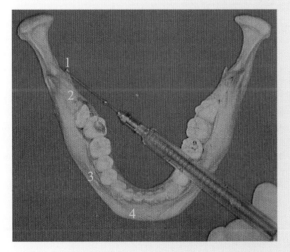

Figure 29.3 Proposed sites of laser application.

Clinical case 29.3 Paresthesia in implantology

A 69-year-old female patient, who was very nervous and angry, presented 1 year after a surgical injury that resulted in inferior alveolar nerve paresthesia.

Surgery was required to fix the implant and lateralization of the alveolar nerve that had lead to the paresthesia. The major complication, fracture of the mandibular bone, occurred during fixation of the prosthesis (Fig. 29.4). Thus the implants had to be removed to allow bone fracture repair. In addition to paresthesia, the patient was left with her face badly deformed by swelling, which lasted until just before the end of treatment with laser acupuncture.

The acupuncture points used were ID3 (small intestine) and B62 (bladder), for recovery of the injured nerve; IG4 (large intestine) and F3 (liver) for circulation of Qi and Xue; PC6 (pericardium) to calm the mind; E36 (stomach) to act on the face and improve the mood of the patient (Fig. 29.5). At these points, 2 J of energy of fluency 50 J/cm^2 were delivered.

Following the very first applications, the results in terms of the patient's emotional state were clearly visible, followed by reduction of facial edema. Fifteen weeks of treatment were required for 100% recovery of paresthesia.

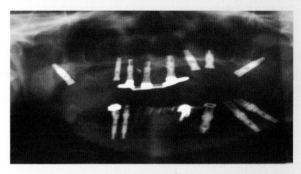

Figure 29.4 Paresthesia in implantology.

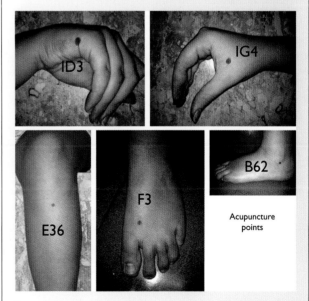

Figure 29.5 Acupuncture points.

sensations similar to those experienced by stimulation of nerve fibers of type A delta (A δ), as occurs in shock and paresthesia.

According to Levine et al.[20] acupuncture applied to areas of skin affected by PHN was not effective, but an analgesic effect may be achieved when puncture points in other areas are used. However, Nurmikko and Bowsher,[21] showed that in PHN the typical sensation produced by stimulation of type A fibers is absent.

The C fibers, which are responsible for the perpetuation of pain, have been found to be more easily stimulated by laser light. Therefore, it was concluded that in the PHN type of pathology, unmyelinated nerve fibers (C) stimulated by light suffer less degradation during the acute phase and/or undergo faster repair.

Paresthesia

Paresthesia is defined as a neurosensitive disorder caused by injury to the nervous tissue. Inferior alveolar nerve paresthesias are the most commonly seen by dentists, often due to injury occurring in procedures such tooth extraction, cystectomy, apicetomy, surgery for implant placement, needle use for anesthesia, as well as several diseases.[22] Extraction of third molars is the most common procedure in surgery and treatment of trauma, and the rate of injury during this procedure that results in paresthesia ranges from 5.5%[5] to 13.4%.[23] The literature on an alternative to B vitamins for the treatment of paresthesia is sparse; laser acupuncture is a possible alternative (see Clinical cases 29.2 and 29.3).

Other disorders, such as mucositis and dental hypersensitivity, as well as those caused by dental procedures (preparation of vital teeth for prosthesis and dentistry, teeth whitening), can also be treated with laser acupuncture, avoiding the redness and pain that can occur with repeated local application of laser therapy.

References

1 Maciocia G. *The Fundamentals of Chinese Medicine.* Sao Paulo: Roca Publisher Ltd, 1996.
2 Whittaker P. Laser acupuncture: past, present, and future. *Lasers Med Sci* 2004; 19: 69–80.
3 Wen TS. *Traditional Chinese Acupuncture.* New York: Cultrix Publisher Ltd, 2006.
4 http://www.maisde50.com.br/artigo.asp? id=5143
5 Shelley M, et al. Preliminary study of low-level laser for treatment of long-standing aberrations in the inferior alveolar nerve. *J Oral Maxillofac Surg* 1996; 54: 2–7.
6 Turner J, Hode L. *Laser Therapy in Dentistry and Medicine.* Prima Books AB Publisher, 1999.
7 Hode L. *Side effects and risks associated with LILT in lasers in medicine and dentistry.* Sweden: Rijeka Vitagraf, 2000: 513–526.
8 Swedish Laser Medical Society. The low-level laser therapy LLLT Internet guide. http://www.laser.nu/lllt/laserworld.htm [accessed 2011].
9 Xinnong C. *Chinese acupuncture and moxibustion [Ednéia Iara Souza Martins, scientific review Lo Sz Hsien].* London: Roca, 1999.
10 Silveira LB. *Checking the behavior of mast cells in the wall of the periodontal pocket is not mineralized bone above subjected to laser radiation of low intensities.* (Study in animal Nobile). Dissertation submitted as part of the requirements for the degree of master professional lasers in dentistry. IPEN/FOUSP, São Paulo, 2001.
11 Almeida LL. Analysis of *in vitro* proliferation of human gingival fibroblasts treated with low power laser. Sao Jose dos Campos. Thesis (MSc). Research and Development Institute of the University of Vale do Paraiba, 1999.
12 Kami T, Yoshimura Y, et al. Effect of low-powered laser diode on flap survival. *Ann Surg* 1985; 14(3): 278.
13 Bradley PF. Pain relief in laser therapy. 5th Congress of the International Society for Laser Dentistry May 5–9 Jerusalem, Israel, 1996.
14 Kwang WT. Laser therapy and Laser acupuncture. Swedish Laser Medical Society. Available at www.laser.nu/lllt/laserworld.htm
15 Chen TS Jirui NW, eds. *Clinical cases of acupuncture in China.* [Rinaldo Koester Santori]. New York: Roca Publisher, 2007.
16 Kemmotsu T, et al. LILT for pain attenuation. Proceedings of the 2nd Congress of the World Association for Laser Therapy, Kansas City, 1998: 7–8.
17 Moore K, et al. LLLT treatment of post herpetic neuralgia. Laser Ther 1998; a: 7.
18 Mckibbin L, et al: Treatment of post herpetic neuralgia using a 904 nm (infrared) low-energy laser: A clinical study. *Laser Ther* 1991; 3(1): 35.
19 Wang KM, Yaos M, Xian YL, Hou Z. A study on the receptive field of acupoints and the relationship between characteristics of needle sensation and groups of afferent fibers. *Scientia Sinica* 1985; 28: 963–971.
20 Levine JD, Gormley J, Fields HL Observations on the analgesic effects of puncture needle (acupuncture). *Pain* 1976; 2: 149–159.
21 Nurmikko T, Bowsher D. Somatosensory findings in post herpetic neuralgia. *J Neurol Neurosurg Psychiatry* 1990; 53: 135–141.
22 Torreira MMG, Lopes MDR, et al. Paresthesia caused by endodontic treatment. *Oral Med* 2003; 8: 299–303.
23 Brann CR, Brickley, MR, Shepherd, JP Factors influencing nerve damage during lower third molar surgery. *Br Dent J* 1999; 186: 514.

Treatment of oral and facial lesions

CHAPTER 30

Papilloma and fibroma

Luiz Alcino Guerios,[1] Igor Henrique Silva,[2] Lucia de Fátima Cavalcanti dos Santos,[3] and Jair Carneiro Leão[1]

[1] Department of Clinic and Preventive Dentistry, Pernambuco Federal University, Recife, PE, Brazil
[2] Maurício de Nassau University Center, Recife, PE, Brazil
[3] Real Center of Systemic Dentistry, Real Hospital Português de Pernambuco, Recife, PE, Brazil

Papilloma (oral squamous papilloma)

Oral squamous papilloma (OSP) is a benign epithelial neoplasia associated with the proliferation of oral epithelium, which promotes a papillary or verrucous surface associated with human papilloma virus (HPV) infection. HPV is a large family of more than 100 subtypes of double-stranded DNA viruses with a remarkable affinity for epithelial cells. Some subtypes of HPV are associated with benign lesions of the oral cavity, and subtypes 6 and 11 are associated with OSP. Verruca vulgaris, condyloma acuminatum, and multifocal epithelial hyperplasia (Heck's disease) are examples of benign lesions associated with other subtypes of HPV.

OSP is clinically characterized as a painless, non-bleeding, pedunculated, exophytic lesion with a verrucous surface forming a cauliflower-like aspect, and microscopically characterized by finger-shaped epithelial projections (see Clinical case 30.1). Oral lesions occur mostly on the tongue, lips, and soft palate, but any site can be affected. The lesions present no gender predilection, and are found at any age, but more commonly in the fourth to fifth decades of life. OSP often presents as a single lesion with a white surface, but coalescent multiple lesions may occur (papillomatosis). Despite the distinctive clinical features, other verrucous or HPV-associated lesions, such as verruciform xanthoma, condyloma accuminatum, oral warts, and oral focal epithelial hyperplasia, should be considered in the differential diagnosis. Therefore, regardless of clinical presentation, biopsy followed by histopathological analysis should always be performed in order to confirm diagnosis. Surgical removal of the lesion is an effective treatment, and recurrence is rarely observed. Laser surgery may also be a suitable treatment option for the management of OSP, reducing surgical time and postoperative complications.

Fibroma (fibrous hyperplasia)

Fibroma or fibrous hyperplasia (FH) is a reactive lesion that originates from the connective tissue and represents a very common lesion of the oral cavity. Although defined by some

authors as a benign neoplasm of connective tissue, it is not believed to represent a benign tumor tissue, but rather a clinical presentation of a reactive hyperplasia. It may occur in any site of the oral cavity, but mostly on the buccal mucosa, lips, and tongue, as an asymptomatic sessile normal colored nodule. Size may vary, but most lesions have a diameter of less than 1.5 cm.

Reactive masses associated with poorly fitting denture edges are called inflammatory fibrous hyperplasia (IFH). Clinically, IFHs are observed as an exophytic lesion with a pleated surface at the edge of the traumatizing prosthesis (see Clinical case 30.2), usually in the buccal fornix and the lingual portion of the lower alveolar ridge. In most cases, both FH and IFH can be diagnosed clinically without the need for additional tests, but microscopic evaluation after exeresis of the lesions is mandatory. Surgical removal is the treatment of choice, and no recurrence is expected if the source of trauma is also removed. In some situations, just removing the local traumatic factor can be an effective treatment. Partial regression of the lesion can be noted after the removal of the source of local trauma, but if complete regression of the lesion does not occur, a surgical procedure is indicated.

Laser treatment

Since the early 1960s when the CO_2 laser was introduced into dental and medical research, several studies using CO_2, diode, Er:YAG, Er,Cr:YSGG, or Nd:YAG lasers for the treatment of oral lesions have been published. Laser surgery is reported to promote minimal bleeding and postoperative pain, diminished scarring and edema, reduced inflammatory reaction, and avoidance of need for suturing.[1] Consequently, laser surgery incurs minimal morbidity and promotes a more conservative surgery, greater hemostasis control, and reduced clinical time. In addition, a precise dissection of tissue allows for adequate microscopic analysis of the specimen and makes the laser an adequate tool for diagnosis and treatment.[2]

On the other hand, delayed repair and tissue necrosis may be observed even when adequate parameters are applied. When the

Lasers in Dentistry: Guide for Clinical Practice, First Edition. Edited by Patrícia M. de Freitas and Alyne Simões.
© 2015 John Wiley & Sons, Inc. Published 2015 by John Wiley & Sons, Inc.

Figures 30.1 and 30.2 show the removal of an OSP and IFH with an Nd:YAG laser (Fotona Fidelis Plus®; Fotona, Liubljana, Slovenia), respectively. Surgeries were performed under local anesthesia. Biosafety protocols were rigorously followed, with consideration given to the risk of smoke contamination and dental team and patient contamination when removing the oral papilloma.

Both patients showed similar clinical results without any recurrence after 6 months of follow-up. For both cases, the Nd:YAG laser was used with an optical fiber with a diameter of 320 μm in the short pulse mode (SP), at 4 W and 60 Hz (power density 5 W/cm^2 and energy density 150 J/cm^2).

Lack of bleeding was noted immediately after complete lesion removal (Fig. 30.2b) and low level laser therapy (LLLT) was performed with the same laser and optical fiber in a unfocused mode (2 mm from the oral mucosa) at 1.25 W and 15 Hz (power density 1.562 W/cm^2) for five sessions of 60 seconds each. After 2 weeks an area of second intention healing was observed at the surgical site without signs of bleeding or inflammation (Fig. 30.1b), and complete healing was observed after 3 (OSP; Fig. 30.1c) to 4 weeks (FPH; Fig. 30.2c).

In summary, the Nd:YAG laser was effective for the surgical treatment of OSP and IFH.

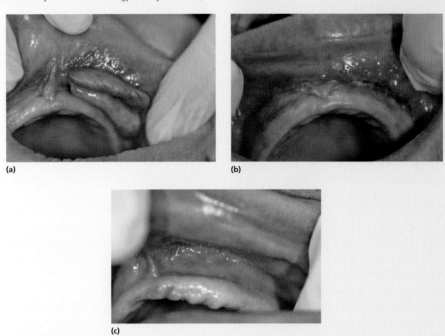

Figure 30.1 (a) Palatal squamous papilloma, with a typical warty surface. (b) Clinical aspect imediately following laser surgery. (c) Complete healing observed 07 days following surgery. No scaring was noted.

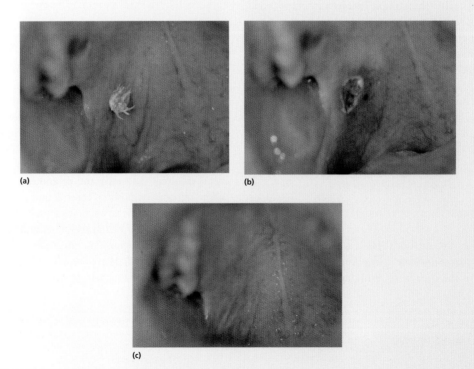

Figure 30.2 (a) Typical aspects of an IFH, located in the anterior buccal sulcus. (b) Clinical postoperative aspect 7 days following laser surgery. (c) omplete healing observed 15 days following surgery. No scaring was noted.

laser beam is in contact with the tissue, it transfers heat, promotes blood clotting (photocoagulation), and has significant advantages for performing oral soft tissue surgery, with greater control of hemostasis and no need for suturing. However, temperatures higher than 100 °C result in volatilization of the tissue, smoke formation, and potential tissue damage. So, the use of high power lasers requires appropriate training for good clinical results and reduced risk of irreversible tissue damage. Postoperative complications such as pain, bleeding, difficulties with speech, obstructive submandibular sialadenitis, and paresthesia of the lingual nerve have been reported after laser surgical treatment of potentially malignant lesions.[1] An extremely rare, but reported, complication is airway fire during operation.[3]

Laser surgery of oral papillomas and fibrous hyperplasia

OSP and FH can be adequately managed with high power lasers. As previously stated, adequate hemostasis at the surgical sites and postoperative comfort can be achieved with laser surgery. Some authors have suggested the feasibility of performing laser removal of OSP and FH under topical anesthesia, mostly when using the Er,Cr:YSGG laser.[4,5] Nevertheless, operative pain may become significant, depending on the lesion size and laser type. Compared to the diode laser (808 nm) and conventional surgery for the removal of oral lesions, the Er,Cr:YSGG laser is less traumatic and provides better healing. The advantages and clinical success of the treatment of oral lesions with a high power laser indicates that it is a safe and effective alternative to conventional surgery. CO_2 laser, high power diode laser, and Nd:YAG laser surgery should be performed under local anesthesia, and similar postoperative results can be obtained. Interestingly, laser surgery of IFH warrants immediate use of an adjusted prosthesis without pain or discomfort during oral function.[6]

Limitations and safety measures
Lesion size

Vescovi et al. evaluated the impact of the laser-associated thermal effect on the histopathological features of FH removed with an Nd:YAG laser.[7] It was demonstrated that lesions with a diameter of less than 7 mm suffer serious thermal effects, regardless of the parameters used, but these do not impair microscopic diagnosis. While the microscopic diagnosis of FH is sound and clear, the diagnosis of other lesions with more complex histopathological features or the grading of epithelial dysplasias may be impaired following their morphological alteration with laser surgery. To avoid compromising the biopsy of small lesions for diagnostic purposes, it can be recommended

that laser surgery is only indicated for the biopsy of lesions larger than 1 cm.

Contamination

The laser removal of OSP is associated with tissue volatilization and risk of HPV contamination. HPV DNA has been identified in the plume generated during CO_2 laser treatment of respiratory tract papillomas and plantar warts, but whether or not these dispersed viral particles are infectious remains elusive. Nevertheless, recurrent respiratory papillomatosis was reported in healthcare workers who performed repeated laser therapies for patients with genital warts.[8] On the other hand, a recent study by Ilmarinen et al. showed that protective equipment, mostly surgical gloves, may become contaminated by HPV, but human viral transmission is unlikely if protective devices are properly used.[9] Rigorous use of protective devices, including laser plume masks, saline irrigation to reduce plume production, and an effective surgical aspirator may diminish the risk of HPV contamination, and are warranted for the safety of the patient and the dental team.

References

1 Goodson ML, Sugden K, Kometa S, Thomson PJ. Complications following interventional laser surgery for oral cancer and precancerous lesions. *Br J Oral Maxillofac Surg* 2012; 50(7): 597–600.
2 Hamadah O, Thomson PJ. Factors affecting carbon dioxide laser treatment for oral precancer: a patient cohort study. *Lasers Surg Med* 2009; 41: 17–25.
3 Brandon MS, Strauss RA. Complications of CO_2 laser procedures in oral and maxillofacial surgery. *Oral Maxillofac Surg Clin North Am* 2004; 16: 289–299.
4 Boj JR, Hernandez M, Espasa E, Poirier C. Laser treatment of an oral papilloma in the pediatric dental office: a case report. *Quintessence Int* 2007; 38(4): 307–312.
5 Trajtenberg C, Adibi S. Removal of an irritation fibroma using an Er,Cr:YSGG laser: a case report. *Gen Dent* 2008; 56(7): 648–651.
6 Paes JT, Cavalcanti SM, Nascimento DF, et al. CO_2 Laser Surgery and Prosthetic Management for the Treatment of Epulis Fissuratum. *ISRN Dent* 2011: 282361.
7 Vescovi P, Corcione L, Meleti M, et al. Nd:YAG laser versus traditional scalpel. *A preliminary histological analysis of specimens from the human oral mucosa. Lasers Med Sci* 2010; 25(5): 685–691.
8 Calero L, Brusis T. Laryngeal papillomatosis—first recognition in Germany as an occupational disease in an operating room nurse. *Laryngorhinootologie* 2003; 82: 790–793.
9 Ilmarinen T, Auvinen E, Hiltunen-Back E, Ranki A, Aaltonen LM, Pitkäranta A. Transmission of human papillomavirus DNA from patient to surgical masks, gloves and oral mucosa of medical personnel during treatment of laryngeal papillomas and genital warts. *Eur Arch Otorhinolaryngol* 2012; 269(11): 2367–2371.

CHAPTER 31

Hemangioma and lymphangioma

Luciane Hiramatsu Azevedo[1] and Cláudia Strefezza[2]
[1]Dentistry Clinic, University of São Paulo (USP), São Paulo, SP, Brazil
[2]Faculdades Metropolitanas Unidas (FMU), São Paulo, SP, Brazil

Hemangioma

Vascular lesions, including both hemangiomas and vascular malformations, are common pathological entities. These lesions can be found in the skin and in the mouth, and rarely cause symptoms. The onset of hemangiomas is at birth; they usually appear in early infancy and then may slowly involute completely by the age of 4 or 5 years.[1] There are many ways to classify hemangiomas. According to Enzinger and Weiss, hemangiomas are broadly classified into capillary, cavernous, and miscellaneous forms like verrucous, venous, and arteriovenous hemangiomas.[2] Capillary hemangiomas further include juvenile, pyogenic granuloma, and epithelioid hemangiomas.[2] The term hemangioma has been commonly misused to describe a large number of vasoformative tumors.[3] However, the International Society for the Study of Vascular Anomalies (ISSVA) has recently provided guidelines to differentiate these two conditions, according to the novel classification first published by Mulliken et al. in 1982.[4] Vasoformative tumors are broadly classified into two groups: hemangiomas and vascular malformations.[4] Hemangiomas are histologically further classified into capillary and cavernous forms.[5,6] A capillary hemangioma is composed of many small capillaries lined by a single layer of endothelial cells supported by a connective tissue stroma of varying density, while a cavernous hemangioma is formed of large, thin-walled vessels, or sinusoids, lined by epithelial cells separated by a thin layer of connective tissue septa. [7]

Vascular malformations are usually noted at birth, grow in concert with body growth, commonly as a single lesion on the ears, face, lips or neck, and do not tend to regress.[1,8] Another common entity of vascular tumors is a venous lake, most frequently in elderly males. These lesions are elevated, usually dome shaped, dark blue to black papules of 1–5 mm in diameter. Except for temporary hemorrhage and compromised cosmesis, their course is uncomplicated.[9]

For the sake of simplicity, this chapter refers to both hemangiomas and vascular malformations as vascular lesions (VLs). This distinction is only made when describing specific cases, as in the study of Vesnaver and Dovsak.[10]

The largest VLs may be liable to injury, causing significant bleeding.[8] For these, surgery is not indicated due to the risk of hemorrhage. Another treatment method is chemical or physical sclerosis. In chemical sclerosis, sclerosing agents are injected into the VL, promoting a decidual necrosis with posterior repair, a reduction of the lumen of the vessels, and a decrease of the local blood flow. Among the substances utilized are monoethanolamine oleate 5%, tedradecil sodium sulfate, and glucose hypertonic solution. Physical sclerosis utilizes agents that freeze the area, with liquid nitrogen being the most commonly used.[10,11]

The mouth, and particularly the lip, may present an aesthetic challenge when surgery and/or sclerosing agents are used, particularly for large lesions. These VLs may be treated efficiently with high power lasers, such as diode lasers, due to the properties of this kind of irradiation (see Clinical case 31.1). The benefit of this treatment is demonstrated by the fact that almost all procedures can be accomplished on an outpatient basis, blood loss is minimal with no requirement for blood replacement, and postoperative pain and edema are virtually non-existent. Argon lasers,[12] Nd:YAG lasers,[10,13] CO_2 lasers,[11,14] and diode lasers[15,16] have all been found to be safe and effective for the treatment of VLs.

Lymphangioma

Lymphangioma, first described in 1828 by Redenbacher, is a relatively rare occurrence and its name is controversial. Considered by many as a congenital malformation of the lymphatic system, others consider it to be a benign vascular tumor of the lymphatic system arising from the proliferation of lymph vessels or a congenital hamartoma.[17,18]

It is histologically benign, but infiltrative features may expand into the surrounding tissue, causing complications. Most lymphangiomas are present at birth (60%), and by the age of 2 years 80–90% are present. It usually occurs in the head and neck, followed by the extremities, trunk, and abdomen. In the head and neck area, the most common location is the submandibular region, followed by the parotid gland. When a lymphangioma

Lasers in Dentistry: Guide for Clinical Practice, First Edition. Edited by Patrícia M. de Freitas and Alyne Simões.
© 2015 John Wiley & Sons, Inc. Published 2015 by John Wiley & Sons, Inc.

occurs in the mouth, the anterior two thirds of the tongue is the most commonly affected region. In the oral cavity, lymphangioma also may involve the palate, gingiva, buccal mucosa, lips, and alveolar ridge of the mandible. Lymphangioma is a rare condition, but among the oral lymphangiomas, tongue involvement is the most common and may be localized or more commonly diffuse. The tongue assumes a granular appearance with multiple cysts filled with transparent lymph. Occasionally, there is bleeding from the vesicles. The tongue increases in size, usually protrudes, and is dry and cracked, which can make chewing, swallowing, and speech difficult as well as causing orthodontic and psychological disorders.[19] The volume increase is due to the process of progressive dilation of the vessels, determined by local changes in flow that can be triggered by trauma or hormonal changes.[4,20]

Lymphangioma persists throughout life with periods of a temporary decrease in total volume. The diagnosis of lymphangioma with superficial infiltration of skin and mucosa by vesicles is

---

Clinical case 31.1 Vascular lesion

A 11-month-old boy was examined for a progressively increasing VL on the right of the lower lip (Fig. 31.1a). A high intensity, 3-W diode laser (Opus10, Tel-Aviv, Israel) was used in a non-contact technique under local anesthesia. Irradiation was delivered using a flexible quartz fiber of 300 μm in diameter, which was kept 2–3 mm away from the lesion, in continuous wave mode, for 10 seconds, with a mean fluency of 20 J/cm², proceeding with quick circular movements. Another two cycles were performed after a 30-second interval to prevent heat damage. The endpoint of treatment was blanching and visible shrinkage of the lesion (Fig. 31.1b). Immediately after laser treatment, the patient developed slight swelling of the treated area that lasted for 3 days. It was necessary to use analgesic medications for 3 days. There was no bleeding. Re-epithelialization was complete by 4 weeks (Fig. 31.1c).

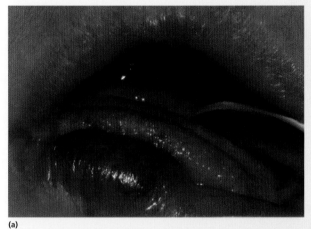

(a)

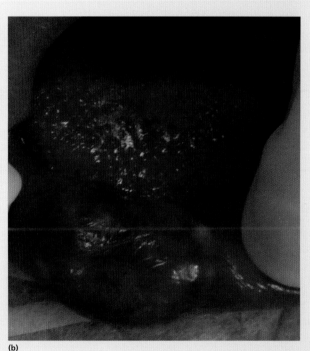

(b)

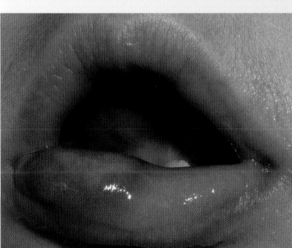

(c)

Figure 31.1 (a) Vascular lesion on the right of the lower lip. (b) Clinical image immediately after photocoagulation. (c) After 4 weeks of follow-up.

clinical. For deeper lesions, Doppler ultrasound, computed tomography, and magnetic resonance imaging may be used to detect the cystic component and low flow that characterizes the lymphangioma.

Various methods have been tried in the treatment of lymphangioma, including surgery, conventional high power laser surgeries (see Clinical case 31.2) radiation, laser therapy, and sclerotherapy. A more conservative surgical approach using radiofrequency ablation has been described in a case of lymphangioma in the right buccal mucosa of the mental foramen area.[6,7] Radiofrequency ablation therapy has a number of advantages for patients with lymphatic malformations. First,

---

Clinical case 31.2 Lymphangioma

An 11-year-old female child reported with multiple papular lesions on the labial mucosa of the left upper lip (Fig. 31.2a). The lesions were present from birth, she had feeding difficulty in the early days, and bleeding occurred frequently. There was no family history of the disease. An incisional biopsy was taken and histopathological examination confirmed a diagnosis of lymphangioma. Vaporization of superficial lesions was performed with a CO_2 laser (8 W, continuous mode) under local anesthesia (Fig. 31.2b). Neither sutures nor dressings were needed after surgery. Only paracetamol and chlorhexidine digluconate mouthwash were prescribed during the postoperative period. There were no postsurgical complaints from the patient. The wound formed due to laser surgery was left open to secondary epithelialization (Fig. 31.2c).

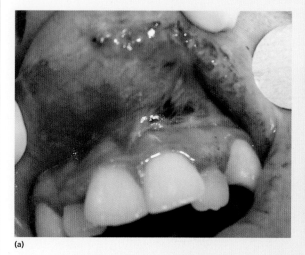
(a)

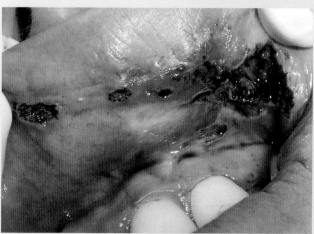
(b)

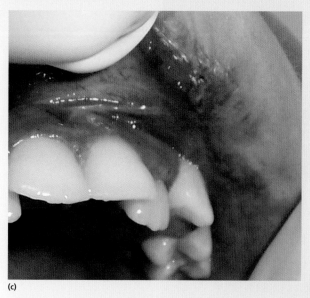
(c)

Figure 31.2 (a) Lymphangioma on the labial mucosa on the left of the upper lip. (b) Clinical image immediately after vaporization. (c) After 4 weeks of follow-up.

the technique can target areas of tissue involvement, sparing critical anatomical neurovascular components and the sensitive mucosal surfaces. Second, the treatment delivered is not limited by the diffusion of injected agents, as in sclerosing therapy (this appears to be a weakness in the use of OK-432). Third, the procedure entails minimal invasive techniques and avoids significant pain and morbidity. This new and effective technique offers clear benefit over the alternative treatments.[21,22]

Although surgical excision is considered as a mode of treatment by most surgeons, this can leave the patient with several morbid conditions, such as nerve injuries, prolonged lymphatic drainage from the wound, recurrent lesions, wound infections, unacceptable scar formation, and incomplete resection due to infiltration of adjacent vital structures. Boiling water, quinine, sodium morrhuate, urethane, iodine tincture, and nitromin have been used as sclerosing agents with low success rates and several side effects. Recently, two sclerosing agents, bleomycin, and OK-432, and α-interferon 2a have been favored by some surgeons in the treatment of lymphangioma.[22,23]

While complete surgical removal has been the treatment of preference, where there is infiltrative lymphangioma, this is difficult and only possible in 10–50% of cases. Because of this, the recurrence rate is a major problem: 0–27% after complete removal and 15–53% after partial removal. Surgery is indicated when lesions are resectable and it does not promote mutilation or sequelae. It is relevant to state that the resection of lymphatic tissue impedes lymphatic flow, causing lymphatic stasis post resection.[24,25]

In complex and extensive lesions of the face, later intervention may be appropriate. Often the growth of the lesion does not follow the child's growth and later removal may be less invasive and more localized. When there is an abrupt increase in the size of a lymphangioma, the use of systemic antibiotic therapy is recommended.

As already mentioned, tongue lymphangioma is a rare malformation that may cause both functional and cosmetic problems for the patient. The challenge is to find a conservative treatment for the pain and other symptoms with low morbidity and better results than those achieved with surgical excision.

Low level laser therapy (LLLT) is a form of phototherapy that involves the application of a low power laser to areas of the body in order to stimulate healing and reduce pain and inflammation. This therapy may be used to reduce tumor size and control pain and inflammation. In a case report,[26] sonography diagnosed lymphangioma in a child with a large hemorrhagic mass on her tongue with a 2-month history of trauma and considerable pain. The base of the lesion was treated with a 2-minute diode laser exposure on every other day for five sessions. After ten sessions of applying LLLT, it was observed that there was a considerable reduction in the size of the lesion and inflammation, and improvement of speaking and swallowing. Tongue tenderness and pain were diminished. There were no side effects. Laser irradiation can decrease pain transmission and stimulate production of morphinic substances.

References

1 Mulliken JB, Glowacki J. Classification of pediatric vascular lesions. *Plast Reconstr Surg* 1982; 70: 120-1.

2 Enzinger FM, Weiss SW. *Soft Tissue Tumors*, 5th edn. St. Louis: Mosby; 2001.

3 Gombos F, Lanza A, Gombos F. A case of multiple oral vascular tumors: the diagnostic challenge on haemangioma still remain open. *Judicial Stud Institute J* 2008; 2: 67–75.

4 Mulliken JB, Glowacki J, Thomson HG. Hemangiomas and vascular malformations in infants and children: a classification based on endothelial characteristics. *Plastic Reconstruct Surg* 1982; 69: 412–422.

5 Shafer WG, Hene MK, Levy BK. *A Textbook of Oral Pathology*. Philadelphia: WB Saunders, 1983.

6 Hall RK. *Paediatric Orofacial Medicine and Pathology*. London: Chapman & Hall, 1994.

7 Neville BW, Damm DD, Allen CM, Bouqot J. *Oral & Maxillofacial Pathology*, 2nd edn. Philadelphia: WB Saunders, 2002.

8 Kaban LB, Mulliken JB. Vascular anomalies of the maxillofacial region. *J Oral Maxillofac Surg* 1986; 44: 203–213.

9 Bondi EE, Jegasothy BR, Lazarus GS. *Dermatology – Diagnosis and Therapy*. California: Appleton & Lange, 1991.

10 Vesnaver A, Dovsak DA. Treatment of vascular lesions in the head and neck using Nd:YAG laser. *J Craniomaxillofac Surg* 2006; 34: 17–24.

11 Niccoli-Filho W, Americo MG, Guimarães-Filho R, Rodrigues NAS. Lip haemangioma removed with CO2 laser: a case report. *Braz J Oral Sci* 2002; 1(2): 89–91.

12 Neumann RA, Knobler RM. Venous lakes (Bean-Walsh) of the lips – treatment experience with the argon laser and 18 months follow-up. *Clin Exp Dermatol* 1990; 15: 115–118.

13 Bekhor PS. Long-pulsed Nd:YAG laser treatment of venous lakes: report of a series of 34 cases. *Dermatol Surg* 2006; 32: 1151–1154.

14 Pozo J. Peña C, Garcia Silva J, Goday JJ, Fonseca E. Venous lakes: a report of 32 cases treated by carbon dioxide laser vaporization. *Dermatol Surg* 2003; 29: 308–310.

15 Angiero F, Benedicenti S, Romanos GE, Crippa R. Treatment of hemangioma of the head and neck with diode laser and forced dehydration with induced photocoagulation. *Photomed Laser Surg* 2008; 26: 113–118.

16 Azevedo LH, Galletta VC, Eduardo Cde P, Migliari DA. Venous lake of the lips treated using photocoagulation with high-intensity diode laser. *Photomed Laser Surg* 2010; 28: 263–265.

17 Ogita S, Tsuto T, Nakamura K, Deguchi E, Iwai N. OK-432 therapy in 64 patients with lymphangioma. *J Pediatr Surg* 1994; 29: 784–785.

18 Molitch HI, Unger EC, Witte CL, VanSonnenberg E. Percutaneous sclerotherapy of lymphangiomas. *Radiology* 1995; 194: 343–347.

19 Reinhardt MA, Nelson SC, Sencer SF, Bostrom BC, Kurachek SC, Nesbit ME. Treatment of childhood lymphangiomas with Interferon-α. *J Pediatr Hematol Oncol* 1997; 19: 232–236.

20 Balakrishnan A, Bailey CM. Lymphangioma of the tongue. A review of pathogenesis, treatment and the use of surface laser photocoagulation. *J Laryngol Otol* 1991; 105: 924–930.

21 Bozkaya S, Dilek Ug, Ceylan SU, et al. The treatment of lymphangioma in the buccal mucosa by radiofrequency ablation: a case report. *Oral Surg Oral Med Oral Pathol Oral Radiol Endod* 2006; 102: e28–e31.

22 Sanlialp I, Karnak FC, Tanyel ME, Senocak N, Büyükpamukçu N. Sclerotherapy for lymphangioma in children. *Int J Pediatr Otorhinolaryngol* 2003; 67: 795–800.

23 Claesson G, Kuylenstierna R. OK-432 therapy for lymphatic malformation in 32 patients. *Pediatr Otorhinolaryngol Int J* 2002; 65: 1–6.

24 Balakrishnan A, Bailey CM. Lymphangioma of the tongue. A review of pathogenesis, treatment and the use of surface laser photocoagulation. *J Laryngol Otol* 1991; 105: 924–930.

25 Lille ST, Rand RP, Tapper D, Gruss JS. The surgical management of giant cervicofacial lymphatic malformations. *J Pediatr Surg* 1996; 31: 1648–1650.

26 Vatankhah Z, Rastgou H. Reduction of pain in lymphangioma by applying low level laser therapy LILT. A case report. Eur J Pain 2011 (Suppl): 146–147.

CHAPTER 32

Non-neoplastic proliferative lesions or soft tissue tumor-like lesions of the oral cavity

Vivian Cunha Galletta Kern,[1] **Edgar Kazuyoshi Nakajima,**[1,2] **Rodrigo Ramos Vieira,**[1,2] **and Luciane Hiramatsu Azevedo**[3]

[1] Special Laboratory of Lasers in Dentistry (LELO), School of Dentistry, University of São Paulo (USP), São Paulo, SP, Brazil
[2] Private Dental Practice, São Paulo, SP, Brazil
[3] Dentistry Clinic, University of São Paulo (USP), São Paulo, SP, Brazil

Introduction

Tissue enlargements of the oral cavity that result from cell proliferation, but are subject to normal control mechanisms, are termed non-neoplastic proliferative lesions or soft tissue tumor-like lesions. Different mechanisms may lead to the development of a soft tissue tumor-like lesion in the oral cavity.[1] Within this group, there is a wide range of lesion subtypes that can be identified according to their etiology, such as cysts, developmental anomalies, and hyperplasias, among others. Hyperplasias are a group of lesions which develop in response to a specific stimulus, usually a chronic injury or inflammation that produces inflamed fibrous and granulation tissues. The most common hyperplasias are inflammatory fibrous hyperplasia (IFH), inflammatory gingival hyperplasia, palatal papillary hyperplasia, pyogenic granuloma, and peripheral giant cell granuloma and peripheral ossifying fibroma.

The aim of this chapter is to introduce the concept of these lesions as well as the treatments commonly used for them, and to demonstrate the benefits of laser treatment.

Inflammatory fibrous hyperplasia

Inflammatory fibrous hyperplasia (IFH) or *epulis fissuratum* is a tissue growth into the oral cavity caused by low intensity chronic trauma, usually from ill-fitting dentures or even parafunctional habits,[2] and may appear in denture wearers over the age of 60 years; it is more common in females.[3,4] The size of the lesion can vary from a localized hyperplasia of less than 1 cm in size to massive lesions that involve most of the length of the alveolar ridges or the soft tissues of the vestibule.[5,6]

Microscopic examination of IFH reveals hyperplasia of the fibrous connective tissue. Often, multiple folds and grooves occur where the denture impinges on the tissue. The overlying epithelium is frequently hyperparakeratotic and demonstrates irregular hyperplasia of the rête ridges. Focal areas of ulceration are not unusual, especially at the base of the grooves between the folds. A variable chronic inflammatory infiltrate is present; sometimes it may include eosinophils or show lymphoid follicles. If minor salivary glands are included in the specimen, then they usually show chronic sialadenitis.[6]

The treatment of choice is surgical excision, but instead of the conventional techniques using scalpels, a reliable alternative is the use of the CO_2 laser (see Clinical case 32.1).[5,7]

Drug-induced gingival overgrowth

Some drugs have an adverse effect on the mouth and periodontal tissues, such as gingival overgrowth. "Gingival enlargement" or "gingival overgrowth" is the preferred term for all medication-related gingival lesions previously termed "gingival hyperplasia" or "gingival hypertrophy," as the earlier terms did not accurately reflect the histological composition of the pharmacologically-modified gingiva.[8]

Drugs associated with gingival enlargement can be divided into three categories: anticonvulsants, calcium channel blockers, and immunosuppressants. Although these drugs have different pharmacological effects on the body, they seem to influence the same tissues in the periodontium, mainly the gingival connective tissues, causing common clinical and histopathological findings.[6] Clinically, the enlargement is confined to the gingiva, beginning in the papillary tissues and extending outward. The color and texture is influenced by the presence of plaque-induced inflammation and the underlying periodontal condition.[9] The main histological features of gingival overgrowth are the predominant fibrotic changes in the connective tissue, especially the collagenous component, with an increase in fibroblasts, an accumulation of

Clinical case 32.1 Inflammatory fibrous hyperplasia

A 62-year-old woman presented with two lesions covering the superior alveolar ridge, and hard and soft palate. One lesion was located on the right side of the alveolar ridge and palate, and the other one on the left side. A diagnosis of IFH was proposed due to an ill-fitting denture. The treatment of choice was the surgical excision of these lesions with a CO_2 laser.

Due to the extent of the lesions (Fig. 32.1a), total excision was performed in two surgical sessions with an interval of 30 days between each surgery.

The excisions were done under local infiltrative anesthesia with a CO_2 laser in focused, continuous mode at 6 W (Fig. 32.1b,c). The specimens

were sent for histopathological analysis (Fig. 32.1d,e) and diagnosis of IFH was confirmed.

Following both surgeries, analgesic and anti-inflammatory medications were prescribed and the prosthesis was rebased. Seven days after both surgical procedures, a fibrin layer was observed at the area where the surgery was performed (Fig. 32.1f,g).

Thirty days after both surgeries, full clinical tissue repair was observed (Fig. 32.1 h,i). One month after the second surgical procedure (Fig. 32.1j), the patient was referred to the dental clinician for the development of a the new superior full denture (Fig. 32.1 k,l).

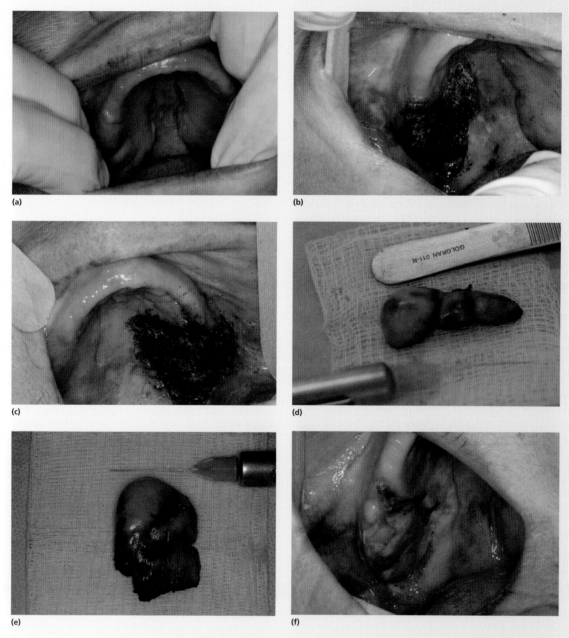

Figure 32.1 (a) Extension of the inflammatory fibrous hyperplasia. (b,c) Immediately post surgery. The excisions were done with CO_2 laser irradiation on both sides. (d,e) The specimens (from the left and right sides) were sent for histopathological study. (f,g) Seven days after both surgical procedures, (h,i) 30 days after both surgical procedures, and (j) 1 month after the second surgical procedure. (k,l) Adapted full denture.

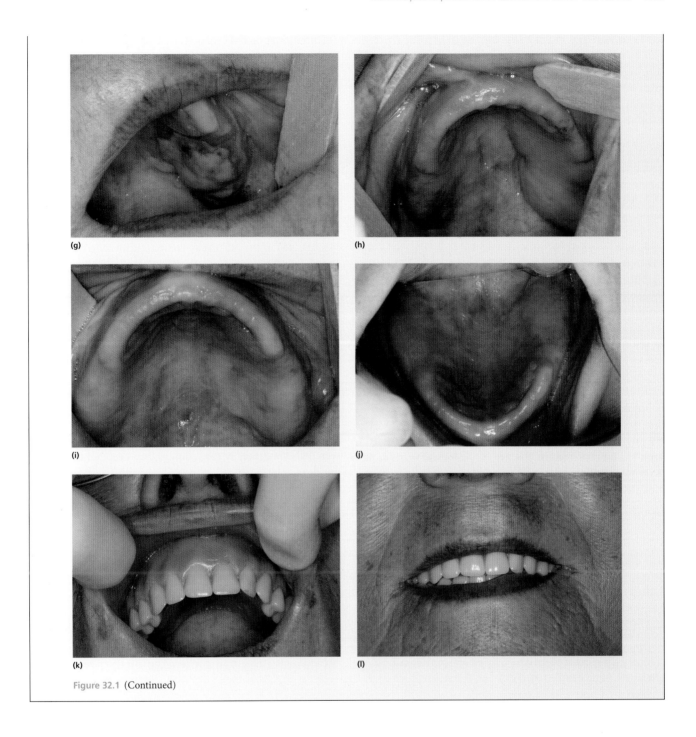

Figure 32.1 (Continued)

extracellular matrix, and various levels of inflammation, thickening of the epithelium with proliferation, and elongation of rête ridges.[9]

The treatment is generally targeted at drug substitution and effective control of local inflammatory factors such as plaque and calculus. When these measures fail to resolve the enlargement, surgical intervention is recommended.[8,10] The use of high power lasers for gingivectomy has proven to be effective in reducing gingival enlargement, providing a fast postoperative hemostasis (see Clinical case 32.2). These treatment modalities, although effective, do not necessarily prevent recurrence of the lesions.[8,11,12]

Inflammatory papillary hyperplasia

Inflammatory papillary hyperplasia of the palate (IPHP) or the granular type of denture stomatitis is a reactive tissue overgrowth, characterized by a hyperemic mucosa with a nodular or papillary appearance, mostly covering the central part of the palate.[13] Although the exact pathogenesis is still unclear, a combination of trauma and *Candida* infection has been suggested in the etiology.[14–16] IPHP is related to ill-fitting dentures, poor denture hygiene, and wearing dentures for 24 hours a day. Old dentures are more frequently associated with IPHP than newer ones, independent of denture quality.[15]

Histopathological examination of IPHP shows papillary projections covered by keratinized stratified squamous epithelium. The underlying connective tissue varies from loose and edematous to densely collagenized, and it is usually infiltrated by chronic inflammatory cells, mainly lymphocytes and plasma cells.[15,16]

Less extensive lesions are resolved by improving hygiene and removing dentures at night. Patients can also benefit from antifungal treatment.[17] In lesions resistant to these treatment measures, removal of the diseased mucosa is required.[18–21] Different techniques have been described, including supra-periosteal excision,[20] the blade-loop technique,[21] or electrosurgery,[19] with or without soft tissue grafts, cryosurgery,[18] and laser vaporization (see Clinical case 32.3).[22] The advantages of the CO_2 laser are minimal bleeding, precise limits for the surgical field, minimal trauma, relative absence of postoperative pain, and accelerated healing.[23]

Once the lesion has been removed, prognosis is good and the lesion does not usually recur if the causative factors and associated risks are corrected: dentures should be replaced and oral hygiene maintained.

Pyogenic granuloma

Pyogenic granuloma (PG) or granuloma pyogenicum is a common tumor-like growth of the oral cavity that traditionally has been considered to be non-neoplastic in nature. The name pyogenic granuloma is a misnomer since the condition is not associated with pus and does not represent a granuloma histologically. PG of the oral cavity commonly involves the gingiva. Extragingivally, it can occur on the lips, tongue, buccal mucosa, and palate. A history of trauma before the development of the lesion is not unusual, especially for extragingival PGs. The etiology of the lesion is not known, although a botryomycotic infection was originally believed to be the cause. It is theorized that PG possibly originates as a response of tissues to minor trauma and/or chronic irritation, thus opening a pathway for invasion of non-specific microorganisms, although microorganisms are seldom demonstrated within the lesion. The pathogenesis of PG is still debated.[24,25]

On intraoral examination, a wide array of clinical appearances, ranging from a sessile lesion to an elevated mass, can be seen. PGs are generally soft, painless, and deep red to reddish-purple in color.[26]

Clinical case 32.2 Drug-induced gingival hyperplasia

A 16-year-old boy presented with extensive hyperplasic lesions, covering the gingival margin of the upper arch. This was a side effect of the continuous and necessary use of several medications for the treatment of cystinosis. The lesions were biopsied and histopathological study confirmed the diagnosis of drug-induced gingival hyperplasia (Fig. 32.2a).

The treatment of choice was excision with a diode laser to improve hygiene and esthetics for the patient. The excisions were done under local infiltrative anesthesia, with a high power diode laser in focused, continuous mode at 3 W (Fig. 32.2b). Only analgesic medication was prescribed. Three months later, the mucosa had epithelialized (Fig. 32.2c).

Nevertheless, due to the continuous use of the medications for treatment of cystinosis, recurrence of the hyperplasic lesions could be observed, but to a lesser degree than before the laser procedure.

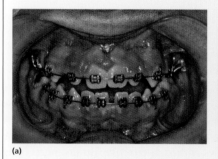 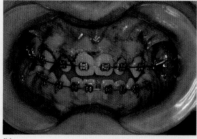 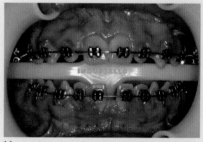

(a)   (b)   (c)

Figure 32.2 (a) Drug-induced gingival hyperplasia. (b) Immediately post surgery. The excisions were done with a Nd:YAG laser. (c) Three months later the mucosa had epithelialized.

Clinical case 32.3 Inflammatory papillary hyperplasia

A 56-year-old woman presented with an extensive papillomatous lesion of the palate. She had had no teeth in the maxilla since she was 20 years old, and wore a complete acrylic maxillary denture all the time. She has smoked 20 cigarettes a day for 40 years. Intraoral examination showed a granular lesion with numerous bulbous projections of between 1 and 3 mm in depth, localized in the hard palate and confined to the limits of

the denture (Fig. 32.3a). Histopathological study of a biopsy specimen confirmed the diagnosis of IPHP.

Treatment was started with 2% miconazole in gel for 15 days. However, the lesion did not heal. The affected area was vaporized with a CO_2 laser in defocused, continuous mode at 6 W (Fig. 32.3b). One month later, the mucosa had epithelialized (Fig. 32.3c).

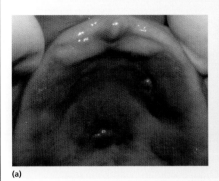 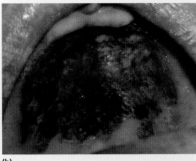 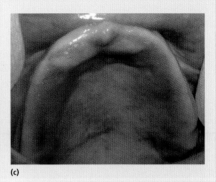

(a) (b) (c)

Figure 32.3 (a) Inflammatory papillary hyperplasia of the palate. (b) Immediately after vaporization with a CO_2 laser. (c) After 4 weeks of follow-up.

There are no radiographic findings in PG. However, Angelopoulos observed localized alveolar bone resorption in rare instances of large and long-standing gingival tumors.[27]

Microscopic examination of PG shows a highly vascular proliferation that resembles granular tissue. Numerous vessels, small and larger endothelium-lined channels, are formed that are engorged with red blood cells. These vessels are sometimes organized in lobular aggregates. The surface is usually ulcerated and this is then replaced by a thick fibrinopurulent membrane. A mixed inflammatory cell infiltrate of neutrophils, plasma cells, and lymphocytes is evident. Neutrophils are most prevalent near the ulcerated surface; chronic inflammatory cells are found deeper in the specimen.[25]

Being a non-neoplastic growth, excisional therapy is the treatment of choice.[28] Although the conventional treatment for PG is surgical excision, a recurrence rate of 16% has been reported.[29] There are also reports of the lesion being excised with an electric scalpel or cryosurgery.[30] Other reported methods include cauterization with silver nitrate, sclerotherapy with sodium tetradecyl sulfate and monoethanolamineoleate ligation,[31] absolute ethanol injection dye,[32] the Nd:YAG[33] and CO_2 lasers,[34] high power diode laser (see Clinical case 32.4),[35] shave excision, and laser photocoagulation.[36]

Peripheral giant cell granuloma and peripheral ossifying fibroma (cementifying fibroma)

Among the frequent focal proliferative lesions of the gingiva are peripheral giant cell granuloma (PGCG) and peripheral ossifying fibroma (POF). Similarly to other fibrous growths of the

oral soft tissue, both lesions are reactive chronic inflammatory hyperplasias caused by minor trauma or irritation of the periodontium.[37]

Although they have a similar clinical appearance (i.e. a sessile or pedunculated nodule of normal or erythematous color located at the interdental papilla of the incisors or canines), their dominant proliferating histological component/cells differ.[38] Roughly, histological examination of PGCG reveals multinucleated giant cells in a background of mononuclear stromal cells and extravasated red blood cells,[39] while POF presents a cellular mass of connective tissue with areas of mineralization consisting of bone, cementum-like material or dystrophic calcifications.[37]

Intraoral radiographs of PGCG and POF may reveal erosion of the crest of bone underlying the lesion area; however, evidence suggests that the nature of bone resorption in PGCG may be due to the osteoclastic activity of the lesion, and POF to long-standing plaque-induced inflammation and constant pressure exerted by the growth.[37,39]

Although the terminology used is similar to that for other pathologies of the oral cavity, POF is not the soft tissue counterpart to a central ossifying fibroma and it is a completely different entity from peripheral odontogenic fibroma and central odontogenic fibroma. It has been considered that at least some cases of POF may arise as a result of maturation of a long-standing PG because of their clinical and histopathological similarity.[37] On the other hand, PGCG microscopically resembles a central giant cell granuloma and is believed to represent its soft tissue counterpart.[39]

Treatment of PGCG and POF is surgical excision along with removal of causative irritants. The extent of excision depends

Clinical case 32.4 Pyogenic granuloma

A 25-year-old female patient in her 24th week of pregnancy was referred to the stomatology clinic of the School of Dentistry, University of São Paulo, with the complaint of localized gingival growth for 3 months. The outgrowing mass was not painful but often bled while eating, rinsing, or sometimes spontaneously. Intraoral examination revealed an oval-shaped, pedunculated mass-like growth of gingiva in the region of tooth 27, measuring approximately 2.5 × 1.5 cm. This nodular, erythematous enlargement did not cover the crown of tooth 27. On palpation, the mass was soft to firm in consistency and readily bled on probing (Fig. 32.4a).

Oral hygiene was well maintained, and no exacerbating factors were identified. Based on the clinical findings, the differential diagnoses were PG, peripheral giant cell granuloma, and peripheral ossifying fibroma.

Removal of the lesion was performed under local infiltrative anesthesia using a diode laser in continuous mode in a contact technique with a power setting of 2 W (Lasering 808, Milan, Italy; 808 nm) (Fig. 32.4b). Histopathological examination confirmed a diagnosis of PG.

Figure 32.4b shows the wound healing after 7 days. No signs of recurrence were observed over 12-month follow-up.

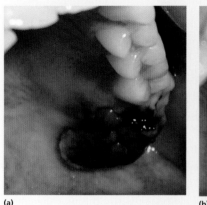
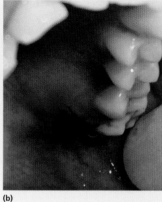
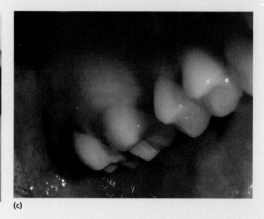

(a)   (b)   (c)

Figure 32.4 Pyogenic granuloma in a pregnant patient. (b) Immediately after excision with a high power diode laser. (c) After 7 days of follow-up.

Clinical case 32.5 Peripheral ossifying fibroma

A 79-year-old female patient was referred to the stomatology clinic of the School of Dentistry, University of São Paulo, with the complaint of localized growth for 2 years. During the anamnesis, the patient reported absence of painful symptoms and that she did not remember having experienced any trauma in this region. On clinical examination, a sessile nodule of firm consistency, approximately 1.3 cm in diameter in the anterior alveolar ridge of the mandible, with no alteration in color, was

observed (Fig. 32.5a). No radiological sign of bone involvement was noted. In view of the anamnesis and clinical and radiographic examinations, removal of the lesion was proposed by means of excisional biopsy. A diode laser in continuous mode in a contact technique with a power setting of 2 W (Lasering 808, Milan, Italy; 808 nm) was used. The histopathological study confirmed the diagnosis of POF. No signs of recurrence were observed over 24-month follow-up (Fig. 32.5b).

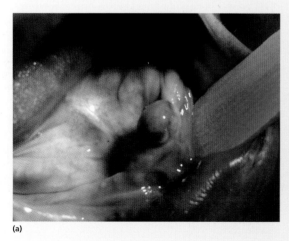
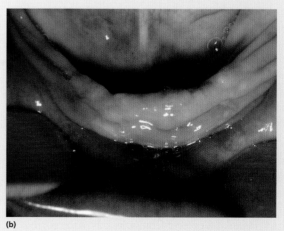

(a)   (b)

Figure 32.5 (a) Clinical intraoral image of the growth; peripheral ossifying fibroma. (b) After 24 months of follow-up.

on the severity of the lesion, since it has a tendency to recur.[38] Curettage as deep as possible and crestal osteoplasty are often performed in order to avoid recurrences.[37] Alternatively to the conventional surgical procedure, high power lasers may be used to remove PGCG and POF. It is important though to highlight that additional curettage might be necessary to achieve complete removal of the lesion and therefore to prevent further recurrence. Bleeding from curettage can be controlled by irradiation with high power lasers. Thermal tissue damage from surgery with a diode laser has been reported to be minimal in lesions larger than 3 mm in diameter, allowing proper histopathological examination of the excised tissue (see Clinical case 32.5).[40] The use of the CO_2 laser has also been reported to be safe regarding thermal damage to the excised oral soft tissue lesion, again not affecting the histopathological diagnosis.[41]

References

1 Pour MAH, Rad M, Mojtahedi A. A survey of soft tissue tumor-like lesions of oral cavity: A clinicopathological study. *Iranian J Pathol* 2008; 3: 81–87.

2 Canger EM, Celenk P, Kayipmaz S. Denture-related hyperplasia: a clinical study of a Turkish population group. *Braz Dent J* 2009; 20: 243–248.

3 Freitas JB, Gomez RS, De Abreu MHNG, Ferreira E. Relationship between the use of full dentures and mucosal alterations among elderly Brazilians. *J Oral Rehabil* 2008; 35: 370–374.

4 Coelho CMP, Sousa YTCS, Daré AMZ. Denture-related oral mucosal lesions in a Brazilian school of dentistry. *J Oral Rehabil* 2004; 31: 135–139.

5 Paes-Junior TJA, Cavalcanti SCM, Nascimento DFF, et al. CO_2 Laser surgery and prosthetic management for the treatment of epulis fissuratum. ISRN Dent 2011: article282361.

6 Neville BW, Damm DD, Allen CM, Bouquot JE. *Soft Tissue Tumors. Oral and Maxillofacial Pathology*, 3rd edn. St Louis: Saunders Elsevier, 2009: 510–512.

7 Pick RM, Pogrel A, Sai Loh H. *Clinical applications of the CO_2 Laser, Lasers in Oral and maxillofacial surgery*. New York: Elsevier: New York, 2000.

8 Dongari-Bagtzoglou A. Academy report. Informational paper. Drug-induced gingival enlargement. *J Periodontol* 2004; 75: 1424–1431.

9 Hallmon WW, Rossman JA. The role of drugs in the pathogenesis of gingival overgrowth. A collective review of current concepts. *Periodontology 2000* 1999; 21: 176–196.

10 Camargo PM, Melnick PR, Pirih FQ, Lagos R, Takei HH. Treatment of drug-induced gingival enlargement: aesthetic and functional considerations. *Periodontology 2000* 2001; 27: 131–138.

11 Marshall RI, Bartold PM. A clinical review of drug-induced gingival overgrowth. *Aust Dent J* 1999; 44: 219–232.

12 Neville BW, Damm DD, Allen CM, Bouquot JE. *Oral and Maxillofacial Pathology*, 3rd ed. St Louis: Saunders Elsevier, 2009: 163–166.

13 Budtz-Jorgensen E. Oral mucosal lesions associated with the wearing of removable dentures. *J Oral Pathol* 1981; 10: 65–80.

14 Bergendal T, Isacsson G. A combined clinical, mycological and histological study of denture stomatitis. *Acta Odontol Scand* 1983; 41: 33–44.

15 Poulopoulos A, Belazi M, Epivatianos A, Velegraki A, Antoniades D. The role of Candida in inflammatory papillary hyperplasia of the palate. *J Oral Rehabil* 2007; 34: 685–692.

16 Kaplan I, Vered M, Moskona D, Buchner A, Dayan D. An immunohistochemical study of p53 and PCNA in inflammatory papillary hyperplasia of the palate: a dilemma of interpretation. *Oral Dis* 1998; 4: 194–199.

17 Salonen MA, Raustia AM, Oikarinen, KS. Effect of treatment of palatal inflammatory papillary hyperplasia with local and systemic antifungal agents accompanied by renewal of complete dentures. *Acta Odontol Scand* 1996; 54: 87–91.

18 Getter L, Perez B. Controlled cryotherapy in the treatment of inflammatory papillary hyperplasia. *Oral Surg Oral Med Oral Pathol* 1972; 34: 178–186.

19 Rathofer SA, Gardner FM, Vermileya SG. A comparison of healing and pain following excision of inflammatory papillary hyperplasia with electrosurgery and blade-loop knives in human patients. *Oral Surg Oral Med Oral Pathol* 1985; 59: 130–135

20 Brown AR, Cobb CM, Dunlap CL, Manch-Citron JN. Atypical palatal papillomatosis treated by excision and full-thickness grafting. *Compend Contin Educ Dent* 1997; 18: 724–726, 728–732, 734.

21 Antonelli JR, Panno FV, Witko A. Inflammatory papillary hyperplasia: supraperiosteal excision by the blade-loop technique. *Gen Dent* 1998; 46: 390–397.

22 Infante-Cossio P, Martinez-de-Fuentes R, Torres-Carranza E, Gutierrez-Perez JL. Inflammatory papillary hyperplasia of the palate: treatment with carbon dioxide laser, followed by restoration with an implant-supported prosthesis. *Br J Oral Maxillofac Surg* 2007; 45: 658–660.

23 Wlodawsky RN, Strauss RA. Intraoral laser surgery. *Oral Maxillofacial Surg Clin North Am* 2004; 16, 149–163.

24 Kamal R, Dahiya P, Puri A. Oral pyogenic granuloma: Various concepts of etiopathogenesis. *J Oral Maxillofac Pathol* 2012; 16: 79–82.

25 Neville BW, Damm DD, Allen CM, Bouquot JE. *Soft Tissue Tumours. Oral and Maxillofacial Pathology*, 3rd edn. St Louis: Saunders Elsevier, 2009: 517–519.

26 Bhaskar SN, Jacoway JR. Pyogenic granuloma – clinical features, incidence, histology, and result of treatment: Report of 242 cases. *J Oral Surg* 1966; 24: 391–398.

27 Angelopoulos AP. Pyogenic granuloma of the oral cavity: Statistical analysis of its clinical features. *J Oral Surg* 1971; 29: 840–847.

28 Jaferzadeh H, Sanadkhani M, Mohtasham M. Oral pyogenic granuloma: A review. *J Oral Sci* 2006; 48: 167–175.

29 Newman MG, Takei H, Carranza FA. In: *Textbook of Carranza's Clinical Periodontology*, 10th edn. The Netherlands: Elsevier, 2006: 176–177.

30 Gupta R, Gupta S. Cryo-therapy in granuloma pyogenicum. *Indian J Dermatol Venereol Leprol* 2007; 73: 14.

31 Matsumoto K, Nakanishi H, Seike T. Treatment of pyogenic granuloma with sclerosing agents. *Dermatol Surgery* 2001; 27: 521–523.

32 Ichimiya M, Yoshikawa K, Hamamoto Y, Muto M. Successful treatment of pyogenic granuloma with injection of absolute alcohol. *J Dermatol* 2001; 31: 342–344.

33 Hammes S, Kaiser K, Pohl L, Metelmann HR, Enk A, Raulin C. Pyogenic granuloma: treatment with the 1,064-nm long-pulsed neodymium-doped yttrium aluminum garnet laser in 20 patients. *Dermatol Surg* 2012; 38: 918–923.

34 Raulin C, Greve B, Hammes S. The combined continuous-wave/ pulsed carbon dioxide laser for treatment of pyogenic granuloma. *Arch Dermatol* 2002; 138: 33–37.

35 Rai S, Kaur M, Bhatnagar P. Laser: a powerful tool for treatment of pyogenic granuloma. *J Cutan Aesthet Surg* 2011; 4: 144–147.

36 Kirschner RE, Low DW. Treatment of pyogenic granuloma by shave excision and laser photocoagulation. *Plast Reconstr Surg* 1999; 104: 1346–1369.

37 Mishra MB, Bhishen KA, Mishra S. Peripheral ossifying fibroma. *J Oral Maxillofac Pathol* 2011; 15: 65–68.

38 Kolte AP, Kolte RA, Shrirao TS. Focal fibrous overgrowths: A case series and review of literature. *Contemp Clin Dent* 2010; 1: 271–274.

39 Tandon PN, Gupta DS, Jurel SK, Saraswat A. Peripheral giant cell granuloma. Contemp Clin Dent 2012; 3(Suppl1): S118–S120.

40 Angiero F, Parma L, Crippa R, Benedicenti S. Diode laser (808 nm) applied to oral soft tissue lesions: a retrospective study to assess histopathological diagnosis and evaluate physical damage. *Lasers Med Sci* 2012; 27: 383–388.

41 Tuncer I, Ozçakir-Tomruk C, Sencift K, Cöloğlu S. Comparison of conventional surgery and CO_2 laser on intraoral soft tissue pathologies and evaluation of the collateral thermal damage. *Photomed Laser Surg* 2010; 28: 75–79.

CHAPTER 33

Oral mucocele

Luciana Corrêa[1] and Luciane Hiramatsu Azevedo[2]

[1] General Pathology Department, School of Dentistry, University of São Paulo (USP), São Paulo, SP, Brazil
[2] Dentistry Clinic, University of São Paulo (USP), São Paulo, SP, Brazil

Introduction

Oral mucoceles are common, benign lesions of minor salivary glands characterized by single or multiple nodules that are generally asymptomatic.[1] The term "mucus extravasation phenomenon" (MEP) is applied to mucoceles that histologically exhibit mucin extravasation to the connective tissue stroma, derived from ductal rupture or transection.[2] Mucoceles may also be characterized by mucus retention in the duct or in the acinus, resulting from ductal obstruction. In these cases, the terms "mucus retention phenomenon" (MRP) or "mucus duct cyst" are preferable.[1,2] MEP is frequently observed in children/adolescents,[1–3] whereas MRP is rare and presents in adults and the elderly.[4] Both lesions are frequently observed in the lower lip, ventral tongue, and floor of the mouth; few cases have been reported in the upper lip, palate, retromolar region, buccal mucosa, and dorsal tongue.[1,2] Generally, mucocele lesions are single, spherical, fluctuant, and painless bluish swellings (see Fig. 33.1a), ranging from 1–2 mm to 1 cm, and even up to 3.5 cm in size.[5] The larger lesions are commonly ranulas, oral mucoceles located in the floor of mouth and involving the sublingual or submandibular salivary glands. The differential diagnosis includes other benign tumors of the salivary glands (i.e. pleomorphic adenoma), lipoma, lymphangioma, and reactive lesions (i.e. fibroma, fibrous hyperplasia lesion). Another aspect of MEP is the occurrence of multiple superficial lesions in the buccal mucosa, retromolar pad, or soft palate, which spontaneously rupture and form a pseudomembrane or ulceration. In this case, the differential diagnosis includes herpes simplex, bullous lichen planus, mucus membrane pemphigoid, or other vesiculobullous disorders.[6]

Standard treatment for oral mucoceles is conventional surgery, but surgical variations and other therapeutic modalities have been described. Table 33.1 shows the main treatments reported in the literature, with a brief description of each modality and its advantages/limitations. Lasers protocols are discussed below.[7–13]

Laser protocols and clinical outcomes

Several clinical reports have described protocols for application of laser irradiation in the excision of oral mucoceles. The large majority have used high power CO_2 lasers for excision or vaporization of the lesions, with a power range from 4 to 10 W. Only four studies have described the use of Nd:YAG, Er:Cr:YSGG, and diode lasers. Table 33.2 summarizes the laser type, parameters, and clinical outcomes of some clinical studies reported in the literature.[14–24]

Considering the English scientific literature, about 163 patients have been submitted to oral mucocele excision using high power lasers. Although the majority of these reports did not describe appropriate monitoring with regard to the recurrence of lesions, the clinical outcomes indicate some advantages of using laser irradiation over the conventional surgical technique:

- Short time of surgery: the procedure of mucocele excision using a CO_2 laser is brief in comparison with that using a scalpel, mainly because sutures are unnecessary.[21,22] This aspect is important, particularly in pediatric patients.
- Immediate hemostasis: during incision and vaporization of the salivary gland, there is no bleeding, which favors clear visualization of the lesion margins.[9,21,22] Some reports have described additional CO_2 laser irradiation in defocused mode on conclusion of surgery, in order to increase hemostasis and shrinkage of the lesion.[21]
- Minor postoperative complications: reported postoperative complications are restricted to prescription of analgesics for a few patients,[20] and transitory local paresthesia at the operative site.[18,21] Good healing and no scar formation were frequently reported.

As regards the limitations described for conventional surgery and other therapeutic modalities to remove oral mucoceles (Table 33.1), excision with a high power laser may be considered safe and advantageous in various clinical situations, and in pediatric patients[20,24] (see Clinical case 33.1).

Lasers in Dentistry: Guide for Clinical Practice, First Edition. Edited by Patrícia M. de Freitas and Alyne Simões.
© 2015 John Wiley & Sons, Inc. Published 2015 by John Wiley & Sons, Inc.

Table 33.1 Main treatment characteristics for oral mucoceles reported in the literature.[7–13]

Treatment modality	Description	Main advantages	Main limitations
Complete surgical excision	Conventional surgery, removing the lesion including the entire minor salivary gland or a part of the sublingual gland in the case of a ranula	Rapid elimination of the lesion	Extensive tissue damage, including nerve injuries High risk of recurrences due lesion rupture during the surgery
Microsurgery	Microdissection of the lesion using magnification and fine microsurgical instruments in order to preserve the lesion wall	Minimizes the risk of the lesion rupturing Less risk of recurrence	Time consuming Requires familiarization with the use of microsurgical instruments
Marsupialization	Unroofing procedure indicated for large lesions	More conservative treatment to avoid damage to neighboring tissues	Recurrences due the early closure of the surgical cavity
Micro-marsupialization	Fine silk suture passed along the internal part of the gland and surgical knot in the widest diameter of the lesion	Less invasive treatment option Low frequency of recurrence	Indicated only for pediatric patients
Cryosurgery	Cycles of topical application of a cryoprobe (i.e. liquid nitrogen at −81 °C) followed by a 1-min thaw	No need for anesthesia Absence of bleeding, infection, and pain	Potential damage to the neighboring tissues, including nerves and sublingual duct in the case of a ranula Cryosurgery equipment is expensive
Sclerosing agent OK-432 (Picibanil)	Single intralesional injection of a lyophilized mixture of a low virulence strain of Streptococcus pyogenes incubated with benzylpenicillin that causes local inflammation and fibrosis	No need for anesthesia No scars	Local discomfort for several days after the injection Side effects of streptococcal preparation Few cases reported in the literature
Administration of homotoxicological drug	Oral administration of nickel gluconate–mercurius heel-potentized swine organ preparation in oral mucoceles of pediatric patients, based on classical medical and homeopathic principles, for resorption of the lesion	No need for anesthesia No scars No side effects	Partial remission of the lesions Few cases reported in the literature
Topical corticosteroids	Topical application of high potency corticosteroid (clobetasol propionate) for multiple, painful, recurrent mucoceles	Impairment of the pain process Total remission of the lesions	Side effects of the corticosteroids Few cases reported in the literature
Systemic administration of gamma-linolenic acid	Prescription of evening primrose oil that is metabolically converted into gamma-linolenic acid, a precursor of prostaglandin E. Indicated for multiple lesions of oral mucocele	No need for anesthesia Partial remission of the lesions	Partial recurrence of the lesions when the therapy was discontinued Few cases reported in the literature

Table 33.2 Laser protocols and clinical outcomes of laser-based excision of oral mucoceles.

Number of patients (age; years)	Laser protocol	Clinical outcomes	Reference
9 (no information)	CO_2 laser, 10 W, cw or pw	Good healing	Frame[14]
1 (55) – multiple lesions	Nd:YAG laser, 10 W, cw	Complete vaporization of the lesions No recurrence after 3 years	Jinbu et al.[15]
1 (13)	CO_2 laser, 6–8 W, cw	Good healing after 1 week	Kopp and St Hilaire[16]
4 (no information) – ranula	CO_2 laser, 4 W, cw	Good healing; no recurrences after 6 months	Niccoli-Filho and Morosolli[17]
12 (no information)	CO_2 laser, 3–9 W, cw or sp	2 (16.6%) recurrences Temporarily diminished sensation in the oral mucosa after the laser excision	Bornstein et al.[18]
1 (12)	Er,Cr:YSGG laser, 11% air, 7% water, 1.5 W	Good healing	Zola et al.[19]
20 (0–15)	CO_2 laser, 3–4 W, cw	11% experienced postoperative pain Good healing	Kato and Wijeyeweera[20]
82 (1–58)	CO_2 laser, 5–8 W, cw	1 (1.21%) patient had transitory local paresthesia at the operative site 2 (2.43%) recurrences after 3 months	Huang et al.[21]
30 (6–65)	CO_2 laser, 5–7 W, cw	Good healing	Yagüe-García et al.[22]
1 (9)	Er,Cr:YSGG laser, 0% air, 0% water, 0.25 W	No scar formation No recurrences after 12 months	Boj et al.[23]
2 (9–10)	Diode laser (810 nm), 2 W, cw, contact technique	Good healing No recurrences after 12 months	Pedron et al[24]

cw, continuous mode; pw, pulsed mode; sp, superpulsed mode.

Clinical case 33.1

A 7-year-old boy was referred to the stomatology clinic of the School of Dentistry, University of São Paulo, presenting with a painless translucent nodule in the lower lip mucosa near the left commissure and approximately 0.5 cm in size, with a duration of 3 months (Fig. 33.1a). Based on the clinical characteristics and history, this lesion was initially clinically diagnosed as a mucocele. Removal of the lesion was performed under local infiltrative anesthesia using a CO_2 laser (UM-L30; Union Medical Engineering Co, Seoul, South Korea: 10 600 nm, continuous mode, power 6 W). Dissection was performed, with the lesion and its associated minor salivary gland separated from the adjacent tissue (Fig, 33.1b). Postoperative care included 0.15% benzydamine hydrochloride mouthwash three times per day for 1 week, and no analgesic medications were necessary. The patient was followed-up until complete healing was achieved, which occurred in 30 days (Fig. 33.1c). No signs of recurrence were observed over a 12-month follow-up. The removed lesion was analyzed and the diagnosis of oral mucocele confirmed (Fig. 33.1d,e). On microscopic analysis, the tissue margins exhibited thermal damage, but this did not interfere with the anatomopathological diagnosis.

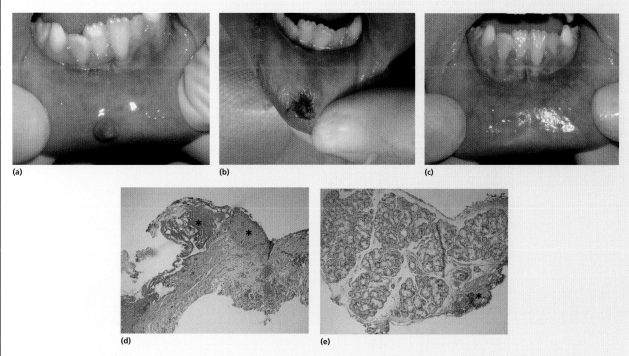

(a)   (b)   (c)

(d)   (e)

Figure 33.1 (a) Nodular lesion in the lower lip mucosa, with a translucent aspect, compatible with diagnosis of an oral mucocele. (b) Clinical image of oral mucocele excision using a high power CO_2 laser. (c) Thirty days post oral mucocele excision. There is complete wound healing and absence of scar. (d,e) Microscopic analysis of the biopsied lesion, confirming the diagnosis of a mucus extravasation phenomenon. (d) Connective tissue showing mucus extravasation sorrounded by granulation tissue and thermal damage in the margins (*). (e) Minor salivary gland parenchyma exhibiting thermal damage restricted to the biospy margins (*). (HE, original magnification ×40 and ×100).

Future perspectives

It is not possible to make comparisons among different types of lasers indicated for oral mucocele excision, due to the low number of reports and the absence of randomized clinical studies. Therefore, further studies must be conducted in order to optimize the laser surgical protocols, and to establish the effectiveness of this therapy for oral mucocele removal, particularly with regard to the level of recurrence and quality of tissue repair.

References

1 Hayashida AM, Zerbinatti DC, Balducci I, Cabral LA, Almeida JD. Mucus extravasation and retention phenomena: a 24-year study. *BMC Oral Health* 2010; 10: 15.

2 Chi AC, Lambert PR 3rd, Richardson MS, Neville BW. Oral mucoceles: a clinicopathologic review of 1,824 cases, including unusual variants. *J Oral Maxillofac Surg* 2011; 69(4): 1086–1093.

3 Sousa FB, Etges A, Corrêa L, Mesquita RA, de Araújo NS. Pediatric oral lesions: a 15-year review from São Paulo, *Brazil. J Clin Pediatr Dent* 2002; 26(4): 413–418.

4 Granholm C, Olsson Bergland K, Walhjalt H, Magnusson B. Oral mucoceles; extravasation cysts and retention cysts. A study of 298 cases. *Swed Dent J* 2009; 33(3): 125–130.

5 Seo J, Bruno I, Artico G, Vechio AD, Migliari DA. Oral mucocele of unusual size on the buccal mucosa: clinical presentation and surgical approach. *Open Dent J* 2012; 6: 67–68.

6 Jinbu Y, Tsukinoki K, Kusama M, Watanabe Y. Recurrent multiple superficial mucocele on the palate: Histopathology and laser vaporization. *Oral Surg Oral Med Oral Pathol Oral Radiol Endod* 2003; 95(2): 193–197.

7 Toida M, Ishimaru JI, Hobo N. A simple cryosurgical method for treatment of oral mucous cysts. *Int J Oral Maxillofac Surg* 1993; 22(6): 353–355.

8 McCaul JA, Lamey PJ. Multiple oral mucoceles treated with gamma-linolenic acid: report of a case. *Br J Oral Maxillofac Surg* 1994; 32(6): 392–393.

9 Garofalo S, Briganti V, Cavallaro S, et al. Nickel gluconate-mercurius heel-potentised swine organ preparations: a new therapeutic approach for the primary treatment of pediatric ranula and intraoral mucocele. *Int J Pediatr Otorhinolaryngol* 2007; 71(2): 247–255.

10 Luiz AC, Hiraki KR, Lemos CA Jr, Hirota SK, Migliari DA. Treatment of painful and recurrent oral mucoceles with a high-potency topical corticosteroid: a case report. *J Oral Maxillofac Surg* 2008; 66(8): 1737–1739.

11 Cecconi D, Achilli A, Tarozzi M, et al. Mucoceles of the oral cavity: a large case series (1994–2008) and a literature review. *Med Oral Pathol Oral Cir Buccal* 2010; 15(4): e551–556.

12 Ohta N, Fukase S, Suzuki Y, Aoyagi M. Treatment of salivary mucocele of the lower lip by OK-432. *Auris Nasus Larynx* 2011; 38(2): 240–243.

13 Tilaveridis I, Lazaridou M, Lazaridis N. The use of magnification and microsurgical instruments for the excision of lower lip mucoceles. *J Oral Maxillofac Surg* 2011; 69(5): 1408–1410.

14 Frame JW. Carbon dioxide laser surgery for benign oral lesions. *Br Dent J* 1985; 158(4): 125–128.

15 Jinbu Y, Kusama M, Itoh H, Matsumoto K, Wang J, Noguchi T. Mucocele of the glands of Blandin-Nuhn: clinical and histopathologic analysis of 26 cases. *Oral Surg Oral Med Oral Pathol Oral Radiol Endod* 2003; 95(4): 467–470.

16 Kopp WK, St-Hilaire H. Mucosal preservation in the treatment of mucocele with CO_2 laser. *J Oral Maxillofac Surg* 2004; 62(12): 1559–1561.

17 Niccoli-Filho W, Morosolli AR. Surgical treatment of ranula with carbon dioxide laser radiation. *Lasers Med Sci* 2004; 19(1): 12–14.

18 Bornstein MM, Winzap-Kälin C, Cochran DL, Buser D. The CO_2 laser for excisional biopsies of oral lesions: a case series study. *Int J Periodontics Restorative Dent* 2005; 25(3): 221–229.

19 Zola M, Rosenberg D, Anakwa K. Treatment of a ranula using an Er,Cr:YSGG laser. *J Oral Maxillofac Surg.* 2006; 64(5): 823–827.

20 Kato J, Wijeyeweera RL. The effect of CO(2) laser irradiation on oral soft tissue problems in children in Sri Lanka. *Photomed Laser Surg* 2007; 25(4): 264–268.

21 Huang IY, Chen CM, Kao YH, Worthington P. Treatment of mucocele of the lower lip with carbon dioxide laser. *J Oral Maxillofac Surg* 2007; 65(5): 855–858.

22 Yagüe-García J, España-Tost AJ, Berini-Aytés L, Gay-Escoda C. Treatment of oral mucocele-scalpel versus CO_2 laser. *Med Oral Pathol Oral Cir Buccal* 2009; 14(9): e469–474.

23 Boj JR, Poirier C, Espasa E, Hernandez M, Espanya A. Lower lip mucocele treated with an erbium laser. *Pediatr Dent* 2009; 31(3): 249–252.

24 Pedron IG, Galletta VC, Azevedo LH, Corrêa L. Treatment of mucocele of the lower lip with diode laser in pediatric patients: presentation of 2 clinical cases. *Pediatr Dent* 2010; 32(7): 539–541.

CHAPTER 34

Potentially malignant disorders of the oral mucosa

Vivian Cunha Galletta Kern,[1] Ana Claudia Luiz,[2] Edgar Kazuyoshi Nakajima,[1,3] Luciane Hiramatsu Azevedo,[4] and Dante Antonio Migliari[5]

[1] Special Laboratory of Lasers in Dentistry (LELO), School of Dentistry, University of São Paulo (USP), São Paulo, SP, Brazil
[2] Cancer Institute of São Paulo (ICESP), São Paulo, SP, Brazil
[3] Private Dental Practice, São Paulo, SP, Brazil
[4] Dentistry Clinic, University of São Paulo (USP), São Paulo, SP, Brazil
[5] Department of Stomatology, School of Dentistry, University of São Paulo (USP), São Paulo, SP, Brazil

Introduction

Potentially malignant disorders (PMDs) of the oral mucosa are pathologies that have an increased potential for malignant transformation at any site in the mouth or oropharynx. According to the most recent classification of the World Health Organization (WHO), the PMDs are oral erythroplakia, palatal lesions in reverse smoking, oral submucous fibrosis, discoid lupus erythematosus, some hereditary disorders (e.g. dyskeratosis congenita, epidermollysis bullosa), actinic keratosis, oral lichen planus, and oral leukoplakia.[1] Some PMDs may be surgically treated by high power lasers, although continuous follow-up is mandatory since oral cancer may arise in any part of the oral mucosa at any given time.

This chapter describes the experience with treatment of oral leukoplakia, actinic keratosis, oral lichen planus, and oral erythroplakia with high power lasers at the Special Laboratory of Lasers in Dentistry (LELO), School of Dentistry, University of São Paulo, Brazil.

Oral leukoplakia

Despite the lack of scientific evidence that treatment for oral leukoplakia can prevent malignant transformation, it is considered safe practice to treat it, irrespective of the absence or presence of epithelial dysplasia.[2] Furthermore, removal of oral leukoplakia may detect early cancer that has been missed by incisional biopsy[3] and decrease the rate of malignant transformation.[4]

Before initiating therapy for oral leukoplakia, it is important to consider that other white diseases of the oral mucosa carry no increased risk for cancer, such as frictional lesions, leukoedema, white sponge nevus, and nicotinic stomatitis. As these have a similar clinical appearance to oral leukoplakia, they must be ruled out for a definitive diagnosis of oral leukoplakia. Clinical assessment of a predominantly white lesion should include lesion inspection and elimination of suspected etiology (e.g. local mechanical trauma, dental restoration materials) or factors that might be associated with the lesion (i.e. superimposed candidosis), followed by biopsy of a persistent lesion. Conventional incisional biopsy (by scalpel) is preferably performed at areas with non-homogeneous features, namely, irregular flat, nodular or reddish appearance, as well as at areas positively stained by toluidine blue. Excisional biopsy should be avoided, although it is preferable if the lesion size is small (i.e. <2 cm) to provide enough material for histopathological analysis. Final removal of the remaining oral leukoplakia lesion should be carried out after histopathological examination of the biopsy has confirmed the suspected oral leukoplakia diagnosis and excluded the presence of carcinoma.[2]

Advantages of surgical excision of oral leukoplakia by high power lasers over conventional method (i.e. scalpel) include bleeding control and less bacteremia, among others, and this can be a particularly favorable technique when large areas of oral mucosa are affected, as wound healing occurs by secondary intention. Usually the laser of choice for oral leukoplakia treatment is the CO_2 laser as it is efficient in cutting oral soft tissues and only produces superficial thermal damage, resulting from the intense energy absorption of this particular wavelength (10 600 nm) by its main chromophore, water, abundant in the oral mucosa.[5] Whenever oral leukoplakia is distributed in areas that are difficult to access with the CO_2 articulated arm, a laser with a flexible optical fiber, such as the diode laser (808–980 nm), can be used in a contact mode.

In our protocol, surgery is performed with the CO_2 laser (UM–L30; Union Medical Engineering Co, USA: continuous mode, 10 600 nm, 5–10 W; see Clinical cases 34.1 and 34.2) or diode laser (GaAlAs, ZAP softlase; ZAP Lasers Inc, USA: continuous mode, 808 nm, 2–3 W) under local anesthesia. Initially, lesions are outlined by vaporization, creating a margin that is 3 mm deep, with a distance of ~5 mm from the lesion border. Following lesion demarcation, the margin is lifted with forceps and excision is carried out by undercutting at a constant depth.[6] Laser excision specimens are submitted to histopathological analysis. Since surgical treatment does not preclude oral leukoplakia from transforming into cancer and does not avoid oral leukoplakia recurrences, a close follow-up must be carried out. There is no evidence of optimal intervals of follow-up after oral leukoplakia treatment. However, lifelong follow-up at intervals of 6 months for non-dysplastic oral leukoplakia and of 3 months for dysplastic oral leukoplakia has been suggested.[2] Our protocol suggests the follow-up of all patients every 3 months, regardless of grade of dysplasia.

Actinic cheilitis

While there is no consensus on surgical treatment of oral leukoplakia, excision of actinic cheilitis has been shown to be effective in preventing cancer progression. While oral leukoplakia is typically not associated with any etiologic factor, except for tobbaco smoking, the etiology of actinic cheilitis is known. UV light induces the occurrence of actinic keratosis in the skin of individuals excessively exposed to sunlight, especially those who are fair skinned, and poses a risk to transformation in a non-melanoma malignant neoplasia of the skin.[7] This condition may affect the lips as well as the skin, involving predominantly the vermilion of the lower lip.[8] Clinically, the appearance of actinic cheilitis of the lip is areas of dry, scaly patches and color change.[9] Atrophy, swelling, loss of vermilion margin or ulceration correspond to signs of severe tissue damage, thus indicating the need for a biopsy.[10]

Actinic cheilitis may be successfully prevented with sunscreen lip balm, along with the recommendation to avoid sun exposure. However, if clinical changes on the lip are noted during follow-up and/or histopathological examination shows dysplasia, the use of topical agents (i.e. imiquimod, trichoroacetic acid or 5-fluorouracil), destruction (i.e. photodynamic therapy or cryosurgery) or removal of the tissue (by scalpel, electrodessication or high power laser) are treatment options that should be considered in order to avoid malignant progression.[8,9] Although vermilionectomy by scalpel is the gold standard treatment for actinic cheilitis, lip contour might be compromised, among other postoperative complications. The use of the CO_2 laser for surgical excision of the entire vermilion lip may be an alternative technique, with satisfactory wound repair and fewer adverse effects (less scarring and paresthesia), yet rendering tissue for histopathological analysis.[9] The surgical technique for the use of high power lasers for actinic cheilitis (excision or vaporization) is similar to that described for oral leukoplakia and oral lichen planus.

Oral lichen planus

Differently from oral leukoplakia and actinic cheilitis, the potential for malignant transformation of oral lichen planus is still a source of controversy.[2] Oral lichen planus is a polymorphous disease that can be classified based on several different features. The reticular and plaque-like are the most common forms, affecting about 60% of patients with oral lichen planus. These forms are symptomless, and do not require treatment but do require periodic evaluation.[11] On the other hand, atrophic and

erosive forms may be painful and require treatment. As a mainstream treatment, topical corticosteroids are widely used, although others therapies can also be used, such as topical retinoids. In some widely spread cases, a short-term treatment with systemic corticosteroids may be necessary.[12]

Oral lichen planus can be difficult to treat and is sometimes refractory to conventional therapies. Surgery is rarely performed, but can be used, especially when the first-line approach is not producing any benefit. Although there is little information in the literature regarding the treatment of oral lichen planus with lasers, some authors have reported that in recalcitrant or refractory cases of oral lichen planus high power lasers should be considered as an option.[13,14] As the CO_2 laser evaporation technique has been shown to be effective in the treatment of superficial mucosal lesions,[15] it can also be applied to oral lichen planus lesions. The technique is similar to the one already described for oral leukoplakia and actinic cheilitis; however, instead of resecting the lesion, the laser beam swipes over the treatment area, penetrating to a depth of ~5mm. In recent case reports, low power lasers (excimer, 308 nm; diode laser, 830 nm, 904 nm, and 630 nm) for recalcitrant cases of oral lichen planus have been shown to be effective for pain control.[13,14,16–18] Only a few studies have investigated the application of different types of lasers or techniques in the treatment of oral lichen planus. Up to now, CO_2 vaporization (see Clinical case 34.4) or low power energy lasers have not been deemed as standard treatment modalities for oral lichen planus. Published reports suggest that low and high power lasers can be used as an option in cases non-responsive to conventional therapy.[13,14,16] It is agreed among these authors that further studies are needed to confirm the efficacy of the laser in the treatment of oral lichen planus, to clarify its biological effect on this disease, and to establish optimal treatment parameters.

In our experience of two cases of oral lichen planus treated with high dose laser surgery, both relapsed after a few months.

Oral erythroplakia

Erythroplakia is a rare lesion that affects the oral mucosa. The prevalence of oral erythroplakia ranges from 0.02% to 0.13%, according to large surveys of the general population. Clinically, oral erythroplakia usually presents as a (bright) red plaque, with signs of atrophy but no specific histopathological features. In most cases (close to 100%), lesions show severe dysplasia or superficial oral squamous cell carcinoma. The differential diagnosis should include erosive and atrophic oral lichen planus, and erythematous candidosis. The histopathological analysis helps the diagnosis by excluding lesions that have specific histopathological features.[19]

In our clinic only one case of oral erythroplakia has been seen over the last decade (see Clinical case 34.5). A surgical laser treatment was proposed and some encouraging postoperative results were obtained. However, 12 months after laser treatment the lesion recurred with an evasive behavior. Eventually the patient was referred to an oncology center.

Clinical case 34.1 Oral leukoplakia

A 60-year-old white man, who reported being a heavy smoker for 46 years, presented to our clinic with a homogenous white plaque, with a smooth, constant texture throughout, affecting the left lateral/ventral tongue (Fig. 34.1a). After incisional biopsy, which revealed hyperkeratosis with moderate dysplasia, removal of the oral leukoplakia lesion was performed with CO_2 laser. The lesion was first outlined by CO_2 laser vaporization (6 W, defocused) (Fig. 34.1b) and then excised (10 W, focused) by lifting the borders with a forceps (Fig. 34.1c), undercutting the connective tissue at a constant depth (Fig. 34.1d). Histopathological examination of the excised oral leukoplakia (Fig. 34.1e) confirmed the previous microscopic examination from the incisional biopsy, showing hyperkeratosis with moderate dysplasia. The healing process was satisfactory, with minimal scarring (Fig. 34.1f,g). The patient was followed up monthly for 5 months, and was free of oral leukoplakia.

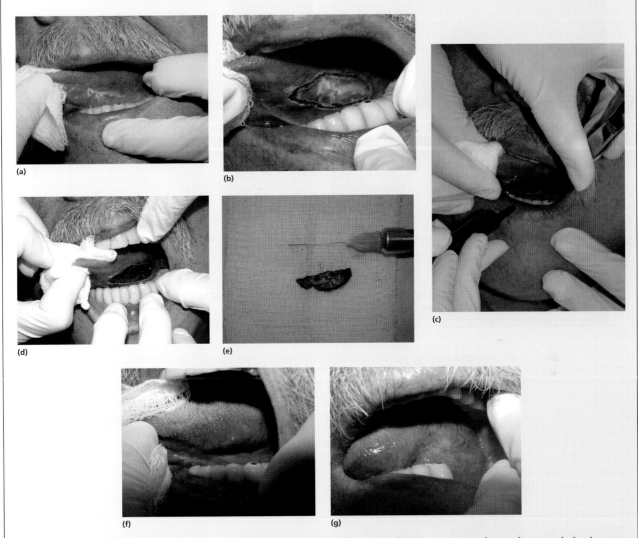

Figure 34.1 (a) Clinical presentation of oral leukoplakia at the lateral border of the tongue. (b,c) Laser surgery technique for removal of oral leukoplakia lesion: (b) the extension of area to be excised was performed by outlining the lesion through vaporization, (c) followed by undercutting the connective tissue within the limited area. (d) Clinical image immediately after laser surgery. (e) Specimen sent for histopathological examination. (f) Clinical appearance 2 weeks and (g) 5 months after the surgical procedure.

Clinical case 34.2 Oral leukoplakia

A 57-year-old white man, who was a non-smoker, was referred to our clinic with a homogenous white plaque, with a corrugated surface, affecting the left buccal mucosa (Fig. 34.2a). At clinical examination, local mechanical trauma was ruled out as a possible etiological factor for the lesion. Histopathological examination of an incisional biopsy showed only hyperkeratosis without cell atypia. The lesion was subsequently treated by surgical excision with a CO_2 laser (Fig. 34.2b). Postoperative evaluation showed complete wound healing within 1 month (Fig. 34.4c,d).

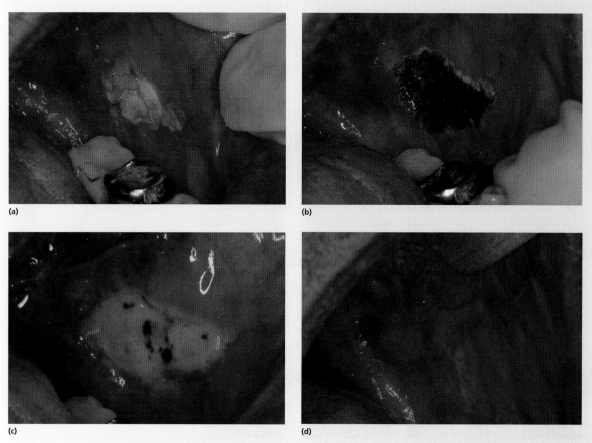

Figure 34.2 (a) Initial clinical presentation of oral leukoplakia at the buccal mucosa. (b) Immediate postoperative clinical appearance after oral leukoplakia removal with a CO_2 laser. (c) A 2-week postoperative clinical examination showed an uneventful healing process; (d) after 4 weeks, the healing was almost complete without any scar.

Clinical case 34.3 Actinic cheilitis

A 66-year-old white man was referred to our clinic for diagnosis and treatment of a lesion on the lower lip that had been present for 3 years. Clinically, there was loss of the vermillion border and an extensive white patch mimicking a leukoplakia-like lesion (Fig. 34.3a). A punch biopsy was performed and the histopathology was that of an actinic cheilitis lesion. Lesion vaporization was performed with a CO_2 laser (Fig. 34.3b). The result was highly satisfactory after a 5-year follow-up (Fig. 34.3c), showing minimal scar on the lower lip, with no recurrence of the lesion.

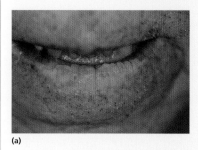 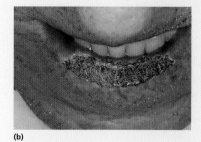 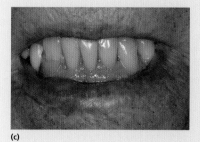

Figure 34.3 (a) Clinical image of actinic cheilitis. (b) Clinical image of lower lip immediately after surgery and (c) 5 years postoperatively.

A 70-year-old male patient presented at the stomatology clinic with oral lichen planus refractory to conventional therapy. Symptomatic lesions were observed on the left buccal mucosa (Fig. 34.4a) and gingival edge (Fig. 34.4b). Management of oral lichen planus was performed with CO_2 vaporization (6 W, continuous mode) at both sites (Fig. 34.4c,d). One week (Fig, 34.4,e,f) and 3 months (Fig. 34.4 g) after the surgical procedure, healing was satisfactory and the patient was asymptomatic. However, 1 year later the lesions had relapsed (Fig. 34.4 h,i).

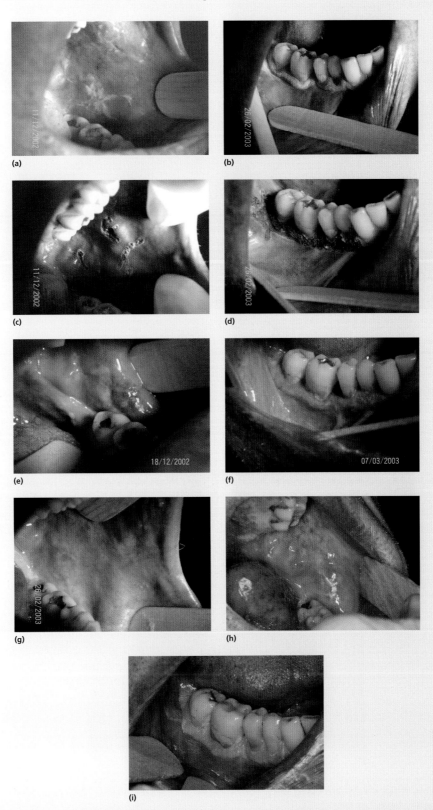

Figure 34.4 Oral lichen planus on (a) the left buccal mucosa and (b) the right gingival edge. (a) Immediate postoperative clinical appearance of the left buccal mucosa and (d) of the right gingival edge. (e,f) Postoperative clinical appearance after 1 week. (g) Clinical image of the buccal mucosa 3 months after oral lichen planus vaporization with a CO_2 laser. (h) Clinical image of the left buccal mucosa and (i) of the gingival edge 1 year after laser vaporization, showing recurrence of oral lichen planus.

Clinical case 34.5 Oral erythroplakia

A 64-year-old white man was referred to our clinic for diagnosis of a lesion on the soft palate, with a 4-month duration. Oral examination showed an extensive erythematous plaque on the posterior area of the soft palate mucosa, extending to the oral pharyngeal mucosa (Fig. 34.5a). The patient reported being a smoker and a chronic alcoholic. A biopsy was performed, confirming the clinical diagnosis of an erythroplakia lesion. The lesion was removed by CO_2 laser irradiation (Fig. 34.5b). Subsequent follow-up appointments were carried over 1 year (Fig. 34.5c,d). Although surgical therapy was successful for 12 months, the lesion recurred with a more aggressive behavior (Fig. 34.5e) and the patient was referred to an oncology center.

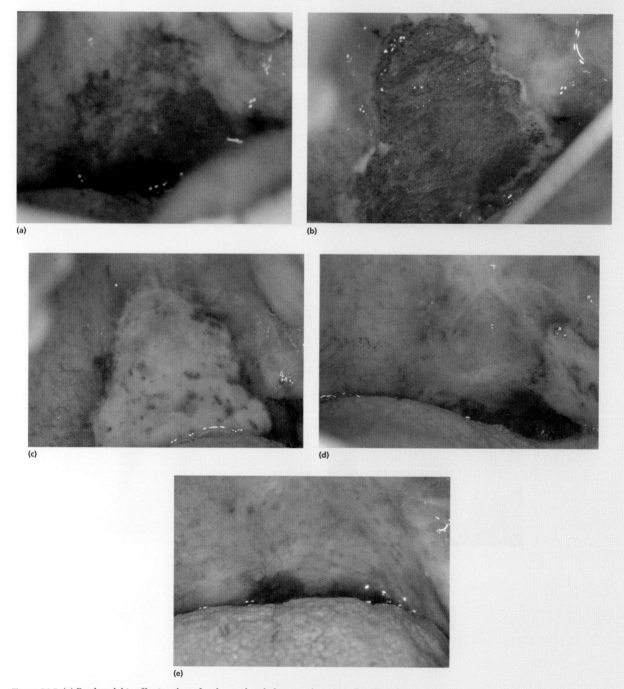

(a)

(b)

(c)

(d)

(e)

Figure 34.5 (a) Erythroplakia affecting the soft palate and oral pharyngeal mucosa. (b) Clinical appearance immediately after erythroplakia excision with a CO_2 laser (6 W), (c) after 2 weeks, and (c) after 6 months of follow-up, when the patient was free of the disorder. (d) Recurrence of oral erythroplakia 1 year after surgical treatment.

References

1 Warnakulasuriya S, Johnson NW, van der Waal I. Nomenclature and classification of potentially malignant disorders of the oral mucosa. J Oral Pathol Med 2007; 36: 575–580.

2 van der Waal I. Potentially malignant disorders of the oral and oropharyngeal mucosa; terminology, classification and present concepts of management. Oral Oncol 2009; 45: 317–323.

3 Lodi G, Porter S. Management of potentially malignant disorders: evidence and critique. J Oral Pathol Med 2008; 37: 63–69.

4 Mehanna HM, Rattay T, Smith J, McConkey CC. Treatment and follow-up of oral dysplasia – a systematic review and meta-analysis. Head Neck 2009; 31: 1600–1609.

5 Meltzer C. Surgical management of oral and mucosal dysplasias: The case for laser excision. J Oral Maxillofac Surg 2007; 65: 293–295.

6 Thomson PJ, Wylie J. Interventional laser surgery: An effective surgical and diagnostic tool in oral precancer management. Int J Oral Maxillofac Surg 2002; 31: 145–153.

7 Del Rosso JQ. Current regimens and guideline implications for the treatment of actinic keratosis: proceedings of a clinical roundtable at the 2011 Winter Clinical Dermatology Conference. Cutis 2011; 88 (Suppl): 1–8

8 Savage NW, McKay C, Faulkner C. Actinic cheilitis in dental practice. Aust Dent J 2010; 55 (Suppl 1): 78–84.

9 Shah AY, Doherty SD, Rosen T. Actinic cheilitis: a treatment review. Int J Dermatol 2010; 49: 1225–1234.

10 Larios G, Alevizos A, Rigopoulos D. Recognition and treatment of actinic cheilitis. Am Fam Physician 2008; 77: 1078–1079.

11 Cheng S, Kirtschig G, Cooper S, Thornhill M, Leonardi-Bee J, Murphy R. Interventions for erosive lichen planus affecting mucosal sites. Cochrane Database Syst Rev 2012; 2: CD008092.

12 Bagan J, Compilato D, Paderni C, et al. Topical therapies for oral lichen planus management and their efficacy: a narrative review. Curr Pharm Des 2012; 18(34): 5470–5480.

13 van der Hem PS, Egges M, van der Wall JE, Roodenburg JLN. CO_2 laser evaporation of oral lichen planus. Int J Oral Maxillofac Surg 2008; 37: 630–633.

14 Jajarm HH, Falaki F, Omid Mahdavi O. A comparative pilot study of low intensity laser versus topical corticosteroids in the treatment of erosive-atrophic oral lichen planus. Photomed Laser Surg 2011; 29: 421–425.

15 Loh HS. A clinical investigation of the management of oral lichen planus with CO_2 laser surgery. J Clin Laser Med Surg 1992; 10: 445–449.

16 Trehan M, Taylor CR. A low-dose excimer 308 nm laser for the treatment of oral lichen planus. Arch Dermatol 2004; 140: 415–420.

17 Cafaro A, Albanese G, Arduino PG, et al. Effect of low-level laser irradiation on unresponsive oral lichen planus: early preliminary results in 13 patients. Photomed Laser Surg 2011; 28: S99–S103.

18 Sivolella S, Berengo M, Cernuschi S, Valente ML. Diode laser treatment is effective for plaque-like lichen planus of the tongue: a case report. Lasers Med Sci 2012; 27: 521–524.

19 Villa A, Villa C, Abati S. Oral cancer and oral erythroplakia: an update and implication for clinicians. Aust Dent J 2011; 56: 253–256.

CHAPTER 35

Herpes

Juliana Marotti

Department of Prosthodontics and Biomaterials, Centre for Implantology, Medical School of the RWTH Aachen University, Aachen, Germany

Introduction

Herpes is a viral disease, caused by herpes simplex virus type 1 (HSV-1) and type 2 (HSV-2). HSV-1 and HSV-2 differ in their site of infection.[1–3] While HSV-1 is responsible for orofacial infections, usually transmitted through kissing and sharing objects contaminated with saliva, HSV-2 is more likely to be detected in genital mucosal disruptions, mainly transmitted sexually or perinatally.[1,2,4] Both are double-stranded DNA viruses type *herpesvirus hominis*, of the Herspesviridae family, which also includes varicella zoster, Epstein-Barr virus, and cytomegalovirus.[1,5] Other disorders such as ocular herpes (keratitis), herpetic whitlow (on fingers or nail cuticle), neonatal herpes, herpes encephalitis, Mollaret's meningitis, and Bell's palsy (facial paralysis) are all caused by HSV.[6,7]

HSV enters the host through skin and mucosal surfaces, commonly the oral cavity, genital tract, and cornea of the eye, by means of direct contact with infected secretions.[4,8] Nevertheless, the majority of primary infections are subclinical.[9] The primary HSV-1 lesions appear as vesicles on the oral mucosa, often associated with pain and fever. After healing of lesions, in around 1–2 weeks, the virus is transported to the trigeminal ganglion and there remains latent until reactivation.[10] The reactivation occurs when there is a decrease in the resistance of the immune system, such as with illness, prolonged exposure to sunlight or cold weather, and most commonly, extended or acute periods of stress.[11] In most cases (around 80%), the recurrent infections cause only salivary asymptomatic infection, but some patients develop a symptomatic process, where vesicles appears on the mucosa and/or skin of the face, usually associated with pain and itchiness.[3,13] The vesicles rupture and coalesce after some days, forming crusts that can take 2 weeks to heal, depending on the lesion extension, and then the virus returns to latency.[10] Figure 35.1 shows the different stages of the infection.

Herpes is one of the most common communicable diseases worldwide.[5] It is colloquially called a cold sore or fever blister. Apart from recurrent and painful disruptions, herpes infection is usually associated with massive psychosocial distress, shame, and uncomfortable feelings, due to a marred esthetic appearance.[5,13]

Herpes was first observed and described by the Austrian pathologist Benjamin Lipschütz in 1921,[14] and since no cure for the disease or vaccine to prevent it has been developed.[4] Several treatment options have been proposed, among them laser therapy; these are discussed in this chapter.

Conventional treatment

The most common treatment for HSV-1 is based on antiviral compounds, such as acyclovir, valacyclovir, and famciclovir.[3] These conventional treatments should be considered to provide symptomatic relief, but not a cure.[15] Despite the emergence of potent agents against HSV-1 during the last decade, the increasing clinical use of medications, such as acyclovir and famciclovir, has been associated with the emergence of drug-resistant virus strains,[16] especially in immunocompromised patients.[17] Moreover, medication is only effective if it is taken when the patient first notices the prodromic symptoms, like itching and pain.[18,19] Furthermore, it was reported that the intermittent administration of medications does not alter the frequency of recurrences.[11,20]

Figure 35.2 shows two clinical cases where the intermittent systemic and topical administration of medication over more than 10 years reduced in effectiveness, possibly due to drug resistance. The patients reported that over time lesions were both more numerous and of greater intensity.

Resistance to the acyclovir family of drugs is caused by deficiency in thymidine kinase (the most frequent cause), decreased thymidine kinase activity, thymidine kinase with altered substrate specificity, or viral DNA polymerase with altered substrate specificity.[9,21,22]

Most current HSV vaccines under development are intended for prevention of HSV-2, as it is a greater public concern than HSV-1. However, because HSV-1 has a similar structure and function to HSV-2, vaccines against HSV-2 may provide cross-protection against HSV-1.[4] The immunization strategies against

Lasers in Dentistry: Guide for Clinical Practice, First Edition. Edited by Patrícia M. de Freitas and Alyne Simões.
© 2015 John Wiley & Sons, Inc. Published 2015 by John Wiley & Sons, Inc.

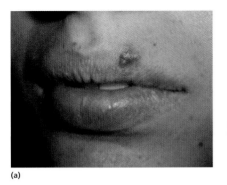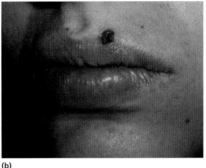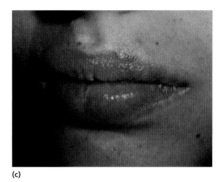

Figure 35.1 Different stages of HSV-1 infection: (a) vesicle, (b) crust (B), (c) prodrome or latent phase.

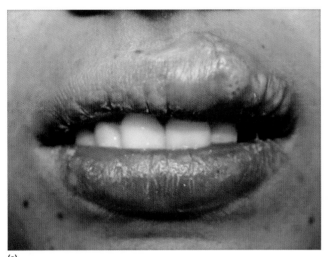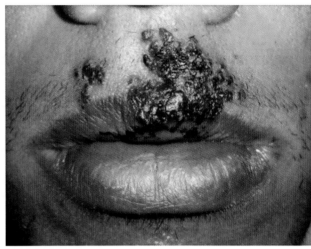

Figure 35.2 (a,b) Severe herpes labialis lesions due to the development of drug resistance.

HSV have been investigated to obtain a better understanding of the basic mechanisms of viral replication and the interplay of the virus with the immune system, in order to develop new approaches to vaccine design.[4]

An effective vaccine could target the primary site of viral entry to prevent viral replication at the initial site of infection, entry into nerve cells, and infection of the sensory ganglion to preclude latency or reactivation by limiting recurrences and spread.[4,8] Although no vaccine has yet been developed, some animal and early human trials seem to be promising.[23–26]

Laser treatment

High power lasers

High power lasers (HPLs) can be used to promote rupture of and to drain herpetic vesicles.[27,28] It is hypothesized that HPL irradiation can reduce the amount of herpes virus present in the fluid, by increasing the local temperature and, consequently, decreasing the frequency and duration of the infection.[29]

The erbium laser is one of the most commonly used HPLs for the treatment of herpes labialis at the vesicle stage. Erbium lasers (Er,Cr:YSGG emitting at 2780 nm; Er:YAG emitting at 2940 nm) are highly absorbed by water and hydroxyapatite, and consequently, also by enamel, dentin, and soft tissue.[30,31] One of their advantages compared to lasers emitting other wavelengths (such as the Nd:YAG and diode lasers) is the possibility of using a water spray, which may reduce the pain experienced during irradiation.[28,32]

While HPLs produce satisfactory results, when used together with low power lasers (LPLs) and photodynamic therapy (PDT), the clinical results and patient response seem to be even better.[27–29,33]

Photodynamic therapy

PDT is based on the interaction of a photosensitizer and light in oxygenated tissue.[34,35] Damaging or killing a biological system by photooxidation is known as "photodynamic inactivation," "photodynamic effect," or "photodynamic therapy." Several studies have reported virus inactivation by means of PDT.[36–38] The antiviral effect is dependent on dye concentration, light source, and substrate.[33] The mechanisms of PDT are described in Chapter 7.

Although the photodynamic effect was demonstrated to be effective against viral targets more than 70 years ago, the use of

Table 35.1 Different laser parameters according to the specific phases of RHL infection.

Phase	Laser	Wavelength (nm)	Parameters	References
Vesicle	HPL	Er,Cr:YSGG: 2780	140–200 µs, 20 Hz, 0.75 W, air/water spray	Marotti et al.[28]
		Er:YAG: 2940	80 mJ/pulse, 2–4 Hz, air/water spray	Bello-Silva et al.[27]
		Nd:YAG: 1064	100 mJ/pulse, 15 Hz, 1.5 W	de Paulo Eduardo et al.[49]
	PDT	660–670 nm (red light)	MB 0.01% 5 min + 100 J/cm², 100 mW, 28 s/point, 2.8 J	Marotti et al.[28], Sperandio et al.[48]
			MB 0.01% 5 min + 120 J/cm², 40 mW, 2 min/point, 4.8 J	Marotti et al.[33]
Crust	LPL	660–670 (red light)	20 J/cm², 40 mW, 14 s/point, 0.5 J/point, 4 sessions in 1 week	Marotti et al.[28]
			3.8 J/cm², 15 mW, 0.15 J/point, 4 sessions in 1 week	Marotti et al.[28]
			3.8 J/cm², 10 mW, 10 s/point, daily during 10 days	Bello-Silva et al.[27]
			4 J/cm², 50 mW	de Paulo Eduardo et al.[49]
			3.8 J/cm², 15 mW, 10 s/point, 3 sessions in 1 week	Marotti et al.[33]
			4.8 J, 40 mW, 2 min	Munoz Sanches et al.[50]
Prodrome/latent	LPL	780–808 (infrared light)	8.75 J/cm², 70 mW, 5 s/point, 2x/week for 5 weeks	de Paulo Eduardo et al.[49]
			2.04 J/cm², 40 mW, 40 s/point, 1.6 J	Munoz Sanches et al.[50]
			4.5 J/cm², 60 mW, 3 s/point, 1 session/week for 10 weeks	de Carvalho et al.[51]

HPL, high power laser; LPL, low power laser; PDT, photodynamic therapy; MB, methylene blue.

photosensitizers as antivirals *in vivo* has been slow to gain acceptance. The reason for this may be the pronounced side effects seen in several cases of the phototreatment of herpes genitalis in the early 1970s.[38] With the development of PDT to treat cancer and localized infections, a great deal of experience has been gained in the targeting and eradication of viruses.[29]

Methylene blue (MB) is one of the photosensitizers that can be used for the treatment of herpes labialis by PDT with satisfactory results.[36] The mechanism of virus inactivation involves binding of the dye to nucleic acid, absorption of light, generation of reactive oxygen species, and guanine oxidation in the viral genome.[39] Some studies have clearly demonstrated the effect of MB against viruses.[36,40] Also, MB shows strong absorption at the red end of the visible spectrum.[33]

Defining protocols for the clinical application of PDT is not an easy task, since this therapeutic modality is affected by several light dosimetry parameters, such as wavelength, power output, exposure time, fluence rate, fluence (dose), number of treatments, and treatment intervals. In addition to the light source parameters, the photosensitizer's chemical and photophysical properties should be considered, as well as the dye concentration and dye solvent used.[29] As PDT is not yet widely used by dentists or physicians, further studies and follow-up clinical reports are required.[33]

Low level laser therapy

Low level laser therapy (LLLT) is a clinical treatment that results in non-thermal effects on tissues. The magnitude of its effects depends on the cells' physiological status and/or the clinical stage of the condition, prior to irradiation.[41–43] Its effectiveness depends on factors such as wavelength, site, duration, and dose. Research into the dose–response profile of LLLT suggests that different wavelengths have specific penetration abilities through human skin. Thus, clinical effects could vary with the depth of the target tissue.[44,45]

Table 35.2 Lasers and irradiation parameters used in each clinical case.

Laser	Protocol	Cases
PDT	(A) MB 0.01% 5 min + 660 nm, 120 J/cm², 40 mW, 2 min/point, 4.8 J/point	35.1, 35.2
	(B) MB 0.01% 5 min + 660 nm, 100 J/cm², 100 mW, 28 s/point, 2.8 J/point	35.3, 35.9
Er,Cr:YSGG	0.75 W, 10% air and 10% water	35.4
Er:YAG	80 mJ, 6 Hz	35.5
Diode	0.75 W, continuous mode	35.6
Nd:YAG	0.75 W, 10 Hz	35.7
LLLT	(A) 660 nm, 3.8 J/cm², 15 mW, 10 s/point, 0.15 J/point	35.1, 35.2, 35.4, 35.6
	(B) 660 nm, 20 J/cm², 40 mW, 14 s/point, 0.56 J/point	35.3, 35.5, 35.7, 35.8, 35.9

PDT, photodynamic therapy; LLLT, low level laser therapy; MB, methylene blue.

LLLT mechanisms are described in Chapters 3–6. As this kind of phototherapy may also have an effect on several immunological reactions, studies have been performed to test the effect of LLLT on HSV-1.[11,46]

HPLs and LPLs, either associated with PDT or not, can be used for the treatment of recurrent herpes labialis (RHL)[27–29,32,33,47–49] (see Clinical cases 35.1–35.8). The therapy should be chosen according to the stage of the lesion. When the lesion is at the vesicular stage, HPL irradiation or PDT is recommended. In the crust phase, LLLT at the red wavelength can be used, aiming to accelerate the healing process (Table 35.1). An infrared laser can also be used at the crusting stage when edema is present, or when there is no infectious process.[29] Various protocols for irradiation are discussed in the literature; however, there is still no consensus among authors.[11,33,52]

Reports in the literature have demonstrated that the use of LLLT combined with HPL or PDT for the treatment of herpes labialis promotes satisfactory results.[27–29,32,33,47–49,53] However, more clinical studies must be performed in order to establish an ideal laser irradiation protocol.

Herpes zoster

Herpes zoster (also known as shingles) is a viral disease, but despite its name and the similarity of its clinical appearance to herpes simplex, it is neither an HSV-1 nor an HSV-2 infection. Herpes zoster is caused by the varicella zoster virus (VZV), or human herpes virus type 3, also responsible for the varicella disease (chickenpox).[54,55] Chickenpox occurs following primary infection, while herpes zoster (usually associated with aging and immunosuppression) is the consequence of reactivation of the latent virus. Post-herpetic neuralgia is the major complication of herpes zoster.[54,55] Approximately 70–80% of patients with herpes zoster complain of prodromal pain in the dermatome, where skin lesions subsequently appear.[55] The prodrome usually last 2–3 days, but longer durations of 1 week have been reported.[55]

Clinical case 35.1 PDT + LLLT

A 25-year-old woman presented with vesicular herpes on the upper lip. The protocol used was PDT (A) followed by LLLT (A). Figure 35.3 shows the treatment steps; the lesion was completely healed after 1 week.

This patient had no pain or discomfort during her clinical care and she had had no recurrence at a 6-month follow-up.[33]

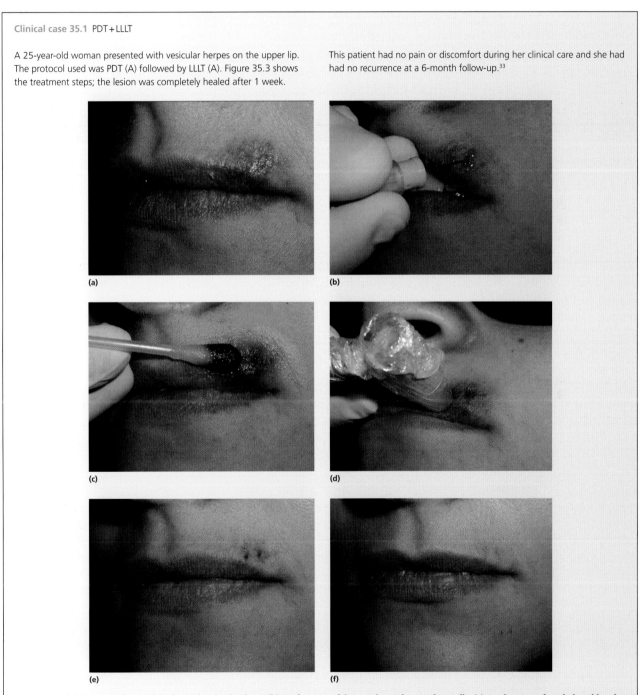

Figure 35.3 (a) Recurrent herpes labialis in the vesicle phase. (b) Perforation of the vesicles with a sterile needle. (c) Application of methylene blue dye solution. (d) After 5 minutes, irradiation with an LPL. (e) Clinical appearance 24 hours post treatment. (f) Complete healing of the lesion after 1 week.

The lesions tend to be grouped, without crossing the middle line, and clusters are often seen where there are branches of the cutaneous sensory nerve. Motor nerves may be involved in 5–15% of cases. Secondary cases of herpes zoster are uncommon in immunologically intact hosts, probably because a herpes zoster episode will boost immunity, and thereby prevent subsequent symptomatic VZV reactivations.[55] Some complications associated with herpes zoster include keratitis, scleritis, central retinal artery occlusion, and cranial nerve palsy.[56]

Conventional treatments for herpes zoster include antivirals (acyclovir, valacyclovir, famciclovir) and analgesics, when there is associated pain.[55] Clinical case 35.9 shows the treatment of herpes zoster infection on the face, with ocular involvement, with PDT.

Clinical case 35.2 PDT + LLLT

A 52-year-old woman showed RHL on the upper lip, and the lesion had a crust due to the topical application of acyclovir. The protocol used was PDT (A) and LLLT (A). Figure 35.4 shows the treatment stepst; the lesion was completely healed after 1 week and the patient had had no recurrences at 10-month follow-up.[33].

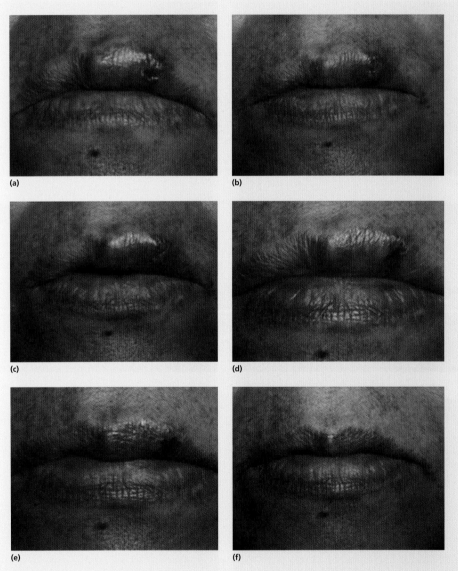

(a) (b) (c) (d) (e) (f)

Figure 35.4 (a) Initial lesion. (b) Vesicle perforation and dye application. (c) Lesion appearance immediately post irradiation. (d) 6 hours post irradiation the crust was formed and there was significant reduction of edema. (e) Advanced healing observed 24 hours post irradiation; slight edema. (f) Complete healing 1 week post treatment.

Final considerations

For successful therapeutic treatment of RHL, it is essential to have a good medical history of the patient's overall health and the historical of clinical disease.[57,58]

The selection of an appropriate type of drug and its delivery (intravenous, oral or topical) can present a dilemma for many practitioners.[12] Additionally, the intermittent administration of acyclovir does not alter the frequency of recurrences and has shown to give a good response only if applied before the onset of vesicles.[59] A cure is still not possible for herpes, but some vaccines in development have shown promising results in animal models.[4] Human vaccines continues to be tested in clinical trials of their efficacy and safety.[4]

Despite the fact that preliminary studies have shown satisfactory results for RHL treatment with lasers, more clinical studies must be performed in order to establish an ideal laser irradiation protocol.

Case reports

The patients considered below presented with lesions on the upper or lower lips, previously diagnosed as RHL, and were referred to the Special Laboratory of Lasers in Dentistry (LELO) at the School of Dentistry, University of São Paulo, Brazil. One of the cases was diagnosed as herpes zoster.

Clinical case 35.3 PDT + LLLT

A 23-year-old woman presented with vesicles on both upper and lower lips, and reported local pain, discomfort, and also an itching sensation that began a day before the scheduled appointment. The protocol used was PDT (B) and LLLT (B). Figure 35.5 shows the treatment steps; the

lesion was completely healed after 1 week. After concluding the treatment, the patient returned once a month, for a period of 6 months, without reporting any recurrence of the lesion.[28]

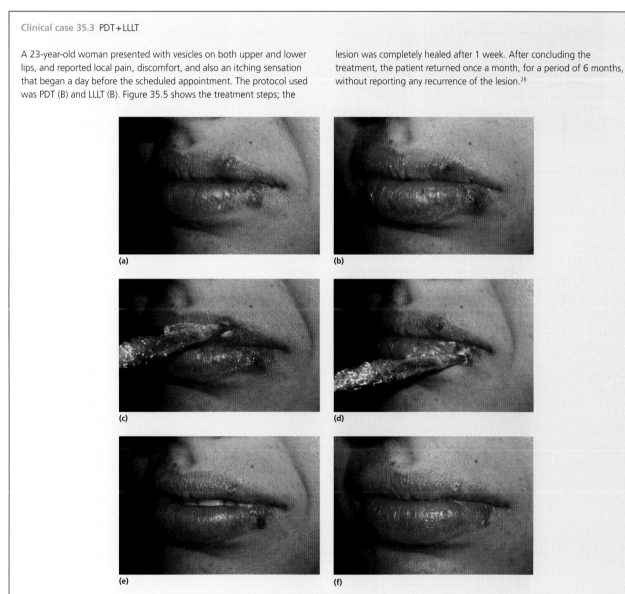

(a) (b) (c) (d) (e) (f)

Figure 35.5 (a) Initial lesions on the upper and lower lips. (b) Application of methylene blue dye. (c,d) After 5 minutes, PDT was performed at three points on each lesion. (e) Lesions 48 hours post treatment. (f) Complete healing was achieved after 1 week.

Clinical case 35.4 Er,Cr:YSGG + LLLT

An 18-year-old man with vesicles on the upper lip (Fig. 35.6a) was treated with an Er,Cr:YSGG laser (Fig. 35.6b) for drainage of the vesicles. Figure 35.6c shows the area immediately after the laser irradiation. A site of crusting was noted 24 hours after HLLT (Fig. 35.6d), and then LLLT (protocol A) was conducted at four points of irradiation (Fig. 35.6e). After 1 week, the patient showed no signs or symptoms related to RHL (Fig. 35.6f). During the 6-month follow-up, no recurrence was observed.[28]

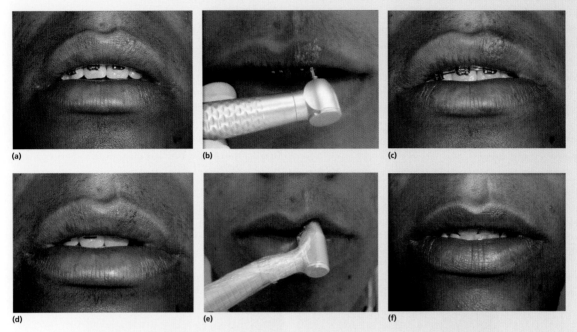

Figure 35.6 (a) Initial lesion on the upper lip. (b) Drainage of vesicles with an Er,Cr:YSGG laser. (c) Vesicles after drainage. (d) LLLT after 24 hours. (e) LLLT at four points on the lesion area. (f) One week after HPL irradiation.

Clinical case 35.5 Er:YAG + LLLT

A 52-year-old woman presented with vesicles on the lower lip. The patient was treated with the Er:YAG laser (Fig. 35.7a–d). After vesicle drainage, pain relief was achieved. After 24 hours, an area of crusting area was noted and LLLT (protocol B) was conducted at five points of irradiation. After 1 week, advanced healing could be observed (Fig. 37.7e). Complete healing was achieved after 10 days (Fig. 35.7f). The patient had had no recurrences at a 6-month follow-up.

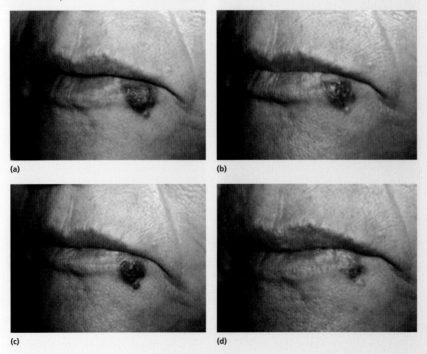

Figure 35.7 (a) Initial lesion after drainage of the vesicles with an Er:YAG laser. (b) A crust was noted after 24 hours; no pain was reported, but edema was present. (c) No edema after 72 hours. (d) Advanced healing after 1 week. (e) LLLT was performed until resolution of the case. (f) Complete healing after 10 days.

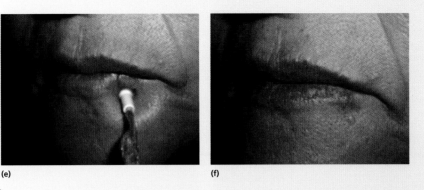

(e)   (f)

Figure 35.7 (Continued)

Clinical case 35.6 Diode+LLLT

A 23-year-old man presenting with vesicles on the upper lip (Fig. 35.8a) was treated with a diode laser (Fig. 35.8b) for drainage of the vesicles. After 24 hours a crust had already formed, with no further edema, pain or itching sensation (Fig. 35.8c). LLLT was performed according to protocol A (Fig. 35.8d) at five points of irradiation. Advanced healing was noted after 48 hours (Fig. 35.8e). Complete resolution was achieved after 1 week (Fig. 35.8f). During the 8-month follow-up, no recurrence was observed.

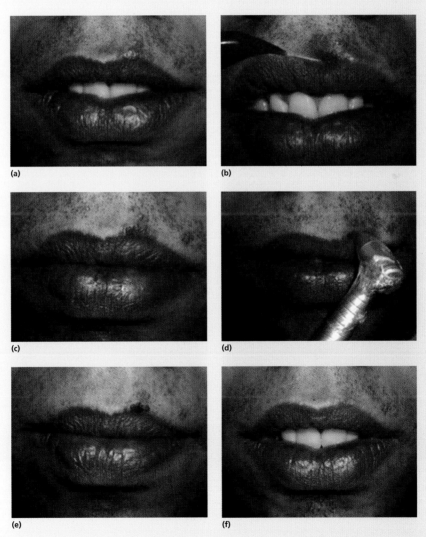

(a)   (b)

(c)   (d)

(e)   (f)

Figure 35.8 (a) Recurrent herpes labialis on the left side of the upper lip. (b) Drainage of vesicles with a diode laser. (c) A crust was present after 24 hours, without edema or pain. (d) LLLT in the crust phase. (e) Advanced healing 48 hours post treatment. (f) Complete healing after 1 week.

Case 35.7 Nd:YAG+LLLT

A 22-year-old woman presented with vesicles on the upper lip (Fig. 35.9a). The vesicles were drained with the Nd:YAG laser (Fig. 35.9b). After 24 hours, an area of crusting was noted and LLLT (protocol B) was conducted at five points of irradiation (Fig. 35.9c–e). After 1 week, complete healing was achieved (Fig. 35.9f). No recurrence was reported at a 6-month follow-up.

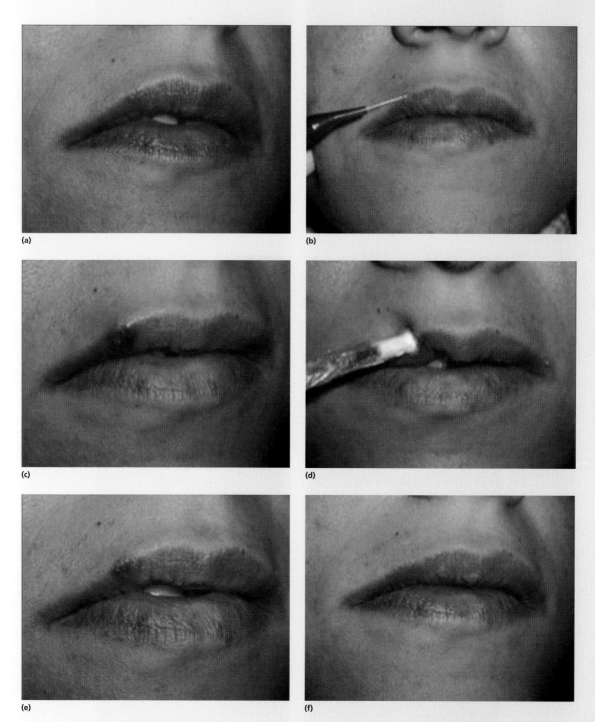

(a)

(b)

(c)

(d)

(e)

(f)

Figure 35.9 (a) Recurrent herpes labialis (RHL) with vesicles on the upper lip. (b) Irradiation with a Nd:YAG laser for drainage of vesicles. (c) A crust was formed after 24 hours and then LLLT was performed (d). (e) Lesion after 72 hours. (f) After 1 week, signs and symptoms related to RHL were no longer present.

Table 35.2 shows the lasers and irradiation protocols used for each clinical case. In all cases, LLLT was conducted at 24, 48, 72 hours, and 7 days after PDT or HPL irradiation for the drainage of the vesicles. The technique of LLLT was punctual, in contact mode. Two different LPLs were used: (1) Twin Flex II® (MMOptics, São Carlos, Brazil), with a spot size of $0.038\,cm^2$; and (2) Photon Lase III® (DMC, Sao Carlos, Brazil), with a spot size of $0.028\,cm^2$. Both lasers were AsGaAl diode lasers, operating in continuous mode.

For the PDT treatment, it was necessary that patients had lesions in the vesicular stage, in order to be able to perforate them. The vesicles had to be carefully perforated with a sterilized needle so that the fluid could flow out. A small cotton ball was soaked in a 0.01% (m/V) MB solution and placed over the lesions for 5 minutes, and then the excess dye was removed. The lesions were irradiated with a 660-nm LPL, using protocol A or B, according to the equipment chosen.

Clinical case 35.8 LLLT

This case illustrates the influence of LLLT on the healing process of RHL. A 26-year-old woman had vesicles on the upper lip a week before this treatment. She reported that the crust fell off when showering. The treatment with LLLT was proposed with the aim of a faster healing process. Irradiation was performed at only one point (protocol B) (Fig. 35.10a). Shrinkage of the lesion could be seen 1 and 2 hours post treatment (Fig. 35.10b,c). Complete healing was achieved after 1 week (Fig. 35.10d).

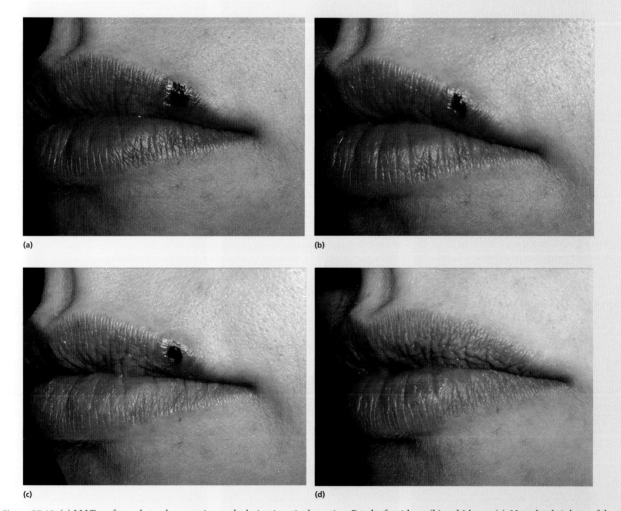

(a) (b) (c) (d)

Figure 35.10 (a) LLLT performed at only one point on the lesion in a single session. Result after 1 hour (b) and 2 hours (c). Note the shrinkage of the lesion. (d) Complete healing after 1 week.

A 35-year-old man presented with herpes zoster (previously diagnosed by a dermatologist) vesicles on the left side of the face, including the eye and head (Fig. 35.11a,b). Pain was reported in the affected area. A multidisciplinary team composed of a dentist, dermatologist, and ophthalmologist supervised this patient.

The treatment of the patient involved conventional therapy with topical acyclovir (only in the affected eye) combined with PDT, performed according to protocol B. Prior to vesicle drainage, the region was isolated to avoid spread of infection to adjacent areas (Fig. 35.11c). PDT was not performed in the eyelid because of the risk of the laser light causing blindness. The patient reported pain relief immediately after PDT treatment (Fig. 35.11d,e). After 24 hours, a significant improvement was observed, but as some vesicles were still present (LLLT in the vesicle phase may worsen the case, according to our clinical experience; Fig. 35.11f), PDT was repeated (Fig. 35.11g). On the following day, after the second session of PDT, the crusts had already formed, with absence of vesicles, so the LLLT (protocol B) could then be performed (Fig. 35.11h). The patient returned after 48 hours for follow-up and LLLT (Fig. 35.11i). After 1 week of the second session of PDT, a satisfactory result was achieved and a last session of LLLT was performed (Fig. 35.11j–l). Topical treatment with acyclovir in the eye under the supervision of an ophthalmologist was also successful. The patient reported no recurrence at a 5-year follow-up.

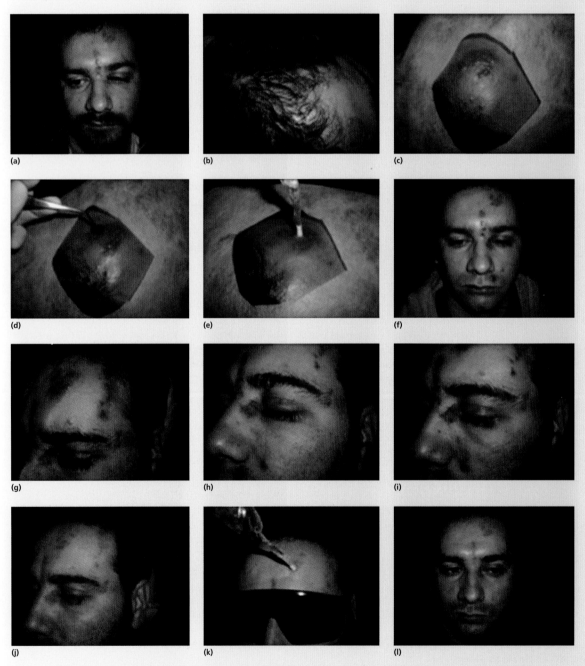

Figure 35.11 (a,b) Herpes zoster affecting the left side of the face, including the eye and head. (c) Before vesicle rupture, the region was isolated. (d) After vesicles drainage, methylene blue dye was applied, and after 5 minutes PDT was performed (e). (f) Vesicles still present. (g) PDT was repeated. (h) Crusts were formed and no vesicles were observed 24 hours after the second PDT session (i), and then LLLT was performed. (j) Fast resolution of the case, with a satisfactory result after 1 week. (k) Last session of LLLT. (l) Clinical appearance 8 days after the first treatment.

References

1 Birek C, Ficarra G. The diagnosis and management of oral herpes simplex infection. *Curr Infect Dis Rep* 2006; 8: 181–188.

2 Buxbaum S, Geers M, Gross G, et al. Epidemiology of herpes simplex virus types 1 and 2 in Germany: what has changed? *Med Microbiol Immunol* 2003; 192: 177–181.

3 De Paula Eduardo C, Aranha AC, Simoes A, et al. Laser treatment of recurrent herpes labialis: a literature review. *Lasers Med Sci* 2014; 29(4): 1517–1529.

4 Chung E, Sen J. The ongoing pursuit of a prophylactic HSV vaccine. *Rev Med Virol* 2012; 22(5): 285–300.

5 Reinheimer C, Doerr HW. Prevalence of herpes simplex virus type 2 in different risk groups: Thirty years after the onset of HIV. *Intervirology* 2012; 55(6): 395–400.

6 Cohen SG, Greenberg MS. Chronic oral herpes simplex virus infection in immunocompromised patients. *Oral Surg Oral Med Oral Pathol* 1985; 59: 465–471.

7 Leigh IM. Management of non-genital herpes simplex virus infections in immunocompetent patients. *Am J Med* 1988; 85: 34–38.

8 Rupp R, Bernstein DI. The potential impact of a prophylactic herpes simplex vaccine. *Expert Opin Emerg Drugs* 2008; 13: 41–52.

9 Woo SB, Challacombe SJ. Management of recurrent oral herpes simplex infections. *Oral Surg Oral Med Oral Pathol Oral Radiol Endod* 2007; 103 (Suppl S12): e11–18.

10 Whitley RJ, Roizman B. Herpes simplex virus infections. *Lancet* 2001; 357: 1513–1518.

11 Schindl A, Neumann R. Low-intensity laser therapy is an effective treatment for recurrent herpes simplex infection. Results from a randomized double-blind placebo-controlled study. *J Invest Dermatol* 1999; 113: 221–223.

12 Arduino PG, Porter SR. Oral and perioral herpes simplex virus type 1 (HSV-1) infection: review of its management. *Oral Dis* 2006; 12: 254–270.

13 Cernik C, Gallina K, Brodell RT. The treatment of herpes simplex infections: an evidence-based review. *Arch Intern Med* 2008; 168: 1137–1144.

14 Lipschütz B. Untersuchungen über die Ätiologie der Krankheiten der Herpesgruppe (Herpes zoster, Herpes genitalis, Herpes febrilis). *Arch Dermatol Syph* 1921; 136: 428–482.

15 Sciubba JJ. Oral mucosal diseases in the office setting--part I: Aphthous stomatitis and herpes simplex infections. *Gen Dent* 2007; 55: 347–354; quiz 355–346, 376.

16 Reusser P. Herpesvirus resistance to antiviral drugs: a review of the mechanisms, clinical importance and therapeutic options. *J Hosp Infect* 1996; 33: 235–248.

17 Piret J, Boivin G. Resistance of herpes simplex viruses to nucleoside analogues: mechanisms, prevalence, and management. *Antimicrob Agents Chemother* 2011; 55: 459–472.

18 Spruance SL, Kriesel JD. Treatment of herpes simplex labialis. *Herpes* 2002; 9: 64–69.

19 Arduino PG, Porter SR. Herpes simplex virus type 1 infection: overview on relevant clinico-pathological features. *J Oral Pathol Med* 2008; 37: 107–121.

20 Whitley RJ, Kimberlin DW, Roizman B. Herpes simplex viruses. *Clin Infect Dis* 1998; 26: 541–553; quiz 554–555.

21 Raborn GW, Grace MG. Recurrent herpes simplex labialis: selected therapeutic options. *J Can Dent Assoc* 2003; 69: 498–503.

22 Morfin F, Thouvenot D. Herpes simplex virus resistance to antiviral drugs. *J Clin Virol* 2003; 26: 29–37.

23 Stanberry LR, Spruance SL, Cunningham AL, et al. Glycoprotein-D-adjuvant vaccine to prevent genital herpes. *N Engl J Med* 2002; 347: 1652–1661.

24 Belshe RB, Leone PA, Bernstein DI, et al. Efficacy results of a trial of a herpes simplex vaccine. *N Engl J Med* 2012; 366: 34–43.

25 Luo C, Goshima F, Kamakura M, et al. Immunization with a highly attenuated replication-competent herpes simplex virus type 1 mutant, HF10, protects mice from genital disease caused by herpes simplex virus type 2. *Front Microbiol* 2012; 3: 158.

26 Kalantari-Dehaghi M, Chun S, Chentoufi AA, et al. Discovery of potential diagnostic and vaccine antigens in herpes simplex virus 1 and 2 by proteome-wide antibody profiling. *J Virol* 2012; 86: 4328–4339.

27 Bello-Silva MS, de Freitas PM, Aranha ACC, et al. Low- and high-intensity lasers in the treatment of herpes simplex virus 1 infection. *Photomed Laser Surg* 2010; 28: 135–139.

28 Marotti J, Sperandio FF, Fregnani ER, et al. High-intensity laser and photodynamic therapy as a treatment for recurrent herpes labialis. *Photomed Laser Surg* 2010; 28: 439–444.

29 Marotti J, Bello-Silva MS, Freitas PM, et al. In: Byrne EK, ed. *Erbium Lasers in the Treatment of Herpes Labialis.* New York: Nova Science, 2010.

30 Bello-Silva MS, Lage-Marques JL, Marotti J, et al. Calcitonin, sodium alendronate and high intensity laser in the treatment of traumatized teeth: a preliminary study. *Lasers Med Sci* 2010; 25: 331–337.

31 Marotti J, Geraldo-Martins VR, Bello-Silva MS, et al. Influence of etching with erbium, chromium:yttrium-scandium-gallium-garnet laser on microleakage of class V restoration. *Lasers Med Sci* 2010; 25: 325–329.

32 Marotti J, Bello-Silva MS, Eduardo CP. Laser em alta e baixa intensidade no tratamento do herpes labial. In: Callegari A, Macedo MCS, Bombana AC, ed. *Atualização clínica em odontologia.* Sao Paulo: Artes Médicas, 2008.

33 Marotti J, Aranha AC, Eduardo Cde P, et al. Photodynamic therapy can be effective as a treatment for herpes simplex labialis. *Photomed Laser Surg* 2009; 27: 357–363.

34 Fisher AM, Murphree AL, Gomer CJ. Clinical and preclinical photodynamic therapy. *Lasers Surg Med* 1995; 17: 2–31.

35 Betz CS, Jager HR, Brookes JA, et al. Interstitial photodynamic therapy for a symptom-targeted treatment of complex vascular malformations in the head and neck region. *Lasers Surg Med* 2007; 39: 571–582.

36 Muller-Breitkreutz K, Mohr H, Briviba K, et al. Inactivation of viruses by chemically and photochemically generated singlet molecular oxygen. *J Photochem Photobiol B* 1995; 30: 63–70.

37 Jones S, Kress D. Treatment of molluscum contagiosum and herpes simplex virus cutaneous infections. *Cutis* 2007; 79: 11–17.

38 Wainwright M. Photoinactivation of viruses. *Photochem Photobiol Sci* 2004; 3: 406–411.

39 Wagner SJ. Virus inactivation in blood components by photoactive phenothiazine dyes. *Transfus Med Rev* 2002; 16: 61–66.

40 Schagen FH, Moor AC, Cheong SC, et al. Photodynamic treatment of adenoviral vectors with visible light: an easy and convenient method for viral inactivation. *Gene Ther* 1999; 6: 873–881.

41 Junior AB. Laser phototherapy in dentistry. *Photomed Laser Surg* 2009; 27: 533–534.

42 Karu T. Photobiology of low-power laser effects. *Health Phys* 1989; 56: 691–704.

43 Karu T. Laser biostimulation: a photobiological phenomenon. *J Photochem Photobiol B* 1989; 3: 638–640.

44 Chow RT, Johnson MI, Lopes-Martins RA, et al. Efficacy of low-level laser therapy in the management of neck pain: a systematic review and meta-analysis of randomised placebo or active-treatment controlled trials. *Lancet* 2009; 374: 1897–1908.

45 Basford JR. Low intensity laser therapy: still not an established clinical tool. *Lasers Surg Med* 1995; 16: 331–342.

46 Schindl L, Schindl M, Polo L, et al. Effects of low power laser-irradiation on differential blood count and body temperature in endotoxin-preimmunized rabbits. *Life Sci* 1997; 60: 1669–1677.

47 Marotti J, Aranha ACC, Eduardo CP, et al. Tratamento do herpes labial pela terapia fotodinâmica. *Rev Assoc Paul Cir Dent* 2008; 62: 309–313.

48 Sperandio FF, Marotti J, Aranha AC, et al. Photodynamic therapy for the treatment of recurrent herpes labialis: Preliminary results. *Gen Dent* 2009; 57: 415–419.

49 Eduardo Cde P, Bezinelli LM, Eduardo Fde P, et al. Prevention of recurrent herpes labialis outbreaks through low-intensity laser therapy: a clinical protocol with 3-year follow-up. *Lasers Med Sci* 2012; 27: 1077–1083.

50 Munoz Sanchez PJ, Capote Femenias JL, Diaz Tejeda A, et al. The effect of 670-nm low laser therapy on herpes simplex type 1. *Photomed Laser Surg* 2012; 30: 37–40.

51 de Carvalho RR, de Paula Eduardo F, Ramalho KM, et al. Effect of laser phototherapy on recurring herpes labialis prevention: an *in vivo* study. *Lasers Med Sci* 2010; 25: 397–402.

52 Eduardo FP, Mehnert DU, Monezi TA, et al. Cultured epithelial cells response to phototherapy with low intensity laser. *Lasers Surg Med* 2007; 39: 365–372.

53 Marotti J, Aranha AC, Eduardo Cde P. A utilização do laser no tratamento do herpes labial. *RPG* 2007; 14: 314–320.

54 Andrei G, Snoeck R. Emerging drugs for varicella-zoster virus infections. *Expert Opin Emerg Drugs* 2011; 16: 507–535.

55 Dworkin RH, Johnson RW, Breuer J, et al. Recommendations for the management of herpes zoster. *Clin Infect Dis* 2007; 44 (Suppl 1): S1–26.

56 Pavan-Langston D. Herpes zoster ophthalmicus. *Neurology* 1995; 45: S50–51.

57 Huber MA. Herpes simplex type-1 virus infection. *Quintessence Int* 2003; 34: 453–467.

58 Fatahzadeh M, Schwartz RA. Human herpes simplex labialis. *Clin Exp Dermatol* 2007; 32: 625–630.

59 Spruance SL, Nett R, Marbury T, et al. Acyclovir cream for treatment of herpes simplex labialis: results of two randomized, double-blind, vehicle-controlled, multicenter clinical trials. *Antimicrob Agents Chemother* 2002; 46: 2238–2243.

CHAPTER 36

Recurrent aphthous ulcers

Leila Soares Ferreira[1] and Daiane Thais Meneguzzo[2]

[1] Biodentistry Master Program, School of Dentistry, Ibirapuera University (UNIB), São Paulo, SP, Brazil
[2] São Leopoldo Mandic Dental Research Center, Campinas, SP, Brazil

Introduction

The recurrent aphthous ulcer (RAU) is the most common ulcerative lesion found in the oral cavity. It is characterized by the appearance of single or multiple ulcerative lesions in the oral mucosa; typically painful, recurrent, small, round or ovoid with circumscribed margins and erythematous haloes.[1] It is usually first observed in adolescence, but it is in adulthood that patients face periods of increased pain and discomfort. Manifestations of RAU impair feeding, swallowing, and speaking, reducing a patient's self-image and quality of life.[2] RAU occurs worldwide and affects 2–66% of the international population. The cause of RAU is unknown, but are thought to be multifactorial with many triggers or precipitating factors.[3] Among patient factors are genetic predisposition, local trauma, medications, allergy, hormonal changes, stress, and immunological abnormalities.[4]

RAU lesions follow a sequence of stages that can be described as: (1) prodromal – presence of symptoms but without any visible clinical signs; (2) preulcerative – initial presentation usually with erythema and slight edema; (3) ulcerative – formation of the epithelial defect; (4) healing – symptom abatement and progressive healing; and (5) remission – no evidence of lesions.[5] Also, RAU has three clinical presentations: minor aphthous ulcers (Fig. 36.1a), major aphthous ulcers (Fig. 36.1b), and herpetiform ulcers (Fig. 36.1c).

Minor RAU is the most common variety and involves every non-keratinized mucosa of the oral cavity. It appears as discrete and painful lesions, covered by a yellow–grey pseudomembrane surrounded by an erythematous halo (Fig. 36.1a). The ulcers are usually smaller than 8–10 mm in diameter and tend to heal within 10–14 days without scarring, but healing is slower than for other oral wounds, possibly because of intense lymphocytic infiltratration.[6,7]

Major RAU is a rare and severe form of RAU. It often produces coalescent ulcers and tends to involve mucosa overlying the minor salivary glands. The lesions are oval, painful, with raised clear defined margins, usually larger than 1 cm in diameter, and tend to involve the mucosa of the lips, soft palate, and throat (Fig. 36.1b). The prodromal symptoms are more intense, and the ulcers usually deeper, larger, and longer lasting than those seen in minor RAU. Fever, dysphagia, and malaise sometimes occur early in the disease process.[6]

Herpetiform aphthous ulcer is the least common variety of RAU. It is characterized by painful ulcers, 1–3 mm in diameter and occurring in crops of 5–100 ulcers at any given time anywhere on the mucosa (Fig. 36.1c). They tend to fuse and produce larger ulcers that last 10–14 days.[7]

The treatment is palliative, since most existing therapies only reduce the symptoms and sometimes the duration of the lesion. Local corticosteroids, antiseptic and antibacterial drugs are used singly or in various combinations.[7] Systemic medication is also used in severe cases or those resistant to topical therapies such as steroids and immunosuppressive systemic agents. However, none of the conventional treatments has been shown to be effective in preventing or even decreasing the incidence of lesions. Low level laser therapy (LLLT), on the other hand, has shown excellent results in the treatment and prevention of RAU.[8]

Low level laser therapy

LLLT is known to modulate the inflammatory process, promote analgesia, and accelerate wound healing (see Chapters 5 and 6),[9–11] and these effects can be expected in the treatment of aphthous ulcers. Zand et al. performed a randomized controlled clinical trial to evaluate the efficacy of a single session of non-ablative CO_2 laser irradiation in reducing pain in minor RAU.[12] The results showed that a low power, non-thermal, single-session of CO_2 laser irradiation reduced pain in RAU immediately and dramatically, with no visible side effects. Another clinical evaluation comparing LLLT and a topical corticosteroid agent demonstrated that 75% of the patients treated with LLLT reported a reduction in pain after LLLT and total regression of the lesion after 4 days, while lesion regression took 5–7 days in the corticosteroid group.[8] Also, LLLT was described to be an

Lasers in Dentistry: Guide for Clinical Practice, First Edition. Edited by Patrícia M. de Freitas and Alyne Simões.
© 2015 John Wiley & Sons, Inc. Published 2015 by John Wiley & Sons, Inc.

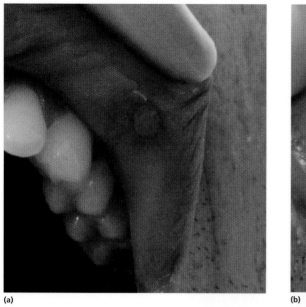

(a)

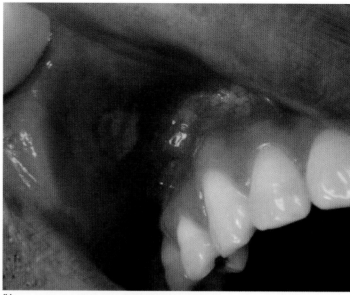

(b)

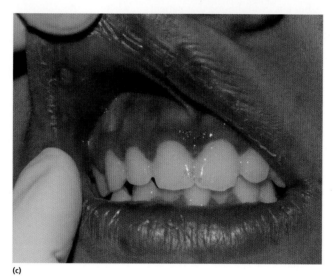

(c)

Figure 36.1 Clinical presentation of recurrent aphthous ulcers (RAU): (a) Minor RAU, (b) major RAU, (c) herpetiform aphthous ulcer.

alternative treatment for primary herpes simplex infection in children, with an immediate positive outcome in severe painful gengivostomatitis lesions.[13]

The immediate analgesic response of phototherapy can be explained by blockage of the neuronal action potential.[10] In addition, the anti-inflammatory response to laser irradiation contributes to the long-term analgesic effects, such as acceleration of the microcirculation, increased natural opioid peptides[14,15]; decreased release of histamine, interleukin-1β (IL-1β), tumor necrosis factor α (TNF-α), and interferon-γ (IFN-γ)[16]; blockage of acetylcholine[15]; and reduction of the synthesis of bradykinin[14,15] and prostaglandin E$_2$.[9] Since the acute inflammatory phase of the lesion is controlled, the tissue is ready to start healing.

The effectiveness of LLLT in the prevention of RAU lesions has not been established yet. However, RAU can be prevented by

treatments that promote the inhibition of endogenous TNF-α, such as thalidomide and pentoxifylline,[17] and the same effect can be achieved by laser irradiation, with no side effects. Therefore, LLLT can be considered a promising approach to the prevention of RAU manifestations.

Laser protocol

The primary goals of therapy of RAU are relief of pain, reduction of ulcer duration, and restoration of normal oral function. The secondary goals include reduction in frequency and severity of recurrences and maintenance of remission.[18,19] Therefore, there are three types of LLLT protocols for RAU management.

Pain relief

As the lesion starts to heal, there are a few days (3–5 days) when the main symptom is severe pain. At this time the patient seeks pain relief. LLLT is the only therapy capable of promoting immediate analgesia with no side effects, being a great clinical differential for dentists and improving patient's perception. Also, when LLLT is performed at this time, the duration of the RAU cycle will also be reduced. The LLLT protocol is daily infrared laser irradiation (2.0–3.0 J per point) until remission of symptoms (Fig. 36.2).

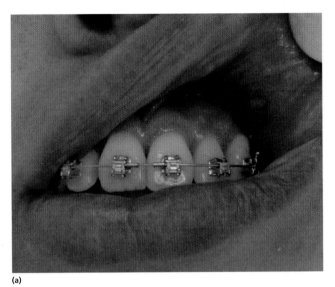
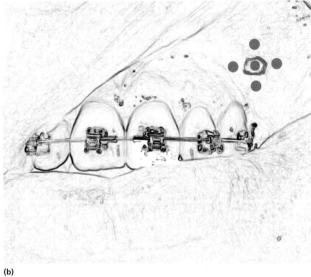

(a)   (b)

Figure 36.2 LLLT treatment of a patient presenting with RAU with traumatic factor: (a) Initial lesion (b) schematic of LLLT irradiation points.

Clinical cases 36.1 Pain in the premolar area

A 22-year-old male patient presented to the Sao Leopoldo Mandic University Laser Center complaining of monthly recurrence of RAU with severe pain in the upper right premolar area (Fig. 36.3a). For pain control treatment, LLLT was applied using the following protocol: red laser irradiation (660 nm) in continuous mode, 100 mW of power, 3 J of energy per point at four points. The patient reported immediate pain relief of about 60%. A second irradiation with the same parameters was applied and 100% pain control was achieved in this session. After 24 hours, the patient returned reporting mild pain and the same LLLT protocol was repeated (Fig. 36.3b). On the following day, the patient reported no more pain and an LLLT protocol was proposed to accelerate healing: red laser, 1 J per point at four points. Complete remission occurred after 7 days (Fig. 36.3c).

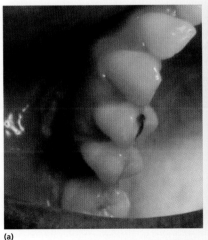
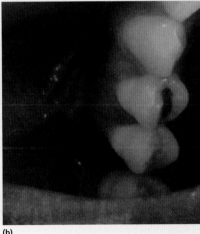
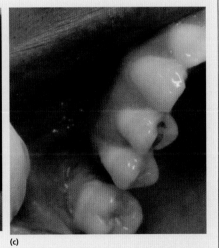

(a)   (b)   (c)

Figure 36.3 Patient with a major RAU in the area of the upper right premolars: (a) Initial lesion (b) appearance of the lesion after 3 days of LLLT (c) complete healing 7 days after the first LLLT session.

Acceleration of wound healing

After pain remission, LLLT can also be performed to accelerate ulcer healing. The LLLT protocol is daily red laser irradiation (0.5–1.0 J per point) until complete lesion healing.

RAU prevention

LLLT can be also used when the patient has no RAU manifestations. LLLT stimulates the immune system and increases the resistance of the mucosa to ulcer formation. The LLLT protocol is weekly infrared or red laser irradiation (2.0–3.0 J per point) for 10 weeks in all regions of high incidence of RAU manifestations (the patient should be asked to indicate the more critical areas).

The following are useful tips for LLLT:

- An anti-inflammatory and analgesic effect dose should be used on and around the lesion;
- The number of points of irradiation can be increased until the patient reports pain relief of at least 90% (the patient should be asked to rate their perception of pain from 0% to 100% before and after irradiation);

Clinical case 36.2 Pain in the lip

LLLT was used to treat a 14-year-old female patient who wore braces and complained of severe pain in the upper right lip (Fig. 36.4a). LLLT was applied using the following protocol: red laser emission (660 nm) in continuous mode, 100 mW of power, 3 J of energy per point in four points (Fig. 36.4b,c). Immediately after laser irradiation, the patient reported pain relief of about 80%. The use of a protective wax on the brackets was recommended to avoid trauma. After 4 days, the lesion had healed completely (Fig. 36.4d).

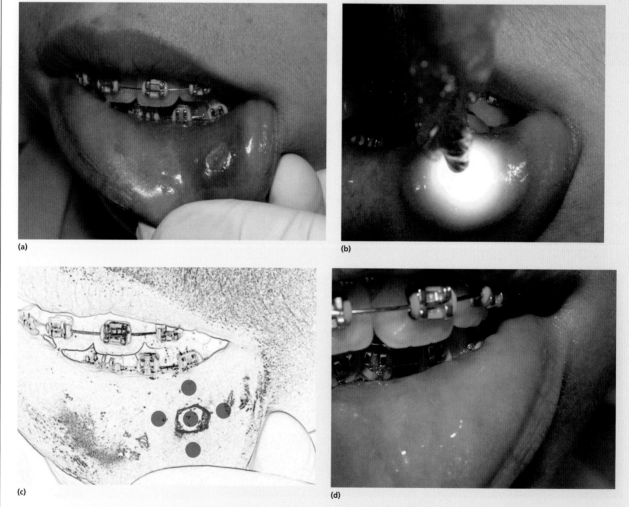

(a)　(b)　(c)　(d)

Figure 36.4 LLLT of an RAU lesion: (a) Initial appearance of the aphthous lesion (b) red laser irradiation at the center of the ulcer, showing light scattering around the lesion (observe that the laser handpiece is not in contact with the tissue) (c) schematic of the LLLT irradiation points: one point in the center and four points around the ulcer (d) remission of the lesion after 4 days.

- As radiation scatters around the lesion, while performing the analgesic protocol this lower scattered energy will also improve the healing process (see Fig. 36.4b);
- Whenever possible, laser irradiation must be perpendicular to avoid loss of energy.

References

1 Jurge S, Kuffer R, Scully C, Porter SR. Mucosal disease series. *Number VI. Recurrent aphthous stomatitis. Oral Dis* 2006; 12(1): 1–21.

2 Mumcu G, Hayran O, Ozalp DO, et al. The assessment of oral health-related quality of life by factor analysis in patients with Behcet's disease and recurrent aphthous stomatitis. *J Oral Pathol Med* 2007; 36(3): 147–152.

3 Wardhana, Datau EA. Recurrent aphthous stomatitis caused by food allergy. *Acta Med Indones* 2010; 42(4): 236–240.

4 Zunt SL. Recurrent aphthous stomatitis. *Dermatol Clin* 2003; 21: 33–39.

5 Boras VV, Savage NW. Recurrent aphthous ulcerative disease: presentation and management. *Aust Dent J* 2007: 52(1): 10–15.

6 Zunt SL. Recurrent aphthous ulcers. *J Pract Hygiene* 2001; 5: 259–264.

7 Scully C. Aphthous ulceration. *N Engl J Med* 2006; 355: 165–172.

8 De Souza TO, Martins MA, Bussadori SK, et al. Clinical evaluation of low-level laser treatment for recurring aphthous stomatitis. *Photomed Laser Surg* 2010; 28 (Suppl 2): S85–88.

9 Bjordal JM, Johnson MI, Iversen V, et al. Low-level laser therapy in acute pain: a systematic review of possible mechanisms of action and clinical effects in randomized placebo-controlled trials. *Photomed Laser Surg* 2006; 24(2): 158–168.

10 Chow RT, Heller GZ, Barnsley L. The effect of 300mW, 830 nm laser on chronic neck pain: a double-blind, randomized, placebo-controlled study. *Pain* 2006; 124: 201–210.

11 Demidova-Rice TN, Salomatina EV, Yaroslavsky AN, et al. Low-level light stimulates excisional wound healing in mice. *Lasers Surg Med* 2007; 39(9): 706–715.

12 Zand N, Ataie-Fashtami L, Djavid GE, et al. Relieving pain in minor aphthous stomatitis by a single session of non-thermal carbon dioxide laser irradiation. *Lasers Med Sci* 2009; 24(4): 515–520.

13 Navarro R, Marquezan M, Cerqueira DF, et al. Low-level-laser therapy as an alternative treatment for primary herpes simplex infection: a case report. *J Clin Pediatr Dent* 2007; 31(4): 225–228.

14 Ohshiro T. An overview of pain. In: Oshiro T, ed. *Low Reactive-Level Laser Therapy: Practical Application*. Chichester: Wiley, 1991: 13–21.

15 Simunovic Z. Pain and practical aspects of its management. In: Simunovic Z (eds). *Lasers in medicine and dentistry*. Zagreb: AKD, 2000: 269–301.

16 Safavi SM, Kazemi B, Esmaeili M, et al. Effects of low-level He-Ne laser irradiation on the gene expression of IL-1beta, TNF-alpha, IFN-gamma, TGF-beta, bFGF, and PDGF in rat's gingiva. *Lasers Med Sci* 2008; 23(3): 331–335.

17 Natah SS, Häyrinen-Immonen R, Hietanen J, et al. Immuno-localization of tumor necrosis factor-alpha expressing cells in recurrent aphthous ulcer lesions (RAU). *J Oral Pathol Med* 2000; 29(1): 19–25.

18 Preeti L, Magesh K, Rajkumar K, et al. Recurrent aphthous stomatitis. *J Oral Maxillofac Pathol* 2011; 15(3): 252–256.

19 James J, Burks W. Food allergies. In: Grammer LC, Greenberger PA, eds. *Pattersons's Allergic Diseases*. 7th edn. Philadelphia: Lippincott Williams & Wilkins, 2009: 315–332.

CHAPTER 37

Burning mouth syndrome

Lucia de Fátima Cavalcanti dos Santos[1] and Jair Carneiro Leão[2]

[1]Real Center of Systemic Dentistry, Real Hospital Português de Pernambuco, Recife, PE, Brazil
[2]Department of Clinic and Preventive Dentistry, Pernambuco Federal University, Recife, PE, Brazil

Introduction

Burning mouth syndrome (BMS) is a distinct clinical condition that causes oral pain and burning in morphologically normal oral mucosa, with patients often complaining of a scalding sensation in the affected areas.[1] Although it may occur in patients of either gender and at any age, BMS most frequently affects middle-aged women in the post-menopausal period.[1,2] However, there is no scientific evidence of a causal relationship between hormonal deficiency and BMS. Usually the distribution of oral burning is bilateral, although it does not follow anatomical structures. The most commonly affected site is the tongue, especially in the anterior region, followed by the lips, hard palate, oral mucosa, and oropharynx.[2,3]

The etiology of BMS is unknown, but some hypotheses have proposed psychogenic, systemic and hormonal factors, local irritants, drugs, and xerostomia.[1] Because of its chronic nature and unknown etiology, BMS is usually treated symptomatically with a combination of several drugs.[4] Recently, low level laser therapy (LLLT) has been described as a possible helpful option, with good results obtained in terms of pain control.[5]

The medical history and clinical examination of each patient should be requested and carefully assessed to exclude burning sensations associated with systemic diseases, such as diabetes mellitus, hematological and thyroid diseases. Serum levels of vitamin B_{12}, iron, glucose, and thyroid hormones should be normal.[1,6] An adequate intra-oral examination should show normal oral mucosa in all patients with a complete absence of injuries that can cause BMS-like symptoms, such as infections, hyposalivation, lichen planus, benign migratory glossitis, allergic reactions, parafunctional habits, and poorly fitting dental prosthetics. Upon confirmation of the above, individuals can then be diagnosed with BMS.[1,2,7]

Treatment

Despite not being classified as a serious or life-threatening disease, BMS is a disorder that forces many of those affected to search for a definitive, unique, and efficient treatment, which unfortunately is still not available.[8] The professional must express interest in elucidating possible causes of the patient's symptoms and offer possible solutions, in an attempt to gain the patient's cooperation. Therapy includes the use of antifungal medication to treat candidiasis, antidepressants in cases of anxiety or depression, and vitamin replacement in cases of nutritional deficiency. Vitamin B replacement is commonly reported to improve symptoms.[1,8]

There is not much scientific evidence for an effective treatment of BMS and a multidisciplinary approach is usually required. A 70% decrease in burning symptoms with clonazepam has been reported.[8] The drug may be administered orally at a dose of 0.25 mg/day (maximum dose of 3 mg/day). A number of psychological disorders can be treated with the potent antioxidant alpha-lipoic acid. Individuals who have not previously used tranquilizers have exhibited an improvement in BMS after receiving this medication.[1]

Capsaicin has also been used as a therapy for BMS since it removes the P substance from nerve endings. It is believed that this substance is associated with the start of the transmission of painful stimuli in different pathologies such as diabetic neuropathy, arthrosis, psoriasis, and BMS.[9]

In BMS, burning and dry mouth are common complaints and, although the therapeutic resources available are not always satisfactory, it is necessary to follow the protocol and to use artificial saliva to protect the mucosa. The patient should be told that the artificial saliva is prepared for frequent use, and although it does not meet the physiological requirements, it can contribute to reducing the symptoms of excessive mucosal dryness.[10]

Thus, despite advances, it is not yet possible to state that BMS control has been defined, although the therapeutic possibilities have provided encouraging results and benefits. However, many BMS patients do not exhibit significant improvements in their symptoms, increasing the need for intensive research into alternatives for adjuvant treatment of this syndrome, such as LLLT.[11–13]

Low level laser therapy

Irradiation protocol

BMS patients should be submitted to a weekly session of LLLT for 10 weeks, totaling ten sessions. The laser irradiation used has a continuous wave length of 660 nm, power of 40 mW, energy of 20 J/cm^2, with 0.4 J per point. Each point of irradiation must be precise, with approximately 1 cm between each point, and an irradiation duration of 10 seconds for each (Fig. 37.1). Before irradiation, the affected area must be cleaned and dried with the aid of gauze. For each affected anatomical area, depending on its size, three to six irradiation points should be used. The burning intensity should be relieved in all sessions according to the visual analog scale (VAS), in which 0 indicates no symptoms and 10 indicates the maximum possible symptoms. The assessment of this intensity should be performed immediately before and immediately after laser irradiation in each LLLT session. A comparison between these two assessments enables assessment of improvement in the BMS patient's symptoms. Results have been encouraging.[5]

Advantages

Laser therapy has been considered one of the greatest technological advances in the field of dentistry. Due to its differential properties, such as monochromaticity, coherence, and directivity, the laser can deposit a large quantity of energy in biological tissues with extreme precision. Many studies have demonstrated that LLLT promotes a cellular biomodulation in healing injuries (proliferation of fibroblasts, collagen synthesis, and the regeneration of bone and nerve tissues), with significant clinical and histological modifications during the inflammatory process, as well as the healing irradiated biological tissues.[11]

Laser irradiation promotes immediate relief in areas affected by burning through the formation of a greater quantity of β-endorphin by the glial cells and a decrease in the production of prostaglandins.[11,13] The action of the laser beam on the cyclooxygenases regulates the transformation of arachidonic acid, as well as providing a biostimulatory effect by increasing mitochondrial ATP and thus optimizing the speed of regeneration in the affected area.

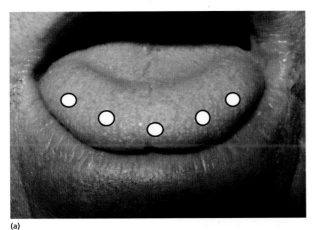

(a)

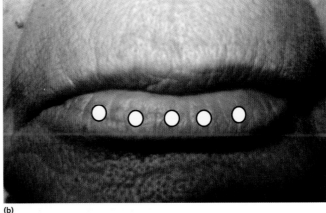

(b)

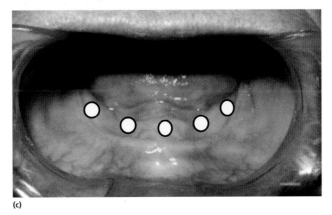

(c)

Figure 37.1 Points of irradiation: (a) On the tip of the tongue (b) on the lower lip (c) on the lower alveolar ridge region.

According to data published to date in the literature, LLLT does not exhibit deleterious effects when used with scientifically proven clinical protocols for specific clinical applications.

Conclusion

From reports in the scientific literature, it is possible to conclude that LLLT is an alternative treatment for BMS, which promises to establish a scientific basis for future treatment of this condition.

References

1 Patton LL, Siegel MA, Benoliel R, De Laat A. Management of burning mouth syndrome: Systematic review and management recommendations. *Oral Surg Oral Med Oral Pathol Oral Radiol Endod* 2007; 103 (Suppl 39): e1–13.

2 Cavalcanti D. *Síndrome de ardência bucal: perfil clínico de pacientese prevalênciade leveduras gênero Cândida (tese de mestrado)*. São Paulo: Faculdade de Odontologia da USP, 2003.

3 Chen Q, Xia J, Lin M, Zhou H, Li B. Serum interleukin-6 in patients with burning mouth syndrome and relationship with depression and perceived pain. *Mediators Inflamm* 2007; 2007: 45327.

4 Gremeau-Richard C, Woda A, Navez NL, et al.. Topical clonazepam in stomatodynia: a randomized placebo-controlled study. *Pain* 2004; 108: 51–57.

5 Santos LFC, Carvalho AAT, Leão JC, Perez DEC, Castro JFL. Effect of low level laser therapy in the treatment of the Burning Mouth Syndrome: a case series. *Photomed Laser Surg* 2011; 29(12): 793–796.

6 Fedele S, Fricchione G, Porter SR, Mignogna MD. Burning mouth syndrome (stomatodynia). *QJM* 2007; 100: 527–530.

7 Hakeberg M, Hallberg LR-M, Berggren U. Burning mouth syndrome: experiences from the perspective of female patients. *Eur J Oral Sci* 2003; 111: 305–311.

8 Grushka M, Epstein J, Mott A. An open-label, dose escalation pilot study of the effect of clonazepam in burning mouth syndrome. *Oral Surg Oral Med Oral Pathol Oral Radiol Endod* 1998; 86: 557–561.

9 Lauritano D, Petruzzi M, Baldoni M. Preliminary protocol for systemic administration of capsaicin for the treatment of the burning mouth syndrome. *Minerva Stomatol* 2003; 52(6): 273–278.

10 López-Jornet P, Camacho-Alonso F, Leon-Espinosa S. Burning mouth syndrome, oral parafunctions, and psychological profile in a longitudinal case study. *J Eur Acad Dermatol Venerol* 2009; 23: 363–365.

11 Yang H-W, Huang Y-F. Treatment of burning mouth syndrome with a low-level energy diode laser. *Photomed Laser Surg* 2011; 29(2): 123–125.

12 Kato IT, Pellegrini VD, Prates RA, Ribeiro MS, Wetter NU, Sugaya NN. Low-level laser therapy in burning mouth syndrome patients: a pilot study. *Photomed Laser Surg* 2010; 28: 835–839.

13 Nakase M, Okumura K, Tamura T, et al. Effects of near-infrared irradiation to stellate ganglion in glossodynia. *Oral Dis* 2004; 10: 217–220.

CHAPTER 38

Nerve repair by light

Felipe F. Sperandio[1,2,3], Ying-Ying Huang,[2–4] Nivaldo Parizotto,[2,3,5] and Michael R. Hamblin[2,3,6]

[1] Department of Pathology and Parasitology, Institute of Biomedical Sciences, Federal University of Alfenas, Alfenas, MG, Brazil
[2] Department of Dermatology, Harvard Medical School, Boston, MA, USA
[3] Wellman Center for Photomedicine, Massachusetts General Hospital, Boston, MA, USA
[4] Aesthetic and Plastic Center, Guangxi Medical University, Nanning, China
[5] Department of Physiotherapy, Federal University of São Carlos, São Carlos, SP, Brazil
[6] Harvard–MIT Division of Health Sciences and Technology, Cambridge, MA, USA

Introduction

Repair of post-traumatic nerve lesions is still a challenge for rehabilitation medicine. If the nerve is permanently damaged, it can result in irreversible motor and sensory disabilities. For this reason, it is particularly important to develop clinical protocols to optimize nerve regeneration. Many reports have been published of the use of low level laser therapy (LLLT) or other kinds of light therapy to improve peripheral nerve repair *in vitro*, in different models, and in animals and humans. The main goal of these studies has been to advance the quality and speed of the nerve repair process. Therapy provides early return of muscle movement and reduces muscle degeneration through prolonged inaction, thereby improving the prognosis of patients suffering from peripheral nerve lesions.[1–3]

There have been some particular applications of light therapy for nerve lesions in the oral and maxillofacial regions: Bell's palsy, trigeminal neuralgia, and postsurgical nerve trauma. In this chapter we will briefly cover the signs and symptoms of all the most common and important neural pathologies that may occur in the head and neck region, and particularly in the oral cavity. We will particularly concentrate on treatment directed at improving the injured nerve responses by stimulating them with light.

The mechanisms that operate in low level laser therapy (LLLT), otherwise known as photobiomodulation (PBM), are becoming better understood at a molecular and cellular level (to some extent at least).[4] LLLT works by initial photon (red or near infrared) absorption by the chromophores of the respiratory chain present in mitochondria, such as cytochrome c oxidase. Increased oxygen consumption, electron transport, mitochondrial membrane potential, and ATP production are the short-term consequences. Changes in intracellular reactive oxygen species, nitric oxide production, and cyclic AMP are also observed. In the longer term, transcription factor activation leads to a large number of cellular changes centered on antiapoptosis, pro-proliferation, increased matrix synthesis, angiogenesis, anti-inflammation, and increased tissue repair. A schematic depiction of these pathways is shown in Figure 38.1.

In fact, light is a very versatile tool when used to treat nerve lesions and its use has been increasing in recent times. Both clinical and experimental results continue to encourage the use of lasers and other light sources to stimulate the process of tissue repair, and to increase function of the muscles innervated by the injured nerves.[5] Tests such as the functional sciatic index[6] and the grasping test[7] in animal models have been used to investigate the functional effect of light in nerve repair.

Oral and maxillofacial neural-related pathologies

Only a few papers cover the use of LLLT in nerve repair of oral and maxillofacial peripheral nerve pathologies; however, when the results of these studies are added to clinical experience of the good results in sciatic nerve repair in rats,[6,8] peripheral mammalian nerves,[9,10] as well as neurorehabilitation,[11] it can be concluded that nerve repair following LLLT in the oral cavity and face also is likely to have very good outcomes. Pinheiro et al. confirmed that LLLT is an effective tool and is beneficial for the treatment of many disorders of the maxillofacial region, including trigeminal neuralgia (TN).[12]

Trigeminal neuralgia

TN is one of the most frequent pathologies that occur in the maxilla or mandible areas. It is a disorder characterized by sudden sharp, shooting, lancinating pain attacks lasting several seconds to several minutes, and localized to one or two branches of the trigeminal nerve.[13] The classic episodes of shooting pain are interrupted by pain-free intervals with remissions that occasionally last for years,[14] and the attacks may begin spontaneously or they can be initiated by stimulation of the so-called trigger zones.[13]

Lasers in Dentistry: Guide for Clinical Practice, First Edition. Edited by Patrícia M. de Freitas and Alyne Simões.
© 2015 John Wiley & Sons, Inc. Published 2015 by John Wiley & Sons, Inc.

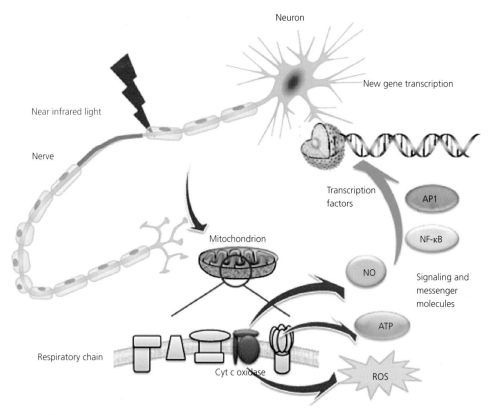

Figure 38.1 Molecular and cellular mechanisms of LLLT. Light is absorbed by cytochrome c oxidase in the mitochondrial respiratory chain of the neurons or their axons. Cell signaling and messenger molecules are up-regulated as a result of stimulated mitochondrial activity, including reactive oxygen species (ROS), nitric oxide (NO), and adenosine triphosphate (ATP). These signaling molecules activate transcription factors including NF-κB and AP-1 that enter the nucleus and cause transcription of a range of new gene products.

Although treatment with LLLT has been utilized as an adjuvant therapy for this disorder,[12] the mechanism of action of the laser light is not well understood. The compression of the nerve by tumors, aneurysms, cysts, and vascular anomalies, as well by normal arteries and veins, is one of the main factors that causes these symptoms. In fact, compression by normal arteries and veins is the most common cause.[13] Vascular compression is found in about 96% of cases of typical TN,[15,16] and only 3% of people without TN display vascular contact with the trigeminal nerve.[17]

There are several treatments proposed for TN. Among the non-invasive methods are drug therapy and gamma knife therapy. If drug therapy is to be prescribed, the gold standard drug is carbamazepine.[13] Besides drugs, percutaneous techniques including glycerol injections, radiofrequency-induced lesions, and balloon compression in or around the Gasserian ganglion are possibilities.[18] The invasive treatment options for TN include percutaneous and surgical interventions, where surgical intervention means mainly microvascular decompression (MVD). MVD has become one of the most important treatment options for TN since its development in the 1970s.[19] On the other hand, the LLLT stimulation of the nerve itself and peripheral areas can be of great help when combined with any of the therapies described above. There are almost no

contraindications for this therapy: only patients who experience stimulated pain reflexes following laser irradiation should be excluded.

Usually TN patients have to deal with episodes of lancinating pain over their entire lifetime. This is why sessions of LLLT along with conventional therapy may improve the quality of the patients' life if carried out with appropriate rigor. It is also worth mentioning that the dentist must be committed to the patient, because the sessions may last for years, and may be undertaken once or twice a week. In addition, it is important for the professional to evaluate the patient periodically, devoting time to modifying the irradiation protocol as needed.

Maeda reported that when light irradiation was performed on rat trigeminal nerves, bradykinin stimulation inhibited the increase in mitochondrial density in the trigeminal nucleus.[20] This was found on the 12th day after irradiation. In this study the site treated was the rat facial skin at the location innervated by the trigeminal branch. The irradiation lasted 15 seconds per point and the wavelength used was 830 nm, with 60 mW, 1.9 W/cm^2, twice a day for 7 days. The light was used in a continuous mode and 12 points of irradiation were used.

Bradykinin is a pro-inflammatory neuropeptide that sensitizes nociceptors and is a key mediator in clinical pain and the associated inflammation.[9,20–22] LLLT stimulation of the trigeminal nucleus of the rat was directly relevant to pain relief. As mentioned, the irradiation consisted of a continuous wave of 830 nm (60 mW) over the bradykinin injection site, which had previously stimulated the nerve. Moreover, continuous wave light of 830 nm (16.2 mW) to isolated neurons blocked the stimulatory effects of bradykinin activity on nociceptors[21] and induced inhibition of somatosensory evoked potentials (SSEPs) in the trigeminal nucleus of rats receiving noxious electrical stimulation of the tooth pulp.[23] Finally, following the injection of pro-inflammatory polysaccharide carrageenan into the rat paw, light irradiation (660 or 684 nm) down-regulated B1 and B2 kinin receptors,[24] which are expressed on nociceptors.[22]

Laser irradiation probably inhibits neural activity in both humans and animals by slowing the conduction velocity in peripheral nerves.[23,25–27] According to a systematic review, visible and near infrared laser irradiation can cause neural impairment, particularly in small diameter Aδ and C fibers, which convey nociceptive stimuli that are very relevant to pain.[9] By this means, other important peripheral neural disorders that occur in the oral and maxillofacial area could be attenuated with LLLT.

Paresthesia

Paresthesia of the inferior alveolar nerve can follow the removal of third molar teeth and has been variously reported in 3%,[28] 5.17%,[29] and 5.5%[30] of such cases. The percentage can also increase to 88.8% during mandibular vestibuloplasty and 100% during sagittal split osteotomy.[31] These disorders can last for over 6 months and generally leave some degree of long-term disability.[32] LLLT has been utilized to help these patients regain partial or complete sensation and feeling in the hemi-mandible, tongue or buccal mucosa.

A subjective improvement of 71.1% according to a visual analog scale in patients suffering from long-standing (>6 months) inferior alveolar or lingual nerve paresthesias after LLLT treatment has been reported.[33] A possible mechanism that may explain the beneficial effects of laser stimulation of nerves, including the effects on injury-induced paresthesias in sensory nerves,[34] is that the laser light reacts with a light-sensitive rhodopsin kinase or a rhodopsin kinase-like protein that occurs in different areas of the nervous system; LLLT would then affect the recovery of neural tissue or the perception of pain in sensory nerves.[35]

To define the correct diagnosis of inferior alveolar nerve paresthesia, the clinician should evaluate the branches of such a nerve and its specific area of innervation. The extent of neural damage that occurs after facial paralysis should also be evaluated. Actually, alveolar nerve paresthesia presents only as sensorial loss, while facial paralysis relates to the facial nerve, affecting its motor counterpart.

Also called Bell's palsy, facial paralysis is in fact a self-limiting, non-fatal, and spontaneously remitting disorder of acute onset due to non-suppurative inflammation of the facial nerve within the stylomastoid foramen.[36] It affects the muscles of facial expression that are unilaterally supplied by the seventh cranial nerve, the facial nerve, causing partial or complete paralysis. Thus, the face is drawn up on the normal side, affecting eating, drinking, and speech.[37] Bell's palsy has an unknown cause, although it can be associated with exposure to cold, trauma, infection, nerve ischemia or autoimmunity.[38]

The primary concern in the treatment of a Bell's palsy patient is restoration of esthetics, function, and comfort.[36] Among the treatments proposed for this disorder are corticosteroids, which are commonly used and show significant short-term and long-term positive effects.[39] Acupuncture, on the other hand, is a safe therapy with a low risk of adverse events in clinical practice,[40] and is one of the most commonly used treatments for Bell's palsy in China.[41] In addition, a Chinese study found that the therapeutic effect of acupuncture combined with HeNe laser irradiation on facial paralysis was better than that of standard medication.[42]

According to the literature, 71% of untreated patients with Bell's palsy will completely recover and 84% will have complete or near-normal recovery.[41] Patients who do not recover will present with persistent moderate to severe weakness, facial contracture, or synkinesis.[43–45] The facial nerve has several branches that innervate the face. Therefore, LLLT should be delivered to each and every branch of the nerve affected by the paralysis, and although there is a lack of studies of this particular application of laser therapy, it should work as well as it works for other peripheral nerve disorders.

Laser and light parameters for treating nerve injuries

Nowadays, the technical concerns with surgical procedures are the use of new materials,[46] and improvements in the dexterity and competence of trained people.[47] In addition for light-based therapies, many factors affect the interaction between light and tissues, such as wavelength,[48] power, frequency,[49] the irradiation regimen,[5] the placement of irradiation,[50] and so on.

There is some agreement about the best wavelengths and range of acceptable dosages to be used (irradiance and fluence), but there is no agreement on whether continuous wave or pulsed light is the best and on what factors govern the pulse parameters to be chosen. The molecular and cellular mechanisms of LLLT are understudied for many kinds of tissue repair, including nerve repair. The type of pulsed light sources available and the parameters that govern their pulse structure are sometimes very important. Studies that have compared continuous wave and pulsed light in both animals and patients have been reviewed by the main group that studies this subject. Frequencies used in other pulsed modalities used in physical therapy and biomedicine have been compared to those used in LLLT. There is some evidence that pulsed light does induce different effects from those of continuous wave light. However, further work is needed to define the best results for different disease conditions and pulse structures.[51]

Figure 38.2 Micrograph of sciatic nerve treated with LLLT (three times a week for 4 weeks) and control evaluated at 28 days after the lesion. The immunomarker is S-100, which stains the Schwann cells. There is greater staining of the laser-treated (c,d) Schwann cells than in the control (sham-treated Schwan cells, a,b) in two magnifications.

One review of the effect of phototherapy on the nerve repair process[52] reported many good results obtained using lasers, light emitting diodes (LEDs),[53] and other kinds of light source.[54] In the review, the authors explain the mechanisms underlying LLLT based on the many previous results.[52] Our group performed a study investigating the effects of 660- and 780-nm LLLT using different energy densities (10, 60, and 120 J/cm^2) on neuromuscular and functional recovery, as well as on matrix metalloproteinase (MMP) activity after crush injury of the rat sciatic nerve.[6] Rats received transcutaneous LLLT irradiation at the lesion site for 10 consecutive days post injury and were sacrificed 28 days after injury. Both the sciatic nerve and *tibialis anterior* muscles were analyzed. Nerve analyses consisted of histology (light microscopy) and measurements of myelin, axon, and nerve fiber cross-sectional area (CSA). S-100 labeling was used to identify the myelin sheath and Schwann cells (Fig. 38.2). Muscle fiber CSA and zymography were carried out to assess the degree of muscle atrophy and MMP activity, respectively. This study showed that 660-nm LLLT with both 10 and 60 J/cm^2 restored muscle fiber, myelin, and nerve fiber CSA compared to the normal group (N). It also increased MMP-2 activity in nerve and decreased MMP-2 activity in muscle and MMP-9 activity in nerve. In contrast, 780-nm LLLT using 10 J/cm^2 decreased MMP-9 activity in nerve compared to the crush group (CR) and N; it also restored normal levels of myelin and nerve fiber CSA. Both 60 and 120 J/cm^2 decreased MMP-2 activity in muscle compared to CR and N. Laser irradiation with 780 nm did not prevent muscle fiber atrophy. Functional recovery in the irradiated groups did not differ from that in the non-irradiated CR. These data suggest that 660-nm LLLT with low (10 J/cm^2) or moderate (60 J/cm^2) energy densities is able to accelerate neuromuscular recovery after nerve crush injury in rats.

These results are particularly interesting because the best results from Rochkind's group[1,50,52,54,55] were obtained with a wavelength in the near infrared band (780 nm), which disagrees with the findings of our group. However, several factors in these applications may explain differences in the results with various types of tissues, including peripheral nerves. In earlier papers,[50,56–58] this same group had good outcomes with laser in the red band (633-nm HeNe laser), confirming the possibility of achieving good results in other spectrum bands.

In a double-blind randomized study, the therapeutic effect of LLLT on peripheral nerve regeneration was evaluated after complete transection and direct anastomosis of the rat sciatic nerve. After this procedure, 13 of 24 rats received LLLT (780-nm laser applied transcutaneously) for 30 minutes daily on 21 consecutive days at corresponding segments of the spinal cord and the injured sciatic nerve. Positive somatosensory evoked responses were found in 69.2% of the irradiated rats, compared to 18.2% of the non-irradiated rats. Immunohistochemical staining in the laser-treated group showed an increase in the total number of axons, and better quality of the regeneration process, due to an increased number of large-diameter axons, compared to the non-irradiated control group. The study suggests that following anastomosis after compete transection, postoperative LLLT enhances the regenerative processes of peripheral nerves.[59]

Growth factors are involved in a variety of responses in the process of nerve regeneration. A study investigated the effects of diode laser (GaAlAs) irradiation at an effective energy density of 5 or $20\,J/cm^2$ on cell growth factor-induced differentiation and proliferation in pheochromocytoma cells (PC12 cells), and whether those effects were related to activation of the p38 pathway. Laser irradiation at $20\,J/cm^2$ significantly decreased the number of PC12 cells, while no difference was seen between the $5\,J/cm^2$ group and the control group. Western blotting revealed marked expression of neurofilament and beta-tubulin, indicating greater neurite differentiation in the irradiated groups than in the control group at 48 hours. Irradiation also enhanced expression of phospho-p38. The decreased number of cells after laser irradiation was reversed by the p38 inhibitor, while neurite differentiation was up-regulated by laser irradiation, even when the p38 pathway was blocked. This results suggests that laser irradiation up-regulated neurite differentiation in PC12 cells, involving p38 and another pathway.[60]

Further evidence of the therapeutic effect of LLLT on neuronal regeneration was provided by the finding of elevated immunoreactivities (IRs) of growth-associated protein-43 (GAP-43), which is up-regulated during neuronal regeneration. The animals received a standardized crush injury of the sciatic nerve, mimicking the clinical situations accompanying partial axonotmesis. The injured nerve received a calculated dose of LLLT immediately after the injury and on four consecutive days thereafter. The walking movements of the animals were scored using the sciatic functional index (SFI). In the laser-treated rats, the SFI was higher at 3–4 weeks, while the SFI of the laser-treated and untreated rats reached normal levels at 5 weeks after surgery. In an immunocytochemical study, although GAP-43 IRs increased both in the untreated control and the LLLT-treated groups after injury, the number of GAP-43 IR nerve fibers was much greater in the LLLT group than in the control group. The elevated numbers of GAP-43 IR nerve fibers reached a peak 3 weeks after injury, and then declined in both the untreated control and the LLLT groups at 5 weeks, with no differences in the numbers of GAP-43 IR nerve fibers in the two groups at this stage. This immunocytochemical study using GAP-43 antibody shows for the first time that LLLT has an effect on the early stages of the nerve recovery process following sciatic nerve injury.[61]

Previous studies have proposed that proliferation and release of certain growth factors by different types of cells can be modulated by LLLT. A study was formulated to demonstrate the effect of laser irradiation on human Schwann cell proliferation and neurotrophic factor gene expression *in vitro*. Human Schwann cells (SCs) were harvested from sural nerve samples obtained from organ donors, followed by treatment with an 810-nm, 50-mW diode laser (two different energies: $1\,J/cm^2$ and $4\,J/cm^2$) over 3 consecutive days. SC proliferation was measured after first irradiation and on days 1, 4, and 7 by the MTT assay. Real-time polymerase chain reaction (PCR) analysis was utilized on days 5 and 20 to evaluate the expression of key genes involved in nerve regeneration: *NGF*, *BDNF*, and *GDNF*. Evaluation of cellular proliferation 1 day after laser treatment revealed a significant decrease in cell proliferation compared to the control group. However on day 7, a significant increase in proliferation was found in both the irradiated groups in comparison with the control group. No significant difference was found between the laser-treated groups. Treatment of SCs with laser resulted in a significant increase in *NGF* gene expression on day 20. Differences between the two treated groups and control group were not significant for *BDNF* and *GDNF* gene expression. These results demonstrate that LLLT stimulates human SC proliferation and *NGF* gene expression *in vitro*.[62] This fact is indicative of laser action on the neural tissue, which could be triggered by stimulation of growth factor expression.

Central nervous system injury (spinal cord injury and traumatic brain injury)

The Rochkind group was the first to study LLLT in the treatment of severely injured peripheral nerves and also injuries to the central nervous system (CNS). The irradiation method first proposed by Rochkind has been modified over recent years. LLLT at specific wavelengths and energy densities is known to maintain the electrophysiological activity of severely injured peripheral nerves in rats, preventing scar formation (at the injury site), as well as degenerative changes in the corresponding motor neurons of the spinal cord, thus accelerating regeneration of the injured nerve. Laser irradiation applied to the spinal cord of dogs following severe spinal cord injury and implantation of a segment of the peripheral nerve into the injured area diminished glial scar formation, induced axonal sprouting in the lesion, and restored locomotor function. Laser therapy has been shown to prevent extensive glial scar formation (a limiting factor in CNS regeneration) between a neural transplant and the host brain or spinal cord. Abundant capillaries were seen to develop in the laser-irradiated transplants and were of crucial importance in their survival. The intraoperative clinical use of laser therapy following surgical treatment of the tethered spinal cord (resulting from myelomeningocele, lipomyelomeningocele, thickened filum terminale or fibrous scar) increases functional activity of the irradiated spinal cord. In a previous experimental work, we showed that direct laser treatment of nerve tissue promotes restoration of the electrophysiological activity of the severely injured peripheral nerve, prevents degenerative changes in neurons of the spinal cord, and induces proliferation of astrocytes and oligodendrocytes. This suggested a higher metabolism in neurons and improved ability to produce myelin following laser treatment. The tethering of the spinal cord causes mechanical damage to neuronal cell membranes, leading to metabolic disturbances in the neurons. For this reason, the Rochkind group believes LLLT may improve neuronal metabolism, prevent neuronal degeneration, and promote improved spinal cord function and repair.[63] The possible mechanisms of LLLT are being investigated by several different centers.

Using electron paramagnetic resonance in cell culture models, the Rochkind group found that at low energy doses, singlet oxygen is produced by energy transfer from porphyrins (not cytochromes as is commonly assumed), which are known to be present at low concentrations in cells. At low concentration, singlet oxygen can modulate the biochemical processes taking place in the cell and trigger accelerated cell division. On the other hand, at high concentration, singlet oxygen is cytotoxic and damages the cell.[64–66] Other groups have introduced LLLT as a method to treat central and peripheral nervous tissue lesions.

Spinal cord injury (SCI) is a severe CNS trauma with no effective restorative therapies. The effectiveness of LLLT on SCI caused by different types of trauma has been studied using two SCI models: a contusion model and a dorsal hemisection model. Near infrared light (810 nm) was applied transcutaneously at the lesion site immediately after injury and daily for 14 consecutive days. A laser diode with an output power of 150 mW was used for the treatment. The daily dosage at the surface of the skin overlying the lesion site was $1589 \, J/cm^2$ (0.3 cm² spot area, 2997 seconds). Functional recovery was assessed by the footprint test for the hemisection model and the open-field test for the contusion model. Rats were euthanized 3 weeks after injury. The average lengths of axonal regrowth in the rats in the LLLT groups with the hemisection (6.89 ± 0.96 mm) and contusion (7.04 ± 0.76 mm) injuries were significantly longer than those in the comparable untreated control groups (hemisection 3.66 ± 0.26 mm; contusion 2.89 ± 0.84 mm). The total number of axons in the LLLT groups was significantly higher compared to that in the untreated

groups for both injury models. For the hemisection model, the LLLT group had a statistically significant lower angle of rotation compared to the controls. For the contusion model, there was a statistically significant functional recovery in the LLLT group compared to the untreated controls. Light therapy applied non-invasively promotes axonal regeneration and functional recovery in acute SCI caused by different types of trauma. These results suggest that LLLT is a promising approach for human SCI.[67]

The Hamblin laboratory has demonstrated that transcranial LLLT can have beneficial effects in two different mouse models of traumatic brain injury (TBI). A study in mice of closed head TBI studied a single post-injury exposure to $36 \, J/cm^2$ delivered at $150 \, mW/cm^2$ from continuous wave lasers emitting at either 665, 730, 810, or 980 nm.[68] The neurological severity score was followed for 4 weeks and showed significant improvement following irradiation with the 660-nm and 810-nm lasers, but not with the 730-nm or 980-nm lasers. A second study using an open skull controlled cortical impact model of TBI compared 810-nm laser irradiation either continuous wave or pulsed at 10 Hz or 100 Hz.[69] Although all three modes of laser delivery were effective compared to the sham treatment control, the 10-Hz pulse frequency was significantly better than either continuous wave or 100 Hz. Furthermore, improvements in the size of the focal brain lesion and in forced swim and tail suspension tests for depression and anxiety were seen. Another study looked at LLLT for cryolesions produced in the rat brain.[70] The most striking finding was that treated lesions showed smaller tissue loss than control lesions at 6 hours. During the first 24 hours the number of viable neurons was significantly higher in the lased group. There was a remarkable increase in the amount of glial fibrillary acidic protein (GFAP) in the control group by 14 days. Moreover, the lesions of the irradiated animals had fewer leukocytes and lymphocytes in the first 24 hours than controls. Considering the experimental conditions of this study, it was concluded that laser phototherapy exerts its effect in wound healing following cryolesion by controlling the brain damage and preventing neuron death and severe astrogliosis, which could indicate the possibility of a better clinical outcome.

Clinical results

Many studies have investigated the effects of phototherapy on nerve regeneration in humans. More time and money needs to be invested to achieve a sufficiently convincing body of data in this field. The nerve repair process is lengthy, and it is difficult to collect data and compare them to regular clinical and surgical treatments. It is known that injury of a major nerve trunk frequently results in considerable disability associated with loss of sensory and motor functions. Spontaneous recovery of long-term severe incomplete peripheral nerve injury is often unsatisfactory.

Clinical case 38.1

A 43-year-old female patient after postsurgical removal of a gemistocytic astrocytoma in the temporobasal region near the cavernous sinus had ptosis, deviation from the central axis of the orbit to adduction, hypoesthesia, and palsy of the left facial muscles (Fig. 38.3a). These neurological deficits were treated with infrared (830 nm) laser therapy 5 days a week for 4 months (120 J/cm²) (Fig. 38.3b–f).

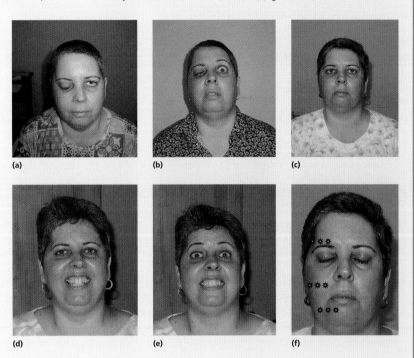

Figure 38.3 (a) Initial presentation; (b) 11 days after the start of the laser treatment (infrared laser 830 nm, energy density 120 J/cm², power density 120 mW/cm², five times per week); (c) after 55 days of treatment; (d,e) outcome of the treatment after 4 months; (f) points of irradiation used to treat the patient, three points on each branch of the facial nerve (courtesy of Prof Luiz Ferreira Monteiro Neto).

A pilot study was conducted to investigate prospectively the effectiveness of LLLT (780 nm) in the treatment of patients suffering from incomplete peripheral nerve and brachial plexus injuries for 6 months up to several years. A randomized double-blind placebo-controlled trial was performed in 18 patients who were randomly assigned to placebo (non-active light: diffused LED lamp) or LLLT (780 nm, 250 mW). Twenty-one consecutive daily sessions of laser or placebo irradiation were applied transcutaneously for 3 hours to the injured peripheral nerve (energy density 450 J/mm²) and for 2 hours to the corresponding segments of the spinal cord (300 J/mm²). Clinical and electrophysiological assessments were done at baseline, at the end of the 21 days of treatment, and 3 and 6 months thereafter. The laser-irradiated and placebo groups had clinically similar conditions at baseline. The analysis of motor function during the 6-month follow-up period compared to baseline showed a statistically significant improvement in the laser-treated group compared to the placebo group. No statistically significant difference was found in sensory function. Electrophysiological analysis also showed statistically significant improvement in recruitment of voluntary muscle activity in the laser-irradiated group compared to the placebo group. This pilot study suggests that in patients with long-term peripheral nerve injury, non-invasive 780-nm laser phototherapy can progressively improve nerve function, which can lead to significant functional recovery.[54]

An example of a successful outcome in a patient who had her peripheral facial nerves affected by trauma or surgery is given in Clinical case 38.1.

There are some examples of good outcomes after phototherapy in specific situations of CNS injury. This is a new field of utilization of LLLT to improve patient quality of life.[71] The use of light as a therapeutic tool has been observed to improve many clinical aspects[71,72]: improvement in cognition in two chronic TBI cases following red and near infrared LED irradiation applied transcranially to the forehead and scalp areas, and significant benefits following application of transcranial LLLT in humans with acute stroke. These are the first case reports documenting improved cognitive function in chronic TBI patients treated with transcranial LED. Treatments were applied bilaterally and to midline sagittal areas using LED cluster heads with 61 diodes (9 x 633 nm, 52 x 870 nm); 12–15 mW per diode; total power 500 mW; 22.2 mW/cm²; 13.3 J/cm² to the scalp (estimated 0.4 J/cm² to the cortex). The patients have since performed nightly home treatments. At the time of this report, both patients are continuing treatment. It can be concluded that transcranial LED may improve cognition and reduce costs of TBI treatment, and can be applied at home. Controlled studies are warranted.[72]

Acknowledgments

Research in the Hamblin laboratory is funded by NIH grants (R01A1050875 and R01CA/AI838801to MRH; R01CA137108 to Long Y Chiang), US Air Force MFEL Program (FA9550-04-1-0079), Center for Integration of Medicine and Innovative Technology (DAMD17-02-2-0006), CDMRP Program in TBI (W81XWH-09-1-0514). FFS was supported by CAPES Foundation, Ministry of Education of Brazil, Brasilia, DF 70040-020, Brazil.

References

1 Gigo-Benato D, Geuna S, Rochkind S. Phototherapy for enhancing peripheral nerve repair: a review of the literature. *Muscle Nerve* 2005; 31(6): 694–701.

2 Moges, H., et al., Effect of 810 nm light on nerve regeneration after autograft repair of severely injured rat median nerve. *Lasers Surg Med* 2011; 43(9): 901–906.

3 Zhang LX, et al. Effects of 660-nm gallium-aluminum-arsenide low-energy laser on nerve regeneration after acellular nerve allograft in rats. *Synapse* 2010; 64(2): 152–160.

4 Chung H, et al. The nuts and bolts of low-level laser (light) therapy. *Ann Biomed Eng* 2012; 40(2): 516–533.

5 Gigo-Benato D, et al. Low-power laser biostimulation enhances nerve repair after end-to-side neurorrhaphy: a double-blind randomized study in the rat median nerve model. *Lasers Med Sci* 2004; 19(1): 57–65.

6 Gigo-Benato D, et al. Effects of 660 and 780 nm low-level laser therapy on neuromuscular recovery after crush injury in rat sciatic nerve. *Lasers Surg Med* 2010; 42(9): 673–682.

7 Santos AP, et al. Functional and morphometric differences between the early and delayed use of phototherapy in crushed median nerves of rats. *Lasers Med Sci* 2012; 27(2): 479–486.

8 Medalha CC, et al. Low-level laser therapy improves repair following complete resection of the sciatic nerve in rats. *Lasers Med Sci* 2012; 27(3): 629–635.

9 Chow R, et al. Inhibitory effects of laser irradiation on peripheral mammalian nerves and relevance to analgesic effects: a systematic review. *Photomed Laser Surg* 2011; 29(6): 365–381.

10 Shen CC, Yang YC, Liu BS. Large-area irradiated low-level laser effect in a biodegradable nerve guide conduit on neural regeneration of peripheral nerve injury in rats. *Injury* 2011; 42(8): 803–813.

11 Hashmi JT, et al. Role of low-level laser therapy in neurorehabilitation. *PM R* 2010; 2(12 Suppl 2): S292–305.

12 Pinheiro AL, et al. Low-level laser therapy is an important tool to treat disorders of the maxillofacial region. *J Clin Laser Med Surg* 1998; 16(4): 226.

13 Oesman C, Mooij JJ. Long-term follow-up of microvascular decompression for trigeminal neuralgia. *Skull Base* 2011; 21(5): 313–322.

14 Dandy W. Concering the cause of trigeminal neuralgia. *Am J Surg* 1934; 24: 447–455.

15 Barker FG, 2nd, et al. The long-term outcome of microvascular decompression for trigeminal neuralgia. *N Engl J Med* 1996; 334(17): 1077–1083.

16 Meaney JF, et al., Demonstration of neurovascular compression in trigeminal neuralgia with magnetic resonance imaging. Comparison with surgical findings in 52 consecutive operative cases. *J Neurosurg* 1995; 83(5): 799–805.

17 Hamlyn PJ, King TT. Neurovascular compression in trigeminal neuralgia: a clinical and anatomical study. *J Neurosurg* 1992; 76(6): 948–954.

18 Nurmikko TJ, Eldridge PR. Trigeminal neuralgia--pathophysiology, diagnosis and current treatment. *Br J Anaesth* 2001; 87(1): 117–132.

19 Jannetta PJ. Arterial compression of the trigeminal nerve at the pons in patients with trigeminal neuralgia. *J Neurosurg* 1967; 26(1) Suppl: 159–162.

20 Maeda T. Morphological demonstration of low re- active laser therapeutic pain attenuation effect of the gallium aluminium arsenide diode laser. *Laser Ther* 1989; 1: 23–30.

21 Jimbo K, et al. Suppressive effects of low-power laser irradiation on bradykinin evoked action potentials in cultured murine dorsal root ganglion cells. *Neurosci Lett* 1998; 240(2): 93–96.

22 Couture R, et al. Kinin receptors in pain and inflammation. *Eur J Pharmacol* 2001; 429(1–3): 161–176.

23 Wakabayashi H, et al. Effect of irradiation by semiconductor laser on responses evoked in trigeminal caudal neurons by tooth pulp stimulation. *Lasers Surg Med* 1993; 13(6): 605–610.

24 Bortone F, et al. Low level laser therapy modulates kinin receptors mRNA expression in the subplantar muscle of rat paw subjected to carrageenan-induced inflammation. *Int Immunopharmacol* 2008; 8(2): 206–210.

25 Snyder-Mackler L, Bork CE. Effect of helium-neon laser irradiation on peripheral sensory nerve latency. *Phys Ther* 1988; 68(2): 223–225.

26 Wesselmann U, Lin SF, Rymer WZ. Effects of Q-switched Nd:YAG laser irradiation on neural impulse propagation: I. *Spinal cord. Physiol Chem Phys Med NMR* 1991; 23(2): 67–80.

27 Kono, T., et al., Cord dorsum potentials suppressed by low power laser irradiation on a peripheral nerve in the cat. *J Clin Laser Med Surg* 1993; 11(3): 115–118.

28 Merrill RG. Prevention, treatment, and prognosis for nerve injury related to the difficult impaction. *Dent Clin North Am* 1979; 23(3): 471–488.

29 Howe GL, Poyton HT. Prevention of damage to the inferior dental nerve during extraction of mandibular third molars. *Br Dent J* 1960; 109: 353–363.

30 Rood JP. Lingual split technique. Damage to inferior alveolar and lingual nerves during removal of impacted mandibular third molars. *Br Dent J* 1983; 154(12): 402–403.

31 Walter JM Jr, Gregg JM. Analysis of postsurgical neurologic alteration in the trigeminal nerve. *J Oral Surg* 1979; 37(6): 410–414.

32 Robinson PP. Observations on the recovery of sensation following inferior alveolar nerve injuries. *Br J Oral Maxillofac Surg* 1988; 26(3): 177–189.

33 Midamba ED, Haanaes RH. Low reactive-level 830 nm GaAlAs diode laser therapy (LLLT) successfully accelerates regeneration of peripheral nerves in human. *Laser Ther* 1993; 5: 125–129.

34 Khullar SM, et al., Preliminary study of low-level laser for treatment of long-standing sensory aberrations in the inferior alveolar nerve. *J Oral Maxillofac Surg* 1996; 54(1): 2–7; discussion 7–8.

35 Somers RL, Klein DC. Rhodopsin kinase activity in the mammalian pineal gland and other tissues. *Science* 1984; 226(4671): 182–184.

36 Somani P, Nayak AK. Restoration of blinking reflex and facial symmetry in a Bell's palsy patient. *IndianJ Dent Res* 2011; 22(6): 857–859.

37 Fogg RA, Radell MH. A removable oral prosthetic appliance for Bell's palsy: report of case. *J Am Dent Assoc* 1977; 94(6): 1169–1172.

38 Muralidhar M, et al. Bilateral Bell's palsy: current concepts in aetiology and treatment. *Case report. Aust Dent J* 1987; 32(6): 412–416.

39 Engstrom M, et al. Prednisolone and valaciclovir in Bell's palsy: a randomised, double-blind, placebo-controlled, multicentre trial. *Lancet Neurol* 2008; 7(11): 993–1000.

40 Zhao L, et al. Adverse events associated with acupuncture: three multicentre randomized controlled trials of 1968 cases in China. *Trials* 2011; 12: 87.

41 Xia F, et al. Prednisolone and acupuncture in Bell's palsy: study protocol for a randomized, controlled trial. *Trials* 2011; 12: 158.

42 Hou YL, et al. [Observation on therapeutic effect of acupuncture combined with He-Ne laser radiation on facial paralysis]. Zhongguo zhen jiu]. *Chinese Acupuncture Moxibustion* 2008; 28(4): 265–266.

43 Holland NJ, Weiner gm. Recent developments in Bell's palsy. *BMJ* 2004; 329(7465): 553–557.

44 May M, Hughes gb. Facial nerve disorders: update 1987. *The Am j Ootol* 1987; 8(2): 167–180.

45 Peitersen E. Bell's palsy: the spontaneous course of 2,500 peripheral facial nerve palsies of different etiologies. Acta Oto-laryngol 2002; (Suppl 549): 4–30.

46 Curtis NJ, et al., Comparison of microsuture, interpositional nerve graft, and laser solder weld repair of the rat inferior alveolar nerve. *J Oral Maxillofac Surg* 2011; 69(6): e246–255.

47 Nectoux E, Taleb C, Liverneaux P. Nerve repair in telemicrosurgery: an experimental study. *J Reconstr Microsurg* 2009; 25(4): 261–265.

48 Barbosa RI, et al. Comparative effects of wavelengths of low-power laser in regeneration of sciatic nerve in rats following crushing lesion. *Lasers Med Sci* 2010; 25(3): 423–430.

49 Chen, Y.S., et al., Effect of low-power pulsed laser on peripheral nerve regeneration in rats. *Microsurgery* 2005; 25(1): 83–89.

50 Rochkind S, et al. Effects of laser irradiation on the spinal cord for the regeneration of crushed peripheral nerve in rats. *Lasers Surg Med* 2001; 28(3): 216–219.

51 Hashmi JT, et al. Effect of pulsing in low-level light therapy. *Lasers Surg Med* 2010; 42(6): 450–466.

52 Rochkind S, Geuna S, Shainberg A. Phototherapy in peripheral nerve injury: effects on muscle preservation and nerve regeneration. *Int Rev Neurobio*, 2009; 87: 445–64.

53 Serafim KG, et al. Effects of 940 nm light-emitting diode (led) on sciatic nerve regeneration in rats. *Lasers Med Sci* 2012; 27(1): 113–119.

54 Anders JJ, Geuna S, Rochkind S. Phototherapy promotes regeneration and functional recovery of injured peripheral nerve. *Neurol Res* 2004; 26(2): 233239.

55 Rochkind S, et al. Efficacy of 780-nm laser phototherapy on peripheral nerve regeneration after neurotube reconstruction procedure (double-blind randomized study). *Photomed Laser Surg* 2007; 25(3): 137–143.

56 Rochkind S, et al. Stimulatory effect of He-Ne low dose laser on injured sciatic nerves of rats. *Neurosurgery* 1987; 20(6): 843–847.

57 Rochkind S, et al. Response of peripheral nerve to He-Ne laser: experimental studies. *Lasers Surg Med* 1987; 7(5): 441–443.

58 Rochkind S, et al. Systemic effects of low-power laser irradiation on the peripheral and central nervous system, cutaneous wounds, and burns. *Lasers Surg Med* 1989; 9(2): 174–182.

59 Shamir MH, et al. Double-blind randomized study evaluating regeneration of the rat transected sciatic nerve after suturing and postoperative low-power laser treatment. *J Reconstr Microsurg* 2001; 17(2): 133–137; discussion 138.

60 Saito K, et al. Effect of diode laser on proliferation and differentiation of PC12 cells. *Bull Tokyo Dent Coll* 2011; 52(2): 95–102.

61 Shin DH, et al. Growth-associated protein-43 is elevated in the injured rat sciatic nerve after low power laser irradiation. *Neurosci Lett* 2003; 344(2): 71–74.

62 Yazdani SO, et al. Effects of low level laser therapy on proliferation and neurotrophic factor gene expression of human schwann cells in vitro. *J Photochem Photobiol B* 2012; 107: 9–13.

63 Rochkind S, Ouaknine GE. New trend in neuroscience: low-power laser effect on peripheral and central nervous system (basic science, preclinical and clinical studies). *Neurol Res* 1992; 14(1): 2–11.

64 Rochkind S, et al. New methods of treatment of severely injured sciatic nerve and spinal cord. An experimental study. *Acta Neurochir (Wien)* 1988. 43 (Suppl): 91–93.

65 Lavi R, et al. Low energy visible light induces reactive oxygen species generation and stimulates an increase of intracellular calcium concentration in cardiac cells. *J Biol Chem* 2003; 278(42): 40917–40922.

66 Lubart R, et al. Low-energy laser irradiation promotes cellular redox activity. *Photomed Laser Surg* 2005; 23(1): 3–9.

67 Wu X, et al. 810 nm Wavelength light: an effective therapy for transected or contused rat spinal cord. *Lasers Surg Med* 2009; 41(1): 36–41.

68 Wu Q, Xuan W, Ando T, et al. Low-level laser therapy for closed-head traumatic brain injury in mice: effect of different wavelengths. *Lasers Surg Med* 2012; 44(3): 218–226.

69 Ando T, et al. Comparison of therapeutic effects between pulsed and continuous wave 810-nm wavelength laser irradiation for traumatic brain injury in mice. *PLoS ONE* 2011; 6(10): e26212–26220.

70 Moreira MS, et al. Effect of laser phototherapy on wound healing following cerebral ischemia by cryogenic injury. *J Photochem Photobiol B* 2011; 105(3): 207–215.

71 Naeser MA, Hamblin MR. Potential for transcranial laser or LED therapy to treat stroke, traumatic brain injury, and neurodegenerative disease. *Photomed Laser Surg* 2011; 29(7): 443–446.

72 Naeser MA, et al. Improved cognitive function after transcranial, light-emitting diode treatments in chronic, traumatic brain injury: two case reports. *Photomed Laser Surg* 2011; 29(5): 351–358.

Laser and antimicrobial photodynamic therapies in cancer patients

CHAPTER 39

Optical diagnosis of cancer and potentially malignant lesions

Cristina Kurachi, Lilian Tan Moriyama, and Alessandro Cosci

Department of Physics and Materials Science, São Carlos Institute of Physics, University of São Paulo (USP), São Carlos, SP, Brazil

Introduction

In the medical sciences, diagnosis refers to the *knowledge* and *discrimination* of the characteristics of the pathology or general condition of a patient. Diagnosis is also considered the procedures used to obtain the information for the identification of the pathology or the metabolism of the tissue. To achieve the diagnosis of a lesion or of the patient's clinical status, the health professional obtains information through anamnesis, clinical examination, and laboratory tests.

In dentistry, the gold standard for diagnosis of cancer, potentially malignant disorders, and other pathologies that affect soft tissues is biopsy and histopathological examination under an optical microscope. Biopsy is indicated only when the dentist suspects, based on the clinical appearance, that the lesion is potentially a carcinoma or severe dysplasia. Depending on the lesion size and its anatomical site, the clinician chooses between a complete excision, mainly for small lesions, and an incisional biopsy. In the latter, a tissue sample is excised and the material sent to a pathology laboratory. Both tissue materials, the whole lesion or the sample, are processed and analyzed under an optical microscope by a certified pathologist. The pathologist will give the diagnosis based on the characteristics seen, especially cell morphology and tissue architecture.

Clinical examination involves palpation inspection and visual identification of lesion characteristics such as color, texture, macroscopic morphology, and surface homogeneity, which must always be compared to the features of the normal tissue. These conventional diagnostic procedures for oral cancer are highly dependent on the clinician's skills and experience in detecting malignant clinical features. Cancer diagnostics in the initial stages of cancer are not simple, since their clinical characteristics are similar to those of the more prevalent benign disorders. The discrimination between dysplasia and carcinoma *in situ* (CIS) is also a clinical challenge.

Another relevant issue is the determination of the biopsy site in a non-homogenous lesion. Distinct surface characteristics result from different histological features that may represent distinct pathological diagnoses. If the clinician does not choose the best site for incisional biopsy, a cancer may be misdiagnosed. It is not feasible to convince the patient to have several biopsies taken from a large lesion. The clinician must perform a detailed clinical diagnosis to enhance the probability of defining the dysplasia and malignant areas, if present.

Optical techniques have been proposed as auxiliary diagnostics tools to clinical examination. These techniques are based on the principle that *light–tissue interactions* change with cancer progression and the analysis of these optical phenomena gives information on biochemical and structural tissue composition. The conventional clinical examination is performed under white light and the re-emitted light visualized at the tissue surface is a result of reflectance, scattering, and absorption interactions in the illuminated region. If the illumination and detection conditions are modified and assembled to optimize the interrogation of some specific light–tissue interactions, some biomolecules and tissue architecture information can be targeted.[1]

Optical techniques are attractive tools since they provide an objective fast response through non-invasive and non-destructive procedures. In this way, the diagnosis is less subjective and dependent on the clinician's expertise.

Light–tissue interactions

When a biological tissue is illuminated, light–tissue interactions take place at the surface and within the tissue. These interactions are modified depending on the light parameters and tissue optical characteristics. The main light parameters that influence these phenomena are: wavelength, spectral bandwidth, and pulse width.[1,2] Biological tissues are composed of several molecules that alter the photon pathways inside the tissue. As a result, the same wavelength will interact differently depending on the biochemical composition and tissue architecture, and the same tissue will interact differently depending on the illumination parameters.

Lasers in Dentistry: Guide for Clinical Practice, First Edition. Edited by Patrícia M. de Freitas and Alyne Simões.

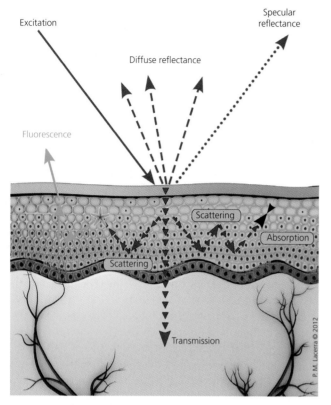

Figure 39.1 Schematic showing the light–tissue interactions taking place in the oral mucosa. The incident light (excitation) is delivered to the tissue surface and the transepithelial photon pathways are shown (diffuse and specular reflectance, scattering, fluorescence, absorption, and transmission (image created by P.M. Lacerra (2012). Provided by Kurachi).

Light–tissue interactions are classified into the following types (Fig. 39.1):
- Reflectance (specular and diffuse);
- Scattering;
- Absorption;
- Transmission;
- Luminescence (fluorescence and phosphorescence).

When photons are delivered to a tissue surface, some are reflected and do not actually interact with the biological molecules. The tissue surface acts as a mirror, reflecting the light without changing its characteristics. This phenomenon is called *specular reflectance* and does not give any information about the tissue. The photons that penetrate the tissue are the ones that provide diagnostic information.

Photons travelling within the tissue will change their direction when they meet a component with a different refractive index. Tissue layers of different biochemical composition and structure show distinct refractive indexes, and if an interface between these layers is in the path of a photon, it will modify the direction in which the photon travels. In oral mucosa, the keratin layer, epithelial tissue, and underlying lamina propria (fibroblasts, connective tissue, small capillaries, inflammatory cells, and

extracellular matrix) have different refractive indexes. Photons travelling from the surface into the inner regions of the oral mucosa will undergo several changes in their direction, a light–tissue interaction known as *scattering*. This phenomenon also takes place at the microscopic level, with photons changing direction as they meet the cell membrane, nuclei, and organelles.

After several scattering interactions, some of the delivered photons will exit from the tissue surface. This light emerging at the tissue surface shows the same wavelength as the incident light, but differs in irradiance and direction. This re-emitted light after multiple scattering is called the *diffuse reflectance*.

Photons that are not absorbed and do not change their direction are transmitted through the tissue layers. When *transmission* occurs, the optical path is not modified by the tissue as the photons have not been influenced by the presence of the biological components.

Absorption is the process that happens when a biological component absorbs the photon energy. This energy can be used for a biochemical reaction or can result in molecular vibration (heat) or in photoemission (luminescence). For most available laser therapies, absorption is the most relevant light–tissue interaction that must take place for the tissue response, such as ablation, vaporization, and carbonization. The main biological absorbers are hemoglobin and melanin.

Some biological chromophores absorb the photon energy and later emit light, through a process called *luminescence*. This photoemission is one of the possible ways that an excited molecule can lose energy to return to its most stable ground electronic state. Luminescence is classified as fluorescence or phosphorescence, according to the length of time that this phenomenon occurs. Most biological luminescent molecules emit light through fluorescence, showing lifetimes in the nanosecond range.

Fluorescence for cancer diagnosis

In optical diagnostics, all these light–tissue interactions provide information about tissue biochemical composition and structure (architecture) and can be used in tissue discrimination. The great majority of the available optical diagnostic systems for dentistry are based on the detection of fluorescence because fluorescence is sensitive to the changes in biochemical composition that occur during malignant development, as well as in other pathological conditions. Structural changes that occur with cancer progression also modify the tissue fluorescence. As a result, the fluorescence emission from a normal oral mucosa is distinct from that from an oral cancer.

The most important biological fluorophores involved with malignant progression are coenzyme nicotinamide adenine dinucleotide (NADH), flavin adenine dinucleotide (FAD), collagen, elastin, and porphyrin. NADH and FAD are molecules involved in important metabolic reactions, and their relative concentrations provide information concerning the metabolic

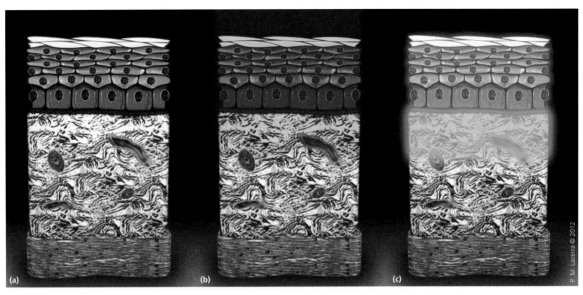

Figure 39.2 Schematic of the optical paths for fluorescence of normal mucosa: (a) Normal mucosa histology; (b) illumination with violet excitation; (c) fluorescence (image created by P.M. Lacerra (2012). Provided by Kurachi).

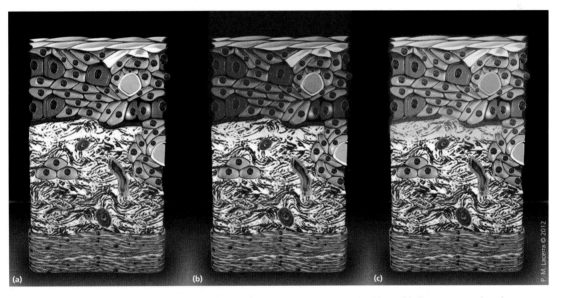

Figure 39.3 Schematic of the optical steps for fluorescence from oral carcinoma: (a) Carcinoma histology; (b) illumination with violet excitation; (c) fluorescence (image created by P.M. Lacerra (2012). Provided by Kurachi).

status of the tissue. Collagen and elastin are structural proteins that are destroyed during carcinoma invasion into deeper tissue layers. When these proteins are destroyed, they stop emitting fluorescence. Porphyrin has higher concentration in malignant cells compared to normal oral epithelium.

The most commonly observed fluorescence behavior related to cancer detection is decreased green emission, due to the diminished collagen emission around 520 nm, and increased red emission around 630 nm, as a result of a higher porphyrin concentration. The main analysis in reported studies of oral cancer is based on the red/green emission rate.

Biological molecules absorb light in the ultraviolet–violet spectrum with higher efficiency, so the available optical systems use light in the spectral region of 380–450 nm for tissue excitation.

Figures 39.2 and 39.3 show the optical paths taken occur at the tissue level for normal and cancer oral mucosa, respectively. Normal epithelium of the oral mucosa is composed of organized layers of epithelial cells, covered by keratin in the keratinized mucosa (Fig. 39.2a). If normal epithelium is illuminated at the surface with a violet light (Fig. 39.2b), all the light–tissue interactions described above take place. Some part of the energy is absorbed by the fluorophores in the optical path, and these re-emit light as fluorescence. The most important fluorophores in the oral mucosa, when excited by light in the violet spectrum, emit light in the green spectrum (Fig. 39.2c). In epithelial cells, the main fluorophore that is excited by light in the violet spectrum is NADH, and in the stroma is collagen. Collagen is the molecule that mainly contributes for the final fluorescence by mucosal cells. The photons of the fluorescence must penetrate the tissue and can be absorbed or undergo multiple scattering before exiting the mucosal surface. Another important fluorophore in the oral mucosa is keratin, which emits an intense green fluorescence.

In comparison to the normal mucosa, oral carcinoma has a disorganized epithelium, increased number of cell layers, and disruption of the collagen cross-links (Fig. 39.3a). These tissue changes, after surface illumination with violet light (Fig. 39.3b), result in decreased green fluorescence (Fig. 39.3c). The increased number of layers enhances the tissue thickness and fewer excitation photons reach the stromal layer, so fewer collagen molecules are excited and emit fluorescence. As a result, fluorescence from a carcinoma shows decreased green fluorescence when compared to normal oral mucosa.

If the mucosa is covered by a thick layer of keratin, the fluorescence will be intense, but the epithelial and stromal layers will not be excited. A false-negative result for carcinoma detection using fluorescence can therefore result if the carcinoma lies beneath this thick keratin layer.

A decreased green fluorescence as a result of an inflammatory benign disorder may lead to a false-positive response in cancer diagnosis. In these inflammatory conditions, an increased microvasculature results in a higher concentration of hemoglobin, enhanced absorption of the excitation light, and increase in fluorescent photons. The final fluorescence collected at the tissue surface will be lower, but in this case is due to a higher absorption and not to decreased collagen fluorescence.

All these factors must be evaluated when using fluorescence diagnostics. No optical technique will be valid for diagnosis without an understanding of the affect of the histological and macroscopic tissue features on light–tissue interactions. The clinician must apply the optical techniques as an auxiliary tool to all the other usual procedures. The advantages of the optical techniques are their objectivity, fast response, as well as being non-invasive procedures.

Optical techniques can be classified into imaging and spectroscopy modalities. The first of these gives a result that can be at the macroscopic or microscopic levels.

Imaging techniques for diagnosis of oral cavity malignancies

Reflectance imaging

Imaging performed with conventional white light (WL) reflectance can be easily improved by selectively focusing on a single feature of the tissue. The images obtained are a superimposition of all the chromatic components of the light reflected by the surface of the sample and the light that has experienced multiple scattering and absorption deep inside the tissue. One way to selectively look at a single feature of the tissue is to use one specific wavelength, by placing a narrow band filter after the WL source emission and before the tissue illumination. For example, the absorption of a specific molecule, such as hemoglobin, can be targeted.[3] In this case, the clinical feature that will be selected is the tissue vasculature. This technique is usually referred to as *narrow band imaging* (NBI).

Another method uses polarized illumination and detection. When reflected from a surface, the polarity of the incident light is preserved, whereas when it is scattered by tissue this polarization is lost. Therefore, using polarized illumination and detection of the reflectance, it is possible to discriminate between light originating from the surface (specular reflectance) – by selectively detecting reflected photons that have the same polarization as the incident light, and light originating from the deeper layers of the tissue (diffuse reflectance) by selectively detecting photons with orthogonal polarization.[4] This technique is referred to as *polarization reflectance imaging*.

The main application of polarization reflectance imaging is to enhance the vessel pattern of the tissue under investigation. The vessel pattern plays an important role in revealing angiogenesis in suspicious areas and may help to discriminate cancer lesions from a false-positive response arising from inflammatory tissue, as has been demonstrated in bladder[5] and colon.[6] Lindeboom et al. used orthogonal polarization reflectance imaging (OPS) to characterize the microcirculatory changes in tongue squamous cell carcinoma (SCC) compared to the normal contralateral side.[7] Using orthogonal polarization detection, with respect to the incident light, the authors were able to achieve better visualization of the vessel pattern beneath the tissue surface. For SCC, dilated and disorganized vessels accompanied by hemorrhagic areas were observed, while the normal contralateral tissue showed no abnormal capillaries or any vessel disarrangement. In another study, Basiri et al. used polarized reflectance imaging to diagnose familial adenomatous polyposis by looking at the vasculature of the oral mucosa, with a sensitivity and specificity of 90.9% and 90.0%, respectively.[8]

Roblyer et al. developed a new set-up that can perform both imaging modalities, narrow band and polarization reflectance.[9,10] A simplified schematic of a system that combines OPS with NBI is shown in Figure 39.4. In their study, Roblyer et al. used OPS, NBI, and fluorescence imaging. Five different types of tissue were investigated: a normal labial mucosa of a healthy volunteer, a leukoplakia at the right gingiva, a leukoplakia at the tongue with confirmed moderate dysplasia, an erythroplakia of the tongue with confirmed severe dysplasia, and a cancer of the lateral tongue. The wavelengths chosen for NBI were 420, 430, 530, and 600 nm as these matched the hemoglobin absorption peaks. Using distinct excitation wavelengths, it was possible to interrogate different tissue depths, since the higher wavelengths penetrate tissue more deeply. Therefore, 420-nm (blue) light

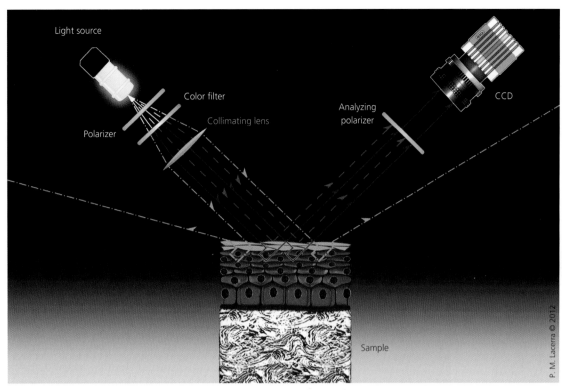

Figure 39.4 System combining OPS and NBI. White light is first polarized. A narrow band filter is used to select the wavelength range of illumination. Reflectance and scattering will occur in the tissue. Specularly reflected photons maintain the incident polarization and, hence, are blocked by the second polarizer to give an orthogonal polarization with respect to the polarization of the incident light. Therefore, only the photons that have lost their initial polarization, that is the ones that suffer multiple scattering and are diffusely reflected at the surface, are detected by the CCD (image created by P.M. Lacerra (2012). Provided by Kurachi).

should probe mainly the superficial layers, while 600-nm (red) light should probe greater depths. Compared to NBI, conventional WL inspection cannot differentiate the vasculature in the more superficial layers from that in the deeper tissue layers. The contrast between the microcirculation patterns is increased using NBI when the wavelengths used match the hemoglobin absorption peak. On the other hand, OPS imaging was found to be helpful in examining leukoplakias. Detection of only the orthogonal component allowed the contribution of the whitish superficial layer to be partly removed; this otherwise would mask important morphological information from the layers beneath.

Reflectance imaging techniques such as OPS and NBI have been shown to enhance the evaluation of the microvasculature evaluation and discriminate between vessels at different depths, providing new important morphological information for lesion assessment.

Fluorescence imaging

Typical WL inspection or reflectance imaging techniques such as NBI and OPS can only give information about tissue reflectance/scattering and absorption features. Besides tissue morphology, an important aspect of the lesion fingerprint arises from its biochemical composition. Under ultraviolet (UV) light

excitation, most tissue chemical components absorb light and re-emit this absorbed energy as an electromagnetic wave, that is they emit a photon. These molecules are referred to as fluorophores. As already mentioned, typical fluorophores in biological tissues are NADH and FAD in epithelial cells and elastin and collagen in the stroma. Each fluorophore has its own characteristic absorption and emission spectra, which influence the fluorescence signal exiting from a tissue. As is the case with reflectance imaging, fluorescence is dependent on the tissue's scattering and absorption properties when transmitting both excitation and fluorescence light. Therefore, fluorescence imaging can provide information on both the biochemical and morphological composition of the tissue.[11,12]

A schematic of a fluorescence imaging set-up is shown in Figure 39.5. Fluorescence imaging uses safe UV–blue light to illuminate the oral cavity. Light penetrates inside the tissue, exciting endogenous fluorophores present in the epithelium and stroma. Re-emitted fluorescence photons travel inside the bulk tissue and may exit the tissue surface. Only these latter photons can be detected by a charge-coupled device (CCD) camera placed near the patient. A longpass filter is placed in front of the camera to block scattered excitation photons. Without this filter, the image would be formed only by the scattered excitation photons, since this light–tissue interaction is much more intense

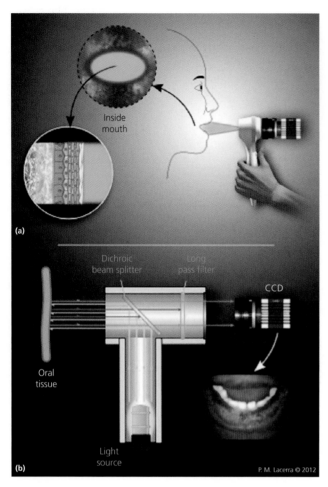

Inside
mouth

(a)

Dichroic
beam splitter

Long
pass filter

CCD

Oral
tissue

Light
source

(b)

P. M. Lacerra © 2012

Figure 39.5 A fluorescence imaging system. (a) A handheld device coupled to a CCD is used for illumination and detection of native tissue fluorescence. (b) This device is composed of a dichroic beam splitter that reflects the excitation light and directs it to the tissue. Re-emitted tissue fluorescence is transmitted by the dichroic mirror and reaches the camera. A longpass filter is placed in front of the CCD for additional blocking of the excitation light (image created by P.M. Lacerra (2012). Provided by Kurachi).

than the induced native tissue fluorescence. Red–green–blue (RGB) images are obtained by placing a Bayer filter mask on the detector.

The spectral information in the widefield image is reduced to three scalar values. This imaging modality provides two-dimensional (2D) biomorphological information: homogeneity, relative fluorescence intensity, distribution pattern for each of the RGB colors. Typical fields of view are of the order of several square centimeters,[9,10] making this modality more suitable for cancer screening than endomicroscopy or fluorescence spectroscopy, which usually provides information for just a few square millimeters.

From a clinical point of view, the widefield fluorescence pattern of the cancer and potentially malignant lesions appears as a dark-brownish area, while healthy tissue shows a pale green

retained fluorescence.[10,13–17] Usually, a contralateral normal tissue, chosen by an expert clinician, is imaged to provide a reference standard. Different studies have attempted to explain the origin of native fluorescence in oral tissue. In two recent studies, Pavlova et al. related the lack of native fluorescence in neoplasia to a loosening of collagen cross-links as a result of cancer cell proliferation inside the connective tissue.[11,12] Typically, loss of native fluorescence in a potentially malignant lesion is accompanied by an increase in red fluorescence, which probably originates from porphyrins.[18]

An important issue in cancer diagnosis is the correct determination of the lesion border in order to avoid only partial removal and reduce cancer recurrence after surgery. For this reason, an extended margin of clinically healthy tissue needs to be defined by the surgeon. Compared to normal WL inspection, better visual contrast between healthy and potentially malignant tissue was achieved by means of fluorescence imaging.[9,14,16,17] Poh et al. observed a loss of fluorescence up to 25 mm away from the detected WL border.[16] Histopathology analysis confirmed the presence of a dysplastic lesion. The dysplasia usually was not isotropically distributed around the lesion, confirming that a safe margin of 10 mm does not ensure total lesion removal. To emphasize the importance of this finding, in a subsequent study Poh et al. screened the recurrence of dysplasia after surgical removal of oral lesions guided by fluorescence imaging. There were no recurrences, compared to a 25% recurrence rate in the control group for whom only WL guidance was used.[19] Fluorescence imaging was also shown to give a higher detection rate for potentially malignant lesion in a study by Paczona et al.[20] In the same study, fluorescence imaging was also shown to be able to reveal occult lesions not detected on normal WL inspection.

The promising results for the clinical assessment by means of fluorescence imaging lead to the development of commercial devices such as VELscope (LED Dental Inc., Burnaby, BC, Canada) and Identafi3000 (DentalEz, Malvern, PA, USA).[21–24] The US Food and Drug Administration (FDA) approved both devices for autofluorescence-based oral mucosal screening. The accessibility of fluorescence imaging devices to hospitals and clinics not necessarily involved in technology development may result in research in low prevalence populations. Indeed, it should be pointed out that most of the clinical studies on the efficacy of fluorescence imaging described above were limited to case reports. When studies are performed in populations with a low cancer prevalence, both specificity and sensitivity decrease. False-positive results are generally ascribed to inflammatory lesions in which epithelium thickening and blood from a trauma can attenuate stroma fluorescence.[14] On the other hand, intense hyperkeratosis produces a bright superficial fluorescence that can mask the presence of a potentially malignant lesion beneath, leading to a false-negative result.[20]

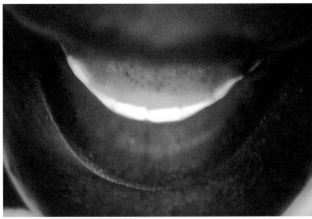

(a)

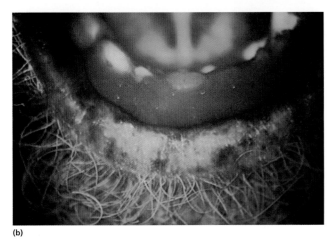

(b)

Figure 39.6 Fluorescence widefield images of (a) the lower lip of a healthy volunteer and (b) of a patient with actinic cheilitis. The normal lip shows a more uniform native fluorescence and the actinic cheilitis lip shows a non-homogenous pattern. It is possible to discriminate areas with high keratinization and areas with loss of fluorescence (b) (courtesy of Drs A. Takahama Jr and R. Azevedo).

From a microscopic point of view, the loss of fluorescence in inflammatory tissue is due to a decrease in fluorescence from epithelial cells and a thickening of the epithelium, which decreases the collection of the signal originating from elastin and collagen within the connective tissue. Cancer epithelial cells are more fluorescent, but there is still a loss of fluorescence due to the weakening of collagen cross-link.[11,12] Collagen is the main contributor to the native fluorescence of the oral mucosa, so when there is no or less emission from this biomolecule, the overall result is a decreased green fluorescence.

The use of digital cameras, and consequently the acquisition of digital data, allows the implementation of an algorithm that scores cancer and potentially malignant lesions.[9,17] The importance of developing computational algorithms relies on the possibility of assessing lesion independently of the level of operator training and experience. Roblyer et al. developed an algorithm in which the ratio of green to red intensity value was used to reveal diseased areas in the oral cavity.[17] The algorithm was based on increase in red fluorescence and loss of green fluorescence inside the lesion area. Using this algorithm, the authors were able to discriminate normal tissue from dysplasia and invasive cancer with 100% sensitivity and 91.4% specificity. These good results lead them to produce a merged image with mapped pixel values indicating greater than 50% risk of the presence of dysplasia/cancer superimposed on the normal WL image, in order to help the surgeon with lesion resection.

As discussed above, fluorescence imaging is a new promising tool in lesion diagnosis, enhancing both discrimination of lesion borders and detection of the initial lesion. Typical sensitivity and specificity are in the order of 90–100% in high cancer prevalence populations, shifting to lower values for low prevalence populations. At the moment, two different devices for fluorescence imaging have already been approved by the US FDA and commercialized. In the future, a lowering of the price of the individual components of the devices, such as the light emitting diode (LED) and CCD, could make this technique cheaper and more accessible.[25]

Figure 39.6 shows fluorescence images of the lower lip from a healthy volunteer and from a patient with actinic cheilitis. It is possible to observe that the healthy lip shows a higher homogeneity in the fluorescence intensity, and in actinic cheilitis it is possible to recognize areas with loss of fluorescence due to epithelium thickening as well areas of hyperkeratinization.

Optical coherence tomography

Biochemical changes inside the malignant lesion are strongly characterized by a peculiar morphology in which neoplastic cells infiltrate the stroma. This disrupts the typical structural layers of the oral mucosa, epithelium, and lamina propria. This feature becomes more evident with lesion progression. On the other hand, inflammation does not interfere with stromal integrity. As already discussed, fluorescence widefield imaging does not easily distinguish the loss of fluorescence caused by epithelium thickening due to inflammation or dysplasia from that caused by collagen cross-link disruption due to cancer cell infiltration.[11,12] Also, an intensely keratinized superficial layer can mask a dysplasia beneath.[20] Therefore, a technique that could resolve, with a precision of the order of tens of micrometers, the different layers of the oral mucosa could give a fingerprint for tissue pathology.[26]

For 20 years a tomography technique based on infrared light has been used as an auxiliary tool for oral lesion diagnosis. This technique uses the same principle as a Michelson interferometer for imaging the different layers inside the tissue. In this system, light is divided into two different paths by a beam splitter (BS). The two beams are back reflected by two mirrors, merge once again at the BS point, and are sent to a detector. If the difference in the pathlength (ΔL) of the two beams is a multiple of the

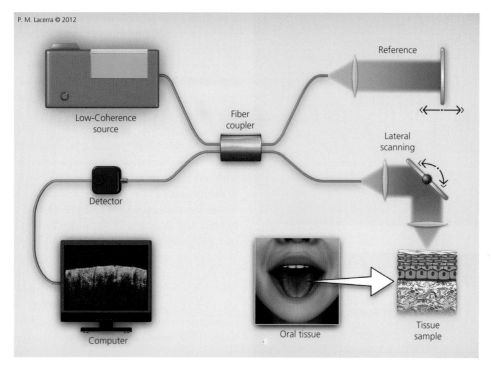

P. M. Lacerra © 2012

Figure 39.7 Schematic of an OCT system. Light from a low-coherence source is sent to a fiber coupler that splits it into two branches. Part of the light is sent to a reference scanning mirror, while the other part is delivered to the sample. A lateral scanning beam is used for lateral scanning. Light from the two branches is mixed once again in the fiber coupler and sent to the detector. The signal from the detector is acquired by the computer to provide a 2D reconstruction of the tissue (image created by P.M. Lacerra (2012). Provided by Kurachi).

photon wavelength (λ), the interference between the two beams will be constructive, leading to an increase in the signal, and vice versa.

In OCT, one mirror is replaced by the tissue, in which every layer is characterized by its own refractive index. The change of refractive index between layers acts as a mirror and partially reflects the light. The photon pathlength and reflectance are dependent on the wavelength. Hence, the interference pattern is dependent on the photon wavelength and the layer's refractive index and scattering properties. A typical OCT system is shown in Figure 39.7. A superluminescent diode in the near infrared range (830–1300 nm) with a bandwidth of 30–50 nm is used as a light source. By scanning the reference arm length and detecting the interference pattern, it is possible to reconstruct the structure and the width of each layer of the tissue. Technically, this scan is referred as an A-Scan, and it represents a vertical section through the tissue.

In order to produce an image of a 2D section of the tissue, a scanning mirror is placed at the tip of the proximal end, related to the light source. With this technique, usually referred to as a B-Scan, it is possible to reconstruct a complete transverse section of the tissue that resembles the vertical sections visible in histology. Compared to histology, OCT has almost the same axial resolution (5–10 μm) and has the advantage of being free of the distortion introduced by fixation.

Examples of OCT images are shown in Figure 39.8. It is possible to recognize the different layers of the tissue investigated: a keratinized epithelial layer, the epithelium, the basement membrane, and the submucosa. The keratinized epithelial layer and the lamina propria are characterized by a strong signal due to the high scattering from keratinized cells and collagen, while the epithelial layer is usually more transparent due to its low optical density. Dark areas could also indicate other structures such as salivary glands,[27] ducts,[28] and blood vessels. More generally, OCT resolution and definition is strongly dependent on the area of the tissue interrogated.[27]

Typical scan lengths and depths of commercial devices are in the order of 10 mm and 2 mm, respectively. B-Scan acquisition time is in the range of 1–20 seconds. New techniques, referred to as Fourier domain and involving sweep laser sources or a spectrometer as the detector, are providing faster imaging acquisition of up to 10 frames per second.[29] In comparison, techniques such as positron emission tomography, magnetic resonance imaging, and ultrasound show a lower resolution (0.5–1 mm) and a longer acquisition time.

When OCT is used for oral cancer diagnosis, the main features to take into account are grade of keranitization, epithelial thickening, epithelial irregular stratification, epithelial proliferation/down growth, and basal hyperplasia.[30] Since changes occur in oral cancer lesions with respect to normal tissue, an

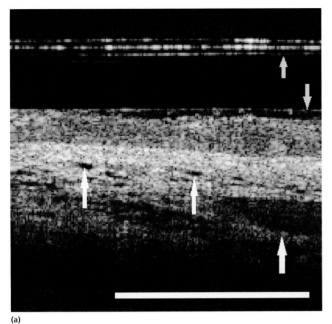
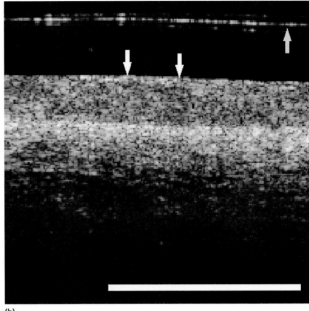

(a) (b)

Figure 39.8 OCT images of (a) a healthy lower lip mucosa and (b) a left buccal mucosa. The epithelial layer and the lamina propria beneath are clearly distinguishable in the two images. The white arrows indicate salivary glands and blood vessels in (a) and the hyperkeratinized superficial layer in (b). The yellow arrows indicate artificial effects due to the protection cup of the fiber tip. Images acquired using Niris from Imalux (Cleveland, OH, USA). Scale bar 1 mm.

additional OCT image is taken from the healthy tissue close to the lesion for comparison.

In mild to severe dysplasia and CIS progression, the epithelial layer will still appear well defined and separated from the connective tissue beneath, but it is usually thicker than normal.[31] In a histological study of larynx biopsies, the epithelial thickening was found to be of a factor of 2 in moderate dysplasia and up to a factor of 3 in CIS,[32] compared to the typical epithelium thickness of different areas inside the oral cavity of healthy volunteer.[33]

In cases of early-stage and well-developed squamous cell carcinoma (SCC), the boundaries between the epithelial layer and the lamina propria and their architecture are disrupted. This peculiar feature is extremely useful in identifying lesion boarders between areas that are clearly stratified and those that are disorganized and in which layers are no longer clearly distinguishable. Another indicator of SCC is a highly heterogeneous appearance of the epithelial layer due to presence of cancer cell nests.[34] Malignancy is also highlighted by the presence of connective tissue papilla (CTP).[31] Early-stage SCC (ES-SCC) is characterized by a high density of CTP, which decreases with cancer progression.

Clinical assessment of oral cavity lesions by OCT has been successfully demonstrated. In a preliminary study involving 50 patients, Wilder-Smith et al. performed OCT immediately after clinical examination. Two blinded, specially trained clinicians diagnosed each lesion based on the OCT images and their features before histopathology analysis.[30] An agreement with the histopathology was observed for 89.6% of lesions, with

a sensitivity and specificity in discriminate SCC versus non-malignant lesions of 93.1% and 93.1%, respectively. Kraft et al., in a prospective study of 193 patients with suspicious larynx lesions, compared the sensitivity and specificity of microlaringoscopy alone and combined with OCT, and found a higher sensitivity with the latter (66%) compared to the former (78%).[35] One of the main limitations of the OCT technique is the need for a trained clinician for a correct diagnosis. Indeed, assessment by OCT is still highly operator dependent.

To achieve a quantitative result and diagnosis by means of OCT images, Tsai et al. developed different imaging parameters[31,34] that could be related to tissue pathology. The evaluation of epithelial thickness could be used as an indicator of the presence of epithelial hyperplasia or moderate dysplasia. They also observed that a high standard deviation of the A-Scan along the epithelial layer highlights the heterogeneity of cell organization, giving a fingerprint for cancer cell nests. The presence of CTP and their density could be scored by looking at the standard deviation of pixel values along a line parallel to the surface at a depth of 350 μm. A high variability indicates high density, hence ES-SCC. On the other hand, a low variability suggests low CTP density and therefore a higher cancer stage. Tsai et al. also observed a higher axial light attenuation in WD-SCC, probably due to the presence of blood capillaries. For this reason, they suggested the exponential decay constant of the average A-scan intensity profile as a parameter to distinguish between well-differentiated (WD)-SCC and ES-SCC.[31]

By using an optical fiber for light delivery, it is possible to make small, compact, and flexible devices. First clinical trials with these have obtained high values for both specificity and sensitivity. One of the main limitations of OCT is its small field of view of just few millimeters, depending on where the clinician decides to place the probe for tissue interrogation. As a result, a cancer can still be misdiagnosed if the probe is not positioned at the right place, as in the punch biopsy procedure. OCT is suited to being coupled to the widefield imaging techniques, such as fluorescence imaging.

Oral tissue microendoscopy

All the imaging techniques described above generally give macroscopic biomorphological information about the tissue. With OCT it is possible to obtain a transverse section that visualizes the tissue layers and their thickness and integrity limits. Cell morphology and nuclear-to-cytoplasmic ratio are well-demonstrated features and provide a powerful fingerprint of tissue malignancy. The main problem with fluorescence widefield imaging is the false-positive results from inflammatory tissue conditions and epithelium thickness.

In the last decade new microscopic *in vivo* techniques for tissue imaging with subcellular resolution have been introduced.[36,37] These techniques use an optical fiber bundle to deliver the light to the tissue. Light can be delivered by a single fiber with a scanning system on the tip[38] or by a special coherent bundle.[37,39,40] In the latter case, each fiber at the proximal end preserves its position at the distal end of the bundle. Systems using a coherent bundle are simple, compact, and low cost.[37]

The optical set-up of a fluorescence microendoscopy system is similar to that used in fluorescence widefield imaging, but with a different fiber bundle and a magnifying objective. The UV–blue light from a source is reflected by a dichroic BS and sent to the fiber bundle using a microscope objective. Light passes through the fibers and reaches the sample. The fluorescence signal is then collected by the same bundle, enters the objective, and passes through the dichroic BS to reach the CDD. A further lens is introduced into the fluorescence optical path in order to give the optimal magnification for the CCD dimensions.[37] The field of view depends on the size of the CCD, which can be up to 1.4 mm. Resolution is in the range of 4–5 µm and depends on fiber size and spacing. With small optical modification, it is possible to transform a fluorescence microendoscope into a reflectance one.[40] The dichroic mirror should be replaced by a 50% BS and two cross-polarized mirrors should be placed in front of the light source and the CCD in a set-up similar to that for OPS.

Unfortunately, the autofluorescence signal from the cells is not strong enough to produce an image with a good signal-to-noise ratio. Therefore, an external fluorophore, acriflavine, should be topically applied. This dye shows affinity for cell nuclei and as a result, the nuclei appear as brilliant structures.

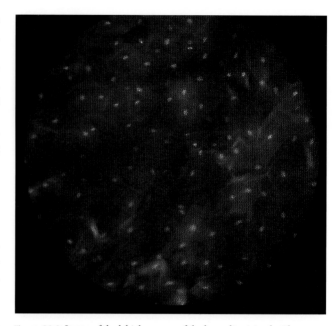

Figure 39.9 Image of the labial mucosa of the lower lip stained with proflavine, acquired using a microendoscope equipped with a coherent bundle, as described by Muldoon et al.[37] The cell nuclei and morphology are clearly distinguishable.

In vivo imaging by microendoscopy has been demonstrated.[37] An *in vivo* image of human labial mucosa, obtained using a microendoscope developed by Muldoon et al.,[37] is shown in Figure 39.9.

The first clinical study on *ex vivo* samples was performed using 150 unique sites from fresh biopsies of 13 patients with confirmed SCC.[39] Two different types of evaluation were used. The first evaluation was accomplished by three observers with long experience in head and neck pathology. Observers were trained by analysis of five microendoscope images for both normal and neoplastic tissues. Images that were out of focus or showed motion artifact were discarded. After training, each observer classified images according to a 5-point scale: 1 for "normal tissue" to 5 for "surely neoplastic." A receiver operator characteristic (ROC) curve was realized, with the threshold varying from 1 to 5. Values for the area under the curve ranged between 0.89 and 0.96.

The second method was based on computational algorithms. For each image, two different parameters were scored: the image entropy, defined as the randomness of pixel values, and the nuclear-to-cytoplasmic ratio. To the 2D scatter plot obtained, a five-fold cross-validation algorithm was applied. The values obtained for sensitivity and specificity were 81% and 77%, respectively. The advantage of using computational algorithms relies on the fact that the result is completely independent of clinician training and expertise.

Microendoscopy has been shown to be a highly promising tool for oral cancer diagnosis, but there are still some limitations. The fiber bundle has to be placed in direct contact with the tissue; therefore, images can only be obtained for the superficial layer. This problem can be solved by optical sectioning or by mechanical bundle penetration by means of a 16-gauge hypodermic needle. Another problem is the small field of view, of just 1.4 mm in the best cases. This means that microendoscopy is not a suitable standalone technique, but must be coupled with a widefield technique. The combination of these techniques could be a promising protocol for oral cancer assessment in which fluorescence imaging could be used for oral screening, while microendoscopy could be used to inspect a suspicious area in order to rule out false-positive results.

Spectroscopy techniques for diagnosis of oral cavity malignancies

Optical spectroscopy refers to the study of the interaction between light and matter and has its origins in the observation of visible light dispersion by a prism. Nowadays the concept of spectroscopy comprises the measurement of radiation intensity as a function of wavelength (λ) or wavenumber (κ), and these quantities are related to each other by the equation:

$$\kappa = 2\pi/\lambda$$

Our knowledge about the structure of atoms and molecules mainly comes from investigations based on spectroscopy. Thus, spectroscopy has made a noticeable contribution to the present state of atomic and molecular physics, chemistry, and molecular biology. The basic devices used for spectroscopic studies are usually called spectrometers, spectrophotometers, or spectrographs.

The value of optical spectroscopy in detecting disease has been known for decades. Spectroscopy techniques can detect biochemical changes in tissue and depending on the technology used to perform tissue evaluation, this can be with high sensitivity and specificity.

The possibility of *in vivo* and real-time spectroscopy measurements relies on the fact that light can be delivered and collected by optical fibers, which can be placed in contact with a tissue surface or inserted into tissues using catheters, needles, and endoscopes.

The main optical spectroscopy techniques used to date for oral cancer diagnosis are fluorescence and Raman spectroscopy.

Fluorescence spectroscopy

Fluorescence spectroscopy is a powerful technique that may identify different molecules. Fluorescence is related to light absorption and results from an electronic transition from the excited state to the ground state of a molecule. Each molecule has a specific emission spectrum and any change in the molecule can, in principle, be detected by changes in the fluorescence spectrum, which depends on the excitation light that is used. Since biological tissues consist of a combination of several different biomolecules, the fluorescence spectrum of a tissue is a combination of the emission spectrum of each of these molecules.

In comparison to the imaging modalities, spectroscopy produces a spectral graph. The fluorescence spectrum is presented as a relative intensity for each emitted wavelength.

The shape of the autofluorescence spectrum of a tissue depends on the presence and quantity of fluorophore, but it is altered by absorption and scattering events. The presence of disease changes the concentration of the fluorophores as well as light scattering and absorption properties of the tissue, due to changes in blood oxygen concentration, nuclear size distribution, collagen content, and epithelial thickness.[41] The fluorescence of collagen and elastin, for example, can be used to distinguish tissues and their pathology, like epithelial and connective tissues.[1]

The possibility of using fluorescence spectroscopy as a technique for non-invasive, real-time, and early detection of oral cancer has been widely explored. In 1998, Gillenwater et al. reported the findings of a clinical study where fluorescence spectroscopy was used to distinguish oral lesions from normal tissue.[42] The excitation wavelength was varied between 337, 364, and 410 nm and the fluorescence emission was acquired between 350 and 700 nm. A decrease in the overall fluorescence spectra of neoplastic and dysplastic tissue was observed. Analysis using peak intensities, spectral line shape, and algorithms was performed and pointed to significant differences in the spectra from normal, dysplastic, and malignant mucosa, and also showed that a better discrimination between normal and abnormal tissue was obtained when using 337 nm and 410 nm as the excitation wavelengths. This study suggested that fluorescence spectroscopy has the potential to improve non-invasive diagnosis of oral cavity neoplasia.

Betz et al. also observed a decrease in the fluorescence intensity when comparing normal and malignant oral mucosa in patients.[43] They used both fluorescence imaging and spectroscopy and measured a reduction of the green autofluorescence at the lesion site in patients. The spectral analysis showed contrasting autofluorescence intensities between tumor and normal tissues in 94.4% of the patients.

Another interesting behavior of the fluorescence spectra of oral cancer was reported in 1999 by Inaguma and Hashimoto.[18] They evaluated 78 oral carcinomas in patients and observed porphyrin-like red fluorescence in 85% of them. The porphyrin-like fluorescent compounds were extracted from the carcinomas and evaluated, showing that, in some cases, a mixture of porphyrins is present in the lesions. The authors suggested the use of this red fluorescence as a criterion for oral cancer optical diagnosis.

Fluorescence can also be used in conjunction with other types of spectroscopy techniques, as described by Muller

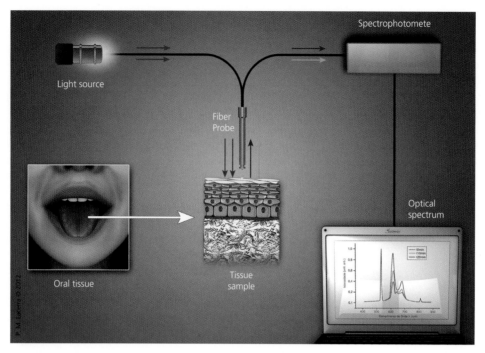

Figure 39.10 Schematic of the set-up of a fluorescence spectroscopy system (image created by P.M. Lacerra (2012). Provided by Kurachi).

et al.[44] These authors correlated biochemical and histological changes in the oral tissue with fluorescence, reflectance, and scattering spectra, introducing an approach called trimodal spectroscopy (TMS). Reflectance and fluorescence spectra were collected from 53 sites in 15 patients with known malignancies, and from 38 sites in eight healthy volunteers. In contrast to the findings of Inaguma and Hashimoto, Muller et al. observed red fluorescence not only in malignant lesions, but also in some oral cavity sites of healthy volunteers, which they suggested was due to bacteria that also produce protoporphyrin IX. With the TMS technique, the authors were able to distinguish cancerous/dysplastic from normal tissue with 96% sensitivity and specificity, and also to discriminate cancerous from dysplastic tissue with 64% sensitivity and 90% specificity.

De Veld et al. combined fluorescence with another optical technique, diffuse reflectance spectroscopy, and evaluated the performance of both spectroscopies in the diagnosis of oral cancer.[45] They evaluated the spectra of 172 lesions and 72 sites in healthy volunteers and compared the techniques individually and combined. When combined, the diffuse reflectance was used to correct the fluorescence spectra for blood absorption. The results showed similar results for raw and corrected autofluorescence, as well as for diffuse reflectance spectra. Their findings also implied that blood absorption and scattering effects are efficient at distinguishing cancerous from normal mucosa. A slight improvement was observed when the two spectroscopy techniques were combined; however, the authors concluded that although lesions of oral mucosa

could be reliably distinguished from healthy mucosa, it was not possible to classify lesion type.

A depth-sensitive optical spectroscopy system was used by Schwarz et al. on oral lesions and normal volunteers, and differences were obtained when comparing autofluorescence and diffuse reflectance of neoplastic versus non-neoplastic sites, keratinized versus non-keratinized tissue, and shallow versus deeper oral tissue.[46] This type of system has four probe channels capable of collecting spectral responses from different tissue depths. One of the channels interrogates the epithelial layer, another both the epithelium and shallow stroma, and the other two primarily the stroma. A loss of fluorescence was once again observed for neoplastic tissue. For non-keratinized oral sites, the sensitivity and specificity were comparable to those achieved with clinical diagnosis by expert observers. This depth-sensitive optical spectroscopy system may be a useful tool in the oral screening examination when performed by a healthcare worker rather than an expert clinical observer.

More recently, Francisco described a study using fluorescence spectroscopy aimed at discriminating oral cavity neoplasia from normal oral tissue[47]; 150 subjects were evaluated, 30 subjects with potentially malignant lesions (leukoplakia and erythroplakia), 50 with neoplasia (confirmed by histology), and 65 normal volunteers. The fluorescence spectra were acquired using 405 nm and 532 nm as the excitation wavelengths. Figure 39.10 shows the optical set-up of the system used in this study, which represents the basic instrumentation used for fluorescence spectroscopy studies.

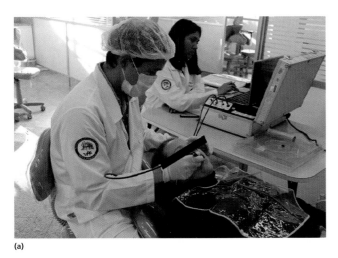

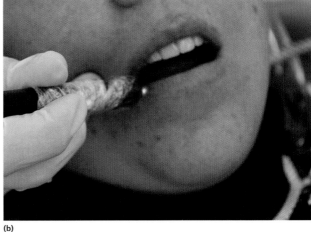

(a)

(b)

Figure 39.11 (a) Fluorescence spectroscopy system and (b) a patient interrogation procedure.

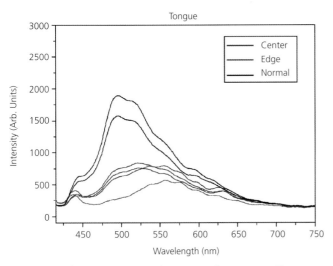

Figure 39.12 Fluorescence spectra of a patient with squamous cell carcinoma of the tongue. The black lines show the fluorescence spectra from the normal contralateral site; the blue lines show the fluorescence spectra from the center of the lesion; and the red lines show the fluorescence spectra from the lesion edges (clinically detected borders). Adapted from Francisco.[47]

This optical system is based on a fiber-optic probe that delivers the excitation light from a laser source to the tissue and also collects the fluorescent emission from the tissue, which is then detected by a spectrometer. Such a system allows fluorescence to be measured non-invasively. The probe tip is placed in direct contact with the tissue surface and the fluorescence spectrum is quickly acquired (Fig. 39.11). The graph shown in Figure 39.12 is an example of the spectral data collected from a patient with an SCC of the tongue. Each line represents the fluorescence spectrum at one interrogated tissue site. It is possible to observe that the shape of the fluorescence spectra differ for normal and malignant tissues. Principal component analysis (PCA) was used to discriminate normal tissue from oral cavity neoplasia. The results showed that fluorescence spectroscopy can discriminate normal tissue from carcinoma, but there is an important variance when considering the anatomical sites.

While fluorescence spectroscopy seems to be a powerful tool for the discrimination between cancerous and normal tissues, a large variation in autofluorescence spectra is often seen, complicating the diagnosis of lesions. Therefore, care needs to be taken with data analysis, because it has been shown that individual characteristics may affect the autofluorescence spectra of healthy oral mucosa. Factors like gender, alcohol consumption, tobacco consumption, wearing of dentures, and importantly skin color may affect the fluorescence emission by tissue.[48] Also, for oral cavity interrogation, the fluorescence spectrum will be affected if the patient has consumed drink or food containing a dye just before optical evaluation.

Raman spectroscopy

Raman spectroscopy is a vibrational spectroscopic technique, that is it uses light to excite vibrational energy states in molecules to get information about the molecular composition, structure, and their interactions in a sample.

Raman spectroscopy is based on Raman scattering, an event that happens when light interacts with a molecule and a small amount of energy is transferred from the photon to the molecule (or vice versa), leading to an excitation of the molecule from its lowest vibrational energy level to a higher one, and causing a shift (usually expressed in wavenumbers) between the incident and scattered photon.[1] The Raman spectra show the scattered light intensity as a function of the energy difference between the incident and scattered photons.

Raman spectroscopy has low sensitivity when compared with infrared spectroscopy or fluorescence spectroscopy because of the relatively low efficiency of Raman scattering. The Raman signals are many orders of magnitude lower that fluorescence signals, which means the fluorescence background overwhelms the Raman bands, limiting the utility of Raman spectroscopy.[2]

Most investigations reported in the literature have used Raman spectroscopy in *ex vivo* specimens obtained by surgical resection. This technique has shown its potential to discriminate between normal, inflammatory, premalignant, and malignant sites in oral cavity tissues.[49] Such discrimination is possible due to differences in the observed Raman bands, which can be attributed to biological compounds such as proteins, lipids, and DNA, as well as to chemical bonds. Variations in the relative intensities, position, and width of the bands are related to the sample composition.[50,51] Complex analysis, like multivariate data analysis, is often used and required to extract the variations in the dataset.

Only a few studies have described the use of Raman spectroscopy *in vivo*. The main reason for this is the fact that the instrumentation for Raman spectroscopy is more complex, less portable, and of higher cost compared to the fluorescence instrumentation. Guze et al. were the first to evaluate the Raman spectra from the oral mucosa of patients to determine if Raman spectra varied for distinct oral mucosal types and to evaluate the clinical applicability or Raman spectroscopy.[52] *In vivo* measurements were taken from 51 human healthy subjects and no clear differences were observed between Asian and Caucasian subgroups. However, in the same ethnic group, significant differences were observed for spectra from different oral sites.

Another *in vivo* study by Bergholt et al. aimed to evaluate differences in normal tissue of oral cavity.[53] They used a system with a 785-nm diode laser as the excitation light source to interrogate the tissue and a fiber-optic Raman probe with a ball lens for maximizing the tissue excitation and collection of the signal. A total of 20 normal healthy subjects were recruited for this study. Data analysis showed that high quality *in vivo* Raman spectra could be acquired from the oral cavity in real time (in about 0.5 seconds) and also that different anatomical sites (hard palate, soft palate, buccal mucosa, inner lip, gingiva, floor of the mouth, and dorsal and ventral tongue) showed variable spectra, indicating the importance of considering the site of investigation in the interpretation of diagnostic algorithms for oral tissue diagnosis and characterization. These results suggest that Raman spectroscopy has the potential to be clinically applied for *in vivo* detection of diseases in the oral cavity, such as oral cancer.

Final considerations

Optical techniques using different light–tissue interactions provide relevant information for cancer diagnosis, concerning the biochemical and structural composition of oral mucosa. Widefield imaging exposes macroscopic surface features, enhancing the visual discrimination of malignant characteristics and lesion borders. Endomicroscopy provides subcellular resolution of morphology similar to histology, such as nuclear-to-cytoplasmic ratio. The information obtained with spectroscopy modalities gives data that may be related to specific fluorophores and absorbers (fluorescence spectroscopy) and to biomolecules such as DNA, proteins, and lipids, or even to specific chemical bonds (Raman spectroscopy).

All this tissue information is quickly obtained through noninvasive and non-destructive procedures. There is less clinician influence on clinical diagnosis when a more objective optical technique is used.

The additional information provided by optical techniques may result in improved resolution and sensitivity for oral cancer diagnosis, but understanding of the light–tissue interactions and the changes induced by cancer development and progression is essential to achieving this.

Optical techniques are relevant auxiliary tools for cancer detection, but must be combined with all the conventional diagnostic procedures.

References

1 Tuchin VV. *Handbook of optical biomedical diagnostics.* Bellingham: SPIE Press, 2002.

2 Prasad PN. *Introduction to biophotonics.* Hoboken, NJ: Wiley-Interscience, 2003.

3 Subhash N, Mallia JR, Thomas SS, Mathews A, Sebastian P. Oral cancer detection using diffuse reflectance spectral ratio R540/R575 of oxygenated hemoglobin bands. *J Biomed Opt* 2006;11(1): 014018.

4 Jacques SL, Ramella-Roman JC, Lee K. Imaging skin pathology with polarized light. *J Biomed Opt* 2002; 7(3): 329–340.

5 Lovisa B, Jichlinski P, Weber BC, Aymon D, van den Bergh H, Wagnieres G. High-magnification vascular imaging to reject false-positive sites in situ during Hexvix (R) fluorescence cystoscopy. *J Biomed Opt* 2010; 15(5): 051606.

6 Wada Y, Kudo S, Misawa M, Ikehara N, Hamatani S. Vascular pattern classification of colorectal lesions with narrow band imaging magnifying endoscopy. *Dig Endosc* 2011; 23: 106–111.

7 Lindenboom JA, Mathura KR, Ince C. Orthogonal polarization spectral (OPS) imaging and topographical characteristics of oral squamous cell carcinoma. *Oral Oncology* 2006; 42(6): 581–585.

8 Basiri A, Edelstein DL, Graham J, Nabili A, Giardiello FM, Ramella-Roman JC. Detection of familial adenomatous polyposis with orthogonal polarized spectroscopy of the oral mucosa vasculature. *J Biophoton* 2011; 4(10): 707–714.

9 Roblyer D, Kurachi C, Stepanek V, et al. Comparison of multispectral wide-field optical imaging modalities to maximize image contrast for objective discrimination of oral neoplasia. *J Biomed Opt* 2010; 15(6): 066017.

10 Roblyer D, Richards-Kortum R, Sokolov K, et al. Multispectral optical imaging device for in vivo detection of oral neoplasia. *J Biomed Opt* 2008; 13(2): 024019.

11 Pavlova I, Weber CR, Schwarz RA, Williams MD, Gillenwater AM, Richards-Kortum R. Fluorescence spectroscopy of oral tissue: Monte Carlo modeling with site-specific tissue properties. *J Biomed Opt* 2009; 14(1): 014009.

12 Pavlova I, Williams M, El-Naggar A, Richards-Kortum R, Gillenwater A. Understanding the biological basis of autofluorescence imaging for oral cancer detection: High-resolution fluorescence microscopy in viable tissue. *Clin Cancer Res* 2008; 14(8): 2396–2404.

13 Betz CS, Stepp H, Janda P, et al. A comparative study of normal inspection, autofluorescence and 5-ALA-induced PPIX fluorescence for oral cancer diagnosis. *Int J Cancer* 2002; 97(2): 245–252.

14 Kulapaditharom B, Boonkitticharoen V. Performance characteristics of fluorescence endoscope in detection of head and neck cancers. *Ann Otol Rhinol Laryngol* 2001; 110(1): 45–52.

15 Poh CF, Ng SP, Williams PM, et al. Direct fluorescence visualization of clinically occult high-risk oral premalignant disease using a simple hand-held device. *Head Neck* 2007; 29(1): 71–76.

16 Poh CF, Zhang LW, Anderson DW, et al. Fluorescence visualization detection of field alterations in tumor margins of oral cancer patients. *Clin Cancer Res* 2006; 12(22): 6716–6722.

17 Roblyer D, Kurachi C, Stepanek V, et al. Objective detection and delineation of oral neoplasia using autofluorescence imaging. *Cancer Prev Res* 2009; 2(5): 423–431.

18 Inaguma M, Hashimoto K. Porphyrin-like fluorescence in oral cancer - In vivo fluorescence spectral characterization of lesions by use of a near-ultraviolet excited autofluorescence diagnosis system and separation of fluorescent extracts by capillary electrophoresis. *Cancer-Am Cancer Soc* 1999; 86(11): 2201–2211.

19 Poh CF, MacAulay CE, Zhang LW, Rosin MP. Tracing the "at-risk" oral mucosa field with autofluorescence: steps toward clinical impact. *Cancer Prev Res* 2009; 2(5): 401–404.

20 Paczona R, Temam S, Janot F, Marandas P, Luboinski B. Autofluorescence videoendoscopy for photodiagnosis of head and neck squamous cell carcinoma. *Eur Arch Oto Rhino Laryngol* 2003; 260(10): 544–548.

21 Awan KH, Morgan PR, Warnakulasuriya S. Evaluation of an autofluorescence based imaging system (VELscope (TM)) in the detection of oral potentially malignant disorders and benign keratoses. *Oral Oncol* 2011; 47(4): 274–277.

22 Farah CS, McIntosh L, Georgiou A, McCullough MJ. The efficacy of autofluorescence imaging (VELScope) in the visualisation of oral mucosal lesions. *Oral Dis* 2010; 16(6): 559.

23 Scheer M, Neugebauer J, Derman A, Fuss J, Drebber U, Zoeller JE. Autofluorescence imaging of potentially malignant mucosa lesions. *Oral Surg Oral Med Oral Pathol Oral Radiol Endodontol* 2011; 111(5): 568–577.

24 Vigneswaran N, Koh S, Gillenwater A. Incidental detection of an occult oral malignancy with autofluorescence imaging: a case report. *Head Neck Oncol* 2009;1: 37.

25 Rahman M, Chaturvedi P, Gillenwater AM, Richards-Kortum R. Low-cost, multimodal, portable screening system for early detection of oral cancer. *J Biomed Opt* 2008; 13(3): 030502.

26 Andrea M, Dias O. *Rigid and Contact Endoscopy in Microlaryngeal Surgery : Technique and Atlas of Clinical Cases*. New York: Raven Press, 1995.

27 Feldchtein FI, Gelikonov GV, Gelikonov VM, et al. In vivo OCT imaging of hard and soft tissue of the oral cavity. *Optics Express* 1998; 3(6): 239–250.

28 Ridgway JM, Armstrong WB, Guo S, et al. In vivo optical coherence tomography of the human oral cavity and oropharynx. *Arch Otolaryngol Head Neck Surg* 2006; 132(10): 1074–1081.

29 Tsai MT, Lee HC, Lu CW, et al. Delineation of an oral cancer lesion with swept-source optical coherence tomography. *J Biomed Opt* 2008; 13(4): 044012.

30 Wilder-Smith P, Lee K, Guo SG, et al. In vivo diagnosis of oral dysplasia and malignancy using optical coherence tomography: preliminary studies in 50 patients. *Lasers Surg Med* 2009;41(5): 353–357.

31 Tsai MT, Lee CK, Lee HC, et al. Differentiating oral lesions in different carcinogenesis stages with optical coherence tomography. *J Biomed Opt* 2009; 14(4): 044028.

32 Arens C, Glanz H, Wonckhaus J, Hersemeyer K, Kraft M. Histologic assessment of epithelial thickness in early laryngeal cancer or precursor lesions and its impact on endoscopic imaging. *Eur Arch Oto Rhino Laryngol* ; 264(6): 645–649.

33 Prestin S, Betz C, Kraft M. Measurement of epithelial thickness within the oral cavity using optical coherence tomography (OCT). *Head Neck* 2012; 34(12): 1777–1781.

34 Tsai MT, Lee HC, Lee CK, et al. Effective indicators for diagnosis of oral cancer using optical coherence tomography. *Optics Express*. 2008; 16(20): 15847–15862.

35 Kraft M, Glanz H, von Gerlach S, Wisweh H, Lubatschowski H, Arens C. Clinical value of optical coherence tomography in laryngology. *Head Neck* 2008; 30(12): 1628–1635.

36 Maitland KC, Gillenwater AM, Williams MD, El-Naggar AK, Descour MR, Richards-Kortum RR. In vivo imaging of oral neoplasia using a miniaturized fiber optic confocal reflectance microscope. *Oral Oncol* 2008; 44(11): 1059–1066.

37 Muldoon TJ, Pierce MC, Nida DL, Williams MD, Gillenwater A, Richards-Kortum R. Subcellular-resolution molecular imaging within living tissue by fiber microendoscopy. *Optics Express* 2007; 15(25): 16413–16423.

38 Thong PSP, Olivo M, Kho KW, et al. Laser confocal endomicroscopy as a novel technique for fluorescence diagnostic imaging of the oral cavity. *J Biomed Opt* 2007; 12(1): 014007.

39 Muldoon TJ, Roblyer D, Williams MD, Stepanek VMT, Richards-Kortum R, Gillenwater AM. Noninvasive imaging of oral neoplasia with a high-resolution fiber-optic microendoscope. *Head Neck* 2012; 34(3): 305–312.

40 Sun JT, Shu CH, Appiah B, Drezek R. Needle-compatible single fiber bundle image guide reflectance endoscope. *J Biomed Opt* 2010; 15(4).

41 De Veld DCG, Witjes MJH, Sterenborg HJCM, Roodenburg JLN. The status of in vivo autofluorescence spectroscopy and imaging for oral oncology. *Oral Oncol* 2005; 41(2): 117–131.

42 Gillenwater A, Jacob R, Ganeshappa R, et al. Noninvasive diagnosis of oral neoplasia based on fluorescence spectroscopy and native tissue autofluorescence. *Arch Otolaryngol Head Neck Surg* 1998; 124(11): 1251–1258.

43 Betz CS, Mehlmann M, Rick K, et al. Autofluorescence imaging and spectroscopy of normal and malignant mucosa in patients with head and neck cancer. *Lasers Surg Med* 1999; 25(4): 323–334.

44 Muller MG, Valdez TA, Georgakoudi I, et al. Spectroscopic detection and evaluation of morphologic and biochemical changes in early human oral carcinoma. *Cancer* 2003; 97(7): 1681–1692.

45 de Veld DCG, Skurichina M, Wities MJH, Duin RPW, Sterenborg HJCM, Roodenburg JLN. Autofluorescence and diffuse reflectance spectroscopy for oral oncology. *Lasers Surg Med* 2005; 36(5): 356–364.

46 Schwarz RA, Gao W, Weber CR, et al. Noninvasive evaluation of oral lesions using depth-sensitive optical spectroscopy. *Cancer* 2009; 115(8): 1669–1679.

47 Francisco ALN. *Espectroscopia de fluorescência para detecção de lesões potencialmente malignas e carcinoma epidermóide da cavidade oral [Masters dissertation]*. Piracicaba: UNICAMP, 2011.

48 de Veld DCG, Sterenborg HJCM, Roodenburg JLN, Witjes MJH. Effects of individual characteristics on healthy oral mucosa autofluorescence spectra. *Oral Oncol* 2004; 40(8): 815–823.

49 Malini R, Venkatakrishna K, Kurien J, et al. Discrimination of normal, inflammatory, premalignant, and malignant oral tissue: a Raman spectroscopy study. *Biopolymers* 2006; 81(3): 179–193.

50 Hu Y, Jiang T, Zhao Z, eds. *Discrimination of Squamous Cell Carcinoma of the Oral Cavity using Raman Spect roscopy and Chemometric Analysis*, IEEE, 2008.

51 Guze K, Short M, Zeng H, Lerman M, Sonis S. Comparison of molecular images as defined by Raman spectra between normal mucosa and squamous cell carcinoma in the oral cavity. *J Raman Spectrosc* 2011; 42(6): 1232–1239.

52 Guze K, Short M, Sonis S, Karimbux N, Chan J, Zeng HS. Parameters defining the potential applicability of Raman spectroscopy as a diagnostic tool for oral disease. *J Biomed Opt* 2009; 14(1): 014016.

53 Bergholt MS, Zheng W, Huang Z. Characterizing variability in in vivo Raman spectroscopic properties of different anatomical sites of normal tissue in the oral cavity. *J Raman Spectrosc* 2012; 43: 255–262.

CHAPTER 40

Low level laser therapy in the prevention and treatment of oral mucositis

Alyne Simões,[1] Fernanda de Paula Eduardo,[2] Cesar A. Migliorati,[3] and Mark Schubert[4,5]

[1] Department of Biomaterials and Oral Biology, School of Dentistry, University of São Paulo (USP), São Paulo, SP, Brazil

[2] Oncology, Hematology and Bone Marrow Transplantation Program, Hospital Israelita Albert Einstein, São Paulo, SP, Brazil

[3] Department of Diagnostic Sciences and Oral Medicine, College of Dentistry, University of Tennessee Health Science Center, Memphis, TN, USA

[4] Oral Medicine – UW School of Dentistry, Seattle, WA, USA

[5] Oral Medicine – Seattle Cancer Care Alliance, Seattle, WA, USA

Oral mucositis

Alimentary tract mucositis is a frequent dose-limiting side effect related to radiotherapy and chemotherapy in patients with cancer. The oral mucosa is a prime target for treatment-related toxicity by virtue of its rapid rate of cell turnover. Studies indicate that up to 50% of patients undergoing conventional or standard chemotherapy, up to 80% of patients receiving high dose chemotherapy/chemoradiotherapy conditioning for a hematopoietic cell transplant, and almost 100% of patients submitted to head and neck cancer radiotherapy will develop some degree of oral mucositis (OM) signs and symptoms at some point during their treatment.[1]

Clinically, OM is characterized by soreness/pain and erythema, and when severe can be characterized by ulcerative lesions. OM occurs frequently on the non-keratinized mucosa, such as that of the buccal mucosa, labial mucosa, lateral/ventral tongue, and floor of the mouth. Depending on the severity of the mucosal breakdown, it is associated with mild to severe pain, which interferes with oral function (eating, drinking, talking, and swallowing) and can severely impact the patient's quality of life. The World Health Organization (WHO) classifies the lesions according clinical presentation and the patient's oral functions, being "0" for no mucositis; "1" for soreness/erythema; "2" for erythema/ulcers, but the patient is able to eat solid foods; "3" for ulcers, but patients requires a liquid diet; and "4" when oral alimentation is not possible (Table 40.1 and Fig. 40.1). Additional OM rating scales are used in research and can provide more precise characterization of mucosal breakdown: the Oral Mucositis Rating Scale (OMRS) and the Oral Mucositis Index (OMI), among others (Table 40.1).

The risk factors for OM development are related to patient characteristics and type of cancer therapy. Patient age, oral health, body mass index, renal function, smoking, and previous cancer treatment are some of the patient-related factors considered to affect mucositis. However, one of the most important patient-related factors appears to be genetic polymorphisms that affect specific pathways that influence the cellular damage initiated by cancer therapies.[5] Clearly, the specific type of therapy administered is associated with the type and severity of the oral mucosal damage. This includes the specific chemotherapy given (e.g. antimetabolites, antitumor antibiotics, and alkylating agents are especially known to be stomatotoxic), dose of agent and administration schedule (e.g. bolus 5-fluorouracil [5-FU] is more stomatotoxic than continuous infusion 5-FU; low dose melphalan is less stomatotoxic than high dose melphalan), and radiation fraction size, frequency, and total radiation dose. When combined radiation–chemotherapy is used, the mucositis is definitely worse.[6]

It is important to know that severe oral mucositis (WHO grade 3–4) can have a significant effect on the course of therapy and efforts should be made as far as possible to prevent it. OM can be associated with treatment delays, treatment interruptions, and even the discontinuation of treatment. OM can increase the frequency and cost of hospitalization of cancer patients.[7] In patients undergoing high dose chemotherapy with hematopoietic stem cell transplantation (HSCT), a 1-point increase in OM, measured with the OMRS mucositis scale, has been found to be associated with a significant increase in the number of days with fever, risk of infection, additional days of total parenteral nutrition, use of intravenous narcotic analgesics, total hospital charges, and 100-day mortality.[8]

With this understanding of what OM is and its importance in cancer treatment, it is now important to understand the biology and mechanisms involved in the development of OM. This will set the stage for understanding how lasers could be used in the prevention and treatment of OM.

Mucosal injury during cancer therapy is a complex process. After radiotherapy and chemotherapy, there is an initiation phase that is characterized by simultaneous injury to epithelial and submucosal tissues, such as those of the endothelium, connective tissue, and extracellular matrix. Initial damage is

Lasers in Dentistry: Guide for Clinical Practice, First Edition. Edited by Patrícia M. de Freitas and Alyne Simões.
© 2015 John Wiley & Sons, Inc. Published 2015 by John Wiley & Sons, Inc.

Table 40.1 National Cancer Institute Common Toxicity Criteria (NCI – CTC) version 3(2), World Health Organization (WHO)[3] and Radiation Therapy Oncology Group (RTOG)[4] scoring criteria for oral mucositis.

	Mucositis grade	Description
NCI – CTC functional/ symptomatic	0	No mucositis
	1	Minimal symptoms, able to eat solids
	2	Symptomatic but can eat and swallow a modified diet (liquid diet)
	3	Oral alimentation not possible
	4	Symptoms associated with life-threatening consequences
	5	Death
NCI – CTC clinical examination	0	No mucositis
	1	Erythema of the mucosa
	2	Patchy ulceration or pseudomembranes
	3	Confluent ulcerations or pseudomembranes, bleeding with minor trauma
	4	Tissue necrosis, significant spontaneous bleeding; life-threatening consequences
	5	Death
WHO	0	Normal
	1	Soreness with or without erythema; no ulceration
	2	Ulceration and erythema: patient can swallow a solid diet
	3	Ulceration and erythema: patient cannot swallow a solid diet
	4	Ulceration and erythema formation of such severity that alimentation not possible
RTOG	0	No change over baseline
	1	Irritation, may experience mild pain, not requiring analgesia
	2	Patchy mucositis that may produce inflammatory serosanguinitis discharge; may experience moderate pain requiring analgesia
	3	Confluent fibrinous mucositis, may include severe pain requiring narcotics
	4	Ulceration, hemorrhage, or necrosis

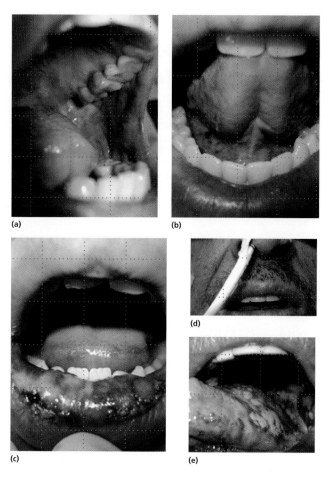

Figure 40.1 Oral mucositis grades according the WHO: (a) grade 1; (b) grade 2; (c) grade 3; (d,e) grade 4.

generally thought to result from the production of reactive oxygen species (ROS). There is a simultaneous promotion of damage due to reactions mediated by the ceramide pathway and the production of a number of transcription factors, including nuclear factor kappa β (NF-κβ). Immediate clonogenic cell death can result from this damage. Additionally, in submucosal tissues, connective tissue degeneration, edema, and inflammatory reactions are noted. NF-κB can also secondarily stimulate the up-regulation of a second set of genes that can cause a "second wave" of damage to affected tissues. The pro-inflammatory cytokines (tumor necrosis factor alpha [TNF-α], interleukin 1β and 6 [IL-1β and IL-6]) produced as a result of the first wave of damage can also signal the "second wave" of damage through their ability to amplify the up-regulation of transcription factors, leading to the production of additional pro-inflammatory cytokines, tissue injury, and apoptosis. Epithelial apoptosis and necrosis exceed the hyperproliferative activity and result in an ulcerative phase that is exacerbated by local bacterial colonization.[8]

Low level laser therapy

The Multinational Association of Supportive Care in Cancer and the International Society for Oral Oncology (MASCC/ISOO) have developed evidence-based guidelines for the prevention and management of alimentary mucositis.[6,8] Basic oral care, patient education, and palliative care (including pain management) are covered. Recommended therapies for palliation of mucositis and acute oral pain include systemic analgesics and other individual agents, palliative mixtures, coating agents, topical anesthetics/analgesics, and oral cryotherapy. In the most recent update of the MASCC/ISOO guidelines, low level laser therapy (LLLT) has been elevated to the level of a recommended therapy.[8]

An increasing number of studies have been reported that support the use of LLLT as an efficacious technique for the prevention and management of OM. The basic effects of LLLT are attributed to biomodulation that results in reduced tissue damage and analgesic effects. This chapter will describe how LLLT can be used as an auxiliary therapy for OM healing and pain relief.

It is well known that almost all cells respond to irradiation with monochromatic radiation from laser and light emitting diodes (LEDs), with changes in their metabolism.[9–11] It is generally accepted that the mitochondrion is the initial site of the response to light in cells, and cytochrome c oxidase is the chromophore for this. This event is a starting point for changes in the cell's metabolism,[12] including the ATP signaling pathway.[13] Apart from being a universal human body fuel, ATP has been described to be a critical signaling molecule that allows cells and tissues throughout the body to communicate with one another.[14] Besides, ATP signaling has been related also to cell proliferation and pain relief,[14] responses which are key in the treatment of OM.

Regarding OM healing, it is known that LLLT increases fibroblast proliferation and collagen production/organization,[15] and reduces cyclooxygenase 2 (COX-2),[16] pro-inflammatory cytokine IL-1β,[17] TNF-α, IL-1β and IL-6 expression,[18] as well as neutrophil infiltration.[15] LLLT also increases angiogenesis[19] and acts on the NF-κB pathway.[20] In addition to analgesia, laser irradiation has been shown to stimulate peripheral nerves by altering the hyperpolarization of the cell membrane and increasing ATP concentration, which could contribute to maintaining the stability of the cell membrane and increase the pain threshold.[21,22] Moreover, laser irradiation can enhance peripheral endogenous opioid production[23] and decrease serum prostaglandin E_2.[24] For more details regarding the mechanism of action of LLLT, see Chapters 4–6.

In addition to LLLT, the use of an LED to treat OM has been studied, with promising results.[25–28] However, more clinical trials are necessary to test the effectiveness of LED in comparison with LLLT in patients with OM induced by cancer therapy. This chapter will focus on the use of LLLT to prevent and treat OM.

LLLT studies and dosimetry

There are many studies addressing the effects of LLLT on OM. However, due to the use of a wide range of laser protocols (energy, energy density, power, irradiation area, etc.), variation in laser dosimetry and laser application mode (contact and non-contact), the use of diverse mucositis scales, as well as differences in patient populations treated, it is difficult to compare the results of these studies and recommend standardized protocols. While the results of the various trials are generally positive, it is imperative that standardized guidelines be established based on the highest level of evidence.

Recently, Bjordal et al. and Bensadoun and Nair published two reviews that discussed the use of LLLT in OM as well as its parameters.[29,30] Both concluded that certain laser treatment recommendations can be recognized for the prevention and/or treatment of OM. In these reviews, the authors suggested daily laser irradiation with a power between 10 and 100 mW.

According to Bjordal et al., the recommended laser energy per point is 3 J for red lasers and 6 J for infrared lasers, and the minimum number of irradiation points and minimum sessions per week during cancer treatment are 6 and 3, respectively. In addition, for OM prevention they suggest 7 days of laser application before the patient starts cancer treatment. On the other hand, Bensadoun and Nair recommended a dose of 2–3 J/cm^2 for prophylaxis and 4 J/cm^2 for therapeutic effect. Nevertheless, as observed in Table 40.2,[31–48] other laser application protocols are also available, showing effective results in the prevention and treatment of OM.

Based on the available reviews it can be observed that there is a great divergence in the suggested parameters for LLLT (e.g. the use of energy density or energy per point?). In their reviews, Bjordal et al. used the energy parameter as a reference for the reader,[29] while Bensadoun and Nair used density of energy.[30] We feel that it is important to mention both parameters. In addition, it is important to consider other irradiation parameters such as the total energy applied (energy per point multiplied by the number of points), power density, anatomic areas receiving the irradiation, wavelength, number of irradiations, and area considered by the software of the equipment (the area of the laser spot or the irradiated surface area). The latter is a significant point of confusion in the literature, as will be discussed later.

Table 40.2 reviews 18 studies of the effect of LLLT on OM. We have included the articles included in Bjordal et al.'s review,[31–36,38,39,42] with exception of two[49,50] that were not mentioned in Migliorati et al.'s systematic review.[51] In addition to these, we included five articles[37,40,41,43,44] published before 2010 and cited by Migliorati et al.[51] and four articles published in 2011 and 2012.[45–48] We used information from the published text and additional information was obtained from the authors or calculated from the data available in the papers (Table 40.2).

According to Table 40.2, the most commonly used wavelengths for biomodulation and analgesia in cancer patients are in the visible and infrared regions of the spectrum, which agrees with the recommendations in the reviews discussed above. The red laser (630–670 nm) is the best option for ulcers due to the poor penetration of these wavelengths and its beneficial effects on wound healing. For pain or deeper tissues, infrared lasers are a better choice. It is important to highlight that other wavelengths can be used, but may not be optimal.[52] A laser parameter for which there is agreement between the results in Table 40.2 and the reviews of Bjordal et al. and Bensadoun and Nair[29,30] is a power range of 10–100 mW.

One point of disagreement between Table 40.2 and the cited reviews relates to the energy suggested per point. As is shown in Table 40.2, there is a decrease in OM severity and incidence when the energy per point is kept between 0.08 J and 0.6 J. Just four of the studies reviewed by Bjordal et al. used a confirmed energy per point higher than 1 J. In addition, an important issue related to this parameter is the number of irradiation points and consequently, the total energy applied. For example, a total energy of 9 J can be delivered by applying 1 J to nine points, or

Table 40.2 Clinical trials characteristics and laser parameters for treatment and prevention of oral mucositis (OM).

Study (year/country)	Patient number (cancer treatment)	Laser (wavelength, nm)	Groups	Power (mW)	OM initial grade	Spot diameter (mm) or area (cm²)
Cowen et al.[31] (1997/France)	30 (BMT – CT+TBI)	HeNe (632.8)	L+(laser) and L– (placebo)	60	0	
Bensadoun et al.[32] (1999/France)	30 (RT)	HeNe (632.8)	L+(laser) and L– (placebo)	60 (1 patient with 25)	0	1.2 mm
Arun Maiya et al.[33] (2006/India)	50 (RT)	HeNe (632.8)	L+(laser) and L– (control)	10	0	
Schubert et al.[34] (2007/USA)*	70 (BMT – CT+TBI)	Diode (780 and 660)	G1: 780 nm G2: 660 nm G3: placebo	60 and 40, respectively for G1 and G2	0	0.04 cm² #
Cruz et al.[35] (2007/Brazil)	60 (BMT/CT)	Diode (780)	G1: BMT G2: CT-ICE or irinotecan G3: previous mucositis in any other CT protocol	60	0	0.04 cm² #
Antunes et al.[36] (2007/Brazil)	38 (BMT)	Diode (660)	L+(laser) and L– (placebo)	46.7	0	0.196 cm²
Jaguar et al.[37] (2007/Brazil)	49 (BMT)	Diode (660)	L+(laser) and L– (retrospective)	10	0	0.04 cm²
Genot-Klastersky et al.[38] (2008/Belgium)	Two prospective studies — 26 (patient with previously OM grade 2 in any other CT protocol) 36 (BMT)	Combination of visible+IR lasers	— L+(laser) and L– (placebo)	Combination of 100 (visible) and 50, 250, and 500 (IR)	0 or 1 (preventive) 2	1.2 mm
Abramoff et al.[39] (2008/Brazil)	13 (CT)	Diode (685)	L+(laser) and L– (placebo)	35		0.6 mm
Simoes et al.[40] (2009/Brazil)	39 (RT)	Diode (low power laser – 660) and diode (high power laser – 808)	G1: low power laser, 3 times per week G2: association of low and high power laser 3 times per week G3: low power laser once a week	40 and 1000 (just for G2)	1–3	0.04 cm²
Eduardo et al.[41] (2009/Brazil)	30 (BMT)	Diode (660)	Just one group but in the same patient, laser was applied to prevent and to treat OM with different protocols (4 or 6 J/cm², respectively).	40	0	0.04 cm²

Irradiation sessions	Irradiated area	Number of points	Dose (J/cm²)	Energy per point (J) and total energy(J)	Time per point (s) or total time (min)	Outcomes and effect
5 consecutive days (from D–5 to D–1)	5 anatomic sites on the right and left side of the oral cavity	15 per anatomic site	1.5	0.6 and 54	10 per point	Laser reduced onset, peak severity, and duration of OM and decreased pain. Duration of morphine administration was reduced by laser applications
35 consecutive days with exception of the weekends	Posterior third of the internal surfaces of the cheeks, soft palate, and anterior tonsillar pillars	9	2		33 per point (for 1 patient it was 80s)	Laser reduced mucositis severity and duration, and pain
5 days per week until the end of RT	Posterior third of the internal surfaces of the cheeks, soft palate, and anterior tonsillar pillars		1.8		3 total	Effective in preventing and treating the OM and reducing pain
From 07 to 13	6 anatomic areas	48	2	0.08 and 3.84	1 and 2 per point for 60 and 40mW, respectively	Laser (660nm) decreased OM severity and pain
From 3 to 5 consecutive days from the initial CT day	5 anatomic areas					NS
D–7–neutrophil recovery	11 anatomic areas	15 per anatomic area	4		16.7 per point	Decreased OM incidence
From first day of conditioning to day+2	8 anatomic areas		2.5	0.1	10 per point	Laser seemed to promote pain relief, reduce the severity of OM, and decrease morphine administration
3 sessions per week	11 anatomic areas		2		33s per site/6 min per session	Laser was effective and safe in preventing and treating OM
Every workday						
3 or more	11 anatomic areas	25 points	72	2 and 50	54 per point	Less OM development, and better recovery as well as pain relief
5–13 G1 received the irradiations (40mW) 3 times per week G2 received combined low and high power laser 3 times per week (40mW and 1W) G3 received the irradiation (40mW) once a week	19 anatomic areas	90	6	0.24 and 21.6	6	Laser phototherapy using low power laser alone or combined with high power laser when applied three times a week maintained the OM grades at 1 and2. Moreover, this fractioned laser phototherapy also prevented pain increase
From the first day of conditioning to neutrophil recovery or total healing	10 anatomic areas	88 points*	4 (to prevent) or 6 (to treat)	0.16 (to prevent) and 0.24 (to treat) per point	4 or 6s per point, respectively	Laser phototherapy tended to maintain mucositis levels at grades 1 and 2, which was a positive effect of this therapy for the treatment of HSCT patients

(*Continued*)

Table 40.2 (Continued)

Study (year/country)	Patient number (cancer treatment)	Laser (wavelength, nm)	Groups	Power (mW)	OM initial grade	Spot diameter (mm) or area (cm²)
Kuhn et al.[42] 2009/Brazil	21 children (CT or BMT)	Diode (830)	Laser and placebo	100	2 or greater	
Lima et al.[43] (2010/Brazil)	25 (RT+CT)	Diode (830)	L+ (laser) and L– (control group – aluminum hydroxide suspension)	15	0	0.2 cm²
Zanin et al.[44] (2010/Brazil)	72 (RT+CT)	Diode (660)	L+ (laser) and L– (control)	30	0	2 mm Considered area: 1 cm²
Silva et al.[45] (2011/Brazil)	42 (BMT)	Diode (660)	L+ (laser) and L- (control)	40	0	0.04 cm²
Carvalho et al.[46] (2011/Brazil)	70 (RT+CT)	Diode (660)	G1 and G2 with different laser protocols	5 for G2) or 15 for G1	0	0.04 cm²
Gautam et al.[47] (2012/India)	121 (CT+RT)	HeNe (632.8)	L+ (laser) and L– (placebo)	24		1 cm²
Lima et al.[48] (2012/Brazil)	75 (RT+CT)	Diode (660)	L+ (laser) and L– (placebo)	10	0	0.04

*Additional data were obtained from the authors.
#MMOptics lasers have a spot area of 0.04 cm².
ICE, iphosphamide, carboplatin, ethoposide and irinothecan. TPN, total parenteral nutrition; CT, chemotherapy; RT, radiotherapy, BMT, bone marrow transplant; IR, infrared; HSCT, human stem cell transplant.

0.25 J to 36 points. Which is the better choice? We believe that higher numbers of points are better for wound healing because a larger area of the mucosa will be stimulated (see Chapter 8 for more details).

Another aspect that needs to be discussed is when to start the LLLT application. Bjordal et al. suggested 7 days of laser application before the patient starts cancer treatment.[29] However, we believe that LLLT should be started immediately after the beginning of radiotherapy or chemotherapy, as no published studies have shown the effectiveness of applying LLLT before the harmful stimulus (radiotherapy and/or chemotherapy). On the other hand, we feel that laser treatment should be provided daily throughout the head and neck radiotherapy and the bone marrow transplantation in order to prevent and treat oral mucositis; however, the reported minimum number of sessions is three times per week for RT patients.[40] LLLT application in patients submitted to chemotherapy depends on the regimen and drugs used. We suggest that the patient be monitored at least once a week and if some mucosal alteration appears, the laser should be started immediately. Table 40.3 gives suggested parameters for use in LLLT protocols.

Tips

It is difficult to establish a single standardized protocol for LLLT because of the variety of laser equipment that has been utilized in published reports and the variation in laser treatment parameters. One must also consider the types of cancer therapies and the toxicities that each one produces. Moreover, as was noted above, it is important to know the area covered by the laser software (calculated from the formula energy density or dose (ED) = power (P) x time (T)/area (A). For example, as the treated surface area is generally 1 cm², the protocols will need to be adjusted if the laser spot area of the equipment is 0.04 cm² and the equipment software does not

Irradiation sessions	Irradiated area	Number of points	Dose (J/cm²)	Energy per point (J) and total energy(J)	Time per point (s) or total time (min)	Outcomes and effect
5 consecutive days	Mucositis lesions		4			LLLT significantly reduced the duration of CT-induced OM
From first day of RT until the end of RT	12 anatomic areas		12	2.4	160 per point	Prophylactic use of both treatments seemed to reduce the incidence of severe OM lesions, but LLLT was more effective in delaying their appearance
Twice a week for 7 weeks	3 points on jugal mucosa, inferior lip internal mucosa; and soft palate 2 points on palatine folds and on sublingual caruncles 5 points on the tongue	Approximately 21 points		2 and 42		The 660-nm diode laser was effective in the prevention and treatment of OM, providing more comfort and a better quality of life
D−4 to D+4	9 anatomic areas	10 per anatomic area	4	0.16 and 12.8	4 per point	Preventive laser therapy was beneficial in reducing the occurrence and intensity of OM in HSCT patients
5 consecutive days per week starting on the first day of RT until the end of RT	8 anatomic areas		G2: 1.3 G1: 3.8	G2: 0.05 per point G1: 0.15 per point	10 per point	Laser (G1) controlled the intensity of the mucositis and pain
	6 anatomic areas		3.5	3.5	145 per point	Laser was effective in preventing and treating OM: decreased incidence of severe oral pain, opioid analgesic use, and TPN in laser group compared to the placebo group
From first day of RT until the end of RT	9 anatomic areas		2.5	0.1	10 per point	Laser therapy was not effective in reducing grade 3 or 4 OM, although a marginal benefit could not be excluded in terms of reducing RT interruptions

Table 40.3 Laser parameters suggested for prevention and treatment of oral mucositis.

Parameter to be considered	Details	Recommendation
Wavelength (nm)	Wound healing Analgesia	630–670 (red) 780–830 (infrared)
Output (mW)	Could be fixed or variable depending on the equipment	10–100
Energy per point (J)	Seems better to have more points with low energy delivered to each, than fewer points with a higher energy delivered to each	0.08–2
Energy density (J/cm²)	It is important to consider that energy density is the energy divided by the area and the area could be the laser spot area or the treated surface area (see "Tips" section). The energy per point needs to be considered	Example (for equipment that takes into consideration a laser spot area of 0.04 cm²): from 2 (being the energy per point of 0.08 J) to 50 (being the energy per point of 2 J)
Area (cm²)	Depends on the equipment software. Could be the laser spot area (e.g. 0.04 cm²) or the treated surface area (generally 1 cm²)	There are no recommendations. The area used by the equipment just needs to be known
Application mode		Perpendicular, in contact with the tissue and punctually – each cm²
Time per point (s)	Depends on the application mode (punctual or scattering)	Calculated using the formula: ED (J/cm²)=[P (W) × T (s)]/A (cm²)
Number of irradiations	During radiotherapy (RT) or chemotherapy (CT)	Daily for RT and once a week (when the patient has oral mucositis grade 0) or daily (when the patient has a mucosal alteration) for CT

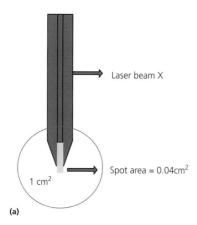

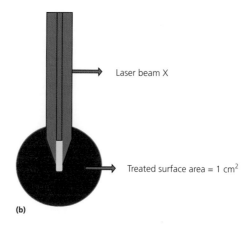

- Dose: 2 J/cm^2

- Power: 0.04 W

- Laser spot area: 0.04 cm^2

- Area used by the laser software - Laser spot area = 0.04 cm^2

- Each treated surface area: 1 cm^2

- Irradiation time: 2 s

- Energy per point: 0.08 J

- Irradiation performed on each cm^2

- Dose: 2 J/cm^2

- Power: 0.04 W

- Laser spot area: 0.04 cm^2

- Area used by the laser software - Treated surface area = 1 cm^2

- Each treated surface area: 1 cm^2

- Irradiation time: 50 s

- Energy per point: 2 J

- Irradiation performed on each cm^2

Figure 40.2 Both lasers (A and B) have a spot area of 0.04 cm^2. However, the software for equipment B uses the "treated surface area" in the formula Energy density or dose = Power × Time)/Area. Observe the alterations to the laser parameters according to the area used by the laser software.

Clinical case 40.1

A 44-year-old women, diagnosed with pulmonary metastases from head and neck cancer, was subjected to high dose chemotherapy (5-FU, cisplatin, and docetaxel). Clinical examination revealed severe oral pain (visual analog scale = 5) and ulceration of the lateral tongue border (WHO mucositis score 3) among others areas (Fig. 30.3a). LLLT was performed daily with a low power diode laser (MMOptics®, Sao Carlos, Brazil), with a spot size of approximately 0.04 cm^2, wavelength of 660 nm, power of 40 mW, and dose of 6 J/cm^2, being 0.24 J of energy per point (6 seconds of irradiation). The continous irradiation was given in contact mode on the entire oral cavity to prevent or treat the ulcerations. A total of 90 points (totaling 21.6 J of energy per session) were irradiated By the sixth day of treatment, the patients showed a great improvement in all oral symptoms, with no pain even though her OM grade was rated as 2 (Fig. 40.3b). Total healing was observed by the ninth day (Fig. 40.3c).

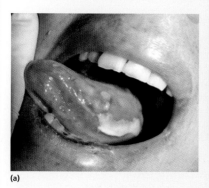
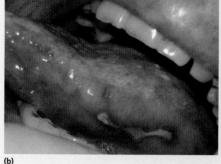
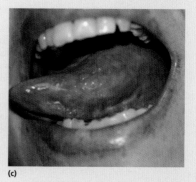

Figure 40.3 (a) Oral mucositis lesions on the tongue border, induced by chemotherapy. Lesions on the fourth (b) and ninth (c) day of laser treatment.

use the "treated surface area" in this formula. This is illustrated in Figure 40.2. Although both lasers (A and B) have the same laser beam and are applied in the same way, the software of laser "A" uses the laser spot area in the formula, while laser "B" uses the treated surface area. While the energy density and the power are the same for both lasers (2 J/cm^2 and 0.04 W, respectively), the others parameters (energy and time per point) are completely different, showing the importance of giving all the laser parameters when reporting LLLT use. The statement that 2 J/cm^2 was applied on its own means nothing, as shown in Figure 40.2.

Final considerations

There is growing evidence in the scientific literature that LLLT can be effective in the prevention of severe mucositis, as well as in OM wound healing and pain relief, improving a patient's quality of life. However, additional well-designed clinical and experimental studies are needed to confirm the effectiveness and mechanism of action of LLLT in the prevention and treatment of OM, as well as to determine ideal protocols for LLLT of OM to provide the best care for patients submitted to high doses of radiation and/or chemotherapy.

Acknowledgments

Some of our studies have received financial support from FAPESP (Fundação de Amparo à Pesquisa do Estado de São Paulo – Grants #2010/03662-6 and #2011/14013-1). In addition, we would like to thank the Special Laboratory for Lasers in Dentistry (LELO) at the School of Dentistry of the University of São Paulo, where the patient described was treated.

References

1 Trotti A, Bellm LA, Epstein JB, et al. Mucositis incidence, severity and associated outcomes in patients with head and neck cancer receiving radiotherapy with or without chemotherapy: a systematic literature review. *Radiother Oncol* 2003; 66(3): 253–262

2 NCI. Common Terminology Criteria for Adverse Events v3.0 (CTCAE). 2006 [2012]; Available from: http://ctep.cancer.gov/protocolDevelopment/electronic_applications/docs/ctcaev3.pdf

3 World Health Organization. *WHO Handbook for Reporting Results of Cancer Treatment.* Geneva: World Health Organization, 1979.

4 Radiation Therapy Oncology Group (RTOG). Acute Radiation Morbidity Scoring Criteria. Available from: http://www.rtog.org/ResearchAssociates/AdverseEventReporting/AcuteRadiationMorbidityScoringCriteria.aspx

5 Pratesi N, Mangoni M, Mancini I, et al. Association between single nucleotide polymorphisms in the XRCC1 and RAD51 genes and clinical radiosensitivity in head and neck cancer. *Radiother Oncol* 2011; 99(3): 356–361.

6 Eilers J, Million R. Clinical update: prevention and management of oral mucositis in patients with cancer. *Semin Oncol Nurs* 2011; 27(4): e1–16.

7 Murphy BA. Clinical and economic consequences of mucositis induced by chemotherapy and/or radiation therapy. *J Support Oncol* 2007; 5(9 Suppl 4): 13–21.

8 Rubenstein EB, Peterson DE, Schubert M, et al. Clinical practice guidelines for the prevention and treatment of cancer therapy-induced oral and gastrointestinal mucositis. *Cancer* 2004; 100(9 Suppl): 2026–2046.

9 Karu TI. O molekuliarnom mekhanizme terapevticheskogo deistviia izlucheniia nizkointensivnogo lazernogo sveta. [Molecular mechanism of the therapeutic effect of low-intensity laser irradiation]. *Dokl Akad Nauk SSSR* 1986; 291(5): 1245–1249.

10 Karu T. Photobiology of low-power laser effects. *Health Phys* 1989; 56(5): 691–704.

11 Karu T. Ten *Lectures on Basic Science of Laser Phototherapy.* Grängesberg: Prima Books AB, 2007.

12 Karu TI. Multiple roles of cytochrome c oxidase in mammalian cells under action of red and IR-A radiation. *IUBMB Life* 2010; 62(8): 607–610.

13 Karu T. Mitochondrial mechanisms of photobiomodulation in context of new data about multiple roles of ATP. *Photomed Laser Surg* 2010; 28(2): 159–160.

14 Burnstock G. Purinergic receptors and pain. *Curr Pharm Design* 2009; 15(15): 1717–1735.

15 Lopes NN, Plapler H, Lalla RV, et al. Effects of low-level laser therapy on collagen expression and neutrophil infiltrate in 5-fluorouracil-induced oral mucositis in hamsters. *Lasers Surg Med* 2010; 42(6): 546–552.

16 Lopes NN, Plapler H, Chavantes MC, Lalla RV, Yoshimura EM, Alves MT. Cyclooxygenase-2 and vascular endothelial growth factor expression in 5-fluorouracil-induced oral mucositis in hamsters: evaluation of two low-intensity laser protocols. *Support Care Cancer* 2009; 17(11): 1409–1415.

17 Gavish L, Perez L, Gertz SD. Low-level laser irradiation modulates matrix metalloproteinase activity and gene expression in porcine aortic smooth muscle cells. *Lasers Surg Med* 2006; 38(8): 779–786.

18 Simunovic-Soskic M, Pezelj-Ribaric S, Brumini G, Glazar I, Grzic R, Miletic I. Salivary levels of TNF-alpha and IL-6 in patients with denture stomatitis before and after laser phototherapy. *Photomed Laser Surg* 2010; 28(2): 189–193.

19 Franca CM, Franca CM, Nunez SC, et al. Low-intensity red laser on the prevention and treatment of induced-oral mucositis in hamsters. *J Photochem Photobiol B* 2009; 94(1): 25–31.

20 Chen AC, Arany PR, Huang YY, et al. Low-level laser therapy activates NF-kB via generation of reactive oxygen species in mouse embryonic fibroblasts. *PloS One* 2011; 6(7): e22453.

21 Kudoh C, Inomata K, Okajima K, Ohshiro T. Low-level laser therapy pain attenuation mechanisms. *Laser Ther* 1990; 2: 3–6.

22 Chow RT, David MA, Armati PJ. 830 nm laser irradiation induces varicosity formation, reduces mitochondrial membrane potential and blocks fast axonal flow in small and medium diameter rat dorsal root ganglion neurons: implications for the analgesic effects of 830 nm laser. *J Peripher Nerv Syst* 2007; 12(1): 28–39.

23 Hagiwara S, Iwasaka H, Okuda K, Noguchi T. GaAlAs (830 nm) low-level laser enhances peripheral endogenous opioid analgesia in rats. *Lasers Surg Med* 2007; 39(10): 797–802.

24 Mizutani K, Musya Y, Wakae K, et al. A clinical study on serum prostaglandin E2 with low-level laser therapy. *Photomed Laser Surg* 2004; 22(6): 537–539.

25 Sacono NT, Costa CA, Bagnato VS, Abreu-e-Lima FC. Light-emitting diode therapy in chemotherapy-induced mucositis. *Lasers Surg Med* 2008; 40(9): 625–633.

26 Lang-Bicudo L, Eduardo Fde P, Eduardo Cde P, Zezell DM. LED phototherapy to prevent mucositis: a case report. *Photomed Laser Surg* 2008; 26(6): 609–613.

27 Corti L, Chiarion-Sileni V, Aversa S, et al. Treatment of chemotherapy-induced oral mucositis with light-emitting diode. *Photomed Laser Surg* 2006; 24(2): 207–213.

28 Freitas AC, Campos L, Brandão TB, et al. Chemotherapy-induced oral mucositis: effect of LED and laser phototherapy treatment protocols. *Photomed Laser Surg* 2014; 32(2): 81–87.

29 Bjordal JM, Bensadoun RJ, Tuner J, Frigo L, Gjerde K, Lopes-Martins RA. A systematic review with meta-analysis of the effect of low-level laser therapy (LLLT) in cancer therapy-induced oral mucositis. *Support Care Cancer* 2011; 19(8): 1069–1077.

30 Bensadoun RJ, Nair RG. Low-level laser therapy in the prevention and treatment of cancer therapy-induced mucositis: 2012 state of the art based on literature review and meta-analysis. *Curr Opin Oncol* 2012; 24(4): 363–370.

31 Cowen D, Tardieu C, Schubert M, et al. Low energy Helium-Neon laser in the prevention of oral mucositis in patients undergoing bone marrow transplant: results of a double blind randomized trial. *Int J Radiat Oncol Biol Phys* 1997; 38(4): 697–703.

32 Bensadoun RJ, Franquin JC, Ciais G, et al. Low-energy He/Ne laser in the prevention of radiation-induced mucositis. A multicenter phase III randomized study in patients with head and neck cancer. *Support Care Cancer* 1999; 7(4): 244–252.

33 Arun Maiya G, Sagar MS, Fernandes D. Effect of low level helium-neon (He-Ne) laser therapy in the prevention & treatment of radiation induced mucositis in head & neck cancer patients. *Indian J Med Res* 2006; 124(4): 399–402.

34 Schubert MM, Eduardo FP, Guthrie KA, et al. A phase III randomized double-blind placebo-controlled clinical trial to determine the efficacy of low level laser therapy for the prevention of oral mucositis in patients undergoing hematopoietic cell transplantation. *Support Care Cancer* 2007; 15(10): 1145–1154.

35 Cruz LB, Ribeiro AS, Rech A, Rosa LG, Castro CG Jr, Brunetto AL. Influence of low-energy laser in the prevention of oral mucositis in children with cancer receiving chemotherapy. *Pediatr Blood Cancer* 2007; 48(4): 435–440.

36 Antunes HS, Ferreira EM, de Matos VD, Pinheiro CT, Ferreira CG. The impact of low power laser in the treatment of conditioning-induced oral mucositis: a report of 11 clinical cases and their review. *Med Oral Patol Oral Cir Bucal* 2008; 13(3): E189–192.

37 Jaguar GC, Prado JD, Nishimoto IN, et al. Low-energy laser therapy for prevention of oral mucositis in hematopoietic stem cell transplantation. *Oral Dis* 2007; 13(6): 538–543.

38 Genot-Klastersky MT, Klastersky J, Awada F, et al. The use of low-energy laser (LEL) for the prevention of chemotherapy- and/or radio-therapy-induced oral mucositis in cancer patients: results from two prospective studies. *Support Care Cancer* 2008; 16(12): 1381–1387.

39 Abramoff MM, Lopes NN, Lopes LA, et al. Low-level laser therapy in the prevention and treatment of chemotherapy-induced oral mucositis in young patients. *Photomed Laser Surg* 2008; 26(4): 393–400.

40 Simoes A, Eduardo FP, Luiz AC, et al. Laser phototherapy as topical prophylaxis against head and neck cancer radiotherapy-induced oral mucositis: comparison between low and high/low power lasers. *Lasers Surg Med* 2009; 41(4): 264–270.

41 Eduardo FP, Bezinelli L, Luiz AC, Correa L, Vogel C, Eduardo CP. Severity of oral mucositis in patients undergoing hematopoietic cell transplantation and an oral laser phototherapy protocol: a survey of 30 patients. *Photomed Laser Surg* 2009; 27(1): 137–144.

42 Kuhn A, Porto FA, Miraglia P, Brunetto AL. Low-level infrared laser therapy in chemotherapy-induced oral mucositis: a randomized placebo-controlled trial in children. *J Pediatr Hematol Oncol* 2009; 31(1): 33–37.

43 Lima AG, Antequera R, Peres MP, Snitcosky IM, Federico MH, Villar RC. Efficacy of low-level laser therapy and aluminum hydroxide in patients with chemotherapy and radiotherapy-induced oral mucositis. *Braz Dent J* 2010; 21(3): 186–192.

44 Zanin T, Zanin F, Carvalhosa AA, et al. Use of 660-nm diode laser in the prevention and treatment of human oral mucositis induced by radiotherapy and chemotherapy. *Photomed Laser Surg* 2010; 28(2): 233–237.

45 Silva GB, Mendonca EF, Bariani C, Antunes HS, Silva MA. The prevention of induced oral mucositis with low-level laser therapy in bone marrow transplantation patients: a randomized clinical trial. *Photomed Laser Surg* 2011; 29(1): 27–31.

46 Carvalho PA, Jaguar GC, Pellizzon AC, Prado JD, Lopes RN, Alves FA. Evaluation of low-level laser therapy in the prevention and treatment of radiation-induced mucositis: A double-blind randomized study in head and neck cancer patients. *Oral Oncol* 2011; 47(12): 1176–1181.

47 Gautam AP, Fernandes DJ, Vidyasagar MS, Maiya GA. Low level helium neon laser therapy for chemoradiotherapy induced oral mucositis in oral cancer patients - A randomized controlled trial. *Oral Oncol* 2012; 48(9): 893–897.

48 Lima AG, Villar RC, de Castro G, Jr, et al. Oral mucositis prevention by low-level laser therapy in head-and-neck cancer patients undergoing concurrent chemoradiotherapy: a phase III randomized study. *Int J Radiat Oncol Biol Phys* 2012; 82(1): 270–275.

49 Chor A, Torres SR, Maiolino A, Nucci M. Low-power laser to prevent oral mucositis in autologous hematopoietic stem cell transplantation. *Eur J Haematol* 2010; 84(2): 178–179.

50 Kuhn A, Vacaro G, Almeida D, Machado A, Braghini PB, Shilling MA. Low-level infrared laser therapy for chemo- or radiation-induced oral mucositis: a randomized placebo-controlled study. *J Oral Laser Appl* 2007; 7: 175–181.

51 Migliorati C, Hewson I, Lalla RV, et al. Systematic review of laser and other light therapy for the management of oral mucositis in cancer patients. *Support Care Cancer* 2013; 21(1): 333–341.

52 Tunér J, Hode L. *The New Laser Therapy Handbook*. Grängesberg: Prima Books AB, 2010: 847.

CHAPTER 41

Cost-effectiveness of laser therapy in hospital practice

Leticia Mello Bezinelli[1] and Luciana Corrêa[2]

[1]Oncology, Hematology and Bone Marrow Transplantation Program, Hospital Israelita Albert Einstein, São Paulo, SP, Brazil
[2]General Pathology Department, School of Dentistry, University of São Paulo (USP), São Paulo, SP, Brazil

Introduction

The cost-effectiveness of health care needs to be studied because of the scarcity of resources in the face of the unlimited needs of society, with a view to satisfying the growing needs of the world population in terms of health promotion, well being, and quality of life.[1]

The comparison between benefits of health care and costs of a new technology, in comparison with available alternatives, is made in studies of cost-effectiveness, cost-utility, and cost-benefit.[2] *Cost-effectiveness* involves a broad spectrum of analyses, mainly based on clinical results, measuring the impact of interventions in a more global manner. The most commonly used units of measurement for these studies are the number of cases avoided, hospitalizations prevented, cases detected, and lives or years of life saved.

Comparisons are made between two or more alternative intervention strategies for prevention, diagnosis or treatment of a certain health condition. Its greatest applicability is in the comparison between two possible strategies that cannot be implemented concomitantly. The cost-effectiveness ratio is the difference between the costs of the two interventions, divided by the difference between their consequences in terms of health (effectiveness). *Cost-utility* is a type of cost-effectiveness analysis in which the measurement of the effects of an intervention considers the improvement in quality of life and increase in longevity.

Lastly, *cost-benefit* (or *cost-minimization*) considers the impact of a health action in terms of monetary values.

The results of these analyses are presented as net benefits (benefits of the intervention less the costs of the intervention).

Measuring cost-effectiveness of laser therapy

Despite the inclusion of the term "cost" in these modalities, cost is not an essential aspect of these analyses; rather it is the manner in which the clinical results with the use of the intervention in a study are obtained.[3]

Considering that laser therapy is a new technology in health care, and that the implementation of this technology generates additional costs, the fundamental question to be answered in economic studies resides mainly in the analysis of the extra cost associated with the extra effect obtained; that is the extra cost-to-extra benefit ratio, or in simpler terms, the cost-effectiveness. Table 41.1 summarizes these measurements.

The extra cost is relatively simple to calculate, since it involves the monetary value of the acquisition and maintenance of laser equipment, the qualification/training of personnel to use laser therapy protocols, and in many cases, the salaries of the professionals who operate this technology. This cost may be divided by the number of sessions in which laser therapy is used. The extra effect, that is the improved clinical results obtained, must consider the indirect as well as the direct effects of laser therapy. Monetary values can be calculated for some of these effects, but not others.

Direct effects of laser therapy

One of the direct effects most discussed in laser therapy is the length of time when the laser is operational, particularly when considering the surgical maneuvers of incision and ablation (in the case of high power laser therapy) and/or biomodulation (in the case of low level laser therapy [LLLT]). Generally, the mean time of a laser therapy session is measured in chronological units and compared with other techniques, commonly of the conventional type. Minimization or maximization of this time may be converted into monetary values using, for example, the unit of number of sessions. It is worth pointing out that in cost-utility studies, in which the monetary value of the intervention is generally not considered, the time taken for sessions may be an important factor, particularly if it interferes with the patient's well being; for example, very long sessions of LLLT may generate discomfort in the patient, which may worsen the morbidity.

The reduction in morbidity is one of the aspects most analyzed in health economics, particularly in cost-effectiveness.

Lasers in Dentistry: Guide for Clinical Practice, First Edition. Edited by Patrícia M. de Freitas and Alyne Simões.
© 2015 John Wiley & Sons, Inc. Published 2015 by John Wiley & Sons, Inc.

Table 41.1 Measurable units in the analysis of the effectiveness of laser therapy, as well as the main characteristics that must be considered in economic analyses.

Measurable unit	Characteristics
Monetary costs	
Number of laser therapy sessions	Includes fixed and variable costs, such as the monetary cost of acquisition/maintenance of laser equipment, qualification/training in the use of laser therapy, professional fees
Direct effects	
Time of sessions	Considered in comparison with other techniques; must be evaluated both in monetary terms and in terms of patient comfort/discomfort
Tissue repair	May be measured from the time taken for surgical repair or repair of lesions, or reduction/increase in lesions or injury, using systems for grading the severity of lesions
Pain	Both postoperative pain (in the case of high level laser therapy) and the analgesic effect (in the case of LLLT) must be measured using, for example, visual pain scales, classifications of loss of function, duration of painful symptoms, or information related to the prescription of analgesics (see "indirect effects"); these have a high impact in cost-utility analyses
Taste and xerostomia	May impact on cost-utility analyses as they contribute to the maintenance of the patient's quality of life; they may also have an influence of the patient's degree of nutrition (see "indirect effects")
Indirect effects	
Prescription of analgesics/anti-inflammatory agents	May be measured in monetary terms, particularly as regards daily costs of prescription and cost of total dose used; may also be considered in cost-utility analyses
Prescription of antimicrobial/antibiotic/antiviral/antifungal agents	May be measured in monetary terms, and also with regards to reduction/increase in risk of sepsis and bacteremia
Nutritional impact	Analysis of body mass gain/loss, nutritional biochemical indices, need for use of artificial nutrition and complementary diet; this type of information should preferably be converted into monetary values; these have a high impact in cost-utility analyses, particularly regarding normal functions of mastication/deglutition and sense of taste
Number of days of hospitalization	One of the main economic indicators at hospital level; must be measured in monetary terms (e.g. daily hospital fee)
Survival of patients	Important indicator of the effectiveness of a technology; not measurable at a monetary level, but is fundamental for analyses concerning social and public policy

In general, the same measurable units are adopted in clinical studies. As the majority of current laser therapy applications aim to promote tissue repair of surgical and other lesions, analysis of the re-establishment of tissue homeostasis is one of the most sensitive indicators in the cost-effectiveness analysis of laser therapy.

As a measurement of time to lesion repair, the reduction/increase in the number of lesions may be adopted, or a classification that measures the severity of signs and symptoms. For example, one way to measure the effectiveness of LLLT in the reduction of oral mucositis is by analyzing both the duration of lesions and their severity. Adoption of the blind method of analysis and standardization of observation are crucial in economic analysis.

When considering morbidity, painful symptomatology also constitutes a crucial aspect of the analysis of cost-effectiveness of laser therapy. The intensity of postoperative pain in the case of high power laser therapy or the analgesic effect of LLLT must be measured with a certain degree of objectivity. Visual pain scales are commonly used in clinical studies, as well as loss of function (e.g. restriction of mandibular movements or facial movements) and duration of painful symptomatology. This information may be complemented in economic analyses by the indirect effect of laser therapy on the prescription of analgesics, which may be attributed a monetary value – the cost of the prescription of opioid or non-opioid analgesics and anti-inflammatory agents.

The units of measurement are variable, ranging from monetary value of a medication prescribed through to daily hospital fees, which may or may not include the cost of medication.

It is important to mention that pain measurement is one of the most important aspects in analyses involving cost-utility, which consider the impact of this symptom at both the individual and society level.

The impact of laser therapy on the reduction of xerostomia and maintenance of taste is also considered. Salivary examinations and inquiries about taste may be important, particularly in cost-utility analyses.

Indirect effects of laser therapy

The indirect effects of laser therapy are mostly observed in hospitalizations that involve a long stay by the patient. In this case, some measurements of the costs of hospitalization and prescription of medications become sensitive.

The impact of laser therapy on tissue repair and its analgesic effect may result in reduction in the prescription of analgesics and anti-inflammatory drugs, as previously mentioned.

If lesions of an infectious nature are involved, or those of a type that may potentially become infected, or increase the risk of bacteremia and sepsis, the early repair of these lesions may result in a reduction in the prescription of antimicrobial agents, antibiotics, antiviral and antifungal medications. Thus, in a cost-effectiveness analysis of laser therapy, the measurement of these items may be important, preferably in monetary terms. Also, particularly in the use of laser therapy in the oral cavity, a reduction in morbidity in this location may have a substantial effect on the patient's nutrition. Maintenance of normal nutritional levels is one of the great challenges to clinical medicine in patients who are hospitalized for long periods of time, and generally results in high treatment costs. Laser therapy may have a positive impact on this aspect. In this sense, consideration of body mass gain/loss, nutritional biochemical indices, need for the use of artificial nutrition and complementary diet are crucial, and must be measured in monetary values. An important point is the impact that the normal ingestion of foods has on the patient's quality of life. Therefore, in a cost-utility analysis of laser therapy, the impact of this technique on the maintenance of the functions of mastication and swallowing, as well as sense of taste can also be useful.

Reduction in the number of days of hospitalization is one of the most important indirect effects in economic analyses of cost-effectiveness, cost-benefit, and cost-utility at the hospital level. It may be considered as one of the monetary items with the greatest impact on the decision of whether or not to adopt the technology in question. As laser therapy may reduce the number of days of hospitalization, particularly due to its impact on morbidity, this information is of fundamental importance in economic analyses.

Lastly, the question of the patient's survival must be considered. Survival is computed as a value that is immeasurable in monetary terms, but substantial in determining the total effectiveness of a technology.

Laser therapy in dentistry: Clinical and economic impact

An important point to be emphasized in economic analyses of laser therapy in dentistry is the association of this technique with overall dental management, that is the technique is performed by an experienced dental surgeon whose actions extend beyond laser irradiation – the cost-effectiveness of laser therapy will depend on the dental surgeon having made the correct decisions regarding diagnosis and treatment. When

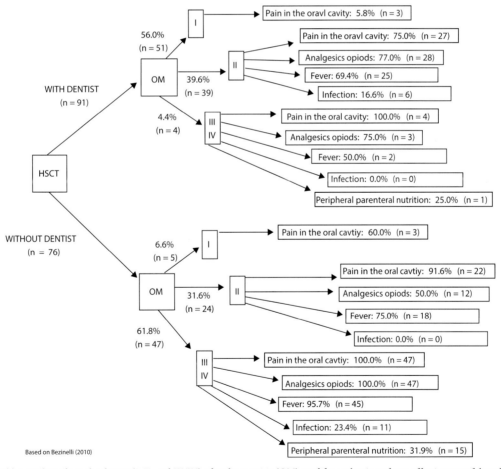

Figure 41.1 Variables resulting from the degree (I, II, and III/IV) of oral mucositis (OM) used for evaluation of cost-effectiveness of dental management associated with laser therapy in patients undergoing high doses of chemotherapy for hematopoietic stem cell transplant (HSCT). The term "with dentist" refers to the group of patients who were under dental management associated with laser therapy, and the term "without dentist" refers to the group of patients without this treatment (based on Bezinelli[4]).

irradiating the oral cavity, the dental surgeon would previously have diagnosed the degree of morbidity of the oral mucosa and teeth, and monitored the degree of oral hygiene. He/she would also have eliminated foci of infection. All these actions must be linked to the laser therapy sessions and their effects must also be measured.

This relationship can be illustrated with a retrospective study of patients hospitalized for hematopoietic stem cell transplantation. This clinical and economic study assessed the degree of morbidity in the oral cavity in two populations of patients: one with dental management performed by a dental surgeon in association with LLLT, and the other without LLLT and specialized oral care.[4] The LLLT was performed daily from the first day after chemotherapy conditioning up to the end of the period of severe neutropenia, without interruption. Some of the variables listed in Table 41.1 were used to analyze the cost-effectiveness of this association. Figure 41.1 illustrates these variables and their frequency in the two populations for oral mucositis. Oral mucositis was chosen as the subject of this study because of its high impact on the quality of life and health of the patient after the transplant.

The cost of hospitalization was partially determined by intermediary monetary analysis of the daily hospital fees, including peripheral parenteral nutrition (PPN) and the prescription of opioids. It was observed that the group without laser therapy and dental management exhibited greater frequency of severe degrees of oral mucositis, with a significant association between this severity and the use of PPN and prescription of opioids, pain in the oral cavity, and fever of greater than 37.8 °C. The hospital costs in this group were up to 159.23% higher. It was concluded that dental management, including laser therapy, performed by a dental surgeon may contribute to the reduction in morbidity resulting from oral mucositis, and consequently to minimizing hospital costs for patients undergoing hematopoietic stem cell transplants.

Final considerations

The analysis of cost-effectiveness may be based on the clinical result alone. Nevertheless, establishing which clinical result is significant in analyzing success may not be easy. The efficacy of laser therapy in various clinical situations has been extensively recorded in the literature; however, there are few economic studies of this technique. As a general rule, it may be concluded that laser therapy entails an increase in costs, but also promotion of clinical effects, with possible impact on morbidity. Further economic investigation is necessary.

Economic analyses objectively measure the clinical effects in conjunction with the costs. This approach allows a direct comparison of the cost-benefit of introducing a new technology or not. However, economic analyses are tools for making estimates and not decisions, since many actions in health care are adopted based on their effect on quality of life, which cannot always be measured in economic terms. Therefore, the decision to use laser therapy or not in certain situations must include an economic analysis, but not be based exclusively on it.

References

1 Nita ME, Secoli SR, Nobre MRC, et al. Visão geral dos métodos em avaliação de tecnologias em saúde. In: Nita ME, Secoli SR, Nobre MRC, et al. *Avaliação de tecnologias em saúde: evidência clínica, análise econômica e análise de decisão*. Porto Alegre: ArtMed, 2010: 225–236.

2 Goodman CS. *Introduction to Health Technology Assessment*. Estados Unidos: National Library of Medicine, 2004.

3 Hoch JS, Dewa CS. An introduction to economic evaluation: what's in a name? *Can J Psychiatry* 2005; 50(3): 159–166.

4 Bezinelli LM. *Dental attendance in bone marrow transplants: clinical and economic impact*. Dissertation. São Paulo: University of São Paulo, Faculty of Dentistry, 2010.

CHAPTER 42

Low Level Laser Therapy for hyposalivation and xerostomia

Alyne Simões, Luana de Campos, Victor Elias Arana-Chavez, and José Nicolau

Department of Biomaterials and Oral Biology, School of Dentistry, University of São Paulo (USP), São Paulo, SP, Brazil

Introduction

The common side effects of head and neck radiotherapy and/or chemotherapy are oral mucositis, hyposalivation/xerostomia, and severe pain. This chapter describes how low level laser therapy (LLLT) can be used as an auxiliary therapy for salivary gland stimulation, improving patient quality of life.

Whole saliva is produced in the major salivary glands (parotid, submandibular, and sublingual glands), which are the main contributors to oral fluid (90%); the minor salivary glands contribute for the remaining 10%. Even though the minor salivary glands produce only 10% of the total volume of saliva, they play an important role in lubricating the mucosa, and consequently their hypofunction can be related to symptoms of dry mouth. The volume of saliva produced per day ranges between 0.5 and 1.0 L in normal physiological conditions, and the physiological pH range for saliva is 6.5–7.4.[1]

It is important to differentiate between xerostomia, which is the subjective feeling of dry mouth, and hyposalivation, which is the objective evidence of reduced saliva flow rate. When patients show a resting saliva flow rate (volume of saliva/collection time) of 0.1 mL/min or less and/or a stimulated whole saliva flow rate of 0.7 mL/min or less, they are diagnosed with salivary gland hypofunction (hyposalivation).[1]

Why is it important to study saliva? Saliva is important for health as it preserves the integrity of teeth and oral soft tissues. Cleansing of the oral cavity, moistening of food, bolus formation, and bacterial and food clearance are other examples of functions at least in part related to saliva. Components of saliva also contribute to a buffering action, an antimicrobial action (i.e. lysozyme and peroxidase enzymes), antioxidant defense (i.e. catalase and peroxidase), and digestion (salivary amylase). Therefore, it is important to study this fluid since patients with salivary gland hypofunction usually are restricted in their daily activities, have poorer general well being, and are handicapped in their social life.

Immunological and rheumatic diseases (see Clinical case 42.1), as well as some genetic disorders, cause a marked reduction in saliva flow rate. Moreover, anticancer therapies, such as head and neck radiotherapy and/or chemotherapy, are inevitably associated with salivary gland injury.

The extent of radiotherapy-induced salivary gland damage depends on the volume of glandular tissue included in the radiation field and on the dose of radiation delivered. Generally, completely irradiated parotid glands exposed to doses of 60 Gy (the standard radiation therapy) sustain permanent damage, with extensive degeneration of acini, as well as inflammation and fibrosis in the interstitium, resulting in hypofunction.[2] A mechanism of action to explain the early effects and the high radiosensitivity of salivary gland cells, in spite of their slow turnover rate (60–120 days), is radiation damage to the plasma membrane, which results in disruption of muscarinic receptor-stimulated water secretion.[2] Furthermore, salivary gland flow rate can be reduced even with relatively low radiation doses (10–15 Gy).[1] Radiation effects on salivary glands are well known and are of particular interest in radiotherapy of head and neck cancer, as the reduced saliva flow rate and altered composition of saliva result in distress, oral dryness, nocturnal oral discomfort, burning mouth, and susceptibility to oral infections and dental caries, as well as hampering oral function and social activities. The saliva also shows increased viscosity, reduced pH and buffering capacity, and altered electrolyte concentrations.

Although many patients treated with chemotherapy also have salivary gland hypofunction, no firm conclusion has been reached in the literature about chemotherapy effects on salivary glands.[3] Some chemotherapeutic agents, including 5-fluorouracil (5-FU), doxorubicin, and cyclophosphamide, can induce salivary gland hypofunction/xerostomia. Although there are few studies of the effect of chemotherapy on salivary glands, reported effects include ductal dilatation, acinar degeneration, cyst formation and inflammation in the glandular tissue, infiltration of inflammatory cells, and swelling and interstitial fibrosis.[4,5] In addition, a small number of

Lasers in Dentistry: Guide for Clinical Practice, First Edition. Edited by Patrícia M. de Freitas and Alyne Simões.

Table 42.1 Clinical studies showing an improvement in xerostomia or saliva flow rate with laser irradiation.

Authors	Number of patients (condition)	Laser and wavelength (nm)	Power (mW)	Energy density (J/cm²)	Laser spot area (cm²)	Energy per point (J)	Total energy (J)	Time per point or area (s)	Irradiation field
Fructuoso and Moset[29]	15 (SS)	GaAs 904	20	6	0.1	0.6	3.0	30 (if the area used in the laser software was 0.1 cm²)	5 points on the parotid glands
Cowen et al.[20]	30 (MSCT)	HeNe 632.8	60	1.5			54	10	5 anatomic sites of the oral cavity
Lopes et al.[21]	60 (RT/CT)	InGaAlP 685	35	2				58	19 points intra- and extra-orally
Campos et al.[11]	1 (RT)	Diode 660	40	6	0.04	0.24		6	Entire oral cavity
Simoes et al.[14]	1 (SS)	Diode 780	15	3.8	0.04	0.15	5.4	10	Major glands
Simoes et al.[12]	22 (RT)	Diode 660	40	6	0.04	0.24	21	6	90 points intraorally
Juras et al.[19]	17 (MD)	Diode Infrared	30	1.8			23		Major glands
Loncar et al.[18]	34 (MD)	GaAs 904	6	29.48	0.02	0.72	4.3	120	Major glands

MSCT, bone marrow transplant; RT, radiotherapy; CT, chemotherapy; SS, Sjögren's syndrome; MD, dry mouth symptom.

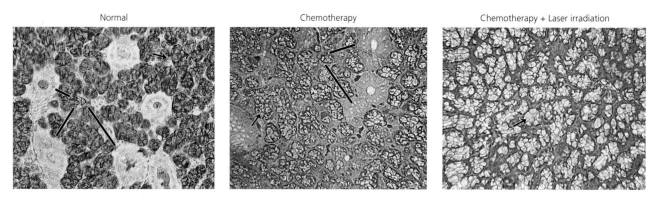

Figure 42.1 Salivary glands from hamsters in the normal control group (Normal), 5-fluouracil (5-FU) chemotherapy group (Chemotherapy), and 5-FU plus LLLT group (Chemotherapy + Laser Irradiation). Animals who received 5-FU (Chemotherapy) showed acinar atrophy with an increase in the intercellular spaces and loss of boundary cells when compared to the Normal and Chemotherapy + Laser Irradiation groups. SD, secretory ducts; arrow, secretory endpieces (original magnifications 40×).

studies show the effect of different chemotherapy regimens on biochemical parameters of saliva (sialic acids, protein and electrolyte content, and saliva flow rate). However, the data are not conclusive since different chemotherapy regimens and study periods were used in relation to the administration of chemotherapeutics.[6,7] Moreover, it is important to highlight that, in contrast to radiation-induced hyposalivation, the damage at salivary gland level after chemoterapy, can return to near-normal levels, depending on, for example, the dose and chemotherapeutic agent used.[8]

Other complications related to hyposalivation induced by cancer treatment include impairment of basic oral functions (such as speech, mastication, swallowing, and taste), as well as oral mucositis, opportunistic infection, fungal infection, and fast progression of caries. Moreover, pain and discomfort associated with hyposalivation and mucositis may affect the quality of life of patients and may be associated with increased morbidity and significant additional hospital costs.[9,10] However, since hyposalivation and/or xerostomia are not life threatening in patients with cancer, they are often described as orphan topics under the heading of supportive care.

Several treatments have been described to minimize the severity of oral side effects induced by radiotherapy and/or chemotherapy. Wetting agents or saliva substitutes have a palliative effect, but are not well accepted by patients. Therapies for hyposalivation also include systemic sialagogues, such as pilocarpine, carbachol, bethanechol, and cevimeline, which stimulate the saliva flow rate; however, they can be associated with side effects. In addition, as described in Chapter 40, LLLT has been used to prevent and treat radiotherapy and/or chemotherapy-induced oral mucositis, as well as hyposalivation and xerostomia.[11–22]

Laser studies on salivary glands

Although few studies have investigated the effect of LLLT on salivary gland hypofunction and xerostomia, their promising results suggest that salivary gland biomodulation following LLLT is likely to give a very good outcome.

One concern about laser application is whether the biostimulation of salivary glands promoted by irradiation

---

Clinical case 42.1[14]

A 60-year-old woman diagnosed with salivary gland hypofunction associated with Sjögren's syndrome was referred to the Special Laboratory of Lasers in Dentistry (LELO) due to symptoms of severe xerostomia. A detailed history and clinical examination were performed, and the following signs and symptoms were observed: dehydrated skin, lack of teeth, xerostomia, xerophthalmia, fissured tongue, angular cheilitis, and parotid gland pain and swelling, which required corticosteroids (Fig. 42.2a).

A semiconductor diode laser (Twin Laser MMOptics®, Sao Carlos, Brazil; 780 nm, 15 mW) was applied to the parotid, submandibular,

and sublingual glands (12, three, and three points on each gland, respectively) (Fig. 42.2b). LLLT was performed in continuous-wave mode; the laser beam spot area was 0.04 cm², the dose was 3.8 J/cm², and, consequently, the laser irradiation time was 10 seconds.[14] The irradiation was performed three times per week for 8 months. The symptom of dry mouth improved during the treatment with LLLT, and parotid and salivary gland pain and swelling were no longer reported (Fig. 42.2c).

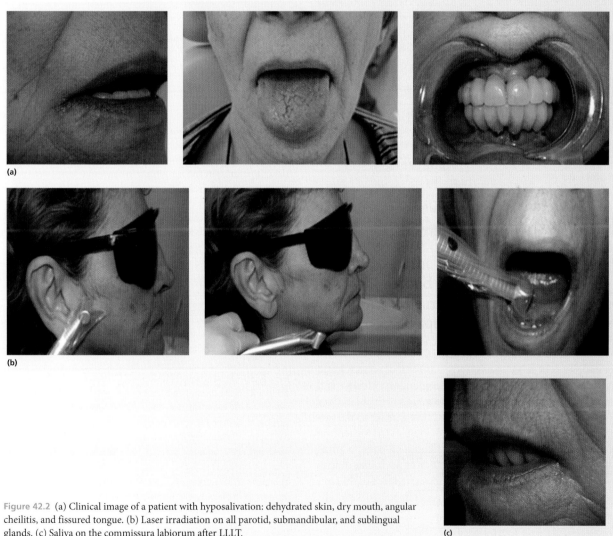

(a)

(b)

(c)

Figure 42.2 (a) Clinical image of a patient with hyposalivation: dehydrated skin, dry mouth, angular cheilitis, and fissured tongue. (b) Laser irradiation on all parotid, submandibular, and sublingual glands. (c) Saliva on the commissura labiorum after LLLT.

results in an increase in saliva secretion or only the relief of symptoms of xerostomia.

The first published works on the effect of laser irradiation on salivary glands demonstrated that laser irradiation can act on the glandular tissue, promoting cellular responses; however, the laser parameters used in these studies are not known in full.[23-28]

Some clinical studies of salivary gland irradiation have demonstrated that LLLT is effective in increasing saliva flow rate,[19,21,29] reducing mouth dryness,[11,12,14,18-20] and biomodulating tissue inflammatory processes[23,25,26] (Table 42.1). In a 1997 study investigating the effect of red LLLT on the prevention of oral mucositis in patients undergoing bone marrow transplant, Cowen et al. also reported improvement in saliva production and in the ability of cancer patients to swallow.[20] In addition, in 2006, Lopes et al. observed an increase in saliva flow rate and a reduction in xerostomia in patients submitted to head and neck radiotherapy (from 45 to 72 Gy total radiation dose) who received red diode laser irradiation to major salivary glands, as well as to some intraoral points to reach the minor salivary glands.[21] In a recent study, we used a combination of objective (sialometry and sialochemistry) and subjective (questionnaires) parameters to examine the effect of red irradiation on salivary glands of patients with salivary gland hypofunction induced by radiotherapy.[12] In that study, we observed that LLLT (three times per week) maintained the saliva flow rate at the same level through to the last radiotherapy session. In addition, an improvement in the symptom of xerostomia was observed, which was caused by an increase in sialic acid, in turn related to lubrication of the oral cavity.

In addition to clinical trials, few laboratory studies were conducted using animals, which demonstrated that infrared LLLT can stimulate salivary glands of rats[13] and change their composition.[30-34] Regarding cell culture, it was observed that laser irradiation of Par-C10 cells (derived from rat parotid acinar cells) promoted cell proliferation and expression of anti-apoptosis proteins in Par-C10 cells.[35]

In addition to these clinical studies, our group is conducting studies on the effect of 5-FU on the salivary glands of hamsters. A clear acinar atrophy of the submandibular glands and an increase in glandular stroma, as well as smaller secretory endpieces of sublingual glands, has been observed. LLLT was shown to prevent the increase in glandular stroma and changes in secretory pieces, and also to maintain the boundary between their cells. Thus, we observed that damage to the salivary gland structure was repaired (Fig. 42.1) when an InGaAIP diode laser, emitting infrared light (780 nm, continuous wave, punctual and contact mode) was used. The output power was 20 mW, with an energy density (dose) of 5 J/cm^2, spot size of 0.04 cm^2, and irradiation time of 10 seconds, totaling 0.2 J of energy per point.

Final considerations

The literature suggests that LLLT is an efficacious method for improving the quality and increasing the quantity of saliva, and thereby improving the quality of life of patients with salivary gland hypofunction. However, the use of LLLT on the salivary glands of cancer patients treated with radiotherapy and/or chemotherapy has not been thoroughly studied, and controlled studies are necessary to confirm whether the stimulation of the salivary glands by LLLT benefits patients treated with radiotherapy and/or chemotherapy.

Acknowledgments

We would like to thank FAPESP (Fundação de Amparo à Pesquisa do Estado de São Paulo - Grants #2010/03662-6 and #2011/14013-1) and CAPES (Coordenação de Aperfeiçoamento de Pessoal de Nível Superior, #1455993) for financial support. In addition, we would also like to thank the Oral Biology Laboratory and the Special Laboratory of Lasers in Dentistry (LELO) at the School of Dentistry of the University of Sao Paulo.

References

1 Jensen SB, Pedersen AM, Reibel J, Nauntofte B. Xerostomia and hypofunction of the salivary glands in cancer therapy. *Support Care Cancer* 2003; 11(4): 207–225.

2 Vissink A, Mitchell JB, Baum BJ, et al. Clinical management of salivary gland hypofunction and xerostomia in head-and-neck cancer patients: successes and barriers. *Int J Radiat Oncol Biol Phys* 2010; 78(4): 983–991.

3 Jensen SB, Pedersen AM, Vissink A, et al. A systematic review of salivary gland hypofunction and xerostomia induced by cancer therapies: prevalence, severity and impact on quality of life. *Support Care Cancer* 2010; 18(8): 1039–1060.

4 Lockhart PB, Sonis ST. Alterations in the oral mucosa caused by chemotherapeutic agents. *A histologic study. J Dermatol Surg Oncol* 1981; 7(12): 1019–1025.

5 Ramaniuk K, Gavin JB, Adkins KF. The effect of methotrexate on salivary glands in the rat. (abstract no 261). *J Dent Res* 1983; 62: 678.

6 Ozturk LK, Emekli-Alturfan E, Kasikci E, Demir G, Yarat A. Salivary total sialic acid levels increase in breast cancer patients: a preliminary study. *Med Chem* 2011; 7(5): 443–447.

7 Jensen SB, Mouridsen HT, Reibel J, Brunner N, Nauntofte B. Adjuvant chemotherapy in breast cancer patients induces temporary salivary gland hypofunction. *Oral Oncol.* 2008; 44(2):1 62–73.

8 Vissink A, Burlage FR, Spijkervet FK, Veerman EC, Nieuw Amerongen AV. Prevention and treatment of salivary gland hypofunction related to head and neck radiation therapy and chemotherapy. *Support Cancer Ther* 2004; 1(2): 111–118.

9 Chambers MS, Garden AS, Kies MS, Martin JW. Radiation-induced xerostomia in patients with head and neck cancer: pathogenesis, impact on quality of life, and management. *Head Neck* 2004; 26(9): 796–807.

10 Brosky ME. The role of saliva in oral health: strategies for prevention and management of xerostomia. *J Support Oncol* 2007; 5(5): 215–225.

11 Campos L, Simoes A, Sa PH, Eduardo Cde P. Improvement in quality of life of an oncological patient by laser phototherapy. *Photomed Laser Surg* 2009; 27(2): 371–374.

12 Simoes A, de Campos L, de Souza DN, de Matos JA, Freitas PM, Nicolau J. Laser phototherapy as topical prophylaxis against radiation-induced xerostomia. *Photomed Laser Surg* 2010; 28(3): 357–363.

13 Simoes A, Nicolau J, de Souza DN, et al. Effect of defocused infrared diode laser on salivary flow rate and some salivary parameters of rats. *Clin Oral Investig* 2008; 12(1): 25–30.

14 Simoes A, Platero MD, Campos L, Aranha AC, Eduardo Cde P, Nicolau J. Laser as a therapy for dry mouth symptoms in a patient with Sjogren's syndrome: a case report. *Spec Care Dentist* 2009; 29(3): 134–137.

15 Simoes A, Eduardo FP, Luiz AC, et al. Laser phototherapy as topical prophylaxis against head and neck cancer radiotherapy-induced oral mucositis: comparison between low and high/low power lasers. *Lasers Surg Med* 2009; 41(4): 264–270.

16 Bensadoun RJ, Nair RG. Efficacy of low-level laser therapy (LLLT) in oral mucositis: What have we learned from randomized studies and meta-analyses? *Photomed Laser Surg* 2012; 30(4): 191–192.

17 Bjordal JM, Bensadoun RJ, Tuner J, Frigo L, Gjerde K, Lopes-Martins RA. A systematic review with meta-analysis of the effect of low-level laser therapy (LLLT) in cancer therapy-induced oral mucositis. *Support Care Cancer* 2011; 19(8): 1069–1077.

18 Loncar B, Stipetic MM, Baricevic M, Risovic D. The effect of low-level laser therapy on salivary glands in patients with xerostomia. *Photomed Laser Surg* 2011; 29(3): 171–175.

19 Juras DV, Lukac J, Cekic-Arambasin A, et al. Effects of low-level laser treatment on mouth dryness. *Collegium Antropol* 2010; 34(3): 1039–1043.

20 Cowen D, Tardieu C, Schubert M, et al. Low energy Helium-Neon laser in the prevention of oral mucositis in patients undergoing bone marrow transplant: results of a double blind randomized trial. *Int J Radiat Oncol Biology Phys* 1997; 38(4): 697–703.

21 Lopes CO, Mas JRI, Zangaro RA. Prevenção da xerostomia e da mucosite oral induzidas por radioterapia com uso do laser de baixa potência. *Radiol Bras* 2006; 39(2): 131–136.

22 Schubert MM, Eduardo FP, Guthrie KA, et al. A phase III randomized double-blind placebo-controlled clinical trial to determine the efficacy of low level laser therapy for the prevention of oral mucositis in patients undergoing hematopoietic cell transplantation. *Support Care Cancer* 2007; 15(10): 1145–1154.

23 Kats AG. Nizkoenergeticheskoe lazernoe izluchenie v kompleksnom lechenii vospaleniia sliunnykh zhelez. [Low-energy laser radiation in the combined treatment of salivary gland inflammation]. *Stomatologiia* 1993; 72(4): 32–36.

24 Kats AG. Vliianie funktsional'nykh prob i nizkoenergeticheskogo gelii-neonovogo lazera na mestnoe krovoobrashchenie v oblasti okoloushnykh zhelez. [The effect of functional tests and of a low-energy helium-neon laser on the local blood circulation in the area of the parotid glands]. *Stomatologiia* 1994; 73(2): 42–44.

25 Kats AG, Belostotskaia IM, Malomud ZP, Makarova LG. Otdalennye rezul'taty kompleksnogo lecheniia khronicheskogo sialoadenita s primeneniem gelii-neonovogo lazera. [Remote results of the complex treatment of chronic sialadenitis using the helium-neon laser]. *Vestnik khirurgii imeni I I Grekova* 1985; 135(10): 39–42.

26 Kats AG, Belostotskaia IM, Zolotareva Iu B, Malomud ZP, Oleinik EM. Primenenie izlucheniia lazera v kompleksnom lechenii bol'nykh sialoadenitom. [Use of laser radiation in the combined treatment of sialadenitis patients]. *Stomatologiia* 1986; 65(2): 66–68.

27 Takeda Y. Irradiation effect of low-energy laser on rat submandibular salivary gland. *J Oral Pathol* 1988; 17(2): 91–94.

28 Plavnik LM, De Crosa ME, Malberti AI. Effect of low-power radiation (helium/neon) upon submandibulary glands. *J Clin Laser Med Surg* 2003; 21(4): 219–225.

29 Fructuoso FJG, Moset JM. Randomized double blind study on biostimulatory effect of laser irradiation of the parotid gland in patients suffering of Sjögren syndrome. *Invest Clinica Laser* 1987; 1: 18–25.

30 Simoes A, Siqueira WL, Lamers ML, Santos MF, Eduardo Cde P, Nicolau J. Laser phototherapy effect on protein metabolism parameters of rat salivary glands. *Lasers Med Sci* 2009; 24(2): 202–208.

31 Simoes A, Nogueira FN, de Paula Eduardo C, Nicolau J. Diode laser decreases the activity of catalase on submandibular glands of diabetic rats. *Photomed Laser Surg* 2010; 28(1): 91–95.

32 Simoes A, Ganzerla E, Yamaguti PM, de Paula Eduardo C, Nicolau J. Effect of diode laser on enzymatic activity of parotid glands of diabetic rats. *Lasers Med Sci* 2009; 24(4): 591–596.

33 Simoes A, de Oliveira E, Campos L, Nicolau J. Ionic and histological studies of salivary glands in rats with diabetes and their glycemic state after laser irradiation. *Photomed Laser Surg* 2009; 27(6): 877–883.

34 Ibuki FK, Simoes A, Nicolau J, Nogueira FN. Laser irradiation affects enzymatic antioxidant system of streptozotocin-induced diabetic rats. *Lasers Med Sci* 2013; 28(3): 911–918.

35 Onizawa K, Muramatsu T, Matsuki M, et al. Low-level (gallium-aluminum-arsenide) laser irradiation of Par-C10 cells and acinar cells of rat parotid gland. *Lasers Med Sci* 2009; 24(2): 155–161.

CHAPTER 43

Antimicrobial photodynamic therapy in cancer patients

Luana de Campos,[1] Cesar A. Migliorati,[2] and Alyne Simões[1]

[1]Department of Biomaterials and Oral Biology, School of Dentistry, University of São Paulo (USP), São Paulo, SP, Brazil
[2]Department of Diagnostic Sciences and Oral Medicine, College of Dentistry, University of Tennessee Health Science Center, Memphis, TN, USA

Antineoplastic treatments, such as ionizing head and neck radiotherapy and chemotherapy, can induce several oral complications in cancer patients. These complications could compromise patient health and quality of life, affect their ability to complete a planned cancer treatment, and also lead to serious systemic infections.[1,2]

Cancer therapy can myelosuppress the patient and put them at risk for infections and bleeding. Common oral complications associated with cancer therapies include pain, damage to the oral mucosa, salivary gland hypofunction, opportunistic infections (herpes, cytomegalovirus, candidiasis, etc.), radiation caries, osteoradionecrosis, and bleeding. Oral complications may be prevented or reduced if the dentist is given the opportunity to examine the cancer patient before the start of cancer treatment. In addition to preventing or reducing the severity of oral complications, the dentist can provide safe, effective, and minimally invasive dental treatment during and after radiotherapy and/or chemotherapy.

Non-invasive therapies to prevent or treat some of these oral complications are of importance. In addition, such therapies may improve oral hygiene, decrease the risk of oral diseases, and make symptomatic patients more comfortable. In this context, there are studies in the literature that show the benefits of the use of low level laser therapy (LLLT) in oral complications induced by antineoplastic treatment. The beneficial effects of LLLT are related to decreasing the healing time of ulcerated lesions, pain relief, and modulation of inflammatory processes. The association of low power lasers with photosensitizers, a process called antimicrobial photodynamic therapy (aPDT) and also known as photoactivated disinfection (PAD), photodynamic inactivation (PDI) or photodynamic antimicrobial chemotherapy (PACT), can be used for reducing microbial contamination and bleeding.[3–5] aPDT involves delivering visible light with an appropriate wavelength into a tissue or microorganism previously exposed to a photosensitizing dye. Their interaction results in a transition from a low energy ground state to a higher energy triplet state. The latter reacts with biomolecules, leading to the production of free oxygen radicals and cell death (for more details, see Chapter 7). Its use is widespread in neoplastic[6,7] and infectious diseases.[8] These features, combined with the fact that LLLT and aPDT are atraumatic and non-invasive techniques, explain why their use in the oral cavity of cancer patients is increasing.

aPDT has been used as a topical antibacterial, antifungal, and antiviral treatment.[8] This technique for delivery of antimicrobial therapy is non-invasive, quick, easy to perform, safe, effective against many species of pathogenic microorganisms, cost-effective, and can also be used to reduce bleeding.[9] Therefore, aPDT is a promising new therapy for cancer patients, with the goal of reducing oral complications of cancer treatment.

To our knowledge, there are only two reported cases of the use of aPDT in patients submitted to radiotherapy and/or chemotherapy (Table 43.1).[3,5] However, our experience suggests that this therapy is effective in cancer patients.

Clinical applications

aPDT should be used as an adjuvant therapy in all dental procedures that have the aim of reducing microorganism load.

Periodontal disease
Patients with compromised immune mechanisms, such as cancer patients, are at increased risk for opportunistic infections. Therefore, it is very important to diagnose such infections at an early stage and to treat them as soon as possible. Periodontal disease in cancer patients is more aggressive due to the systemic compromise. aPDT may be a useful method for the control of periodontopathogens, complementing and accelerating the healing post conventional periodontal treatment, which includes dental plaque removal (when possible), descaling, and root planing.

Lasers in Dentistry: Guide for Clinical Practice, First Edition. Edited by Patrícia M. de Freitas and Alyne Simões.
© 2015 John Wiley & Sons, Inc. Published 2015 by John Wiley & Sons, Inc.

Table 43.1 Case reports of the use of PAD in oral complications of oncology patients

Authors (year)	Number of patients (cancer therapy)	Wavelength (nm)	Laser output (mW)	Spot size (cm²)	Dose (J/cm²)	Irradiation time (s)	Treatment
Campos et al.[3] (2009)	1 (radiotherapy)	660	40	0,04	120	120	Periodontitis
Simões et al.[5] (2009)	1 (chemotherapy)	660	40	0,04	120	120	Herpes

The goal of using aPDT in patients with periodontal disease is to reduce the bacterial load in periodontal pockets (see Clinical case 43.1). It can be performed immediately before and after the conventional periodontal treatment. When cancer patients are severely compromised and conventional periodontal therapy cannot be used because of the risk of infection and severe bleeding, aPDT is the only alternative available to help improve oral health prior to cancer treatment.

Herpes lesions

Oral mucosal infections in cancer patients may also be caused by fungal and viral organisms. Recurrent herpes simplex virus 1 infection can be triggered by a number of factors, including stress and immunocompromise. The aim of aPDT treatment is to produce free oxygen radicals in tissue, resulting in virus elimination, acceleration of tissue healing, and pain relief (see Clinical case 43.2).

Infected oral mucositis

Oral mucositis, which is a common lesion in cancer patients submitted to radiotherapy and/or chemotherapy, can be treated with LLLT (see Chapter 40 for further details). However, sometimes these lesions appear to be contaminated, making healing difficult. These contaminated lesions are common on the lips and aPDT is a possible treatment for such infected lesions (see Clinical case 43.3).

Tissue bleeding

Bleeding may occur during chemotherapy-induced thrombocytopenia. The oral manifestations of acute leukemia are usually represented by gingival enlargement, mucosal ecchymosis, and gingival bleeding,[10,11] due to the defective bone marrow. Although oral findings may be present when the diagnosis of leukemia is confirmed,[12] there is little discussion in the literature about the oral monitoring of these patients by the dentist.

Non-invasive therapies in the oral cavity of these individuals may improve hygiene, decrease oral disease, and make symptomatic patients more comfortable. In this context, aPDT can also be used to reduce microbial contamination of periodontal pockets and infected ulcerative lesions, and to control bleeding (see Clinical case 43.4).[3,4]

Surgery

In addition to soft tissue injuries, changes in the bone matrix are expected when patients are treated with radiation therapy. Radiation injury to the fine vasculature of bone and its surrounding tissues first leads to hyperemia, followed by endarteritis, thrombosis, and a progressive occlusion and obliteration of the small vessels.[13] Therefore, irradiated bone is likely to respond poorly to trauma and infection.[13]

Patients receiving radiation therapy are at risk for the severe complication of osteoradionecrosis. Osteoradionecrosis is an infectious process, which progresses rapidly and spreads throughout the bone and then cannot be walled off because of compromised vascularity and minimal regenerative capabilities. The source of trauma may include denture irritation, sharp or hard food particles, and sharp bony ridges. Tooth extraction is said to be the most common cause of trauma, suggesting that the underlying problem in osteoradionecrosis is compromised wound healing that can be aggravated by infection.

In some cases, "trauma" to the oral tissues cannot be avoided. When head and neck radiation patients are not treated by the dentist prior to the start of radiation therapy, because of the severe xerostomia secondary to the radiation of the major salivary glands, there is an increased risk of caries and periodontal involvement. Patients may develop extensive decay and teeth may need to be extracted after radiation has been delivered. aPDT can be used to decrease the risk of infection and bleeding during tooth extraction. Studies with aPDT have demonstrated that this technology can be used to stimulate healing with acceptable success (see Clinical case 43.5).[14,15]

Final considerations

Based on the clinical anecdotal reports in this chapter, we would like to suggest that aPDT is a safe and effective treatment to control infection and bleeding, as well for the stimulation of wound repair. It improves the quality of life of the cancer patient. However, the use of aPDT technology in cancer patients is new and not scientifically tested: controlled studies are necessary to confirm whether or not the effect of aPDT is beneficial to cancer patients.

Clinical case 43.1 Periodontal disease

A 15-year-old girl diagnosed with palate mucoepidermoid carcinoma underwent surgical excision of the tumor followed by radiotherapy. Gingivitis was diagnosed in her anterior lower gums, which was a consequence of her difficulty brushing her teeth due to the presence of mucositis in this area (Fig. 43.1a). Oral hygiene orientation and aPDT were performed as auxiliary therapy to decrease gingival bleeding and to promote plaque removal (Fig. 43.1b–d). MB (0.01%) was applied to the periodontal pockets 5 minutes before laser irradiation. Low power diode laser continuous irradiation (MMOptics®, São Carlos, Brazil) was performed in contact mode at a dose of 120 J/cm², divided between four points (30 J/cm² per tooth; two in the buccal and two in the lingual area), 30 seconds per point, 40 mW, and 1.2 J of energy per point, with a spot size of 0.04 cm². One week later, after a single aPDT application, clinically the gingival tissues had improved considerably (Fig. 43.1e).

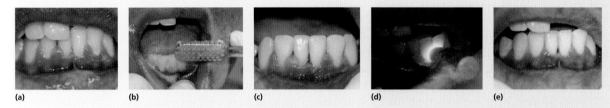

(a)   (b)   (c)   (d)   (e)

Figure 43.1 aPDT on the periodontium. (a) Clinical image before aPDT. Note the severe gingival inflammation and enlargement. (b) Oral hygiene orientation and tooth brushing under supervision. (c) MB dye applied to the periodontal pockets for 5 minutes; (d) phototherapy with a low power laser in contact mode; (e) clinical image 1 week after the single aPDT treatment.[3]

Clinical case 43.2 Herpes lesions

This patient with head and neck cancer developed oral mucositis secondary to radiotherapy. The mucositis was treated with LLLT. However, a painful palatal lesion did not heal in the expected time. Herpes simplex virus (HSV) infection was suspected from the clinical characteristics of the lesion and the fact that it was located on keratinized oral mucosa (Fig. 43.2a). aPDT was used in an attempt to treat the ulcers. Low power continuous diode laser irradiation (MMOptics®, São Carlos, Brazil) was performed in contact mode, with a dose of 120 J/cm², 120 seconds per point (three points), 40 mW, and spot size 0.04 cm². MB (0.01%) had previously been applied to the lesion with the use of a cotton swab for 5 minutes before the laser irradiation. Five days following aPDT application, the lesion had healed without complication (Fig. 43.2b–d).

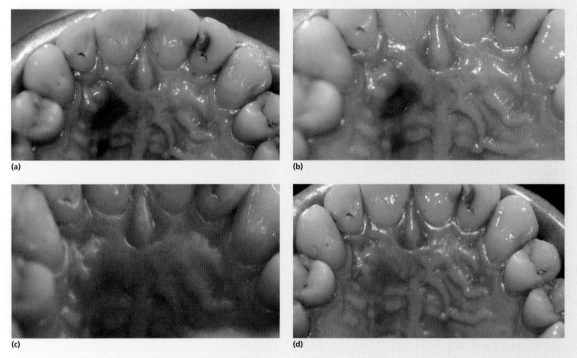

(a)   (b)

(c)   (d)

Figure 43.2 (a) HSV infection of the palatal mucosa in a head and neck cancer patient treated with radiotherapy. The ulcers were covered with MB for 5 minutes prior to laser irradiation. (b) The day after the first aPDT treatment there was considerable improvement and the lesion was painless (c) clinical image 5 days after aPDT(d) clinical image 13 days after aPDT.[5]

Clinical case 43.3 Infected oral mucositis

A 57-year-old male was diagnosed with intestinal cancer and subjected to high dose chemotherapy. Clinical examination revealed severe oral pain and ulceration on the inferior lip with no conclusive diagnosis (WHO mucositis grade 3 or HSV infection) (Fig. 43.3a). This infected lesion was frequently traumatized by the patient. After 20 laser phototherapy sessions to treat the oral mucositis, this had healed with the exception of this area on the lower lip. The patient was educated about keeping his hands away from the area to prevent further trauma and contamination. We suspected that this lesion was infected and initiated aPDT to eliminate the infection and accelerate wound repair.

Two sessions (with a 1-week interval between) were performed with MB (0.01%) applied for 5 minutes before continuous irradiation LLLT in contact mode (660 nm, 40 W, 120 J/cm², 4.8 J of energy per point) (Fig. 43.3b,c). A few minutes after the first session of aPDT, the patient reported an analgesic effect. The initial healing of the lesion became evident on the following day, indicated mainly by a reduction in the size and the appearance of a dry crust. Fifteen days after the first aPDT session, the lesion was completely healed (Fig. 43.3d–f).

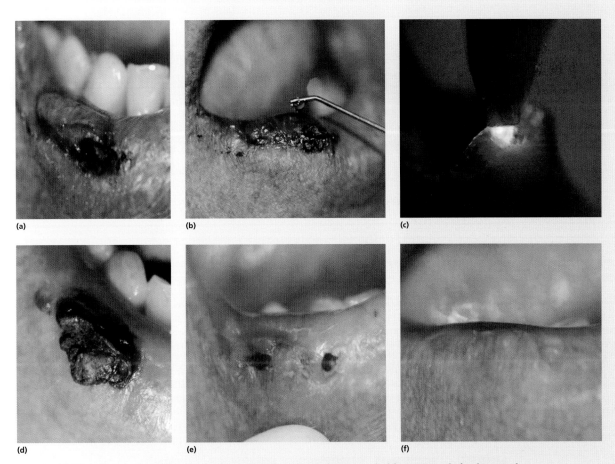

Figure 43.3 (a) Clinical image of an infected oral lesion before aPDT. (b) MB (0.01%) applied for 5 minutes before laser irradiation. (c) Irradiation with a red low power laser in contact mode. (d) Clinical image 7 days after treatment; a second aPDT session was then performed (same parameters); (e) clinical image 10 and (f) 15 days after the first aPDT session.

Clinical cases

Patients in the clinical cases presented below attended the Special Laboratory for Lasers in Dentistry (LELO) at the School of Dentistry of the University of São Paulo. All of them were treated with a LLLT (red diode laser) combined with methylene blue (MB) (0.01%), which is a phenothiazine dye that has been used in medical practice for more than 100 years.

Acknowledgments

Some of our studies have received the financial support of FAPESP (Fundação de Amparo à Pesquisa do Estado de São Paulo – Grants #2010/03662-6 and #2011/14013-1) and CAPES (Coordenação de Aperfeiçoamento de Pessoal de Nível Superior, #1455993). In addition, we would like to thank the Special Laboratory for Lasers in Dentistry (LELO) at the School of Dentistry of the University of São Paulo, where the patients were treated.

Clinical case 43.4 Tissue bleeding

A 13-year-old girl diagnosed with recurrent acute myeloid leukemia was submitted to chemotherapy. She arrived at the dental clinic with a complaint of intermittent fever that had been present for 4 days and gingival enlargement in the maxilla and mandible, with many areas of spontaneous gingival bleeding and pain (Fig. 43.4a). These were making oral hygiene difficult. Blood test results were hemoglobin 8.3 g/dL, hematocrit 24.6%, leukocytes 100 cells/mm³, no lymphocytes, and platelets 2000/mm³. After the clinical examination, an extramedullary leukemic infiltrate was suspected. A panoramic X-ray showed no evidence of periodontal pockets. Although extramedullary leukemic infiltrate is not locally treated, the excessive bleeding has to be compensated for by transfusion.[16] In this case, despite chemotherapy and blood transfusion, an increase in platelets could not be achieved and the oral bleeding and pain continued to cause discomfort to the patient. aPDT was performed to help improve the patient's quality of life and the hope that by reducing the inflammation, the bleeding could be controlled.

Careful local debridement was performed and the patient given oral hygiene instruction. Biofilm removal was performed carefully with soaked cotton balls and without abrasive toothpaste (Biotene®). Next, the photosensitive dye (MB 0.01%) was applied to the periodontal pockets for 5 minutes (Fig. 43.4b), followed by laser irradiation (Fig. 43.4c). Red low power continuous laser irradiation with a diode laser (MMOptics®, São Carlos, Brazil), spot size of approximately 0.04 cm², 660 nm, 40 mW, 120 J/cm², was performed. Unlike the usual contact mode, the laser irradiation was performed approximately 1.0 cm away from the tissues to avoid any trauma that could lead to bleeding. Immediately after the treatment, the patient reported pain relief. One week after a single aPDT application, the patient was pain free. The procedure was repeated and 15 days later there was no bleeding. It is important to highlight that though the patient did not receive blood transfusions, levels of platelets were maintained.

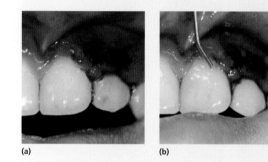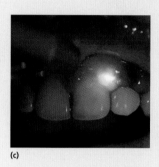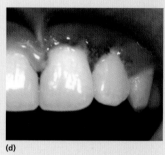

Figure 43.4 (a) Gum before treatment. (b) Dye carefully applied to the periodontal pockets after biofilm removal. (c) Laser irradiation with no contact. (d) Clinical image 15 days after oral treatment.

Clinical case 43.5 Surgery

A 58-year-old male with a diagnosis of nasopharyngeal carcinoma was subjected to high doses of radiotherapy (70.4 Gy). Oral mucositis (WHO mucositis grade 3) associated with severe periodontitis was found. LLLT for treatment of oral mucositis was performed and a panoramic radiograph was taken.

The panoramic radiograph confirmed general bone loss, affecting all teeth (Fig. 43.5a). Dental treatment included dental plaque removal and root planing. Two months after the end of radiotherapy, teeth extractions were carried out (Fig. 43.5b–d). To decrease the risk of osteoradionecrosis, this surgery was performed in steps, with a few teeth removed at a time.

Oral hygiene orientation and aPDT were performed before the surgery as an auxiliary therapy to decrease bleeding and to promote plaque removal (the same protocol as used for Clinical case 43.1). After dental extraction, curettage of the alveolus was performed and all bony ridges were removed. Next MB (0.01%) was applied to the alveolus for 5 minutes (Fig. 43.5e), and then continuous laser irradiation with a red low power diode laser (MMOptics®, São Carlos, Brazil) was performed at a dose of 120 J/cm², 2 minutes per point, 40 mW, 4.8 J of energy per point, and spot size of 0.04 cm² (Fig. 43.5f). Three points was irradiated. Three months after aPDT, the surgical wound was completely healed (Fig. 43.5 g–i).

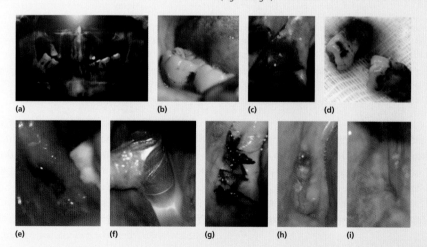

Figure 43.5 (a) Panoramic radiograph showing severe bone loss; (b)clinical image before dental extractions; (c) alveolus after curettage; (d) image after teeth removal; (e) dye applied for 5 minutes; (f) laser irradiation; (g) mass suture; (h) clinical image 2 months after extractions, showing the epithelialized area; (i) clinical image 3 months after the extractions, showing total tissue repair.

References

1 de Castro G Jr, Guindalini RS. Supportive care in head and neck oncology. Curr Opin Oncol 2010; 22(3): 221–225.

2 Jones DL, Rankin KV. Management of the oral sequelae of cancer therapy. Tex Dent J 2012; 129(5): 461–468.

3 Campos L, Simoes A, Sa PH, Eduardo Cde P. Improvement in quality of life of an oncological patient by laser phototherapy. Photomed Laser Surg 2009; 27(2): 371–374.

4 de Paula Eduardo C, de Freitas PM, Esteves-Oliveira M, et al. Laser phototherapy in the treatment of periodontal disease. A review. Lasers Med Sci 2010; 25(6): 781–792.

5 Simoes A, Campos L, Freitas PM, Eduardo CP, Nicolau J. Laser as a therapy for oral complications induced by chemotherapy and radiotherapy Jornal Brasileiro de Laser 2009; 2(10): 18–23.

6 Hopper C, Kubler A, Lewis H, Tan IB, Putnam G. mTHPC-mediated photodynamic therapy for early oral squamous cell carcinoma. Int J Cancer 2004; 111(1): 138–146.

7 Lee J, Moon C. Current status of experimental therapeutics for head and neck cancer. Exp Biol Med 2011; 236(4): 375–389.

8 Kharkwal GB, Sharma SK, Huang YY, Dai T, Hamblin MR. Photodynamic therapy for infections: clinical applications. Lasers Surg Med 2011; 43(7): 755–767.

9 Sperandio FF, Simões A, Aranha AC, Corrêa L, Orsini Machado de Sousa SC. Photodynamic therapy mediated by methylene blue dye in wound healing. Photomed Laser Surg 2010; 28(5): 581–587.

10 da Silva Santos PS, Fontes A, de Andrade F, de Sousa SC. Gingival leukemic infiltration as the first manifestation of acute myeloid leukemia. Otolaryngol Head Neck Surg 2010; 143(3): 465–466.

11 Gallipoli P, Leach M. Gingival infiltration in acute monoblastic leukaemia. Br Dent J 2007; 203(9): 507–509.

12 Santos FA, Pochapski MT, Pilatti GL, Kozlowski VA Jr, Goiris FA, Groppo FC. Severe necrotizing stomatitis and osteomyelitis after chemotherapy for acute leukaemia. Aust Dent J 2009; 54(3): 262–265.

13 Vissink A, Jansma J, Spijkervet FK, Burlage FR, Coppes RP. Oral sequelae of head and neck radiotherapy. Crit Rev Oral Biol Med 2003; 14(3): 199–212.

14 Jefferis AF, Chevretton EB, Berenbaum MC. Muscle damage and recovery in the rabbit tongue following photodynamic therapy with haematoporphyrin derivative. Acta Oto-Laryngol 1991; 111(1): 153–160.

15 Stern SJ, Flock ST, Small S, Thomsen S, Jacques S. Photodynamic therapy with chloroaluminum sulfonated phthalocyanine in the rat window chamber. Am J Surg 1990; 160(4): 360–364.

16 Parisi E, Draznin J, Stoopler E, Schuster SJ, Porter D, Sollecito TP. Acute myelogenous leukemia: advances and limitations of treatment. Oral Surg Oral Med Oral Pathol Oral Radiol Endod 2002; 93(3): 257–263.

CHAPTER 44

Photodynamic therapy in cancer treatment

Juliana Ferreira-Strixino[1] and Elodie Debefve[2]
[1] University of the Vale of Paraíba, São José Campus, São Paulo, SP, Brazil
[2] Swiss Federal Institute of Technology (EPFL), Lausanne, Switzerland

Introduction

Oral cancers are the sixth most common cancers in the world, with 6% affecting young people under the age of 45 years. Moreover, survival rates are moderate (about 50% over 5 years) despite the recent advances in surgery and radiotherapy.[1]

Oral cancers, which are subtypes of head and neck cancers, include any cancerous tissue located in the lips, buccal mucosa, gingiva, tongue, and hard palate or floor of the mouth.[2] The tumor size and its localization are important factors to be considered when determining the prognosis, diagnosis, and choice of treatment. The treatment choice is ablative surgery, radiotherapy and chemotherapy, or palliative care, as well as a combination of these therapies.[3]

Surgery is a common treatment for oral cancers, but it is an invasive and mutilating treatment. Indeed, surgical removal of head and neck cancers can be unesthetic and can also damage normal structures like nerves, collagen fibers, and blood vessels, thus affecting important functions such as swallowing, taste and speech, and often necessitating reconstructive surgery. Radiotherapy is a very effective localized treatment; however, it sometimes induces irreversible side effects when oral tissue is irradiated.[4,5] Moreover, radiotherapy cannot be repeated. Indeed, re-irradiation leads to an increased risk of serious side effects because surrounding tissues have already received the maximum tolerable dose of ionizing radiation.[6] Chemotherapy, currently used for example for nasopharyngeal cancer (NPC), involves the non-selective inhibition of cell proliferation. This standard systemic treatment often induces side effects such as nausea, loss of appetite, loss of hair, vomiting, and increased infection risk. Tumor cells can also be resistant to these chemotherapies. These limitations create a serious need for new treatment modalities, particularly when re-treatment is necessary. In this respect, photodynamic therapy (PDT) seems to be a very good candidate.[7]

Photodynamic therapy

PDT is a local rather than a systemic treatment; it is only suitable for localized disease. It is based on the activation of the photochemical properties of substances called photosensitizers (PS), resulting in cellular or vascular damage (Fig. 44.1).

Initially, a PS is administered to the patient, either locally or systemically. Some time after PS administration, the treatment site is irradiated with visible or near infrared light of a specific wavelength. Absorption of light by the PS initiates photochemical reactions with the local oxygen, generating cytotoxic oxygen species and free radicals, which can directly kill tumor cells or damage tumor vasculature. This highly toxic singlet oxygen can only diffuse $0.02\,\mu m$. Tissue damage is therefore restricted to the localization of the PS and the penetration depth of the light used to activate the PS.[8,9]

There are different types of PS available for PDT. In the porphyrin family, Photofrin®, Photogem®, Photosan®, Levulan®, ®Kerastick®, Metvix®, and Visudyne® have been approved for clinical applications. Foscan®, Photodithazine®, and Radachlorin in the chlorin family and Photosen® in the phtalocyanin family have also been approved.[10] New PS or new formulations of the existing PS are currently being assessed in clinical or preclinical trials.

Light sources that activate the PS are lasers, light emitting diodes, and xenon lamps. Lasers are the most convenient and controllable source as they deliver coherent and monochromatic light. Furthermore, they can be easily handled and directed using optical fibers that allow irradiation into hollow organs and of deep-seated tumors, during surgery or interstitial irradiation. The anatomy of the oral cavity and oropharynx usually allows for good visualization of the cancer, and therefore exposure of the tumor by the laser light as well as accessibility.[6] Oral cancers are thus good candidates for PDT.

PDT has several advantages; one important factor for oral cancer is the relative double selectivity of the treatment. Indeed, the PS itself has no toxicity when not irradiated and the light by itself is non-thermal and does not affect the tissue. Only the PS

Lasers in Dentistry: Guide for Clinical Practice, First Edition. Edited by Patrícia M. de Freitas and Alyne Simões.
© 2015 John Wiley & Sons, Inc. Published 2015 by John Wiley & Sons, Inc.

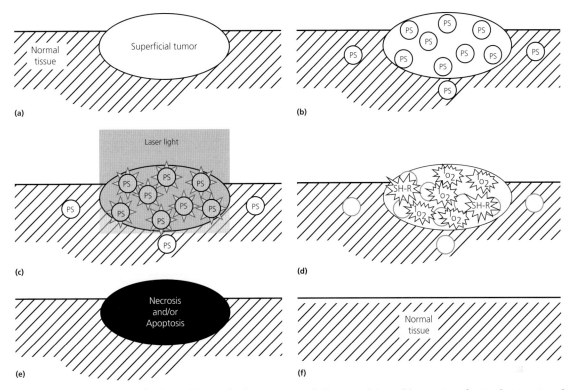

Figure 44.1 Schematic of the basic principle of PDT. (a) Superficial tumor surrounded by normal tissue; (b) some time after its administration, the photosensitizer (PS) preferentially accumulates in the target tumor tissue; (c) the target site is irradiated by laser light at a specific wavelength, exciting the PS. The penetration of this light is limited and depends on its wavelength; (d) activated PS induces photochemical reactions with the local oxygen, generating mainly singlet oxygen ($^1O_2$), other cytotoxic oxygen species, and free radicals (SH-R); (e) tissue damage (apoptosis and/or necrosis) is restricted to the tumor; (f) normal tissue after destruction of the tumor by PDT.

Table 44.1 Parameters for the photosensitizer, drug–light interval, and light source to consider and optimize to define a PDT protocol adapted for each type of oral cancer.

	Parameter	Dependence
Photosensitizer (PS)	Molecule	*
	Formulation/vehicle (PEG, liposomes, etc.)	*
	Drug dose	*
	Infusion method (IV versus topical)	Localization and accessibility of the cancer
Drug–light interval (DLI)		PS chosen and its distribution
		Target tissue (after intravenous drug administration: short DLI for vascular; long DLI for cellular)
Light	Source (laser, LED, etc.)	Localization and accessibility of the cancer, PS chosen
	Wavelength (nm)	PS chosen, depth of target area
	Fluence (mW/cm²)	*
	Time of irradiation (e.g. continuous or fractionated)	Calculated according to fluence and fluence rate
	Fluence rate (J/cm²)	*

*Parameter for which there is a relatively large freedom of choice, depending on the target tissue and expected effects of PDT. However, there is a limited choice for several parameters, because they are interdependent; for example, the wavelength of the excitation light depends on the choice of PS.

activated by the appropriate light wavelength will induce local tissue damages. Thus, a PS can be chosen with physicochemical properties that ensure it selectively accumulates in the target tumor, and the area comprising the tumor can be selectively irradiated, thus limiting the activation of the PS and its toxic effects to inside the tumor, without affecting the normal surrounding tissues. The anatomy of the mouth cavity can be expected to be better preserved than with ablative surgery. PDT is a minimally invasive technique that, unlike ionizing radiation, can be repeated several times, even for recurrent disease after chemo-radiation, postoperative radiotherapy or ablative surgery. It can be applied as an adjuvant therapy before, during or after surgery, radiotherapy or chemotherapy,[6,7,11] without compromising future treatment options.

According to numerous representative clinical studies,[5,12–20] PDT has the potential to be a very effective local treatment modality for head and neck cancer, including NPC and other oral cancers, especially in patients with recurrent, residual or second primary squamous cell cancer of the head and neck (SCCHN).[18]

However, a few problems remain, depending on the PS used and the protocol followed. Side effects include generalized phototoxicity and necrosis-related pain, but these are not long lasting. Pain can be controlled by a combination of opiate, opioid, and non-steroidal anti-inflammatory drug (NSAID) analgesia. The tumor localization has to be accessible to laser light. The lack of penetration of the PS and light limits the application of PDT to superficial tumor with an infiltration depth of less than 1 cm;[6] deeper tumors can be irradiated interstitially and internal organs by surgical techniques. Nowadays, available PS do not yet have optimal specificity. Foscan® is one of the best available for the treatment of head and neck cancers. It has several advantages: (1) a short period of photosensitivity (about 2 weeks); (2) activation at longer wavelengths, allowing lights to be used that emit wavelengths that penetrate deeper into the target tissue; (3) higher yields of singlet oxygen, producing an efficient phototoxicity; and (4) better tumor selectivity, thus avoiding collateral damage to normal tissues.[21]

Clinical case 44.1 Squamous cell carcinoma of the tongue

In a male patient diagnosed with squamous cell carcinoma of the tongue (Fig. 44.2a), one session of PDT was applied as first treatment. After 1 month, the lesion had healed completely and there was no relapse (Fig. 44.2b,c). The PS used was intravenous Photogem® at 2 mg/kg. After 24 hours, the lesion was irradiated using a laser at 630 nm with a coupled optical fiber to direct light, a fluence of 200 mW/cm², and a fluence rate of 200 J/cm².

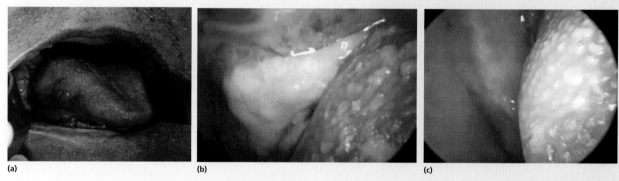

(a) (b) (c)

Figure 44.2 (a) Initial lesion: squamous cell carcinoma of the tongue; (b) 5 days after PDT; (c) 1 month after PDT (courtesy of IFSC/USP – Optical Group, Biophotonics Laboratory, Brazil).

Clinical case 44.2 Squamous cell carcinoma of the lip

In a male patient with squamous cells carcinoma of the lip (Fig. 44.3a), PDT was applied as first treatment. After 1 month the lesion had healed completely and there was no relapse (Fig. 44.3b,c). The PS used was intravenous Photogem® at 2 mg/kg. After 24 hours, the lesion was irradiated using a 630-nm laser with a coupled optical fiber to direct the light. Inside the lip the fluence used was 200 mW/cm² and the fluence rate was 250 J/cm², and outside the lip the fluence used was 250 mW/cm² and the fluence rate 300 J/cm².

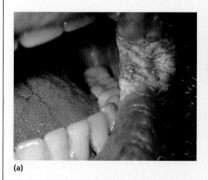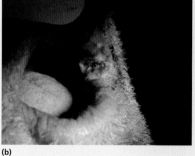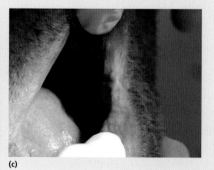

(a) (b) (c)

Figure 44.3 (a) Initial lesion: squamous cell carcinoma of the lip; (b) 1 month after PDT; (c) 1 year after treatment (courtesy of IFSC/USP – Optical Group, Biophotonics Laboratory, Brazil).

Clinical case 44.3 Squamous cell carcinoma of the cheek

In a male patient with squamous cell carcinoma of the cheek (Fig. 44.4a), one session of PDT was applied as first treatment. The PS used was intravenous Photogem® at 2 mg/kg. After 1 month the lesion had healed completely and there was no relapse (Fig. 44.4b,c). After 24 hours, the lesion was irradiated using a 630-nm diode laser with an optical fiber coupled to direct light, with a fluence of 200 mW/cm² and a fluence rate between 200 and 250 J/cm².

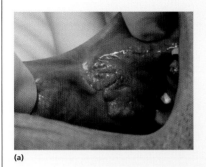
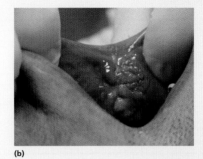
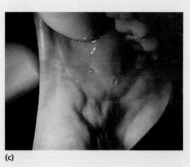

(a)   (b)   (c)

Figure 44.4 (a) Initial lesion: squamous cells carcinoma of the cheek; (b) immediately after PDT; (c) 5 months after treatment (courtesy of IFSC/USP – Optical Group, Biophotonics Laboratory, Brazil).

As summarized in Table 44.1, there are many other parameters than the choice of PS to consider and optimize to define the PDT protocol best adapted to each type of oral cancer.

Conclusion

In conclusion, PDT in the head and neck region, particularly in oral cancer treatment, is still regarded as an emerging treatment modality, despite the very promising clinical results. For PDT to be broadly accepted by clinicians, uniformly accepted protocols need to be developed.[11]

In the Clinical cases 44.1, 44.2, and 44.3, the inflammation (edema), erythema, swelling, pain, and vascular damage were observed immediately after treatment. During the first week after treatment, some analgesics, antibiotics, and/or anti-inflammatory drugs can be administrated and the lesion must be cleaned properly. Depending on the local lesion, mucosa or skin, necrosis and scab were observed after 7 and 15 days, respectively. New epithelialization occurred 1 or 2 months after PDT.

References

1 Jemal A, Bray F, Center MM, Ferlay J, Ward E, Forman D. Global cancer statistics. *CA Cancer J Clin* 2011; 61: 69–90.

2 Bagan JV, Scully C. Recent advances in Oral Oncology 2007: epidemiology, aetiopathogenesis, diagnosis and prognostication. *Oral Oncol* 2008; 44: 103–108.

3 Jerjes W, Upile T, Hamdoon Z, Mosse CA, Morcos M, Hopper C. Photodynamic therapy outcome for T1/T2 N0 oral squamous cell carcinoma. *Lasers Surg Med* 2011; 43: 463–469.

4 Fleming TJ. Oral tissue changes of radiation-oncology and their management. *Dent Clin North Am* 1990; 34: 223–237.

5 Grant WE, Hopper C, MacRobert AJ, Speight PM, Bown SG. Photodynamic therapy of oral cancer: photosensitisation with systemic aminolaevulinic acid. *Lancet* 1993; 342: 147–148.

6 Nyst HJ, Tan IB, Stewart FA, Balm AJ. Is photodynamic therapy a good alternative to surgery and radiotherapy in the treatment of head and neck cancer? *Photodiagn Photodyn Ther* 2009; 6: 3–11.

7 Hopper C. Photodynamic therapy: a clinical reality in the treatment of cancer. *Lancet Oncol* 2000; 1: 212–219.

8 Souza CS, Neves AB, Felicio LA, Ferreira J, Kurachi C, Bagnato VS. Optimized photodynamic therapy with systemic photosensitizer following debulking technique for nonmelanoma skin cancers. *Dermatol Surg* 2007; 33: 194–198.

9 Wilson BC, Patterson MS. The physics, biophysics and technology of photodynamic therapy. *Phys Med Biol;* 2008; 53: R61–109.

10 Allison RR, Sibata CH. Oncologic photodynamic therapy photosensitizers: a clinical review. *Photodiagn Photodyn Ther* 2010; 7: 61–75.

11 Bredell MG, Besic E, Maake C, Walt H. The application and challenges of clinical PD-PDT in the head and neck region: a short review. *J Photochem Photobiol B* 2010; 101: 185–190.

12 Biel MA. Photodynamic therapy and the treatment of head and neck neoplasia. *Laryngoscope* 1998; 108: 1259–1268.

13 D'Cruz AK, Robinson MH, Biel MA. mTHPC-mediated photodynamic therapy in patients with advanced, incurable head and neck cancer: a multicenter study of 128 patients. *Head Neck* 2004; 26: 232–240.

14 Fan KF, Hopper C, Speight PM, Buonaccorsi G, MacRobert AJ, Bown SG. Photodynamic therapy using 5-aminolevulinic acid for premalignant and malignant lesions of the oral cavity. *Cancer* 1996; 78: 1374–1383.

15 Fan KF, Hopper C, Speight PM, Buonaccorsi GA, Bown SG. Photodynamic therapy using mTHPC for malignant disease in the oral cavity. *Int J Cancer* 1997; 73: 25–32.

16 Hopper C, Kubler A, Lewis H, Tan IB, Putnam G. mTHPC-mediated photodynamic therapy for early oral squamous cell carcinoma. *Int J Cancer* 2004; 111: 138–146.

17 Kubler AC, Scheer M, Zoller JE. Onkologie. *Photodynamic therapy of head and neck cancer* 2001; 24: 230–237.

18 Lee J, Moon C. *Exp Biol Med (Maywood)* 2011; 236: 375–389.

19 Stranadko EF, Garbuzov MI, Zenger VG, et al. (2001) [Photodynamic therapy of recurrent and residual oropharyngeal and laryngeal tumors]. Vestn Otorinolaringol 2001; 36–39.

20 Yoshida T, Tokashiki R, Ito H, et al. Therapeutic effects of a new photosensitizer for photodynamic therapy of early head and neck cancer in relation to tissue concentration. *Auris Nasus Larynx* 2008; 35: 545–551.

21 Jerjes W, Upile T, Hamdoon Z, Mosse CA, Akram S, Hopper C. Photodynamic therapy outcome for oral dysplasia. *Lasers Surg Med* 2011; 43: 192–199.

Index

Note: Page numbers in *italics* refer to Figures; those in **bold** to Tables.

Lasers in Dentistry: Guide for Clinical Practice, First Edition. Edited by Patrícia M. de Freitas and Alyne Simões.
© 2015 John Wiley & Sons, Inc. Published 2015 by John Wiley & Sons, Inc.